NURSING CARE IN THE COMMUNITY

SECOND EDITION

NURSING CARE IN THE COMMUNITY

JOAN M. COOKFAIR, RN, MSN, EdD

Professor

Division of Nursing
D'Youville College
Buffalo, New York

Illustrated

M Mosby

St. Louis Baltimore Boston Carlsbad Chicago Naples New York Philadelphia Portland
London Madrid Mexico City Singapore Sydney Tokyo Toronto Wiesbaden

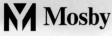
Mosby

Dedicated to Publishing Excellence

A Times Mirror Company

Publisher: Nancy L. Coon
Editor: Loren Wilson
Associate Developmental Editor: Brian Dennison
Project Manager: Mark Spann
Production Editor: Elizabeth Fathman
Designer: David Zielinski
Manufacturing Manager: Betty Richmond

A NOTE TO THE READER:

The author and publisher have made every attempt to check dosages and nursing content for accuracy. Because the science of pharmacology is continually advancing, our knowledge base continues to expand. Therefore we recommend that the reader always check product information for changes in dosage or administration before administering any medication. This is particularly important with new or rarely used drugs.

Printed in the United States of America
Composition by Progressive Information Technologies
Printing/binding by R.R. Donnelley

Mosby – Year Book, Inc.
11830 Westline Industrial Drive
St. Louis, Missouri 63146

Library of Congress Cataloging-in-Publication Data

Nursing care in the community / [edited by] Joan M. Cookfair. -- 2nd
  ed.
      p.   cm.
    Includes bibliographical references and index.
    ISBN 0-8151-1538-5
    1. Community health nursing.   I. Cookfair, Joan M.
RT98.N855   1996
610.73'43 -- dc20   95–300
                                                  CIP

96 97 98 99 00   /   9 8 7 6 5 4 3 2 1

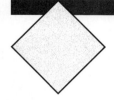

CONTRIBUTORS

Carol Batra, RN, PhD
Professor and Chairperson
Division of Nursing
D'Youville College
Buffalo, New York

Elizabeth Johnson Blankenship, RN, BSN, CNA
Director of Nursing
Briarwood Nursing Center
Little Rock, Arkansas

Arthur S. Cookfair, BA, EdD
Instructor
American Chemical Society
Buffalo, New York

Diane L. Cookfair, MS, PhD
Department of Neurology
School of Medicine
State University of New York at Buffalo
Buffalo, New York

Janice Cooke Feigenbaum, RN, PhD
Professor and Coordinator of Community
    Addictions Program
D'Youville College
Buffalo, New York

John Flannery, RN, MS
Executive Director
Casey House Hospice
Toronto, Ontario, Canada

Carole A. Gutt, RN, EdD
Associate Professor
Director of Graduate Program
D'Youville College
Buffalo, New York

Dorothy Hoehne, RN, MED, PhD
Associate Professor
D'Youville College
Buffalo, New York

Margaret R. HoSang, RN, MS
Clinical Instructor
Ryerson University
Toronto, Ontario, Canada

Janet T. Ihlenfeld, RN, PhD
Professor
Division of Nursing
D'Youville College
Buffalo, New York

Janet E. Jackson, RN, MS
Faculty, Department of Nursing
Bradley University
Peoria, Illinois

Linda Janelli, RNC, EdD
Assistant Professor
State University of New York at Buffalo
Buffalo, New York

Katherine Jones, RN, MS
Professor
Ryerson Polytechnic University
Toronto, Ontario, Canada

Karen Cassidy King, RN, EdD
Assistant Professor
University of Kentucky
School of Nursing
Louisville, Kentucky

Diane K. Kjervik, JD, RN, MS, FAAN
Professor and Associate Dean for Community
  Outreach
University of North Carolina
Chapel Hill, North Carolina

Ruth N. Knollmueller, RN, PhD
Visiting Professor
University of Kentucky College of Nursing
Center for Rural Health
Hazard, Kentucky

Margo MacRobert, RN, MS, CNAA
Director of Nursing Research and Development
Children's Hospital
Oklahoma City, Oklahoma

Susan K. Markel, BSN, CRNI, CNSNS
Senior Director of Clinical Services
Option Care, Inc.
Bannockburn, Illinois

Patricia A. O'Hare, DrPH, MS, RN, A-CCC
Associate Professor
Georgetown University School of Nursing
Washington, DC

Karen Piotrowski, RNC, MSN
Assistant Professor of Nursing
Division of Nursing
D'Youville College
Buffalo, New York

Mary Rea, BS, MS
School Integration Consultant
Community Health Services
Toronto, Ontario, Canada

Christine L. Rubadue, RN, MN, COHN
Director of the Division of Federal Health
U.S. Public Health Service
Region X
School of Nursing
Washington, DC
  Information given is the author's own and not
  the responsibility of the U.S. Public Health
  Service.

Don Sabo, PhD
Professor of Sociology
Division of Liberal Arts
D'Youville College
Buffalo, New York

Mary K. Salazar, RN, EdD, COHN
Director of Occupational Health
Assistant Professor
School of Nursing
University of Washington
Seattle, Washington

Elizabeth Schenk, RN, MSN, MDiv
Pastor
Plymouth United Methodist Church
Ashtabula, Ohio

June A. Schmele, RN, PhD
Associate Professor
College of Nursing
University of Oklahoma
Oklahoma City, Oklahoma

Sandra L. Termini, RN, MS
Practice Manager
University Physicians' Office
State University of New York at Buffalo
Buffalo, New York

P. Susan Wagner, RN, ABSC, MSC (Nursing)
Associate Professor
College of Nursing
University of Saskatchewan
Saskatoon, Saskatchewan, Canada

William E. Wilkinson, JD, DrPH, COHN
Attorney at Law
Ibáñez and Wilkinson
Tucson, Arizona

Martha J. Yingling, RN, BSN, MS
Associate Professor
Division of Nursing
D'Youville College
Buffalo, New York

FOREWORD

Community health nurses are the care coordinators for communities and their members. They are actively involved both socially and politically to empower residents, high-risk aggregates, families, and communities as an entirety to initiate and maintain health-promoting environments. Health care in the community is at its peak at the present time with the creation of new programs, residential facilities, services, and agencies to meet the needs of community residents. Community health nurses are becoming leaders in the health care industry and will, without doubt, carry their innumerable skills and talents into the twenty-first century to continually strive to better the health of the citizens of the world.

During the twentieth century, community health nursing has changed from its beginnings, during which most of the home visiting was concentrated on newborn infants, to the present day when nursing interventions involve the delivery of highly technological care in the homes of acutely and terminally ill clients. No matter what the crisis or need in the community, community health nursing is always willing to make changes to appropriately respond to the need.

The overall well-being and health of the community is the primary focus of all nursing intervention within the community setting. Individuals are cared for in their home environments, the goal being to restore them to their highest functional level. In addition to treating and facilitating health within the individual, the community health nurse assists the family to understand and cope with the care needed. Community health nurses are constantly involved in assessment of the community to identify areas where nursing can educate and support clients within the community. It is the community health nurse who is best equipped with assessment knowledge to pinpoint where intervention is needed.

As activists dedicated to the health and well-being of the community, the keen observations of community health nurses are utilized in the establishment of well-child conferences, senior citizens clinics, screening clinics for chronic illnesses, sexually transmitted disease clinics, and seasonal immunization clinics to meet the needs of the people. Mobile units are used to transport community health nurses to areas where the individuals cannot travel or cannot afford to travel to stationary clinical sites. Migrant workers and immigrants are cared for by community health nurses. Wherever and whenever there is a need for health care delivery, the community health nurse makes an attempt to respond.

There appears to be a reciprocal relationship between community health nursing and the community. At the present time, with health care dollars dramatically decreasing, and populations rapidly increasing, the needs for professional nursing care that is effective, beneficial, and cost effective are imperative. In the future it can be postulated that the leaders and coordinators of the health care industry in the community will be community health nurses. As populations continue to expand, the needs for community health nurses will also expand, new and different challenges will await the community health nurses of tomorrow, who, like their predecessors, will respond with the utmost efficiency.

Nursing Care in the Community, second edition, readily serves both the novice and experienced community health nurse to meet the everyday challenges of nursing in the community. This volume is formatted to easily demonstrate the use of nursing theoretical models in community nursing practice. It contains chapters authored by experts in their fields and demonstrates the smooth and necessary integration of the multidisciplinary approach to caring for individuals, families, groups, and communities. The volume contains valuable and readily accessible information on all the stages of life from infancy through the golden-aged years of senior citizens. The prevention and control of communicable and social disease through the use of epidemiologic practices, the care of the pregnant woman, the care of the newborn, and the care of the HIV/AIDS aggregate, to mention a few, are presented in easily read, meaningful formats. Complete guidelines and examples of total community assessments are given, as well as the ethical and legal aspects of nursing communities.

I am honored to have had the opportunity to write this foreword and am enthusiastic over the publication of this edition, which will serve the immediate as well as long-range needs of community health nursing. I visualize its use in both educational and practice settings, where its factual and sensitive wisdom will be appreciated.

Patricia A. Anderson, RN, PhD
Associate Professor
D'Youville College
Buffalo, New York

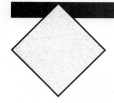

PREFACE

Nurses providing care to those in the community need to be prepared with a broad knowledge base that provides them with the ability to give skilled care to clients while teaching families and other aggregates how to actively participate and learn to care for themselves. The community health nurse often needs to collaborate with other health care professionals in the community to provide total care of the client. Managing the total care of the client is often the most time consuming and challenging aspect of the community health nurse's role.

Nursing Care in the Community is a comprehensive, introductory text that provides undergraduate nursing students with a basic foundation for the practice of community health nursing. This concise text has been written to help students understand the impact of factors such as societal influences, community, and family on the health of the individual. The book focuses on how to plan care for individuals, families, and communities with an emphasis on prevention at every level. The expanded roles of the nurse in the community are also included, as are methods of primary prevention. Students are also provided with information that will enable them to be accountable and fiscally responsible in health care systems that are becoming increasingly complex and expensive to maintain.

ORGANIZATION

The second edition is divided into eight parts. Part I describes historical events that have influenced the development of health care and the emergence of nursing theory. Nursing theory is included and integrated into nursing process. The health care delivery system is presented as an interacting dynamic phenomenon that is influenced by culture and economics.

Part II lays the foundation for health promo-

tion in the community by focusing on health education, research, leadership, and accountability. The part provides an understanding of the concept of wellness in the community and presents the student with methods of teaching health at primary, secondary, and tertiary levels.

Part III supplies information that will assist the nurse in caring for clients at different developmental stages. Care of the maternal-infant client, children, women, and men are discussed. The special needs and risks of the adolescent and elderly are also outlined.

Part IV helps the student focus on families as a unit of service and shows the importance of health promotion in both functional and dysfunctional families. Health of the client within the context of the family is emphasized.

Part V deals with caring for aggregates at risk. Communicable diseases and methods of prevention are described. The special needs of clients with chronic illness, developmental disabilities, and chemical dependencies are contained within this part. A special chapter that deals with health risks experienced by high-risk aggregates concludes the part.

Part VI provides the student with specific information about the changing face of contemporary home health care. Discharge planning and collaborative practice methods are discussed, as are the complexities of case management and client-centered nursing care.

Part VII describes specific practice roles to introduce the student to the diversity present in community health nursing. Separate chapters are devoted to the roles of occupational health nurses and school health nurses. The chapters explain the importance of each role and the issues they encounter.

Part VIII focuses on issues and concerns relevant to community health nursing practice today. Environmental concerns, legal and ethical issues, and professional issues that may affect community health nursing are discussed.

NEW TO THIS EDITION

Numerous new features have been added to the second edition to give students the information they need to provide care in the community setting. New to this edition is an emphasis on the health care delivery system from a broad perspective. Students are encouraged to develop a perception of the health care delivery system as an interacting, dynamic phenomenon that is influenced by various societal factors, including economics and culture. The culture chapter (Chapter 3) has been rewritten with a focus on culturally congruent care and expanded to include Bloch's classic assessment guide.

A new chapter (Chapter 9), "Management Concepts in Community Health Nursing" includes a discussion on case management and collaboration with other members of the health care team.

School health is discussed in a new chapter (Chapter 28) and presents the role and functions of the nurse in this specialized community setting.

Separate chapters on women's health (Chapter 15) and men's health (Chapter 16) are included in this new edition to reflect the growing understanding of gender-specific health issues and concerns. Maternal–infant care is also discussed in a separate chapter (Chapter 12) to discuss the role of the community health nurse in caring for newborns and new mothers.

In Chapter 5, the discussion of nursing theories and nursing process has been expanded to include a variety of nursing theories and several examples of how they are applied to the nursing process.

The chapter on quality assessment (Chapter 11) has been significantly revised to include current information on continuous quality improvement (CQI) and total quality management (TQM).

PEDAGOGICAL FEATURES

To facilitate the teaching-learning process, a number of pedagogical aids are included in the text. Chapter objectives and key terms are included at the beginning of each chapter to assist the student in focusing on important content. Key terms are printed in bold throughout the text to help reinforce the content. Numerous new research highlights are integrated throughout the text to illustrate the application of research to community health nursing practice. Case studies throughout the text demonstrate the application on concepts to practice. Chapter highlights review and reinforce important content in each chapter. New critical thinking exercises at the end of each chapter help students apply content to the practice setting. A glossary of key terms used in the text facilitates understanding of complex or unfamiliar terms.

An Instructor's Resource Manual, prepared by Janet T. Ihlenfeld, is available to qualified adopters and provides chapter summaries, objectives, key terms, topical lecture outlines, teaching strategies, application, and additional critical thinking exercises, and over 450 test questions. The manual will also include 24 transparency masters for class use.

I have always viewed community health nursing with enthusiasm and excitement. I hope that some of that enthusiasm and excitement will be conveyed to students who will then choose to work in the community. I am certain that the emerging, expanding role of the community health nurse will profoundly affect health care in the future.

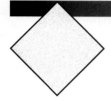

ACKNOWLEDGEMENTS

I would like to express my sincerest thanks to the reviewers who provided feedback for the second edition of *Nursing Care in the Community:*

Gwendolyn F. Foss, MSN, RNC
Point Loma Nazarene College

Janice Giltinan, MSN, RN, CS
Edinboro University of Pennsylvania

Mary Barb Haq, PhD, RN, CS
Seton Hall University

Gail J. Smith, RN, MSN, EdD
Miami–Dade Community College

Roselena Thorpe, PhD, RN
Community College of Allegheny

I also want express appreciate to Dorothy Hoehne, D'Youville College, for contributing new research highlights for Chapters 3, 4, 7, 9, 10, 15, 17, 18, 19, 20, 21, 22, and 26. I also thank Art Cookfair for providing many of the fine photos for the text.

My special thanks to my family for the support and many contributions to this textbook and my students who provided the incentive to write it.

Joan M. Cookfair

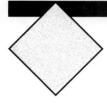

CONTENTS

PART ONE   **INTRODUCTION TO COMMUNITY HEALTH NURSING**

1   **Historical Overview of Community Health Nursing, 3**

Historical Roots, 4
Religious Figures, 6
Seminal Figures, 8
Military Service, 14
Nursing Theory and Community Health Nursing, 15

2   **Community as Client, 19**

Definitions of Community, 20
Conceptual Framework, 21
Assessing the Level of Wellness in a Community, 28

3   **Community Health Nursing in a Multicultural Society, 38**

The Cultural Diversification of North America, 39
Definitions of Culture, 40
The Link between Culture, Health, and Illness, 41
Issues in Cultural Categorization, 41
The Community Health Nurse in a Multicultural Society, 42
Communication, 43
Barriers to Effective Care, 44
Developing Cultural Sensitivity, 45
Using the Nursing Process in a Multicultural Society, 48
Culture and Nursing Education, Administration, and Research, 61
The Leading Edge of Transcultural Community Health Nursing, 62

4   **Health Care Delivery Systems, 65**

The United States Health Care System, 67
The Canadian Health Care System, 74
The Norwegian Health Care System, 78
Health Care in the United Kingdom, 78
The World Health Organization, 78
Health Service Issues in Underdeveloped Nations, 81

5   **Nursing Theory and Nursing Process in the Community, 85**

Nursing Process and the Standards of Community Health Nursing
    Practice, 87

The North American Nursing Diagnosis System (NANDA), 89
Problem Classification Scheme, Visiting Nurse Association, Omaha,
    Nebraska, 89
Guidelines for Writing Community Nursing Diagnosis Statements, 89
Iowa Intervention Project: Nursing Intervention Classification (NIC), 99
Nursing Process Frameworks, 102

PART TWO   STRATEGIES AND TOOLS FOR HEALTH PROMOTION

    6   Epidemiology in Community Health Nursing, 125

         Historical Evolution of Epidemiology, 127
         Key Biologic and Epidemiologic Concepts, 128
         Measures of Disease Frequency, 131
         Sources of Data, 133
         Methods Used in Epidemiologic Research, 133
         Statistical Concepts, 135
         Causality, 137
         Investigating a New Disease, 138
         Applications of Epidemiologic Concepts to Community Health Nursing, 139

    7   Health and Wellness in the Community, 143

         Historical Development of the Wellness Movement, 144
         Prominent Individuals in the Wellness/Health Movement, 146
         Terms Used in the Wellness Movement, 147
         Models of Wellness, 149
         Assessment of Wellness Behavior, 158
         Alternative or Complementary Treatment Modalities, 162
         Wellness Components, 164

    8   Health Teaching in the Community, 175

         Historical Background, 176
         Legal Issues in Health Teaching, 178
         Teaching/Learning Theories, 178
         Types of Learning, 179
         Principles of Teaching/Learning, 182
         The Teaching/Learning Process and the Nursing Process, 182

    9   Management Concepts in Community Health Nursing, 200

         Developing Management Theory, 201
         Organization, 207
         Application of Management Concepts, 210
         Organizing the Home Visit, 213
         Organizational Management, 214

   10   Working with Groups in the Community, 217

         Definition of Group, 218
         Functions of Groups, 219

Characteristics of Groups, 220
Group Development, 220
Role Differentiation, 221
The Group Leader, 221
Shared Leadership, 223
Social Power and Group Conflict, 223
Group Cohesion, 224
Motivational Theory, 224
Type of Groups, 225
Initiating a Small Group, 227

11   Quality Assessment and Improvement in the Community, 231

Environmental Context, 233
Social Context, 234
Quality, 236
Quality Assessment and Improvement in Health Care, 236
The Quality Improvement Movement, 237
Models of Quality Assessment and Improvement, 238
Data Sources and Methods, 247
Quality Management Roles, 249
Research, 250

PART THREE   **CARING FOR THE INDIVIDUAL IN THE COMMUNITY**

12   Caring for the Maternal-Infant Client, 257

Roles of the Community Health Nurse in Maternal-Infant Care, 260
Biostatistical Data Related to the Maternal-Infant Client, 261
Maternal-Infant Health Care Services in the Community, 265
Secondary Prevention, 276
Tertiary Prevention, 279

13   Caring for Children, 285

Growth and Development, 286
Immunizations, 289
Accidents and Accident Prevention, 290
Dental Problems, 294
Acquired Immunodeficiency Syndrome (AIDS), 294
Nutrition, 296
Iron Deficiency Anemia, 297
Lead Poisoning/Plumbism, 298
Violence, 300
Child Abuse and Neglect, 302
Poverty, 303

14   Caring for Adolescents and Young Adults, 307

Major Causes of Mortality and Morbidity in Adolescence, 308
Nutritional Status in Adolescence, 309
Puberty, 311

Health Concerns of Adolescents and Young Adults, 314
Emotional Concerns of Adolescents and Young Adults, 315
Adolescent Sexual Development, 316
Adolescents and Sports, 317
Substance Abuse in Adolescence, 318
Risk Taking Behavior in Adolescence, 320
Social Concerns Relating to Adolescents and Young Adults, 321

15   Caring for Women, 324

Historical, Social, and Political Factors Influencing Women's Health Care, 325
Women's Entry into the Health Care System, 327
The Nursing Process and Women's Health Care, 329
Meeting Women's Health Care Needs in the Community, 330
Preventive Health Care and Women's Health, 331
Self-Concept and the Role of the Nurse in Promoting a Positive Self Image, 335
Sexuality, 337
Violence and Abuse of Women, 341

16   Caring for Men, 345

Men's Health and the Study of Gender, 347
Men's Overall Health Status, 348
Theories of Men's Health and Illness, 350
Masculinities and Men's Health, 352
Men's Health Issues, 357
HIV/AIDS, 359

17   Caring for Older Adults, 366

The Aging Process, 367
Psychosocial Theories of Aging, 370
A Psychoanalytic Theory of Aging, 372
Normal Physical Changes, 372
Normal Cognitive Changes, 373
Health Promotion in the Senior Citizen Center, 373
The Frail Elderly, 377
Spiritual Nursing Care, 384
Social Concerns for the Elderly, 385

PART FOUR   CARING FOR THE FAMILY IN THE COMMUNITY

18   The Family as a Unit of Service, 391

What is a Family?, 393
Types of Families, 393
The Evolving Family Structure, 393
Roles Within the Family, 395
The Functional Family, 395
Adaptive Family Coping Patterns, 396

Conceptual Frameworks for Studying the Family, 397
Family Health, 399
Nursing Care of the Family, 399
The Family/Community System, 407

19   The Family Copinzg with Multiple Stressors, 413

Characteristics of Families with Multiple Stressors, 414
Nursing Concerns, 416
Assessment, 416
Nursing Diagnosis, 426
Planning and Intervention, 426
Implementation, 428
Evaluation, 432

PART FIVE   **CARING FOR CLIENTS AT RISK**

20   Clients with Communicable Diseases, 439

What is a Communicable Disease?, 440
Mode of Transmission, 440
Incubation Period, 443
Period of Communicability, 443
Immunity, 443
Surveillance, 445
Primary Prevention, 445
Secondary Prevention, 445
Tertiary Prevention, 445
Problematic Communicable Diseases, 445
HIV/AIDS, 451
Infection Control, 466

21   Clients with Chronic Illnesses, 472

Context, 473
Assessment of Families, 476
Planning, 485
Implementation, 489
Evaluation of Care, 491

22   Clients with Developmental Disabilities, 496

What is a Disability?, 497
Brief History of the Disability Movement, 498
Developmental Disability across the Lifespan, 498
Selected Developmental Disabilities, 502
Health Promotion and Prevention of Developmental Disabilities, 504
Nursing Process, 504
Communication Skills in Nursing Care of Individuals with a Disability, 507

23   Clients with Chemical Dependencies, 509

Issues and Trends in Substance Abuse, 510
Scope of the Problem, 511
Theories of Causation, 512
Factors that Place Populations at Risk, 512
Common Substances of Abuse, 516
Chemical Dependency, 522
Use of the Nursing Process, 523

24   High-Risk Aggregates in the Community, 532

The Homeless, 534
Migrant Agricultural Workers, 537
Refugees, 543

PART SIX   **HOME HEALTH CARE**

25   Discharge Planning and Continuing Care, 551

Historical Perspective, 552
Current Perspectives, 553
The Process of Discharge Planning, 554
Components for Providing Continuity of Care, 557
Review of Critical Process Information, 558
Discharge Planning Roles, 559

26   Care of Clients in the Home, 565

Definition of Home Health Care Nursing, 567
Definition of Home Health Care, 568
Medicare, 568
Medicaid, 568
Private Insurance, 568
The Interdisciplinary Team, 568
Collaborative Interdisciplinary Care, 570
High-Tech Home Care, 570
Hospice Care, 572
Caseload Management, 573
Future Trends, 575

PART SEVEN   **SPECIAL ROLES AND SETTINGS**

27   Occupational Health Nursing, 581

History, 583
Work-Related Injuries and Illness, 586
Maintenance of Health in the Workplace, 587
Major Categories of Hazards in the Workplace, 588
Roles and Functions of the Occupational Health Nurse, 594
The Occupational Health History, 597

Occupational Disease: Difficulties in Determination, 598
The Nursing Process in the Occupational Setting, 602
Occupational Safety and Health Programs, 602

28   School Health Nursing, 607

History Perspective, 609
Current Issues, 609
Educational Preparation and Classification, 610
Outlines and Standards Developed by the American Nurses' Association, 612
Role and Functions of the School Nurse, 612
Primary Prevention, 615
Secondary Prevention, 619
Tertiary Prevention, 623
Future Considerations, 626

PART EIGHT   **ISSUES AND CONCERNS IN COMMUNITY HEALTH NURSING**

29   Environmental Concerns, 633

The Population Effect, 635
Waste Disposal and Dispersal, 636
Water Pollution, 645
Noise Pollution, 646
Air Pollution, 648
Radiation in the Environment, 650
Environmental Disasters, 652
Pollution in the Home, 655
Nursing Interventions, 659

30   Legal and Ethical Issues, 663

The Legal System, 664
Ethical Theories, 666
The Relationship Between Ethics and Law, 668
Ethics, Law, and Community Health Nursing Standards, 669
Major Ethical and Legal Issues in Community Health Nursing, 671

31   Professional Issues, 681

Empowerment Through the Change Process, 682
Empowerment Through Participation in Organizations, 685
Empowerment Through Political Activity, 688
Community Health Nursing Issues, 694
The Future of Community Health Nursing, 698

Glossary, 704

Index, 733

Nursing Care in The Community

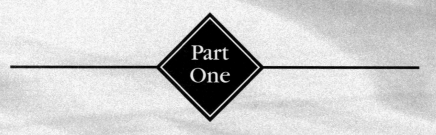

Part
One

Introduction to Community Health Nursing

Sickness and suffering have always been part of the human experience, and from the very earliest times there have been men and women who have cared about the welfare of the afflicted. The first semblance of "nursing" probably was practiced by family members as they attempted to soothe and protect the ill and the injured. As knowledge accumulated and moral codes evolved, a class of dedicated individuals, who belonged mainly to religious orders, focused their energy on the alleviation of suffering and of helping those in need of care. Chapter 1 describes some of the historical events that have helped to shape our modern system of community health nursing.

Defining the community as the client enables nurses to acquire a sense of the influence that a total population has on the health of a community. It also equips the nurse to identify aggregates in a population that can be targeted for care. Chapter 2 views the community as a client and provides case studies to help students understand how to assess the overall health of a community.

Nursing care in North America is a multicultural experience in which nurses are required to interact with persons whose values and belief systems may differ from their own. Methods of practicing in a multicultural society are described in Chapter 3.

In the United States the system for health care services to the community has become increasingly complex during the last few decades. This is due, in part, to the accelerating accumulation of information about the causes of ill health and disease and the rapid growth of sophisticated technology available to health care providers. However, health care needs are not always met in the United States, and much of the population remains underserved. Health care providers and legislators in the United States need to provide a more equitable method of distribution of services. (Canada provides universal health care, as do most other developed countries.) Nurses need to have a global view of health care systems. Chapter 4 deals with this concept.

Nursing has begun to define itself as an autonomous profession. A body of theoretical knowledge is available that assists nurses in making decisions about their practice and in objectively analyzing the needs of their clients. Community health nurses are using this knowledge to become more effective health care providers and advocates for their clients in the community setting. The application of nursing theory to community health nursing is presented in Chapter 5.

1

HISTORICAL OVERVIEW OF COMMUNITY HEALTH NURSING

Joan M. Cookfair

Change is the process by which the future invades our lives, and it is important to look at it closely, not merely from the grand perspectives of history, but also from the vantage point of the living, breathing individuals who experience it.

Alvin Toffler

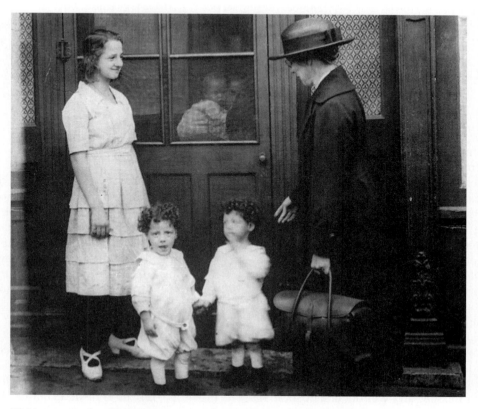

Visiting nurse, circa 1900. *(Reprinted with permission of the Visiting Nurses' Association of Western New York.)*

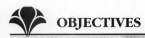

OBJECTIVES

At the conclusion of this chapter, the student will be able to:

1. Define the key terms listed.
2. Describe various historical events that have influenced the development of community health nursing.
3. Identify selected individuals who have contributed to the development of community health nursing.
4. Describe the development of organized public health.
5. Define public health nursing and community health nursing.
6. Describe the standards of community health nursing practice.

KEY TERMS

Community health nurses
Community health nursing
District nursing service

Frontier nursing service
  (FNS)
Florence Nightingale

Lillian Wald
Public health nursing

For community health nurses to understand the present, it is imperative that they review the past. Since before antiquity, special men and women have attempted to heal and cure. Even in the Neolithic age some individuals were viewed as having the ability to promote healing. Beginning in antiquity and continuing to the present, patterns of caring and caretaking have emerged. As a result of understanding the influence the environment has on the health of communities involved, caring persons shifted their focus to improving living conditions for populations in communities and providing access to care. This chapter will describe the contributions of selected individuals who have helped to develop the practice of what is now known as community health nursing, and will document some historical events that have enabled humankind to become healthier.

HISTORICAL ROOTS
Neolithic Age (ca. 10,000 BC)

Archeologists hypothesize that during the Neolithic age, a belief in supernatural forces dominated humankind's attempts to cope with sickness and death. Artifacts collected from this period indicate that this was the case. Physical anthropologists have discovered human remains that show that a surgical procedure was performed by boring a hole in the head (trephination), perhaps to let out evil spirits.

The Egyptians

It was not until the Egyptians invented a method of writing around 3000 BC that records were kept concerning care of the sick. According to Lucas (1953, p. 62), an ancient manuscript from that time period, the *Book of Surgery,* documented the observations of a court physician who made the following assessment concerning diagnosis and treatment:

If thou examinist a man having a crushed vertebrae in his neck and thou findest that one vertebrae has fallen into the neck, while he is voiceless, and cannot speak, his one vertebrae crushed into the next one; and shouldest thou find that he is unconscious of his two arms and legs because of this diagnosis, thou shouldest say concerning him, one having a crushed vertebrae in his neck, he is unconscious of his two arms and legs, he is speechless, he has an ailment not to be treated.

Record keeping and documentation increased knowledge about the care of the sick and helped spread this accumulated information. Evidence exists that medicines were prescribed in ancient times. The following remedy, also noted in the Book of Surgery, was prescribed for crying children: "Pods of poppy plant/Fly dirt which is on the wall/Make it into one, strain, give for four days" (Lucas, 1953, p. 62). One wonders how many children survived the cure.

The Hebrews

Around 2000 BC the Hebrew people kept written records and instructed as to what was safe to eat and drink. Considering the lack of refrigeration at that time and the prevalence of parasites, the following advice was excellent:

Ye are the children of the Lord your God.
Thou shalt not eat any abominable thing.
Ye shall not eat of them that chew the cud as the camel, the hare or the swine.
Ye shall eat of all that are in the waters, all that have fins and scales.
All clean birds ye shall eat, but not the vulture or his kind.
Ye shall not eat of anything that dieth of itself.
(Deuteronomy 12:7-21).

Ancient Greece

The Greeks developed a society that took great interest in healing disease and preventing illness. This is evident in the writings of two of the famous Greek physicians who lived in ancient times.

Hippocrates, who is believed to have lived between 460 and 375 BC, documented his work with his associates, all of whom were collectively called the Guild of Healers. They studied anatomy and classified diseases. They encouraged rest, fresh air, diet, and cleanliness as prevention against disease (Lucas, 1953).

Galen, who lived in the second century AD, wrote numerous treatises on anatomy and physiology. He was the first person to write about the study of animals, and he documented his experiments with them (*The Columbia Encyclopedia*, Vol 8, 1969).

Christianity (30 AD to present)

The teachings of Jesus Christ, which form the basis of the Christian religion, emphasized empathy and concern for others. Jesus commanded his followers to "love thy neighbor as thyself" (Mark 12:31). This gentle approach to human relationships still influences the way that Christian religious groups, many of which still exist today, provide care to the sick.

Rome (79 AD to 476 AD)

The Roman culture made a major contribution to the advancement of sanitation. When the city of Pompeii was excavated, archaeologists found the Roman methods of water distribution and drainage systems to be quite sophisticated. The Romans also established hospitals and health organizations. One excavated hospital contained 40 wards, vestibules, administration rooms, and apothecary shops (Lucas, 1953).

Islam (600 AD to present)

In the Koran, believers in the teachings of Mohammed are instructed that they "must not eat the flesh of animals that die a natural death, blood, and pigs' meat; also the flesh of strangled animals and of those beaten or gored to death" (Darwood, 1968, p. 376).

Middle Ages (500 AD to 1400 AD)

After the fall of Rome, the Western world moved into the Dark Ages. Constant warfare and plague depleted energy and creative thought. Scientific and rational thought became eroded by folk practices. The Celts, Germans, and Slavs relied on spells and incantations to cure disease. Lucas (1953, p. 280), mentions the following example taken from German folklore:

Balder and Woden fared to a wood there was Balder's foal's foot sprained. Then charmed Woden as well he know how for bone sprain for blood sprain for limb sprain bone to bone, blood to blood, limb to limb as though they were glued.

Vestiges of this kind of folk remedy still surface in today's society, particularly when medical science has no effective treatment for an incurable disease, and people feel hopeless and helpless as they did during the early Middle Ages.

The early Crusades, which took place over a 54-year period (1096 to 1149), were an attempt to rid Jerusalem and the surrounding area of so-called infidels or people who did not believe in Jesus Christ. To accomplish this task, knights and nobles from France and England journeyed from their homes to Palestine. Their adoption of some Greek and Arabic concepts of science is believed to have contributed to scientific thought in the Western world.

St. Thomas Aquinas (1225-1274), a Dominican monk, developed a concept of cause and effect, which resulted in a method of logical reasoning that is rational and linear in character. It led to a tendency to treat the body and the mind separately. Although nursing has taken a more holistic approach in recent years, this philosophical approach still is apparent in medical practice today.

Bubonic plague (Black Death), typhus (the plague), smallpox, scarlet fever, and diphtheria occurred in epidemic proportions throughout Europe during the fourteenth century. It is estimated that in the year 1394, two thirds of the European population died during an outbreak of the Black Plague. This widespread occurrence of disease contributed to the lack of scientific development during the so-called Dark Ages. During this period, the concept of quarantine evolved. Quarantine was officially legislated in Marseilles in 1383 (Anderson, Morton, & Green, 1978).

The Renaissance (1400-1700)

From the fifteenth through the seventeenth centuries, a period of rebirth occurred. A group called the humanists encouraged reading, art, and literature, and there was renewed interest in pursuing a scientific approach to curing illness and preventing disease. Much of the work by scientists such as Copernicus, Galileo, and Sir Isaac Newton was accepted. Copernicus' discovery that the earth was only part of a planetary system, and not central to the universe, Galileo's work in astronomy and physics, and Newton's proof of the laws of gravity stimulated reflection, scientific methods, and logical reasoning in other fields. The events of the Renaissance ushered in the Age of Enlightenment in the 1700s.

Table 1-1 describes historical events and mentions individuals who have influenced the health of humankind from antiquity until the latter part of the nineteenth century.

RELIGIOUS FIGURES

St. Francis of Assisi (1181-1226) was a Christian monk who founded an order that included men and women, called brothers and sisters, who cared for the sick and helped the destitute. Some of the hospitals in the United States are still administered by the Franciscan order.

St. Vincent de Paul (1581-1660) founded the Sisters of Charity. His society of missioners and *dames de charite* went from cottage to cottage giving food, medicine, and care to the sick. He encouraged the brothers and sisters in the order to help people help themselves (Dolan, 1973).

Theodur Fliedner founded the deaconesses of Germany in the seventeenth century who created hospices to provide care for the sick and destitute.

St. D'Youville (1701-1771). (See Figure 1-1.) In Montreal, Canada, Saint D'Youville founded an order called the Grey Nuns of the Sacred Heart. These women provided a home for orphans and unwed mothers. They also began a program that included visiting the sick in their homes. A branch of the order moved to Buffalo, New York, and continued ministering to the needs of the community. This group, which still exists, provides family care, job training, and education to community residents. In 1908, the nuns started a school in Buffalo that included a nursing program. Branches of the order exist in other parts of the United States and in Canada.

Mother Teresa (1910-present). Mother Teresa founded the Missionaries of Charity in 1955. These missionaries minister to the needs of the dying, abandoned children, and starving adults.

TABLE 1-1   Historical events influencing the development of nursing and medicine

Time	Place	Historical event	Cultural event
Antiquity:			
3000 BC	Eqypt	Written records	System of diagnosis
2000 BC	Canaan	Old Testament	Standards of conduct and behavior
500 BC	Greece	Hippocrates' papers	Scientific method
Anno Domini (AD):			
First century	Jerusalem, Rome, Greece	New Testament	Spread of moral code
79	Rome	Pliny's Historia Naturalis (Natural History)	Record of medical practice
130	Greece	Galen's study of physiology	Scientific approach
200	Rome	Central distributing system for water	Sanitation
400	Rome	Fall of Western Roman Empire	Cultural decline
500	Byzantium	Written records	Preservation of knowledge
610	Mecca	Koran	Standards of conduct and behavior
The Middle Ages:			
500	Europe	Continuous warfare	Folklore, unscientific approach
1096-1149	Middle East	Crusades	Cultural exchange
1181-1286	Rome	St. Francis of Assissi's Order of Friars Minor	Organized care of sick
1225-1274	Rome	Thomas Aquinas' papers on cause and effect	Logical reasoning
1390-1400	Europe	Epidemics	Cultural decline
The Renaissance:			
1400	Europe	Humanism	Emphasis on classics
1492	Western Hemisphere	Columbus discovers America	Expansion of world view
1517	Europe	Protestant Reformation	Diminished influence of Catholic Church
1530	Europe	Girolamo Fracastoro names syphilis	Beginning of germ theory
1581-1660	Belgium	Sisters of Charity	Hospices established
1591-1600	Europe	Beginnings of rationalistic approach	Scientific method
1628	England	William Harvey's study	Understanding of blood circulation
1646	England	Invention of microscope	Scientific research possible
1649	England	Watch with second hand	Ability to count pulse and respiration
Age of Enlightenment:			
1749	England	Variolation (Jenner's discovery of vaccination)	Concept of prevention of disease
1781	Vienna	Rene Laennec's invention of stethoscope	Ability to listen to heart and breath sounds
Nineteenth century: Beginning of modern scientific age			
1852	France	Louis Pasteur's discovery of pasteurization	Prevention of growth of bacteria
1855	England	John Snow's discovery of mode of cholera transmission	Prevention of disease spread
1870	Germany	Robert Koch's germ theory	Prevention of disease
1870	Scotland	Joseph Lister's principle of antisepsis	Use of antiseptics

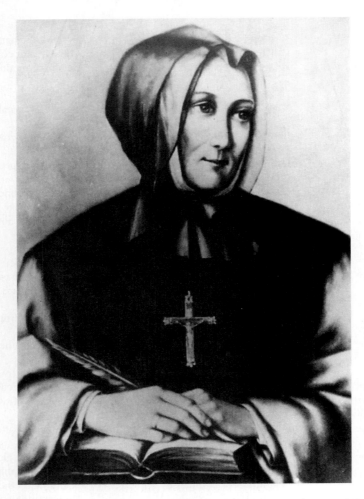

FIGURE 1-1   Saint D'Youville (1701-1771), founder of the Grey Nuns of the Sacred Heart. The nuns visited the sick at home and provided a home for orphans and unwed mothers. *(Reprinted with permission from D'Youville College archives, Buffalo, NY.)*

Mother Teresa's work began in Calcutta and has spread to Rome, Australia, Latin America, Holland, and New York City.

SEMINAL FIGURES

William Harvey (1578-1657), an English physician and anatomist, discovered blood circulation. His book, *Anatomical Exercises and Motions of the Heart in Animals,* provided health professionals with information that helped them understand blood circulation in human beings (Lucas, 1953).

Edward Jenner (1749-1823), who proved that cowpox provided immunity against smallpox, laid the foundation for modern immunology as a science (Lucas, 1953).

Florence Nightingale (1820-1910). **Florence Nightingale** was employed as superintendent of the Home for Invalid Ladies in England until 1854 (see Figure 1-2). When England became involved in the Crimean War in 1853, she was asked to take a group of nurses to the war zone to care for the wounded.

Nightingale went to Scutari in the Crimea with 38 nurses. She reported that the barracks were "filthy, dilapidated, and had no sanitation"

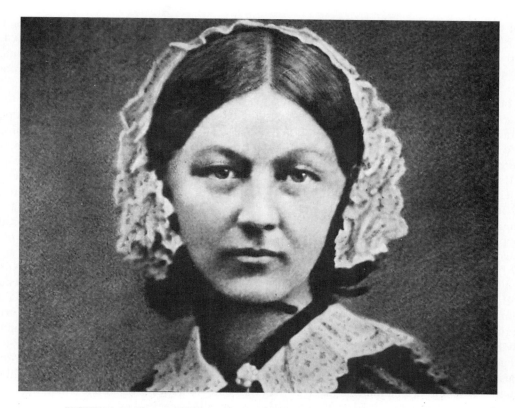

FIGURE 1-2 Florence Nightingale (1820-1910). *(From the Bettman Archives.)*

(Baly, 1986, p. 5). The small group of nurses had to plan cooking arrangements, "organize the hospital, and give care, at times, to four miles of patients" (Baly, 1986, p. 6). In addition, despite the lack of cooperation from the military physicians, the nurses' work made a measurable difference in the mortality rate from secondary infection and disease experienced by the soldiers.

Nightingale believed that sanitation, ventilation, and the proper foods would prevent a good deal of sickness. She also believed that nursing was an art as well as a science. These beliefs were put into practice during her work in the Crimean War.

Nightingale's experience left her physically ill and emotionally drained, but she returned home a national heroine. A grateful English public collected a large sum of money, which was placed into a fund called The Nightingale Fund, for her use in supervising a hospital nursing school. She used the fund to establish a training school for nurses at St. Thomas Hospital in London. She never directly supervised or taught the nurses, but she set up the program and hired the staff that provided these functions. She also helped finance the Nurses' Home near Liverpool Hospital, where nurses were trained to provide home nursing care. This institution became a model that was used to establish branches of the District Nursing Service throughout England. Nightingale insisted that in addition to nursing the patient, "a home nurse should show the family how to achieve sanitary conditions, keep the patient's room healthy, and improvise appliances in the home for patient care" (Baly, 1986, p. 132). Florence Nightingale's ability to organize and influence the development of nursing had a profound effect on the profession, and it is still felt today.

Queen Victoria (1819-1901). In 1887 Queen Victoria appropriated a large sum of money to found the Queen Victoria Jubilee Institute for nursing the poor and sick in their homes. This began a system of organized home nursing in England. By the end of the century, 539 nurses had formed the **District Nursing Service,** which was modeled after the Nightingale home nursing plan. These nurses lived in a nursing home and were responsible to a home supervisor. They were trained in the hospitals for 1 year and then received 13 months of additional training in public health. Similar district nursing services were set up throughout the United Kingdom (Ravenol, 1921). There began an effort to standardize community health nursing services. The distribution of material goods and many charitable activities were separated from nursing care. Religious proselytizing was prohibited (Clark, 1992).

Clara Barton (1821-1912). Clara Barton was inspired by the work of Jean Henri Durant, who founded the International Red Cross in 1863. Its guidelines state that it mobilizes services to assist soldiers and civilians during time of war, and assists civilians and soldiers who have been caused suffering during the war. In peacetime it helps individuals who have been affected by personal or community disaster. It maintains a Red Cross nursing reserve that may be called on in times of emergency (Griffin & Griffin, 1973).

Barton spent years studying the organization of the Red Cross in other countries. She returned to the United States and in 1881 persuaded government officials to organize the American Red Cross. She became its first president in 1882.

American Red Cross nurses served in Cuba during the Spanish-American war in 1898. In 1900 the Red Cross received its first federal charter, with William Howard Taft proclaiming himself ex officio president of the organization (Griffin & Griffin, 1973).

Jane Delano (1862-1919). In the late nineteenth century, Jane Delano organized the American Red Cross Nursing Service and became president of the Associated Alumni of Nurses, which was later named the American Nurses' Association. As a result of her administrative experience, she was asked in 1909 to become superintendent of the Army Nurse Corps reserve. Her main goal was to improve the quality of nurses who would be reserve members of the Corps. She succeeded in building up the reserve list to 3000 nurses before she resigned as superintendent in 1912 (Fitzpatrick, 1983). Her successors, Isabel McIsaac and Doris Thompson, continued her work.

Delano, as head of nursing for the American Red Cross, and Doris Thompson, as superintendent of the Army Nurse Corps, organized base hospitals and staffed them with members of the Army Nurse Corps before and during World War I (Fitzpatrick, 1983). The leadership and organizational abilities of these two women were responsible for saving many lives during the war.

Lillian Wald (1867-1940). **Lillian Wald** was a prominent figure in the organization of public health care in the United States. She graduated from the New York State School of Nursing in 1891. After graduation, she and a friend, Mary Brewster, rented a tenement in New York City and established a center called the Henry Street Settlement, where Wald employed nurses to work on a fee-for-service basis. She wrote of her experiences in *The House on Henry Street* and noted the many obstacles her nurses had to overcome to reach the families that needed home care. Wald developed a detailed and comprehensive method of keeping records and statistics regarding the incidence and prevalence of disease in the neighborhoods in which the nurses worked. The nurses in her employ taught families how to care for sick members, promote good hygiene, encourage prevention of disease, and raise healthy children (see Figure 1-3). The nurses also were encouraged to delve into the social causes of the illnesses that affected families. The poor of New York City, for example, were victims of tuberculosis, cholera, scarlet fever, and diphtheria.

Wald worked closely with health administrators, physicians, and legislative officials. It was largely through her efforts that a children's bureau was formed to facilitate care of sick children in New York City. Wald also was instrumental in organizing the Town and Country Service of the American Red Cross. In addition, the nursing division of the Metropolitan Life Insurance Company was formed at her urging (Griffin & Griffin, 1973). Wald convinced the Metropolitan's executives that it was more economical to use the ser-

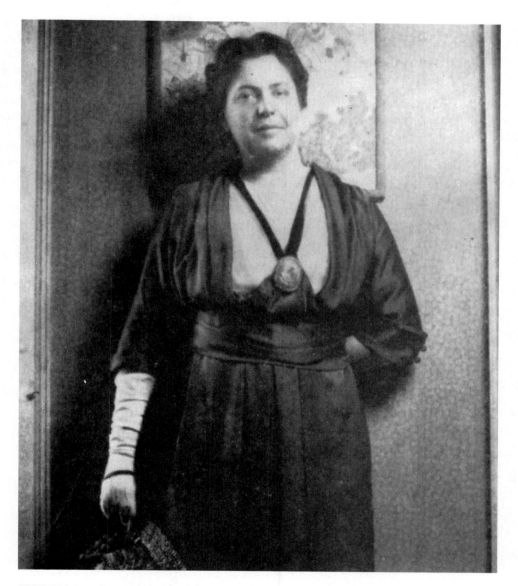

FIGURE 1-3 Lillian Wald (1867-1940). *(From* Lillian Wald: Neighbor and Crusader *by R.L. Duffus, 1938, New York: Macmillan Publishing Co. Used with permission.)*

vices of her nurses than to employ their own. According to Birnbach and Levenson (1991, p. 318), Wald maintained that:

Among the many opportunities for civic and altruistic work pressing on all sides, nurses, having superior advantages in their practical training, should not rest content with being only nurses, but should use their talents wherever possible in reform and civic movements.

Wald also believed that public health nurses had to know more about teaching and prevention than did hospital nurses. She and her friend Mary Gardner were instrumental in organizing the National Organization for Public Health Nursing (NOPHN). The purpose of the new society was to standardize public health efforts and coordinate all efforts in the field (Griffin & Griffin, 1973). The NOPHN stressed collaboration with physicians, legislators, and public health officials. Lillian Wald became its first president. This group, probably more than any other, influenced the development of organized public health nursing in this country until it was absorbed by the National League of Nurses (NLN) in 1952, which also incorporated the following organiza-

tions: the National League for Nursing Education, the Association of Collegiate Schools of Nursing, the Joint Committee of Practical Nurses and Auxiliary Workers in Nursing Services, the Joint Committee on Careers in Nursing, and the National Accrediting Service. (Table 1-2 lists nursing organizations in the United States chronologically from 1894 to 1953.)

Mary Breckinridge (Figure 1-4) founded the **Frontier Nursing Service (FNS)** in Lexington, Kentucky. The organization began as a small

TABLE 1-2   Development of nursing organizations in the United States

Year	Society	Purpose and function
1894	National League for Nursing Education	• To expand American Society of Superintendents of Training Schools • To establish minimum entrance requirements • To improve living and working conditions • To increase opportunities for postgraduate and specialized training
1900	American Red Cross	• To maintain a reserve list of nurses who can serve in war and disaster • To instruct the public in hygiene and care of the sick
1911	American Nurses' Association (ANA)	• To establish and maintain a code of ethics • To elevate standards of nursing education • To promote interests of the nursing profession
1912	National Organization of Public Health Nurses (NOPHN)	• To standardize public health nursing • To coordinate efforts in the field
1952	National League of Nurses	• To expand NOPHN • To provide examination and related services for use in licensing professionals • To accredit educational programs for nurses • To promote continued study and educational curricula to meeting changing needs • To define standards for organized nursing services and education
1952	Reorganized American Nurses' Association	• To work for continuing improvement of professional practice • To define functions and promote standards of professional nursing practice • To provide professional counseling • To serve as a national lobby for professional nurses • To implement the international exchange of nurses' program
1953	National Student Nurses' Association	• To represent student nurses • To provide counseling • To interact with ANA to promote improvement of professional practice

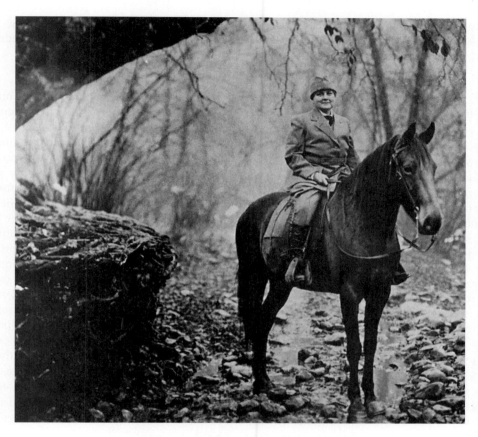

FIGURE 1-4 Mary Breckinridge founded the Frontier Nursing Service in Lexington, Kentucky. *(Reprinted with permission from the Frontier Nursing Service, Wendover, KY.)*

group whose purpose was to provide basic health care for mothers and babies in the hills of southeastern Kentucky. It soon became evident that it was impossible for a nurse to enter a home without providing care for the entire family. For example, a nurse would enter a home to check on an expectant mother and would be asked to give advice about an ulcer on a grandmother's leg. Soon Mary Breckinridge's nurses on horseback were providing a broad program of preventive and curative care for all family members. After 68 years in operation in one of the economically poorest regions of the United States, the program is responsible for the delivery of more than 23,000 babies, with a loss of only 11 mothers in childbirth throughout its entire history (Breckinridge, 1981).

Today the FNS includes a hospital that has a primary health clinic, three district nursing clinics, a home health agency, and a school of midwifery that is the largest in the nation.

Over the years, the FNS has evolved into a model of decentralized health care in a rural setting. It is known worldwide as an exceptional example of family-centered health care. Graduates from the school of midwifery at FNS have served all over the world, and each year professionals from other countries come to observe the program.

In the beginning, nurses rode their horses through blizzards, fog, and floods on mountain paths and trails (Figure 1-4). Today, nurses ride in four-wheel drive vehicles on roads that are at least passable. They still emphasize prevention and family care, which is consistent with the focus of public health nursing since Florence

Nightingale's time when nurses began visiting the sick in the home. The family was then and remains now the unit of care for the public health nurse.

MILITARY SERVICE
World War I

American casualties in World War I numbered over 318,000. Of this number, 50,280 were killed in battle, 62,000 died of disease, and 206,000 were wounded despite the work of the Army Nurse Corps and the American Red Cross. Nurses worked close to the battlefield under grueling conditions. They were exposed to danger from disease and from enemy bombardment. At times the nurse-patient ratio was 1:50, and a total of 101 nurses died (Surgeon General of the United States, 1919).

There was a nursing shortage in the war zone and at home. In 1918, Annie Warburton Goodrich, who had worked with Lillian Wald at the Henry Street Settlement, recommended the establishment of an army school of nursing to supply hospitals with needed personnel. The budget to support the school was approved in June 1918, and Goodrich became dean of the Nursing Department of the United States Army. In 1921, 500 nurses were graduated from the school and entered the Army Nurse Corps.

Julia Stimson, director of the American Expeditionary Force during World War I, believed that the Army Nurse Corps should be a progressive organization. After the war, she replaced Annie Goodrich as dean of the army nursing school. She advocated that nurses become teachers of health, a role she believed was part of the nurse's responsibility (Griffin & Griffin, 1973).

Post-World War I

The Army Nurse Corps had distinguished itself during the war, and under the direction of Annie Goodrich and Julia Stimson had developed quite a sophisticated curriculum that included both theoretical knowledge and technical skills. It was not until 1920 that nurses were given relative rank in the army, although physicians continued to have supervisory status. The army nursing school was closed in 1932 as an economic measure by the government (Griffin & Griffin, 1973),

and membership in the Army Nurse Corps declined until about 1940 when a second world war appeared unavoidable.

World War II

Although the United States did not enter World War II until December, 1941, the Council for National Defense was organized in 1940, with Julia Stimson as president. The organization immediately began to recruit nurses in preparation for the nursing needs created by another world war. The council was instrumental in forming the Cadet Nurse Corps. In World War I the army had its own nursing school. In World War II the government provided tuition, fees, uniforms, and stipends for interested young women to attend existing schools of nursing. Many nurses graduated from this program and entered military service at home or abroad (Fitzpatrick, 1983).

During this war, the mobile army surgical hospital (MASH) was formed. Nurses helped convert transport planes into flying ambulances and organized the loading and unloading of the sick and wounded. After the ill and injured were placed on board, the nurses were responsible for their care. The nurses' record of only five deaths per 100,000 casualties is evidence of their excellent work.

Post-World War II

After the war, army nurses benefited from the GI Bill of Rights, which awarded veterans funds for education. This opportunity encouraged some nurses to return to school to obtain Baccalaureate degrees.

The Korean War

During the Korean War, the mobile Army hospitals operated only 8 to 10 miles from the front line. Rapid evacuation of the wounded by helicopter considerably decreased the mortality rate of the combat troops (Fitzpatrick, 1983).

The Vietnam War

During the Vietnam War, the concept of mobile hospital units was changed because there were no front lines. A medical unit, self-contained and transportable, was devised. This unit (MUST) was equipped with medical supplies and staffed by physicians and nurses. They operated so close to the combat zones that medical personnel were themselves in danger. Four navy nurses sustained wounds in a bombing in Saigon, and one Army nurse was killed at an evacuation hospital at Chu Lai (Fitzpatrick, 1983).

Desert Shield/Desert Storm

Self-contained units were used in this confrontation as well; however, war in the desert necessitated down-sizing some units to "forward surgical elements" (FSE) to enhance mobility. These units consisted of 140 medical personnel who could be rapidly transported to areas where they might be needed. FSEs included nurses trained in advanced trauma life support, nurse anesthetists, operating room nurses, and intensive care nurses. Enduring excessive heat, sand storms, rain, and an unfamiliar culture, nurses in these units cared for wounded Americans, Iraqi soldiers, and Iraqi civilians.

Operation Restore Hope

The goal of the United States medical forces in Somalia was to support the U.S. forces. Nurses who served on hospital ships off the coast of Somalia were primarily operating room nurses caring for patients undergoing surgery. Army nurses worked as flight nurses to assist in the transportation of soldiers and civilians who needed care. Nurses from many nations worked and continue to function in humanitarian relief agencies sponsored by the International Medical Corps, The International Committee of the Red Cross, and others. In Somalia, the nurses worked under extremely austere and harsh conditions and witnessed the results of anarchy, starvation, and lack of sanitation. Sometimes in remote villages they provided care with limited support systems. For example, one young intensive care nurse from Belgium worked in a Red Cross–sponsored hospital with no physicians. She was "treating gunshot wounds and other illnesses with the best care that could be provided" (Cowan, 1993, p. 1).

Somalia was dramatic and required nurses and other medical personnel to work under extreme conditions. It was just one of many emergencies the Red Cross and others responded to and continue to respond to. Emergencies that may be caused by natural disaster, such as Hurri-

cane Andrew, or internal violence, such as that which has caused such extreme suffering in Somalia, continue to need immediate intervention.

NURSING THEORY AND COMMUNITY HEALTH NURSING

The development of a theory of nursing has helped to legitimize nursing as a profession. Nursing scholars have analyzed the nature and scope of nursing knowledge and practice in an attempt to define the role of the nurse and to explain its unique contribution to the individual person, to health, and to the environment. Nursing theory helps to guide practice, to stimulate research, and to upgrade professional education. Chapter 5 describes the work of several nurse theorists who have influenced community health nursing.

Public Health Nursing

Public health nursing was redefined by the American Public Health Association (1980, p. 4), to incorporate the impact of nursing theory on public health nursing practice. The redefinition is as follows:

Public health nursing synthesizes the body of knowledge from the public health sciences and professional nursing theories for the purpose of improving the health of the entire community. This goal lies at the heart of primary prevention and health promotion and is a foundation for public practice.

Public health nurses may be generalists employed by state and provincial governments. They may work in health departments and provide services in homes, clinics, schools, and workplaces within a specified geographic region. Those employed in the private sector are often responsible for a caseload of families within a designated area.

Nurses working in the community have always been able to associate the affects of the environment on individuals, groups, and families with health states of a given community. Lack of sanitation, poor housing, harsh weather, and poor nutrition all contribute to possible impaired health states (see the discussion on environment in Chapter 30).

Community Health Nursing

Community health nurses have an expanded role that is broader than that of the public health nurse. Their responsibility is to the population as a whole. It is not episodic but continuous (Northrop & Kelly, 1987). Community health nurses may function in discharge planning and infection control, management of home care, nurse-managed centers, and other community settings.

The American Nurses' Association (ANA) (1980, p. 2), defined community health nursing as follows:

Community health nursing is a synthesis of nursing theory and public health practice applied to promoting and preserving the health of populations. Health promotion, health maintenance, health education and management, coordination, and continuity of care are utilized in a holistic approach to the management of the health care of individuals, families, and groups in the community.

This definition includes the following assumptions:

1. The health care system is complex.
2. Primary, secondary, and tertiary prevention are components of the health care system.
3. Nursing, as a subsystem of the health care system, is the product of education and practice based on research.
4. The provision of primary health care predominates in community health practice with lesser involvement in secondary and tertiary health care (ANA, 1980, p. 2).

The ANA has set standards of community health nursing practice in an attempt to clarify the functions of the nurse's role (see the box at right).

In 1928, the Goldmark report pointed out the need for advanced preparation for community health nursing. The Brown report of 1948 emphasized the importance of educating nurses specifically to meet the needs of the community as regards health care (Benson & McDevitt, 1976). There was continued concern that nurses working in the community needed special preparation, and in 1964 the ANA stated that public health nurses needed a Baccalaureate degree to

STANDARDS OF COMMUNITY HEALTH NURSING PRACTICE

Standard I: theory

The nurse applies theoretical concepts as a basis for decisions in practice.

Standard II: data collection

The nurse systematically collects data that are comprehensive and accurate.

Standard III: diagnosis

The nurse analyzes data collected about the community, family, and individual to determine diagnoses.

Standard IV: planning

At each level of prevention, the nurse develops plans that specify nursing actions unique to client needs.

Standard V: intervention

The nurse, guided by the plan, intervenes to promote, maintain, or restore health, to prevent illness, and to effect rehabilitation.

Standard VI: evaluation

The nurse evaluates responses of the community, family, and individual to interventions in order to determine progress toward goal achievement and to revise the data base, diagnoses, and plan.

Standard VII: quality assurance and professional development

The nurse participates in peer review and other means of evaluation to ensure quality of nursing practice. The nurse assumes responsibility for professional development and contributes to the professional growth of others.

Standard VIII: interdisciplinary collaboration

The nurse collaborates with other health care providers, professionals, and community representatives in assessing, planning, implementing, and evaluating programs for community health.

Standard IX: research

The nurse contributes to theory and practice in community health nursing through research.

Adapted from American Nurses' Association, *Standards of Nursing Practice* (1986).

be certified. Many educational programs now include Masters' and Doctoral programs in community health.

Community Nursing Centers (CNC) provide a wide range of health services, from basic health services such as physical care, to services for the acutely ill, the chronically ill, and the terminally ill.

During the 1980s, new reimbursement policies encouraged hospitals to provide care that included outpatient surgery and discharge before completion of the healing process. As a result, the home care industry experienced phenomenal growth. Consumer concerns led the NLN to establish a community health accreditation program (CHAP). In 1987, this became an independent subsidiary of the NLN. CHAP accredits home and community-based agencies in the United States. This group includes volunteer, not-for-profit, proprietary, and publicly financed organizations. The organization's goal is to assure the availability of high quality home care services and allay consumer concerns. CHAP's standards are based on the following four quality management principles:

1. The organization's structure and function consistently support a consumer-oriented philosophy and purpose.

2. The organization must consistently provide services and products of the highest quality.

3. The organization must have adequate human, financial, and physical resources to accomplish its stated purpose.

4. The organization must be positioned for long-term viability.

A private organization, the Joint Commission of Home Care Organizations, also accredit community health agencies. Agencies may request them to do so on a voluntary basis to assure their consumers that they are providing quality care.

Chapter Highlights

- Historical events have contributed to the well-being of humankind and the changing roles of nurses in the community. Written records since 2000 BC trace the attempts of men and women to heal and cure. Selected religious figures who influenced the development of community health nursing include Saint Margarite D'Youville and Mother Teresa.

- Florence Nightingale's nurses' home care organization was the model for the District Nursing Service of England.

- Lillian Wald's influence on the development of community health care in the United States was achieved through her work in settlement houses.

- Seminal figures who played a strong role in the development of community health nursing include Jane Delano, who organized the American Red Cross Nursing Service, and Mary Breckinridge, who founded the Frontier Nursing Service.

- Nurses have served effectively in the military from World War I to Operation Restore Hope.

- Community health nursing synthesizes nursing theory and public health practice to promote and preserve the health of populations. Health promotion, health maintenance, and continuity of care are incorporated into a holistic approach and applied to the management of the health care of individuals, families, and groups in the community.

- The NLN has established an accreditation body (CHAP) to ensure that the availability of quality care will be given by home health care agencies.

CRITICAL THINKING EXERCISE

The attempts, by thinking men and women, to avoid illness can be traced back to antiquity. The beginnings of a system for diagnosing illnesses, standards of conduct for behavior, and the use of the scientific method are examples of some of these attempts.

In recent times, the standards of community health nursing emphasize health promotion, mainte-

nance of wellness, and prevention of illness.

1. Historically, what nursing leaders have influenced the development of these standards?
2. How would you integrate the thinking of these individuals into your practice today?

REFERENCES

American Nurses' Association, Division on Community Nursing. (1980). *A conceptual model of community health nursing* (ANA Publication No. Ch-102M, 5/80). Kansas City, MO: Author.

American Nurses' Association. (1986). *Standards of community health nursing practice.* Kansas City, MO: Author.

American Public Health Association, Nursing Section. (1980). *The definition and role of public health nursing in the delivery of health care.* Washington, D.C.: Author.

Anderson, C.L., Morton, R.F., & Green, L.W. (1978). *Community health* (3rd ed.). St. Louis: Mosby.

Baly, M.B. (1986). *Florence Nightingale and the nursing legacy.* Beckenham, UK: Croom Helm.

Bennett, P. (1991). One army nurse's experience in a forward surgical unit during the ground offensive. *Journal of Emergency Room Nursing, 17*(5), 27A-34A.

Benson, E.R., & McDevitt, J.Q. (1976). *Community health and nursing practice.* Englewood Cliffs, NJ: Prentice-Hall.

Birnbach, N., & Levenson, S. (1991). *First words: Selected addresses from the National League for Nursing, 1894-1933.* New York: National League for Nursing Press.

Birnbach, N., & Levenson, S. (1993). *Legacy of leadership.* New York: National League for Nursing Press.

Breckinridge, M. (1981). *Wide neighborhoods.* Lexington, KY: The University Press of Kentucky.

Clark, M.J. (1992). *Nursing in the community.* Norwalk, CT: Appleton & Lange.

Community Health Accreditation Program, Inc. (CHAP). (1993). *Quality through accreditation.* New York: National League for Nursing Press.

Cowen, M.L. (1993). Reminiscences of operation restore hope. *Navy Medicine, 84*(2), 1-8.

Darwood, N.J. (Trans). (1968). *The Koran.* Great Britain: The Penguin Classics.

Dolan, J. (1973). *Nursing in society.* New York: Saunders.

Falco, S. (1980). *Nursing theories: The base for professional nursing practice.* Englewood Cliffs, NJ: Prentice-Hall.

Fitzpatrick, L. (1983). *Prologue to professionalism: A history of nursing.* London: Prentice-Hall International.

Frontier Nursing Service, Development Office, Wendover, KY, 41775.

Giff, P. (1986). *Mother Teresa: Sister to the poor.* New York: Viking Press.

Griffin, G.J., & Griffin, J.K. (1973). *History and trends of professional nursing* (7th ed.). St. Louis: Mosby.

Hall, J., & Weaver, B.R. (1986). *A systems approach to community health.* Philadelphia: JB Lippincott.

Henderson, V. (1966). *The nature of nursing: A definition and its implications for practice, research and education.* New York: Macmillan.

King, I. (1981). *A theory of nursing: Systems, concepts, process.* New York: Wiley.

Leininger, M. (1984). *Care: The essence of nursing and health.* Thorofare, NJ: Slack.

Lucas, H.S. (1953). *A short history of civilization* (2nd ed.). New York: McGraw-Hill.

Northrop, C.E., & Kelly, M.E. (1987). *Legal issues in nursing.* St. Louis: Mosby.

Ravenol, M. (1921). *A half century of public health.* New York: American Public Health Association.

Stowe, H. (1992). Into Iraq nursing: Organization in a combat support hospital. *Journal of Nursing Administration Quarterly, 22*(2), 49-53.

Surgeon General of the United States. (1919). *Report of the Surgeon General.* Washington, D.C.: United States Army Historical Unit.

Toffler, A. (1970). *Future Shock.* New York: Random House.

Visiting Nurses' Association, 4230 Lea Road, Amherst, New York, 14226.

2

COMMUNITY AS CLIENT

Joan M. Cookfair

We must now emphatically refuse to deal with single components, but instead relate to the concept of wholeness.

Betty Neuman

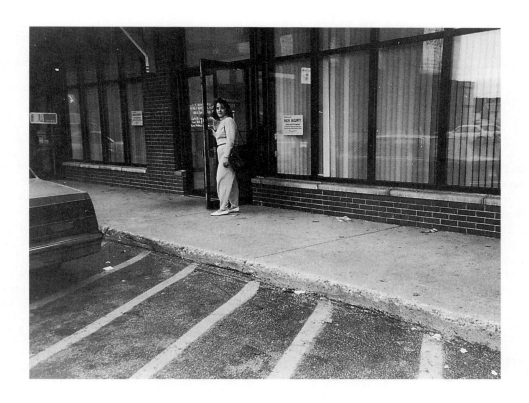

OBJECTIVES

At the conclusion of this chapter, the student will be able to:

1. Define key terms listed.
2. Define community.
3. Use nursing process within a nursing theorist framework to assess a geopolitical community.
4. Compare a community with a low level of wellness to a community with a high level of wellness.

KEY TERMS

Aggregates	Geopolitical community	Secondary prevention
Community as a client	Neuman Systems Model	Tertiary prevention
Community assessment	Primary prevention	Statistical analysis
Conceptual framework		

Chapter 1 describes many of the roles and functions of the community health nurse. It also contains a definition of community health nursing as described by the American Nurses' Association. This second chapter will present selected definitions of community that may be used by the community health nurse in practice. It will also describe assessments of a high-risk community and a well community. Each assessment is organized within a four-step nursing process framework and uses selected portions of Betty Neuman's systems model.

DEFINITIONS OF COMMUNITY

According to the dictionary, community is defined as the people living in a specific area. This is consistent with the definition of the community as a place. This focus is helpful if a community health nurse is conducting a **statistical analysis** of a selected geographical area. Most statistics are recorded relative to person, place, and time. This type of community might be called a **geopolitical community.**

Communities can also be defined as **aggregates.** This term would apply to individuals who share similar characteristics or experience common factors. Aggregates may be ethnic communities, religious communities, developmental communities, or communities of need; for example, high-risk aggregates (see Chapter 24).

A community may also be defined as a social system. This implies some type of interaction. People interact formally or informally within the broader system, and they form networks that operate for the benefit of the individuals within the group. The group may evolve as a result of a shared need, for example, support groups or parents' groups, or a group may be based on a shared interest. In some cases, the interest is purely social; in others it is not.

The nursing theorist Betty Neuman views the community as a practice setting, a target of service, or a small group within the larger community. "The client is an interacting open system in total interface with both internal and external forces or stressors" (Neuman, 1989, p. 12). This definition allows the nurse to focus on the client as a geopolitical community (a practice setting) or an aggregate group (a target of service).

The operational definition used by the nurse needs to be consistent with the role of that nurse in the community.

CONCEPTUAL FRAMEWORK

The use of the nursing process to plan client care in the community allows the nurse to integrate the Standards of Community Health Nursing Practice into the plan of care (see Chapter 1). Data collection, diagnosis, planning, intervention, evaluation, and the application of nursing theory are all recommended by the American Nurses' Association as a way to clarify the nurse's role in the community. The five processes described in the standards have been consolidated into four steps by authors Yura and Walsh (1983). These steps are defined as follows:

1. Assessment: Assessing is the act of collecting data about a situation for the purpose of diagnosing a client's actual or potential health problems.

2. Planning: Careful planning and thoughtful goal setting should occur. The nurse must validate the plan with the data assessment.

3. Implementation: During this phase, the nurse implements and completes the actions necessary to carry out the plan.

4. Evaluation: Appraisal of the client's behavioral changes, or possibly lack of change, as a result of the action occurs during evaluation.

Neuman's Nursing Process Format

Betty Neuman (1989) presents a nursing process format, as follows, in three steps:

1. Nursing diagnosis: This includes a data base that assesses the physiological, psychological, sociocultural, developmental, and spiritual variables comprising the client system. This step is concluded when a nursing diagnosis has been formulated.

2. Nursing goals: The goals of the plan include a negotiation with the client to correct variances with wellness. Intervention strategies to maintain the client system are a part of this step.

3. Nursing outcomes: Intervention strategies that use one or more preventive interventive modalities are included in this step. The results of the interventions or outcomes are evaluated to confirm the attainment of nursing goals.

The Neuman Systems Model

Neuman (1989) has developed a model that demonstrates her approach to patient problems. This model uses a systems approach (Figure 2-1). In the **Neuman Systems Model,** health is viewed as a condition in which all parts and subparts are in harmony. Disharmony reduces the wellness state. Environment is believed to be all those factors that affect or are affected by the person or that influence that person's wellness state or normal line of defense. "The goal of nursing is to facilitate for the client optimum wellness through retention, attainment, or maintenance of client system stability" (Neuman, 1989, p. 72).

The normal line of defense is an adaptive state that has been developed by an individual or community over time. This state is considered normal for that individual or community. Surrounding the normal state in the model is a broken circle that represents the flexible line of defense. This represents a protective buffer that can change. It can strengthen and help prevent stressors from breaking through the normal line of defense. On the other hand, poor nutrition and lack of sleep can weaken this line of defense and penetrate the normal line of defense. This may threaten the lines of resistance.

Lines of resistance are the individual's internal factors that help to defend against a stressor. For example, the body's innate immune response would be the last line of defense against a stressor's breaking through to the basic core. The basic core is the energy resource that enables the individual to fight against a stressor; for example, normal temperature, genetic structure, or ego structure.

In Neuman's system, primary prevention is aimed at reducing the possibility of encounters with stressors and strengthening the flexible line of defense. Secondary prevention relates to early case finding and treatment of symptoms. Tertiary prevention focuses on readaptation, education to

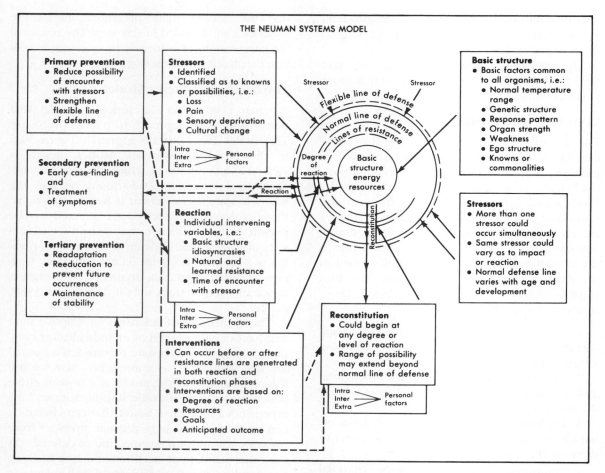

FIGURE 2-1   The Neuman Systems Model. *(From* The Neuman systems model *by B. Neuman, 1989, Norwalk, CT: Appleton & Lange.)*

prevent further occurrences, and maintenance of stability. Figure 2-2 demonstrates Neuman's format for primary, secondary, and tertiary interventions.

Applications of the Neuman Model

Nurses who are beginning a **community assessment** might find it helpful to use Neuman's approach in viewing the **community as a client.** This approach, which is illustrated in a model by Anderson, McFarlane, and Helton (1986) (Figure 2-3), expands Neuman's systems model, which is based on the nursing process as a framework to activate her view of the commu-

nity as a system that affects target groups. The total population is assessed, and the impact of stressors that affect its health status is analyzed. The interventions are planned at primary, secondary, and tertiary levels. Evaluation of the health plan is included. The following eight interacting subsystems are included: health and safety, sociocultural, education, communication and transportation, recreation, economics, law and politics, and religion (Anderson et al., 1986). This model is useful in identifying high-risk aggregates in a community. As with any systems model, the nurse must avoid collecting irrelevant data in the assessment process. Although all data may have

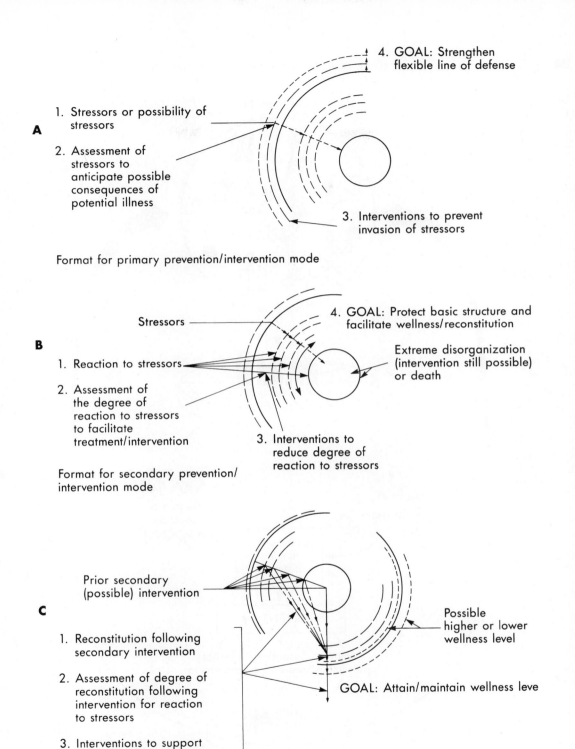

A 1. Stressors or possibility of stressors

2. Assessment of stressors to anticipate possible consequences of potential illness

4. GOAL: Strengthen flexible line of defense

3. Interventions to prevent invasion of stressors

Format for primary prevention/intervention mode

B Stressors

1. Reaction to stressors

2. Assessment of the degree of reaction to stressors to facilitate treatment/intervention

4. GOAL: Protect basic structure and facilitate wellness/reconstitution

Extreme disorganization (intervention still possible) or death

3. Interventions to reduce degree of reaction to stressors

Format for secondary prevention/intervention mode

C Prior secondary (possible) intervention

1. Reconstitution following secondary intervention

2. Assessment of degree of reconstitution following intervention for reaction to stressors

3. Interventions to support internal/external resources for reconstitution

Possible higher or lower wellness level

GOAL: Attain/maintain wellness leve

Format for tertiary prevention/intervention mode

FIGURE 2-2 **A,** Primary prevention/intervention mode. **B,** Secondary prevention/intervention mode. **C,** Tertiary prevention mode. *(From* The Neuman systems model *by B. Neuman, 1989, Norwalk, CT: Appleton & Lange.)*

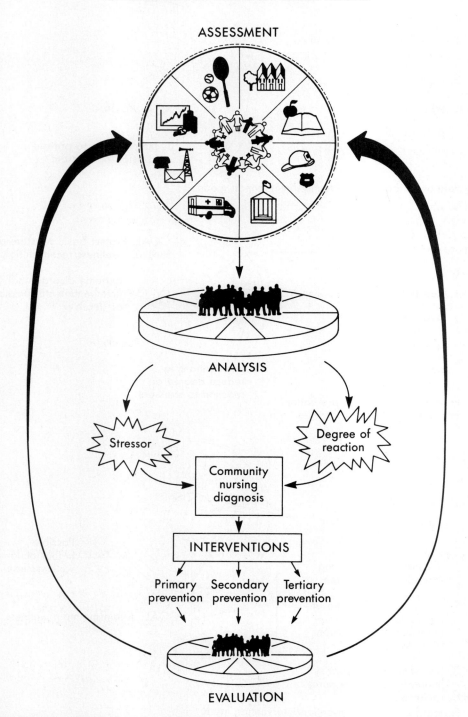

FIGURE 2-3   The community-as-client model. *(From Community-as-client: A model for practice by E. Anderson, J. McFarlane, & A. Helton, 1986, Nursing Outlook, 34(5), p. 22. Reprinted with permission.)*

TABLE 2-1 The Neuman Community—Client Assessment Guide*

Aggregate client	Geopolitical client
Intrasystem	
System boundary; client defined	Same as for aggregate client
Physiological	
1. Physical assessment as appropriate	Same as for aggregate client
2. Specific maturational stage data; for example, Apgar scores of newborns	
Psychological	
1. Emotional health of aggregate members: prevalence of isolation and depression, divorce, and crime rates	1. Emotional health of community
2. Communication patterns: response patterns to feedback from other systems	2. Same as for aggregate client
Developmental	
1. Maturational stage of aggregate	1. Maturational stage of community
2. Age range and median of aggregate	2. Age range and median of population
Sociocultural	
1. Demographic characteristics: sex, age, education level, income, and ethnicity	Same as for aggregate client
2. Health beliefs: immunization levels, child rearing practices	
3. Lifestyles, including risk-taking behaviors	
4. Consumer participation in community programs	
Spiritual	
Religious affiliation	Same as for aggregate client
Client perceptions	
—	Perceived problems
—	Perceived solutions
Intersystem	
Primary caregiver system	System boundary — geographical or political
Health and safety	
1. Personnel: number, education, and experience	1. Health indicators: morbidity, life expectancy, etc.
2. Case load of personnel	2. Resource allocation and utilization
3. Occupational health programs	3. Facilities: hospitals, health department, outpatient clinics
4. Agency programs and clientele served: — Services to strengthen families — Services for special groups	4. Safety services: — Official services, such as police, fire — Volunteer services, such as block parent, neighborhood watch
5. Environmental conditions and safety hazards within the building	5. Sanitation services, such as garbage and sewage disposal
	6. Case loads of professionals

Continued

TABLE 2-1   The Neuman Community—Client Assessment Guide*   cont'd

Aggregate client	Geopolitical client
	7. Environmental conditions and safety hazards: — Air, water, and soil inspection — Abandoned or unkempt buildings, trash and garbage, broken sidewalks
Sociocultural	
1. Ethnic composition of personnel and languages 2. Membership in associations and professional organizations	1. Culture composition of population and languages spoken 2. Guiding values 3. Positions and roles 4. Associations and clubs 5. Services to strengthen families, such as preschool and senior day care 6. Services for special groups, such as handicapped and new immigrant
Education	
1. Education level and experience of personnel 2. Continuing education for employees: journal subscriptions, inservice education	1. Personnel: education level of residents 2. Facilities: universities, colleges, schools, libraries 3. Personnel: number, education, and experience
Communication and transportation	
1. Communication patterns within agencies: formal and informal systems 2. Communication methods to intrasystem and extrasystems: pamphlets, posters, home visits, and mass media 3. Accessibility: — Location: accessibility and acceptability — House of service — Cultural interpretation and translation services	Same as for aggregate client
Recreation	
1. Facilities: lunchrooms, lounges, etc. 2. Activities: planned and informal	1. Facilities: schools, library, museums, ice rinks, etc. 2. Personnel: number, education, and experience 3. Programs: adult, children, and special needs 4. Accessibility
Economics	
1. Resources: funding, personnel, buildings, equipment, supplies 2. Health and welfare benefits for employees: health and dental insurance, pension plans, etc. 3. Paid continuing education programs	1. Employment: employment status and income levels of residents 2. Income assistance: percentage of the population 3. Education levels, literacy rate 4. Housing: quality and types 5. Industry and occupational health programs

TABLE 2-1 The Neuman Community—Client Assessment Guide* cont'd

Aggregate client	Geopolitical client
Law and politics	
1. Policy formulation: decision and problem-solving patterns	1. Power: sanctions and making legislation as sanctions relate to health of community
2. Positions and roles	
3. Contracts	
Religion	
1. Agency philosophy	1. Number and types of churches
2. Beliefs and values of employees	2. Church programs and activities
Client perceptions	
—	Perceived problems
—	Perceived solutions
Extrasystem description	
Same as the geopolitical intersystem	System boundary: location, climate, urban or rural, topography, square miles
	— Population: number per square mile, mobility
	— History
Subsystem data	
Same as the geopolitical intersystem	Collect data selectively about subsystems at a federal level, or state or provincial level, or both, as it pertains specifically to the needs of the geopolitical community

From *The Neuman systems model* (2nd ed., pp. 371-373) by B. Neuman, 1989, Norwalk, CT: Appleton & Lange.
* The list of assessment data and examples of the type of data collected serve only as a guide and are not exhaustive.

an indirect connection in terms of this model, information may be outside the nurse's range of influence.

For simplicity and clarity, a community assessment may need only to incorporate selected concepts from the Neuman model. In the community, basic structure includes all the variables that keep the community functioning as a unit. The normal line of defense may be the coordinated efforts of the city mayor, city council, and the health department. The flexible line of defense might be a special nutrition program for low-income pregnant women that might suddenly be discontinued (Neuman, 1989).

It is possible that a community may have health problems that require intervention at primary, secondary, and/or tertiary levels. **Primary prevention** calls for the prevention of disease by altering susceptibility or reducing exposure of susceptible individuals. It is accomplished by health promotion through teaching and advocacy, or specific protection through immunizations and altered environment. **Secondary prevention** is the early detection and treatment of disease by such techniques as case finding, screening surveys, and prevention of the spread of communicable disease. **Tertiary prevention** is the alleviation of disability that results from disease and the attempt to restore effective functioning. Tertiary prevention may be achieved by means of rehabilitation, or palliative methods if rehabilitation is impossible (Leavell & Clark, 1965).

On the basis of Neuman's terminology, primary prevention in a community would be aimed at strengthening the flexible line of defense. Secondary prevention would be directed toward strengthening the lines of resistance, and the tertiary prevention would be directed toward promoting maximum wellness by protecting the basic core in a target group or practice setting already identified as having a compromised level of wellness. The nurse may find it helpful to refer to the client community assessment guide (Table 2-1) in applying Neuman's model.

ASSESSING THE LEVEL OF WELLNESS IN A COMMUNITY

One hundred nursing students in a baccalaureate program were asked by local community leaders to assess the health of a selected urban community close to their school. The students used selected parts of Neuman's assessment tool (Table 2-1) to conduct their investigation. They chose a

four-step nursing process framework to organize the data, shown as follows:

I. Assessment
  A. Community boundaries
  B. Statistical data
  C. Education
  D. Economy/occupations
  E. Environment
  F. Community resources
  G. Vital statistics
  H. Morbidity data
  I. Health resources
  J. Other
II. Community diagnosis
III. Nursing goals (plans and interventions)
IV. Nursing outcomes (evaluation)

The case study that follows is a compilation of the nursing students' work.

■ CASE STUDY 1

Assessment

Community boundaries. The community was located in a low-income urban area. Its boundaries were established within a specific census tract that encompassed approximately 4 square miles.

Demographic data. Students collected statistical

data from the 1980 census taken by the local county government and interviewed approximately 250 families and some community leaders. The total population was 5329 and, according to statistics, was fairly stable. The estimated percentage of newcomers during the previous 5 years was 16.6%. Slightly fewer than half

TABLE 2-2   Age and race distribution of community studied

Age distribution			Ethnic distribution		
Year	Number	Percent	Race	Number	Percent
5	614	11.5	White	1131	21.2
5-9	615	11.5	Black	1783	33.5
10-14	551	10.3	Indian	241	4.5
15-19	612	11.5	Hispanic	1935	36.3
25-34	892	16.8	Other	239	4.5
35-44	529	9.9	TOTAL	5329	100.0
45-54	573	10.8			
55-64	600	11.3			
65-74	343	6.4			
TOTAL	5329	100.0			

From Community project: Class of 1987 by J. Dzimian, N. Schoelkopf, K. Spalti, L. Waldowski, and M. Zimmerman, 1987, unpublished manuscript, D'Youville College, Buffalo, NY.

TABLE 2-3 Children attending school in the community

Type of school	Number	Percent
Nursery	144	5.9
Kindergarten	153	6.3
Elementary (1-8)	1789	73.9
High school (9-12)	336	13.9
TOTAL	2422	100.0

From Community project: Class of 1987 by J. Dzimian, N. Schoelkopf, K. Spalti, L. Waldowski, and M. Zimmerman, 1987, unpublished manuscript, D'Youville College, Buffalo, NY.

TABLE 2-4 Income levels in the community

Earnings	Number	Percent
Below $5,000	1207	55.2
$5,000-7,499	395	18.1
$7,500-9,999	238	10.9
$10,000-14,999	345	15.8
TOTAL	2185	100.0

From Community project: Class of 1987 by J. Dzimian, N. Schoelkopf, K. Spalti, L. Waldowski, and M. Zimmerman, 1987, unpublished manuscript, D'Youville College, Buffalo, NY.

the residents were white; the remainder of the population was mostly black or Hispanic. The age and ethnic distribution of the population is described in Table 2-2. According to local officials, some Native Americans refused to participate in the census because they considered themselves members of the Indian nation. It was therefore believed that more native Americans resided in the area than the statistics indicated. The 1980 census tract information indicated that there were 780 households headed by women in this community.

Education. The distribution of children who attended school the year before the assessment is recorded in Table 2-3. The level of education in the community showed that fewer than half of all adults older than 25 years had any high school education. A very small group, 6%, had finished college.

Economy/occupations. The average income was low; more than half the families had an annual income below $5000. Many were receiving public assistance. Of the adults older than 16 years, 26% were unemployed (Table 2-4). The majority of the labor force, those individuals age 16 years and older, were employed in clerical positions or service jobs. A small group, 16%, was engaged in lower-level managerial positions.

Environment. The community was located in a temperate climate that had very harsh winters, which were sometimes accompanied by deep snow. Summers were warm and pleasant, and spring and fall are cold and damp. There were few trees and flowers, and the living quarters were crowded together. The neighborhood was an urban area, bordered on one side by a main street leading to a downtown shopping section, a middle-income housing district on the other side, and lower-income housing districts on the other two sides. Houses generally were run down and in need of repair (Figure 2-4). Many fences were broken and yards untended. Playgrounds were not usable because of broken equipment (Figure 2-5).

Parents in three of the families interviewed said they kept their children in the (home) yard and away from the playground because it was a "drug drop." Another drug drop, according to neighbors, was the corner in front of the local day-care center. Residents voiced concern about the lack of police surveillance in spite of a high incidence of crime in the area. Residents complained that the city fire department was slow to answer calls for assistance and that snow removal in the winter often took much longer in their neighborhood than in surrounding neighborhoods.

Students reported that communication was difficult because many of the residents of the community did not speak English and the students did not speak Spanish, which was the primary language in most of the homes in which students attempted to obtain information.

Dogs and cats roamed the streets in great numbers. Some people said they needed the dogs for protection and the cats to keep the rat population down. According to residents, there was no attempt made by local authorities to enforce a leash law or to impound dogs that roamed free.

Some area residents were concerned about individuals attracted to the area by a neighborhood food pantry. Students expressed feelings of anxiety when

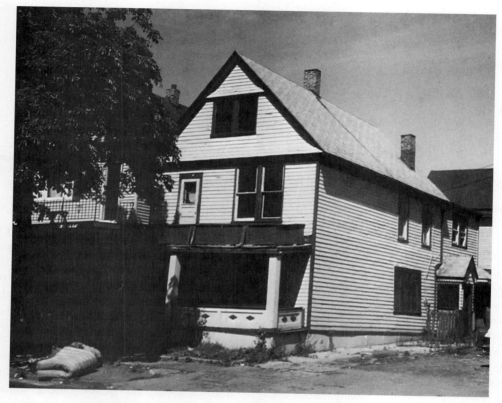

FIGURE 2-4   Houses generally run down and in need of repair.

they walked past some groups of men who stood around and talked in front of stores and on street corners and were verbally abusive to them.

Community resources. The area is governed by the city, and the local councilman seemed aware of the needs of the residents. When students interviewed him, however, they found that he did not have a plan to respond to those needs. Among the community resources were a library, a city college, and a hospital, all of which could be reached by public transportation. A local newspaper helped to enhance a sense of community.

Vital statistics. Statistics from the 1980 census tract survey concerning infant mortality were compared with city, county, and state norms (Table 2-5). The infant mortality rate in a community can predict the general wellness state of the community.

Local records indicated that the incidence of neonatal death was 3.9 times higher than in the surrounding county. The incidence of post neonatal death was 3.6 times higher.

Morbidity data. Data were not available for the census tract studied.

Health resources. Students reported that there was one private physician in the area and that an ambulatory care clinic and a large county hospital were available by bus.

TABLE 2-5   Infant mortality statistics

Area	Number of deaths/1000
Local neighborhood	25.4
City	15.2
County	11.7
State	10.5

From Community project: Class of 1987 by J. Dzimian, N. Schoelkopf, K. Spalti, L. Waldowski, and M. Zimmerman, 1987, unpublished manuscript, D'Youville College, Buffalo, NY.

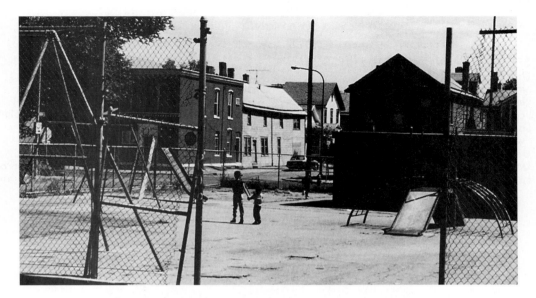

FIGURE 2-5　Playground unusable because of broken equipment.

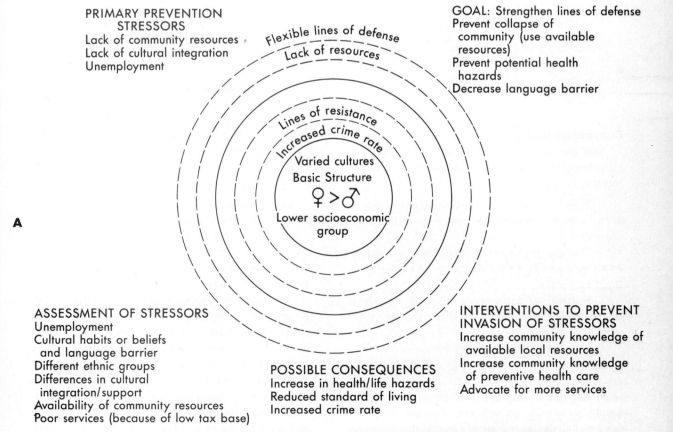

PRIMARY PREVENTION STRESSORS
Lack of community resources
Lack of cultural integration
Unemployment

Flexible lines of defense
Lack of resources

Lines of resistance
Increased crime rate

Varied cultures
Basic Structure
♀ > ♂
Lower socioeconomic group

GOAL: Strengthen lines of defense
Prevent collapse of community (use available resources)
Prevent potential health hazards
Decrease language barrier

ASSESSMENT OF STRESSORS
Unemployment
Cultural habits or beliefs and language barrier
Different ethnic groups
Differences in cultural integration/support
Availability of community resources
Poor services (because of low tax base)

POSSIBLE CONSEQUENCES
Increase in health/life hazards
Reduced standard of living
Increased crime rate

INTERVENTIONS TO PREVENT INVASION OF STRESSORS
Increase community knowledge of available local resources
Increase community knowledge of preventive health care
Advocate for more services

A

FIGURE 2-6　Application of Neuman's model to a community at risk. **A,** Primary prevention.

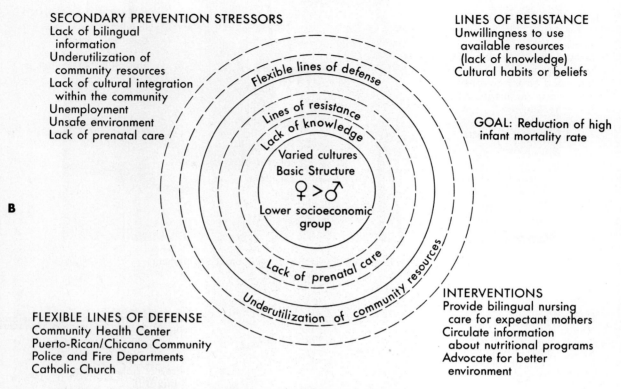

SECONDARY PREVENTION STRESSORS
Lack of bilingual
 information
Underutilization of
 community resources
Lack of cultural integration
 within the community
Unemployment
Unsafe environment
Lack of prenatal care

LINES OF RESISTANCE
Unwillingness to use
 available resources
 (lack of knowledge)
Cultural habits or beliefs

GOAL: Reduction of high
 infant mortality rate

Flexible lines of defense

Lines of resistance

Lack of knowledge

Varied cultures
Basic Structure
♀ > ♂
Lower socioeconomic
group

Lack of prenatal care

Underutilization of community resources

B

FLEXIBLE LINES OF DEFENSE
Community Health Center
Puerto-Rican/Chicano Community
Police and Fire Departments
Catholic Church

INTERVENTIONS
Provide bilingual nursing
 care for expectant mothers
Circulate information
 about nutritional programs
Advocate for better
 environment

FIGURE 2-6, cont'd. Application of Neuman's model to a community at risk. **B,** Secondary prevention.

Community Diagnosis

After analyzing the data, the students prioritized the elements of the community diagnosis in the following manner:

1. Potential weakness in the flexible line of defense of the community related to low income and unemployment.

2. Potential weakness in the flexible line of defense related to communication difficulties as a result of the language barrier.

3. Potential hazard to normal line of defense related to state of community health; for example, infant mortality.

4. Potential hazard to line of resistance related to hazardous and inaccessible playground in the community (Figure 2-5).

5. Potential weakness in the line of resistance resulting from unsafe environment in the community; for example, abandoned homes, drug traffic, increased crime rate.

6. Potential penetration of the basic structure of the community related to high infant mortality, 25.4/1000.

Nursing Goals

Students planned interventions at primary, secondary, and tertiary levels and integrated their plans with Neuman's (1989) model. Figure 2-6 illustrates assessment, nursing diagnosis, goals, interventions, and expected outcomes at all three levels.

Nursing Outcomes

The students' evaluative outcome projected that the infant mortality rate would decrease over a 3-year period. The students also concluded that a community health nurse could provide health education through the schools and a Puerto Rican community center and could encourage the use of an ambulatory care clinic for prenatal care. There could also be an attempt to raise the level of awareness of public officials with regard to the plight of this community by making the students' research available.

TERTIARY PREVENTION STRESSORS
Lack of community resource
 information
Decreased use of community resources
Decreased cultural support
Decreased community involvement
Lack of cultural integration within
 the community
Unemployment
High infant mortality rate

LINES OF RESISTANCE
Unwillingness to use
 available resources
 (lack of knowledge)
Cultural habits or beliefs

GOAL: Reduction of high
 infant mortality rate

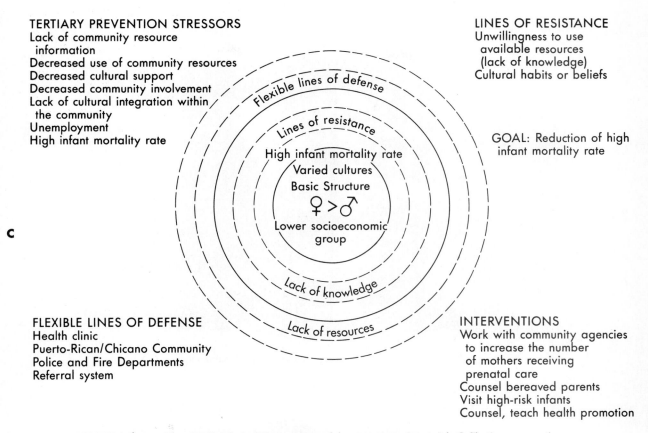

C

FLEXIBLE LINES OF DEFENSE
Health clinic
Puerto-Rican/Chicano Community
Police and Fire Departments
Referral system

INTERVENTIONS
Work with community agencies
 to increase the number
 of mothers receiving
 prenatal care
Counsel bereaved parents
Visit high-risk infants
Counsel, teach health promotion

FIGURE 2-6, cont'd.   Application of Neuman's model to a community at risk. C, Tertiary prevention.

■ CASE STUDY 2

Another group of students conducted an assessment of the health of a suburban community as a course requirement. They used the same definition of community as that used by the students in case study 1 and confined their study to one census tract.

Assessment

Community boundaries. The community was located in an upper middle-class suburban area. The boundaries were within a single census tract spread over an area of about 8 square miles that included a small park. The total population of the census tract was 5110.

Demographic data. The statistical data were obtained primarily from the most recent census (1985: about 2 years previously) taken by the county govern-

ment and from information on record at the county court house and at the local school district office.

The population of the community (5110) had been increasing steadily for about 5 years. The residents were predominantly white (97%); 73% of the population was older than 18 years; and 12% was older than 65 years. The most recent census information indicated that there were fewer than 100 households headed by women.

Education. Exact statistics concerning education were not readily available because the boundaries of the census tract did not coincide with the boundaries of the local school districts. It was established, however, that there were approximately 2250 students in the tract, including about 180 kindergarten students,

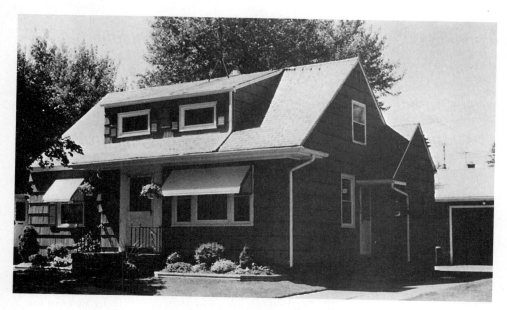

FIGURE 2-7 Houses and yards clean and well maintained.

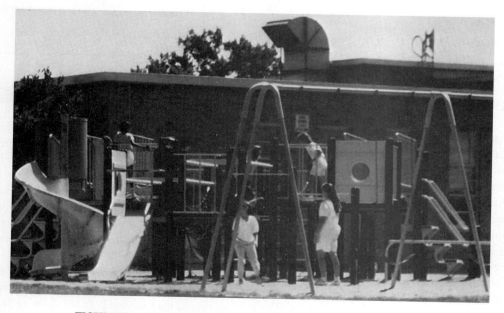

FIGURE 2-8 Playground with new equipment is used by area children.

PRIMARY PREVENTION STRESSORS
Aging
Lack of knowledge
  of methods of prevention
  of cardiovascular disease
  and malignant neoplasms

GOAL:
Strenghten lines of resistance
Prevent potential health hazards

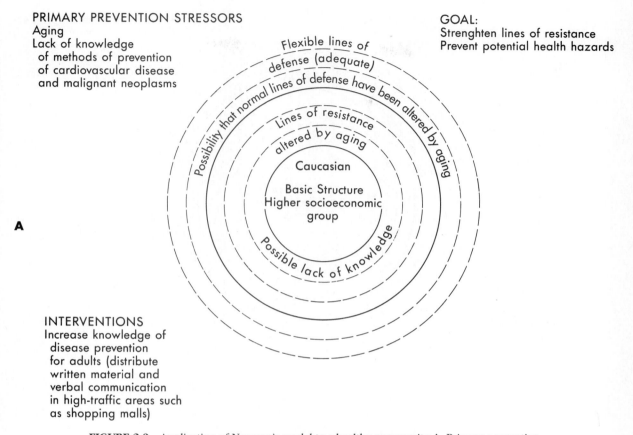

A

INTERVENTIONS
Increase knowledge of
disease prevention
for adults (distribute
written material and
verbal communication
in high-traffic areas such
as shopping malls)

FIGURE 2-9   Application of Neuman's model to a healthy community. **A,** Primary prevention.

1800 elementary students, and 280 secondary school students. Approximately 75% of the adults older than 25 years were high school graduates, and approximately 25% had completed at least 4 years of college.

Economy/occupations. There was a high percentage of white collar workers in the community, and the average family income level was more than $20,000. Unemployment was low at the time of the study, about 6%, and many households had two incomes.

Environment. The community was located in a temperate climate (the same as that of the community of case study 1), with harsh winters; cool, damp springs and falls; and warm, pleasant summers. The area was well kept, and the houses were neat and well maintained. No garbage or trash was observed except that which was placed at the curb on garbage pick-up days (Figure 2-7). The residential streets were characterized by well-kept lawns, neat flower gardens, and

young trees. The residents who were interviewed all spoke English and voiced no concern about public services. A leash law was enforced to keep pets off the streets.

Community resources. The community had a library, two nearby hospitals, many private physicians, and a senior citizens' center. The community was within a township, and members of the town board interviewed by the students seemed to be firmly committed to working on the problems of the community. A playground had recently been donated by a local community group for area children (Figure 2-8).

Vital statistics. Infant mortality in this suburban community was 7.3 per 1000 compared with 15.2 per 1000 in the nearby city and 11.7 per 1000 in the surrounding county.

Morbidity data. Morbidity data were not available. However, interviews with several local physicians indi-

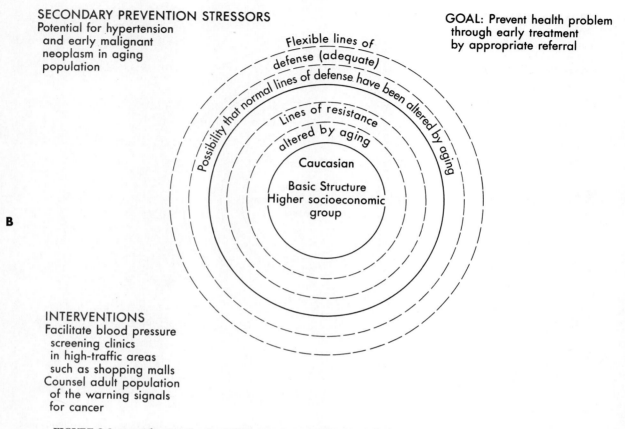

SECONDARY PREVENTION STRESSORS
Potential for hypertension
and early malignant
neoplasm in aging
population

GOAL: Prevent health problem
through early treatment
by appropriate referral

B

INTERVENTIONS
Facilitate blood pressure
screening clinics
in high-traffic areas
such as shopping malls
Counsel adult population
of the warning signals
for cancer

FIGURE 2-9, cont'd. Application of Neuman's model to a healthy community. **B,** Secondary prevention.

cated that the leading and possibly major causes of mortality in the community were cardiovascular disease and malignant neoplasms, both in the over-65 population.

Health resources. Health resources were ample and included a number of private physicians, a well-baby clinic, and two private hospitals nearby.

Community Diagnosis

Students evaluated this area as having a strong normal line of defense, adequate flexible lines of defense, and a high level of wellness. Students hypothesized that lines of resistance could be compromised in the over-65 population (12%) because of aging and a consequent lowering of immunity to selected disease states. Their community diagnosis consisted of the following analysis:

1. Alteration of lines of resistance in a specific target group (older than 65 years) to cardiovascular disease and malignant neoplasm as a part of the aging process.

2. Potential high risk of cardiovascular disease and malignant neoplasm in the over-65 population.

Nursing Goals and Outcomes

The students' goals focused on primary and secondary prevention in terms of Neuman's health care systems model (Figure 2-9). Their projected outcome was that knowledge of method of prevention of cardiovascular disease and malignant neoplasms and early diagnosis of altered health states would decrease the incidence of cardiovascular disease and malignant neoplasms in the target population (persons older than 65 years).

Chapter Highlights

- Communities can be defined as selected geographical areas, aggregates, groups, or interactive systems.

- Betty Neuman defines the client in a community as an interacting open system in total interface with both internal and external forces or stressors.

- The use of the nursing process to organize a plan of care facilitates the implementation of the Standards of Community Health Nursing Practice.

- Neuman's systems model uses a total client approach that considers all of the factors that may affect the client's level of wellness: physiological, sociological, psychological, or developmental.

 CRITICAL THINKING EXERCISE

A rural area of southern California is characterized by large farms, a predominately permanent resident population of upper-income persons, and a seasonal population of migrant workers. During harvest season, the local hospital emergency room receives an influx of persons with stomach problems, rashes, and serious upper respiratory infections. Most of the patients are migrant workers and the nurses are aware that some of the symptoms could be the result of exposure to pesticides used on the farms.

1. Are the migrant workers considered a part of the community?
2. What would the nurses need to know to plan appropriate interventions for them?

REFERENCES

American Nurses' Association. (1980). *Nursing, a social policy statement.* Kansas City, MO: Author.

American Nurses' Association Council of Community Health Nurses. (1980). *A conceptual model for community health nursing* (ANA Publication No. CH-102M, 5/80). Kansas City, MO: Author.

American Public Health Association, Division of Nursing. (1980). *The definition and role of public health nursing in the delivery of health care.* Washington, D.C.: Author.

Anderson, E., McFarlane, J., & Helton, A. (1986). Community-as-client: A model for practice. *Nursing Outlook, 34*(5), 220-224.

Dzimian, J., Schoelkopf, N., Spalti, K., Waldowski, L., & Zimmerman, M. (1987). Community project, class of 1987. Unpublished manuscript, D'Youville College, Buffalo, N.Y..

Griffith-Kenney, J., & Christensen, P. (1986). *Nursing process: Application of theories, frameworks, and models.* St. Louis: Mosby.

Leavell, H.R., & Clark, E.G. (1965). *Preventive medicine for the doctor in his community: An epidemiologic approach* (3rd ed.). New York: McGraw-Hill.

Muecke, M. (1984). Community health diagnosis in nursing. *Public Health Nursing, 1*(1), 24.

Neuman, B. (1989). *The Neuman systems model* (2nd ed.). Norwalk, CT: Appleton & Lange.

Smith, J. (1988). Public health and the quality of life. *Family Community Health, 10*(4), 49-57.

Tinkham, C., Voorkies, E., & McCarthy, N. (1984). *Community health nursing.* Norwalk, CT: Appleton-Century-Crofts.

World Health Organization, Regional Office for Europe. (1985). Targets for health for all two thousand: Targets in support of the European strategy for health for all. Geneva: WHO.

Yura, H., & Walsh, M. (1983). *Nursing process* (4th ed.). New York: Appleton & Lange.

3

COMMUNITY HEALTH NURSING IN A MULTICULTURAL SOCIETY

Margaret R. HoSang

To seek, to know, and to understand designated cultures—with their values, beliefs, and daily living patterns—is probably one of the greatest challenges for students of human behavior.

Madeleine Leininger

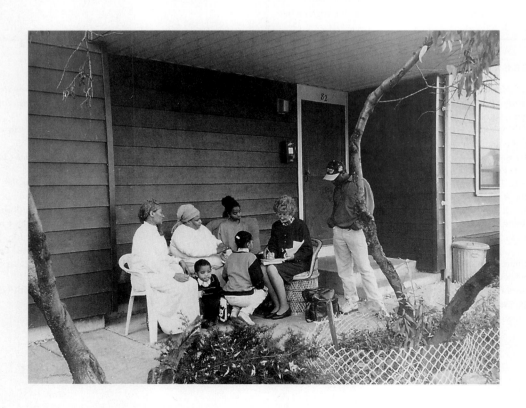

OBJECTIVES

At the conclusion of this chapter, the student will be able to:

1. Define the terms listed.
2. State how culture influences health beliefs and practices.
3. Discuss the implications of stereotyping, ethnocentrism, and cultural imposition.
4. Use the process of development of cultural sensitivity.
5. Discuss the role of the community health nurse in the provision of culturally appropriate care.
6. Use various assessment tools to conduct a cultural assessment.
7. Apply the nursing process in the provision of culturally appropriate care.
8. Examine the importance of culture as an essential component of nursing education, research, and administration in community health nursing.

KEY TERMS

Cultural assessment

Cultural care
  Accommodation
  Preservation

Repatterning

Cultural imposition

Cultural sensitivity

Culturally congruent care

Ethnocentrism

Stereotyping

Nursing in North America today is a multicultural experience in which nurses interact with and are required to provide effective nursing care for persons from diverse cultural backgrounds. The values and belief systems of these clients may differ from the nurse's own, but these influence the clients' perceptions of health and learned patterns of response to illness and treatment of illness. Concomitantly, nurses' own values and beliefs are reflected in the care they attempt to provide to clients. For such care to be effective, it is essential that care be meaningful to the client within a familiar context. To ensure the provision of effective client-centered nursing care in a multicultural society, it is imperative that nurses know about the essential roles of culture and cross-cultural interactional skills in the provision of care.

This chapter will examine some of the concepts of culture pertaining to nursing. In addition, there will be a discussion of the importance of the development of cultural sensitivity that guides nurses to explore their own culture. The nursing process will be reviewed using Leininger's theory of cultural care diversity and universality. Finally, in addition to the practice issues described herein, consideration will be given to importance of culture in education, research, and administration in community health nursing.

THE CULTURAL DIVERSIFICATION OF NORTH AMERICA

North America is a common destination for immigrants seeking a change in lifestyle and opportunities. Whether this change is voluntary or is a result of traumatic displacement due to war, famine, religious and political persecution, or disaster, many immigrants leave their homeland to settle in the United States and Canada, which they perceive as offering relative safety, freedom, and opportunities for personal success. International events such as wars may bring victims of war to North America and at the same time may expose North American residents to the culture of the regions at war. This exposure may occur as personnel travel to the affected regions to provide military service or media coverage. Exposure may occur locally as relatives and friends maintain contact and vigil for those living in or serving in the affected regions. Persons with no direct link with the region are also exposed as instantaneous news reports are transmitted throughout the world via satellite. Consider the local effect of the world wars, wars in Vietnam and the Middle East, turmoil in South Africa and other African nations, Europe, China, South America, Mexico, and the Caribbean. As persons leave the countries affected, North America becomes one of their destinations. Now consider the effect of economic growth and trade with countries and regions such as Japan, the Middle East, Mexico, Canada, and the United States. Local population shifts now include temporary or permanent residents from around the world who wish to enjoy a measure of economic success. The relative ease of world travel and the popularity of tourism have also brought together people from around the world.

Societies are becoming more diverse, not less so, and thus it is incumbent on nurses to acquire knowledge and to be prepared to respond appropriately and effectively to any person who may require care, regardless of cultural background. Astute nurses find that culture influences all areas of one's life, and this influence is particularly pronounced in a multicultural society. If cultural concepts are not applied in appropriate context, clients will not be receptive to care offered, and ineffective outcomes may result in which clients are perceived to be, and inappropriately labelled as, resistive, ignorant, or noncompliant.

Nurses who are not knowledgeable about cultural influences use their own familiar value-based interventions when dealing with new and unfamiliar practices. This mode of intervention and the clients' unfamiliarity with the dominant health care values and practices of the community are partly responsible for the frustrations encountered when values conflict. In such in-

stances nurses might find it difficult to empower clients whose values are not familiar to them. Cultural sensitivity and application of the principles of transcultural nursing reduce the frustrations that impede the provision and receipt of care (Murphy & Clark, 1993).

Anderson (1987) stated that cultural variations in the client population increase the complexity of caring and demand an understanding that usually goes beyond our normal preparation as nurses. Proactive nurses can develop their knowledge by learning about new client cultures as they first arrive in the community and by anticipating needs and planning for them before the clients enter the health care system. By learning about the culture of incoming clients, nurses can develop rapport with key representatives of the group to learn about the culture from the essential *emic* (within-culture) perspective (Leininger, 1991). Initiatives such as health fairs in public settings may serve to attract the attention of members of the target community to health promotion activities.

DEFINITIONS OF CULTURE

According to Madeleine Leininger (1978), culture refers to the learned, shared, and transmitted values, beliefs, norms, and life practices of a particular group that guide thinking, decisions, and actions in patterned ways. Leininger (1978, p. 491) cites anthropologist E.B. Tyler's (1874) classic definition of culture as "a complex whole which includes knowledge, belief, art, morals, law, custom, and any other capabilities and habits acquired by man as a member of society."

Anthropologists Mead and Metráux (1959, p. 22) defined culture as

. . . the total learned, shared behavior of a functionally autonomous society that has maintained its existence through a sufficient number of generations so that each stage of the life span of an individual can be included in the system. Such learned behavior, when studied, has been found to be systematic, and this systemization can be referred to the uniformities in the structure, and the functioning of the human beings who embody the culture.

These definitions describe how culture influences our total way of life. It is not a simple artistic or exotic concept. Herskovits (1955) postulates that culture is universal in the experience of humanity while possessing unique local or regional manifestations. There is a stable yet dynamic element to culture that results in constant change. Finally, culture pervades and directly influences the course of one's life, yet it is rarely present in conscious thought.

THE LINK BETWEEN CULTURE, HEALTH, AND ILLNESS

Culture encompasses all facets of our lives, including beliefs and practices pertaining to health and illness. Leininger (1988) states that people are born, live, become ill, and die within a cultural belief and practice system but are dependent on human care for growth and survival. As providers of care, it is essential that community health nurses explore their own cultural belief systems and compare them with the clients' so the clients' values can be acknowledged, accepted, respected, and included in the assessment and planning of care. The understanding of differences and similarities facilitates the provision of effective, meaningful client-centered care.

Knowledge based on transcultural nursing facilitates nurses' identification of their own values, and those of other health professionals and the clients. Common beliefs pertaining to health and illness include the belief that illness may result from stress, environmental factors such as pollution and the depleting ozone layer, and sociological and economic factors such as poverty and inadequate nutrition. In this instance, cultural groups subscribing to these beliefs might attempt to reduce or manage stress by engaging in fitness programs to enhance health and might engage in protective or restorative environmental measures such as recycling programs and the protection of forests. Attempts to address health concerns caused by poverty include the existence of social assistance and food stamp programs, and meal programs in schools or charitable organizations.

Other beliefs might be that illness is the result of punishment or a message sent from a deity (Roberson, 1987). In this instance, health behaviors may include prayer or rituals intended to appease the deity. Yet another commonly held belief is the importance of balance in the body in the form of the *yin* and *yang* of certain traditional Chinese cultures (Chen-Louie, 1983), also known to some Vietnamese groups as the *am* and *duong* (Calhoun, 1986). In this instance substances that are considered hot or cold are manipulated in order to restore balance. Hot and cold reflect the therapeutic character, not the temperature of foods. Although these beliefs originated from the Orient, they have recently been adopted by the North American new age movement, which shuns the allopathic model of health care. Common beliefs of nurses reflect not only their culture of origin but also the culture of nursing and the culture of the North American model of health and illness care.

Cultures also subscribe to two domains of health care according to Leininger (1978). There is the *folk* or *generic* form of health care, which takes place outside the dominant organized professional health care system, and the *professional* form, which encompasses the Western allopathic health care system in North America. The preceding paragraph contained examples of *generic* care, additional examples of which are well-known self care practices such as over-the-counter remedies or bed rest and chicken soup for the flu.

Kleinman (1978) described three domains of health care similar to Leininger's. In addition to the professional domain, he describes the folk domain as nonprofessional healers and the popular domain as the family, social network, and community, in which 70% to 90% of health care takes place. Most illness episodes are addressed in the popular domain, where persons seek help and advice from family, friends, or lay sources. When illness requires treatment in the professional domain, decisions about treatment and care are made primarily in the popular domain, most commonly in the family context with advice from acquaintances and lay sources.

ISSUES IN CULTURAL CATEGORIZATION

Our cultural values are also influenced by the values and practices of the many cultures to which we are exposed in our local home environment, and for this reason the common current practice of categorizing people should be reconsidered and approached with caution. Current practices by the United States Census Bureau and Statistics Canada use a *pigeonhole* approach to describe persons in North America. Categories such as African-American or Chinese-Canadian do not give credence to the lifeways of Oriental or black immigrants from the West Indies who now reside in North America. Instead, such labels create excessively broad categories that can lead to overgeneralization and stereotyping if accepted uncritically by the novice nursing practitioner in a multicultural society.

These labels and categories are not only limited in accuracy in identifying persons but can also be hazardous to health if certain issues are not addressed. As the practitioners of the art and science of human care, nurses need to recognize and surmount the inadequacies of the standard categories.

The category of Hispanic-American is another that is too broad to allow the careful consideration of the clients' culture necessary to give effective, culturally appropriate care. The category Asian is another of concern. Many people of "Asian" origin can be found living throughout the world, where they have adopted the customs of that country for many generations. For example, the Chinese immigrated to the West Indies many generations ago, settling primarily in Jamaica and Trinidad. Europeans, East Indians, and others immigrated as well, and interracial marriages have always been common. Yet in the case of the Chinese, many of their children speak only English with a local accent and know no other culture but that of the island. However, when these persons immigrate to the United States or Canada, it is not uncommon for them to be judged according to their Oriental appearance and to be ascribed with unfamiliar values and expectations of the Chinese who have moved directly from China.

To complicate matters further, Chinese who move to North America may have lived in India, Europe, or Africa before migrating here. When they immigrate to North America, they have already been acculturated to some of the values of each society in which they lived, and when they meet each other or others in North American society, differences abound. This scenario is not unique to the Chinese.

Because the goal is to determine the clients' cultural beliefs and practices to incorporate them into health care, it is probably wise to avoid the use of labelling terms. Ask the client to identify the culture with which they associate themselves most closely, as well as their racial or ethnic origin, to identify issues such as possible lactose or alcohol intolerance, thalassaemia, or sickle cell traits in persons of mixed racial background. For example, second- or third-generation Chinese who were born in Jamaica may identify with the Jamaican rather than Chinese or North American cultures, but they may still refer to themselves as Chinese. At the same time, physiological characteristics of race should not be overlooked for relevance to health status. The person of Chinese heritage may carry a thalassaemia trait or may be lactose or drug intolerant regardless of their place of birth or cultural association.

A further example is that of persons commonly referred to as South Asians. Although the majority are said to originate from India and Pakistan, this group has also travelled and relocated extensively. Persons of so-called South Asian background may have resided in China, Africa, the former Soviet Union, or the West Indies where they have acquired values of the resident community. When met in their new community of residence in North America, they are often dismayed at and resentful of the unfamiliar title of South Asian that has been given to them. In addition, recent practice has been to expand the categories to include groups called Asians, South Asians, East Asians, and South East Asians. Confused? So are many persons who find themselves addressed by these labels.

THE COMMUNITY HEALTH NURSE IN A MULTICULTURAL SOCIETY

Community health nurses cannot always predict the cultural background of their clients before meeting them. Ever-changing patterns of migration and increasing diversity require that nurses be equipped to respond with cultural sensitivity to anyone who might require care, regardless of cultural background. At the same time community health nurses require culture-specific knowledge about aggregate populations in the community in order to provide culturally congruent care.

Even within North America, economic upheaval caused by recession and the North American free trade agreement has resulted in the migration of local residents from one part of the country to another, and across the Canadian-United States-Mexican borders, in search of more desirable economic conditions. How are community health nurses educated and prepared to respond to clients of diverse cultural backgrounds, in particular, to those whose values are unfamiliar or divergent from their own values? Furthermore, how do nurses proceed to give effective, meaningful client-centered care if the beliefs, practices, and values of the client group conflict with those of the nurses?

Community health nurses are in a unique position to perform proactively as they observe and meet these diverse clients in community settings. The nature of community health nursing affords the opportunity for nurses to "scan the field," or to conduct a visual assessment of new residents of the community. Nurses may then establish rapport with key informants (Leininger, 1992) to gain culture-specific knowledge. Nurses might assist in the group's adjustment to the community and could assess the need for health protection and promotion in the context of the group's culture. Nurses might learn about the group's culture before the members of the group suffer illness, while empowering the group as possible consumers of the professional health care system. Such knowledge would benefit both clients and nurses; nurses would have the opportunity to learn about the health beliefs, practices, and responses within the culture, and then would be ready to incorporate these into client care as needed.

COMMUNICATION

Effective communication is essential in the development of the nurse-client relationship and the provision of culturally appropriate nursing care. If the client's first language is not English, or if there is a pronounced accent, it is unwise to as-

sume that the client does not understand basic English. English is heard and taught worldwide to varying degrees, and it is rare to find someone who does not understand at least a few words of greeting to establish rapport.

Terminology requires careful choice, such as when inquiring about seemingly personal or sensitive issues. Technical terms such as *void* may confuse persons from diverse backgrounds who might believe that somehow, perhaps in order to be a "good patient," they ought to know the meaning of *void*. Clients whose culture places value on harmony might answer affirmatively so as not to appear to disagree with the nurse. In the most recently observed situation, the term *void* was unfamiliar to an elderly man from an Anglo background who was embarrassed to admit that he did not know its meaning.

In addition, if someone appears to be from a non-English speaking culture, it is unwise to assume that he or she was born outside of the North American continent. Superficial assessments and false assumptions can be condescending in the least and dangerous at the worst. Consider the interaction between a client and a nurse who had immigrated from Australia, her country of birth. Upon observing the nurse's physical characteristics and after a brief conversation, the client remarked: "You speak English very well for a Chinese." The scenario could very easily have been reversed with the nurse making the comment to the client. If resentment results, communication will be impeded as the therapeutic relationship is damaged. It is more appropriate to ask questions such as: What is your mother tongue (first language)? Where were you born? Which culture have you adopted? Clients and nurses may speak many languages, such as the Vietnamese who may be fluent in Chinese, French, and English, or persons from the European continent who commonly speak three languages. Persons from the West Indies may speak in dialects that may sound like a foreign language but are actually English with a unique grammatical form.

Nonverbal communication techniques can be used while taking cues from the client. If the client does not establish eye contact, the reasons may be varied. Perhaps it is considered rude to make eye contact with someone who is considered to be in a position of authority, or perhaps it is believed that if eye contact is established, one's soul will be taken away, or perhaps the client is shy. In some instances touching the client may signify disrespect or invasion of personal space, while in other instances touching may signify caring. The most effective course of action should be guided by client response because these behaviors are not culture-bound; there are as many differences within cultural groups as among groups.

Caution is advised when using translators or interpreters. Hatton's (1992) study suggests that translators may perceive their work as interpreting, and they may wield enormous power in conveying quantity and quality of information between client and care provider. Translators from a similar cultural background may adjust information to protect the dignity of their culture if the information could be embarrassing. They may also advise the client while explaining a treatment plan. In one instance it was discovered through a second translator that although the first translator was asked to explain a procedure to obtain consent, the translator had actually told the client to decline permission to avoid being used as a "guinea pig."

Accordingly, it would be prudent to select translators carefully, to clarify their role, to request a review of information translated to assess accuracy and clarity, and to address ethics, imposition, and confidentiality. If children of clients are asked to translate, information may be edited if the client finds it inappropriate for children to hear the issues being discussed.

Terminology to be avoided includes the expressions *minority, lower class* or *underprivileged,* and *underdeveloped countries* or *third world.* Such terms are perceived to be negatively value laden and ethnocentric, placing the persons described in a subordinate position. Along with the discomfort and risk involved in extending oneself to communicate cross-culturally, errors can also occur. Kavanagh and Kennedy (1992) describe resistance that may occur in communication if trust is not established. In addition, communication errors will occur cross-cul-

turally just as they do intraculturally, but the development of recovery skills (Pederson, 1988) facilitates effective repair of any damage done when communication errors threaten the nurse-client relationship.

BARRIERS TO EFFECTIVE CARE

Although many barriers exist, three common ones are ethnocentrism, stereotyping, and cultural imposition. **Ethnocentrism** is defined by Leininger (1978) as the tendency of an individual (or group) to believe that one's own lifeways are the most desirable, acceptable, or best and to act in a superior manner to the lifeways of other culture groups. An example of ethnocentrism is the longstanding paternalistic approach to patient care that has been prevalent in traditional health care settings in the United States and Canada, where the relationship with the client is determined by the value system present in the health care setting.

All persons are members of at least one cultural group, and as such all subscribe to a set of values, beliefs, and practices that are believed to be desirable or correct. This provides a sense of identity and a positive self-image. When the unfamiliar is experienced or observed, it is compared with one's own value system, which serves as a reference point against which to judge new actions. When new actions are judged to be inferior according to one's own values, that is called ethnocentrism. If new experiences are seen as a variation rather than a deviation from one's own, then cultural sensitivity can develop. If, however, an ethnocentric stance is adopted, clients become aware that their values are not respected. This contributes to a climate of resistance and mistrust, and care will be rejected or will be ineffective.

Furthermore, ethnocentrism can prompt **cultural imposition** defined by Leininger (1978, 1991) as "the tendency of an individual or cultural group to impose their beliefs, values, and patterns of behaviour upon another culture for varied reasons." Such has been the case of the traditional health care system, which imposes expectations on the client and family to abide by its rules and regulations, schedules, expectations of dress, conduct, and visitation.

Stereotyping can be defined as the tendency to ascribe the values, attributes, or behaviors of a small number of people to all members in the group. An example is the stereotype of Orientals as being highly stoic and tolerant of pain, thus requiring very little pain medication. Although stoicism is a commonly observed attribute, it is a response that is not universal to all members of the community; stoicism is not a measure of pain perception or tolerance, nor is it an indicator of the lack of need for pain relieving therapies. Hence the danger in the dissemination and uncritical dependency on "cookbook style" literature describing attributes and values of particular groups.

DEVELOPING CULTURAL SENSITIVITY

The development of **cultural sensitivity** facilitates the communication process between health personnel and the client and is an essential first step in providing culturally appropriate health care. Through the development of cultural sensitivity, nurses first explore and affirm their own cultural identity. It then becomes easier to demonstrate acceptance, respect, and interest in learning more about clients' culturally based needs, particularly as they pertain to health and illness (see box below).

The development of cultural sensitivity on the part of the nurse enhances the nurse-client relationship and facilitates the caring process. In the nurse-client relationship, the values of both the nurse and client come into play because both are members of cultural groups. When these values differ, it is important for the nurses to be able to perceive the clients' values as a variation rather than a deviation from those values to which the nurse is accustomed. Nurses' values are a product of their own cultural backgrounds, and they are also a product of the culture of the health care system in North America, in general, and of the local region, in particular.

Although the nurse may experience surprise or disagreement at the disparity between the

---

AN EXERCISE FOR DEVELOPING CULTURAL SENSITIVITY

1. Begin by engaging in self-reflection and values to identify and explore your own culture as it is expressed in your values, your beliefs, and your practices. This step will be difficult; one's own values are usually assumed and are not usually perceived as unique until a comparison is presented.
2. Clarify which values came from your home environment (indigenous values) and which ones were adopted as a result of exposure to other environmental influences such as social, professional, academic, and clinical settings.
3. Explore some of the ideas you value and have adopted and some of the ideas you did not agree with and have not adopted.
4. Explore your thoughts on dealing with persons whose values you do not agree with. This is a crucial step because resistance, ethnocentrism, and cultural imposition might reveal themselves here no matter how well-intentioned the nurse might be. Acknowledge and explore any negative feelings you may have as a way of allowing yourself to clarify and respect your own point of view. This makes it easier to acknowledge and

respect another person's viewpoint even as you continue to hold your own.
5. Develop a way of accepting, respecting, and allowing the other party to continue their own way. It is not implied that the nurses need to adopt or seem to adopt the clients' values as their own; however, the clients' values should not be challenged. Collaborate with a peer or colleague. Review an example of a situation in which you disagreed with another party, perhaps a sibling, classmate, or colleague. You might recall feelings of resistance to the other person's viewpoint. Perhaps you gave no credence to their ideas or felt angry or impatient as they disagreed with your point of view. Now review the resolution. Conflict management theory might be useful here. If the resolution was not favorable for both sides, replay the situation while examining options for obtaining agreement or compromise. Be prepared to back down or compromise. If the outcome is not a mutual-win situation, then the client and nurse will be dissatisfied with the therapeutic relationship or intervention, and care will not be effective.

client's values and his or her own, it is important to acknowledge these feelings without challenging the client's values. If the nurse does not acknowledge and challenge his or her own response when away from the client later, his or her position in the therapeutic relationship may be perceived as being superficial. In the presence of the client it is important to show respect, acceptance, and willingness to be involved with the client's culture. Curiosity is generally acceptable, enabling the nurse to learn more by asking about the meaning of a particular behavior.

Nurses need to be clear about their own values and their effect on the nurse's life and professional practice. It is then that nurses are able to appreciate the clients' values and their effect on the health and illness response. The consideration of personal values helps prevent ethnocentric forms of "health teaching" that try to repattern client response when it might be appropriate to preserve or accommodate the clients' practices.

Cultural values are not bound by race, ethnicity, or nationality. Persons who live in poverty, the homeless, and those who choose nontraditional lifestyles should not be overlooked in deference to ethnic origin. Values and norms are learned and upheld by members of such groups who commonly endure stereotyping as well.

On a wider societal level, the development of cultural sensitivity by all persons would be of benefit in reducing tension created by contact with new and unfamiliar persons and customs. Once a nurse has developed cultural sensitivity, she or he will find that these principles can be applied to other areas of life. Cultural sensitivity is not restricted to an academic exercise or a nursing intervention. It changes one's way of thinking, and relationships are approached from a broader perspective.

Cultural sensitivity allows the nurse to be receptive to the clients' different perspective and to appreciate the meaning and implications of life processes to the clients from their (emic) standpoint (Kavanagh and Kennedy, 1992). Bennett (1986) described six stages of development of cultural sensitivity. According to this model, learners, or in this instance nurses, progress from ethnocentrism to increased cultural sensitivity in a stepwise fashion (Figure 3-1).

Stage 1. Denial In this stage, nurses do not recognize the existence of cultural differences. The nurse's own culture is believed to be the only culture, resulting in cultural blindness. Ethnocentrism prevails, whether consciously or unconsciously, and variant behavior may be interpreted and labelled in suspicious or deviant terms such as "Pt claims . . .", "refuses to . . .", "non-compliant", "resistive", "demanding", and other similarly charged terms.

Stage 2. Defense In this stage cultural differences are recognized, but they are defended by the belief in the superiority or correctness of the nurse's own culture. This conscious state of eth-

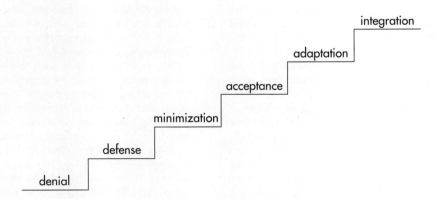

FIGURE 3-1 Bennett's stages of development of cultural sensitivity. (*From A developmental approach to training for intercultural sensitivity by M.J. Bennett, 1986,* International Journal of Intercultural Relations, 10, *179-196.*)

nocentrism, as well as the denial stage, present the challenge for nurses to be vigilant against stereotyping and cultural imposition.

Stage 3. Minimization Cultural differences are recognized, but the magnitude of their influence is minimized (Henderson, Sampselle, Mayes, & Oakley, 1992). This is often evident in the unjudicious application of nutritional guidelines such as the U.S. Department of Agriculture's Food Guide Pyramid or Canada's Food Guide, which serve as client education resources but do not reflect the dietary habits of various cultural groups. Nurses can act effectively in this stage by eliciting the emic or insider's view (Leininger, 1978) or meaning of a situation. Perhaps the group's diet is different, but if there is evidence of adequate nutrients, why is there a need to change it?

Stage 4. Acceptance The nurse may now begin to acknowledge the existence and also the validity of other cultural beliefs and practices. The current interest in *alternative therapies* and their practices, which include traditional Chinese and Aboriginal or Native American healing prac-

tices, are examples of acceptance. It is noteworthy that such practices gain easier acceptability when adopted by members of the dominant cultural group. When used by the Chinese or Aboriginal persons, these therapies may be perceived differently than when they are used by the Anglo culture. The stage of acceptance is the first one in which effective transcultural nursing care can be delivered.

Stage 5. Adaptation The nurse can adapt to another culture. This is believed to occur rarely, unless learners have had extensive exposure to another culture. In this stage nurses recognize that clients who have lived in other countries may have adopted a multiplicity of health beliefs and effective practices; accordingly, stereotyping and cultural imposition will be minimal here.

Stage 6. Integration Integration is believed to occur very rarely, as learners move comfortably among cultures while recognizing variations in cultural practices.

The following case study illustrates the care delivered by a community health nurse in the adaptation stage of cultural sensitivity.

■ CASE STUDY 1

The nurse arrived at the home of a Chinese-speaking client, whereupon the client's granddaughter arrived to translate. The client had an outbreak of herpes zoster and the nursing care plan called for the application of a commonly used antiviral ointment. The client requested that the ointment not be applied as it caused a great deal of pain. The nurse's first thought was to respond by explaining the importance of the ointment to the healing process. The client's granddaughter then explained that they had visited a nearby Chinese medicine shop where they had shown the lesions to the herbalist who then sold them the appropriate Chinese treatment, a red powder that was made into a paste and applied to the lesions by the client's husband. On further assessment, the nurse, who was from a similar culture but unfamiliar with traditional medicine, determined that there had been improvement of the lesions over the days since the family caregivers had initiated generic care. She also assessed that

the family had received appropriate instructions from the herbalist about protecting the client's husband from infection. The nurse assessed the client family's emic health care practices and concluded that they were effective in treating the client's condition. She then conducted telephone consultations with the nursing supervisor and referring physician, reported her assessment of efficacy and safety, advocated for the client to continue her preferred regimen, and received support from both parties. As a result the client did not require a daily nurse's visit, thereby saving health care costs and preserving the clients' effective pattern of health care. The client remained empowered because respect was shown for her belief, and there was no disapproval or ridicule by the health care team. Furthermore the family received supportive care when they were given the option of requesting the nurse's return or to follow up with their family physician in subsequent days.

USING THE NURSING PROCESS IN A MULTICULTURAL SOCIETY

As societies that are as multicultural as Canada and the United States rapidly increase in diversity, development of cultural sensitivity has become essential basic knowledge for all nurses to facilitate their response to the client community through the provision of culturally sensitive care. Continued development of knowledge, competence, and expertise in the area of transcultural nursing assists nurses in developing culture-specific knowledge to provide culturally congruent care (Leininger, 1992).

Leininger's (1978) model of ongoing development of the field of transcultural nursing enables nurses to develop knowledge and skill in the acquisition and use of culture-specific knowledge. This model undergoes rigorous development and application and is most compatible with a qualitative mode of inquiry. It is suggested that the reader supplement the information in this section with one of the primary sources since the model is not simplistic, linear, or positivistic.

The Sunrise model (Figure 3-2) depicts the theory of cultural care diversity and universality. The fan-shaped portion represents the world view, cultural, and social structure dimensions that provide the overall context within which the client or aggregate exists. The nurse assesses the influence of each component from the emic point of reference to determine health patterns and practices. The next step is to act as liaison between the client's generic care system and the professional system. The client's lifeway is retained to the maximum extent, with the selection of nursing actions designed to incorporate the client's generic care practices.

Assessment Enablers

Many assessment tools exist that can assist nurses in conducting a **cultural assessment.** Leininger's assessment tool (Figure 3-3) and Bloch's ethnic/cultural assessment guide (Table 3-1) are considered to be seminal. Others have been described by Anderson (1987), Boyle and Andrews (1989), Fong (1985), Graison, O'Leary, and Wagner (1984), Rosenbaum (1991), and Tripp-Reimer, Brink, and Saunders (1984).

When conducting the assessment it is important to elicit the emic viewpoint, and to conduct the interview in a culturally relevant context. In addition to the application of cultural sensitivity and communication issues as described above, cultural communication and interaction patterns should be noted and preserved. This may occur in cases in which a spokesperson answers questions on behalf of the client, or the grandmother makes the decisions, or the entire family needs to be in attendance.

Leininger's (1991) list of transcultural care constructs is included in the box on page 58. These findings reflect exhaustive application of the ethnonursing methodology and are not to be used in a positivistic manner as a cookbook approach. The inclusion of these findings demonstrates the extensive application of principles of transcultural nursing in the communities studied. The study of care constructs yields information about cultural values of the target communities (Leininger, 1978).

The lists contain prevalent dominant cultural values identified among persons ranging in age from 20 to 85 years. Slight intergenerational and gender differences were noted. Informants belonged to and practiced the culture studied and were interviewed in a natural (emic) context. Leininger's (1978) culture care theory was used to study expressions, meanings, and patterns of culture care.

Goal Setting and Interventions

Anderson (1987) supports the application of a mutual participation model in which the beliefs and expectations of the nurse and client are legitimate and respected, even if it means the client chooses to defer to the nurse. Self-care is not necessarily expected or imposed in this model. It would be appropriate for the nurse to ask, "How would you normally deal with this situation?" to elicit the client's expectations. Here it is also important to consider the meaning of cultural concepts to the client.

Leininger (1990) discussed major American cultural values of optimal health, democracy, individualism, achievement, cleanliness and its associated values of optimum health, beauty and aesthetics, time and schedule-driven activities, and

Text continues on p. 59.

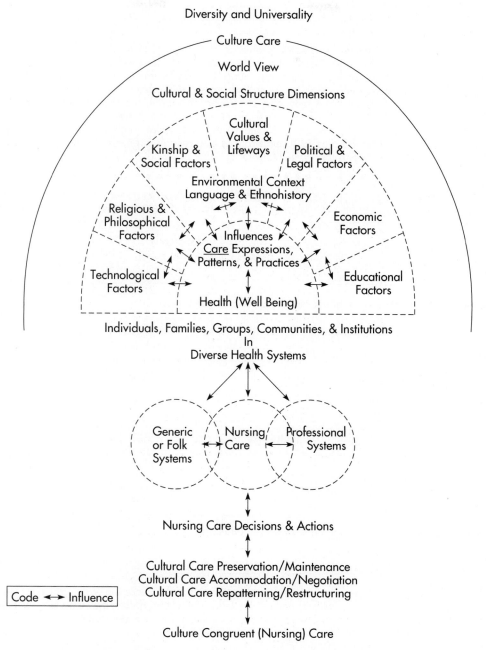

FIGURE 3-2   Leininger's sunrise model to depict theory of cultural care. (*From* Culture care and diversity: a theory of nursing by *M. Leininger, 1991, New York: National League for Nursing.*)

Name of Assessor _____   Date: _____

Informants or Code No. _____ Sex: _____ Age: _____

Place or Context of Assessment: _____

Directions: This tool provides a general qualitative profile or assessment of traditional or non-traditional orientation of informants of their patterned lifeways. Health care influencers are assessed with respect to world view, language, cultural values, kinship, religion, politics, technology, education, environment, and related areas. This profile is primarily focused on emic (local) information to assess and guide health personnel in working with individuals and groups. The etic (or more universal view) may also be evident. In Part I, the user observes, records, and rates behavior on the scale below from 1 to 5 with respect to traditionally or non-traditionally oriented lifeways. Numbers are plotted on the summary in Part II to obtain a qualitative profile to guide decisions and actions. The user's brief notations on each criterion should be used to support ratings and reliable profile. This tool is not designed to be a quantitative measurement tool, but is rather a qualitative tool.

• •

Part I: RATING OF CRITERIA TO ASSESS TRADITIONAL AND NON-TRADITIONAL
PATTERNED CULTURAL LIFEWAYS OR ORIENTATIONS

Rating Indicators:	Mainly Traditional 1	Moderately Traditional 2	Average 3	Moderately Non-Traditional 4	Mainly Non-Traditional 5	Rater Value No.

Cultural Dimensions to Assess Traditional or Non-Traditional Orientations

1. Language, Communication, & Gestures (Native or non-native). Notations: _____
_____
_____

2. General Environmental Living Context (Symbols, material & non-material signs).
Specify: _____
_____
_____

3. Wearing Apparel & Physical Appearance. Notations: _____
_____
_____

4. Technology Being Used in Living Environment. Notations: _____
_____
_____

5. World View (How person looks out upon the world). Notations: _____
_____
_____

* Note: This tool has been developed, refined, and used for three decades (since the early 1960s) by Dr. Madeleine Leininger. It has been frequently in demand by anthropologists, transcultural nurses, and others. It has been useful to obtain informant's orientation to traditional and non-traditional lifeways. It provides qualitative indicators to meet credibility, confirmability, recurrency, and reliability for qualitative studies.

FIGURE 3-3 Leininger's acculturation health care assessment tool for culture patterns in traditional and non-traditional lifeways. (*From Becoming aware of types of health practitioners and cultural imposition by M. Leininger, 1991,* Journal of Transcultural Nursing, 2(2), 40-43.)

6. Family Lifeways (Values, beliefs, and norms). Notations: _____

7. General Social Interactions and Kinship Ties. Notations: _____

8. Patterned Daily Activities. Notations: _____

9. Religious (or Spiritual) Beliefs and Values. Notations: _____

10. Economic Factors (Rough cost of living estimates and income). Notations: _____

11. Educational Values or Belief Factors. Notations: _____

12. Political or Legal Influencers. Notations: _____

13. Food Uses and Nutritional Values, Beliefs, & Taboos. Specify: _____

14. Folk (Generic or Indigenous) Health Care-Cure Values, Beliefs & Practices. Specify: _____

15. Professional Health Care-Cure Values, Beliefs, & Practices. Specify: _____

16. Care Concepts or Patterns that guide actions, i.e., concern for, support, presence, etc. Specify: _____

17. Caring Patterns: _____

18. Views of Ways to: a) Prevent illnesses: _____
    b) Preserve or maintain wellness or health: _____
    c) Care for self or others: _____

19. Other Indicators to support more traditional or non-traditional lifeways: _____

FIGURE 3-3, cont'd.

Part II: ACCULTURATION PROFILE FROM ASSESSMENT FACTORS

Directions: Plot an **X** with the value numbers rated on this profile to discover the orientation or acculturation gradient of the informant. The clustering of numbers will give information of traditional or non-traditional patterns with respect to the criteria assessed.*

Criteria	1 Mainly Traditional	2 Moderately Traditional	3 Average	4 Moderately Non-Traditional	5 Mainly Non-Traditional
1. Language & Communication Modes					
2. Physical Environment					
3. Physical Apparel & Appearance					
4. Technology					
5. World View					
6. Family Lifeways					
7. Social Interaction & Kinship					
8. Daily Lifeways					
9. Religious Orientation					
10. Economic Factors					
11. Educational Factors					
12. Political & Legal Factors					
13. Food Uses					
14. Folk (Generic) Care-Cure					
15. Professional Care-Cure Expressions					
16. Caring Patterns					
17. Curing Patterns					
18. Prevention/Maintenance Factors					
19. Other Indicators					

*The assessor will total numbers to get a summary orientation profile. Use of these ratings with written notations provides a holistic qualitative profile. Detailed notations are important to substantiate the ratings.

TABLE 3-1 Bloch's Ethnic/Cultural Assessment Guide

Data categories	Guideline questions/instructions	Data collected
Cultural		
Ethnic origin	Does the patient identify with a particular ethnic group (e.g., Puerto Rican, African)?	
Race	What is the patient's racial background (e.g., Black, Filipino, American Indian)?	
Place of birth	Where was the patient born?	
Relocations	Where has patient lived (country, city)? During what years did patient live there and for how long? Has patient moved recently?	
Habits, customs, values, and beliefs	Describe habits, customs, values, and beliefs patient holds or practices that affect patient's attitude toward birth, life, death, health and illness, time orientation, and health care system and health care providers. What is degree of belief and adherence by patient to his or her overall cultural system?	
Behaviors valued by culture	How does patient value privacy, courtesy, respect for elders, behaviors related to family roles and sex roles, and work ethics?	
Cultural sanctions and restrictions	*Sanctions* — What is accepted behavior by patient's cultural group regarding expression of emotions and feelings, religious expressions, and response to illness and death? *Restrictions* — Does patient have any restrictions related to sexual matters, exposure of body parts, certain types of surgery (e.g., hysterectomy), discussion of dead relatives, and discussion of fears related to the unknown?	
Language and communication processes	What are some overall cultural characteristics of patient's language and communication process?	
Language(s) and/or dialect(s) spoken	Which language(s) and/or dialect(s) does patient speak most frequently? Where? At home or at work?	
Language barriers	Which language does patient predominantly use in thinking? Does patient need bilingual interpreter in nurse-patient interactions? Is patient non–English-speaking or limited–English-speaking? Is patient able to read and/or write in English?	
Cultural healers	Does patient rely on cultural healers (e.g., medicine men for American Indian, Curandero for Raza/Latina, Chinese herbalist, hougan [voodoo priest], spiritualist, or minister for Black American)?	
Nutritional variables or factors	What nutritional variables or factors are influenced by the patient's ethnic/cultural background?	
Characteristics of food preparation and consumption	What types of food preferences and restrictions, meaning of foods, style of food preparation and consumption, frequency of eating, time of eating, and eating utensils are culturally determined for patient? Are there any religious influences on food preparation and consumption?	

Continued

TABLE 3-1   Bloch's Ethnic/Cultural Assessment Guide   (cont'd)

Data categories	Guideline questions/instructions	Data collected
Cultural (cont'd)		
Influences from external environment	What modifications, if any, did the ethnic group patient identifies with have to make in its food practices in White dominant American society? Are there any adaptations of food customs and beliefs from rural setting to urban setting?	
Patient education needs	What are some implications of diet planning and teaching to patient who adheres to cultural practices concerning foods?	
Sociological		
Economic status	Who is principal wage earner in patient's family? What is total annual income (approximately) of family? What impact does economic status have on life style, place of residence, living conditions, and ability to obtain health services?	
Educational status	What is highest educational level obtained? Does patient's educational background influence his ability to understand how to seek health services, literature on health care, patient teaching experiences, and any written material patient is exposed to in health care setting (e.g., admission forms, patient care forms, teaching literature, and lab test forms)? Does patient's educational background cause him to feel inferior or superior to health care personnel in health care setting?	
Social network	What is patient's social network (kinship, peer, and cultural healing networks)? How do they influence health or illness status of patient?	
Family as supportive group	Does patient's family feel need for continuous presence in patient's clinical setting (is this an ethnic/cultural characteristic)? How is family valued during illness or death? How does family participate in patient's nursing care process (e.g., giving baths, feeding, using touch as support [cultural meaning], supportive presence)?	
Communication process	What are rules (linguistics) and modes (style) of communication process (e.g., "honorific" concept of showing "respect or deference" to others using words only common to specific ethnic/cultural group)? Is there need for variation in technique of communicating and interviewing to accommodate patient's cultural background (e.g., tempo of conversation, eye-body contact, topic restrictions, norms of confidentiality, and style of explanation)? Are there any conflicts in verbal and nonverbal interactions between patient and nurse? How does patient's nonverbal communication process compare with other ethnic/cultural groups, and how does it affect patient's response to nursing and medical care?	

TABLE 3-1 Bloch's Ethnic/Cultural Assessment Guide (cont'd)

Data categories	Guideline questions/instructions	Data collected
Sociological (cont'd)		
	Are there any variations between patient's interethnic and interracial communication process or intracultural and intraracial communication process (e.g., ethnic minority patient and White middle-class nurse, ethnic minority patient and ethnic minority nurse; beliefs, attitudes, values, role variations, stereotyping [perception and prejudice])?	
Healing beliefs and practices		
Cultural healing system	What cultural healing system does the patient predominantly adhere to (e.g., Asian healing system, Raza/Latina Curanderismo)? What religious healing system does the patient predominantly adhere to (e.g., Seventh Day Adventist, West African voodoo, Fundamentalist sect, Pentacostal)?	
Cultural health beliefs	Is illness explained by the germ theory or cause-effect relationship, presence of evil spirits, imbalance between "hot" and "cold" (*yin* and *yang* in Chinese culture), or disequilibrium between nature and man?	
	Is good health related to success, ability to work or fulfill roles, reward from God, or balance with nature?	
Cultural health practices	What types of cultural healing practices does person from ethnic/cultural group adhere to? Does he use healing remedies to cure *natural* illnesses caused by the external environment (e.g., massage to cure *empacho* [a ball of food clinging to stomach wall], wearing of talismans or charms for protection against illness)?	
	How does ethnic/cultural family structure influence patient response to health or illness (e.g., roles, beliefs, strengths, weaknesses, and social class)?	
	Are there any key family roles characteristic of a specific ethnic/cultural group (e.g., grandmother in Black and some American Indian families), and can these key persons be a resource for health personnel?	
	What role does family play in health promotion or cause of illness (e.g., would family be intermediary group in patient interactions with health personnel and making decisions regarding his care)?	
Supportive institutions in ethnic/cultural community	What influence do ethnic/cultural institutions have on patient receiving health services (i.e., institutions such as Organization of Migrant Workers, NAACP, Black Political Caucus, churches, schools, Urban League, community clinics)?	
Institutional racism	How does institutional racism in health facilities influence patient's response to receiving health care?	
Psychological		
Self-concept (identify)	Does patient show strong racial/cultural identity? How does this compare with that of other racial/cultural groups or to members of dominant society?	

Continued

TABLE 3-1   Bloch's Ethnic/Cultural Assessment Guide   (cont'd)

Data categories	Guideline questions/instructions	Data collected
Psychological (cont'd)		
	What factors in patient's development helped to shape his self-concept (e.g., family, peers, society labels, external environment, institutions, racism)?	
	How does patient deal with stereotypical behavior from health professionals?	
	What is impact of racism on patient from distinct ethnic/cultural group (e.g., social anxiety, noncompliance to health care process in clinical settings, avoidance of utilizing or participating in health care institutions)?	
	Does ethnic/cultural background have impact on how patient relates to body image change resulting from illness or surgery (e.g., importance of appearance and roles in cultural group)?	
	Any adherence or identification with ethnic/cultural "group identity" (e.g., solidarity, "we" concept)?	
Mental and behavioral processes and characteristics of ethnic/cultural group	How does patient relate to his external environment in clinical setting (e.g., fears, stress, and adaptive mechanisms characteristic of a specific ethnic/cultural group)? Any variations based on the life span?	
	What is patient's ability to relate to persons outside of his ethnic/cultural group (health personnel)? Is he withdrawn, verbally or nonverbally expressive, negative or positive, feeling mentally or physically inferior or superior?	
	How does patient deal with feelings of loss of dignity and respect in clinical setting?	
Religious influences on psychological effects of health/illness	Does patient's religion have a strong impact on how he relates to health/illness influences or outcomes (e.g., death/chronic illness, cause and effect of illness, or adherence to nursing/medical practices)?	
	Do religious beliefs, sacred practices, and talismans play a role in treatment of disease?	
	What is role of significant religious persons during health/illness (e.g., Black ministers, Catholic priests, Buddhist monks, Islamic imams)?	
Psychological/cultural response to stress and discomfort of illness	Based on ethnic/cultural background, does patient exhibit any variations in psychological response to pain or physical disability of disease processes?	
Biological/physiological		
Consideration of *norms* for different ethnic/cultural groups		
Racial-anatomic characteristics	Does patient have any distinct racial characteristics (e.g., skin color, hair texture and color, color of mucous membranes)?	
	Does patient have any variations in anatomical characteristics (e.g., body structure [height and weight] more preva-	

TABLE 3-1   Bloch's Ethnic/Cultural Assessment Guide   (cont'd)

Data categories	Guideline questions/instructions	Data collected
Biological/physiological (cont'd)		
	lent for ethnic/cultural group, skeletal formation [pelvic shape, especially for obstetrical evaluation], facial shape and structure [nose, eye shape, facial contour], upper and lower extremities)?	
	How do patient's racial and anatomical characteristics affect his self-concept and the way others relate to him?	
	Does variation in racial-anatomical characteristics affect physical evaluations and physical care, skin assessment based on color, and variations in hair care and hygienic practices?	
Growth and development patterns	Are there any distinct growth and development characteristics that vary with patient's ethnic/cultural background (e.g., bone density, fatfolds, motor ability)? What factors are important for nutritional assessment, neurological and motor assessment, assessment of bone deterioration in disease process or injury, evaluation of newborns, evaluation of intellectual status, or capacity in relationship to motor/sensory development in children? How do these differ in ethnic/cultural groups?	
Variations in body systems	Are there any variations in body systems for patient from distinct ethnic/cultural group (e.g., gastrointestinal disturbance with lactose intolerance in Blacks, nutritional intake of cultural foods causing adverse effects on gastrointestinal tract and fluid and electrolyte system, and variations in chemical and hematological systems [certain blood types prevalent in particular ethnic/cultural groups])?	
Skin and hair physiology, mucous membranes	How does skin color variation influence assessment of skin color changes (e.g., jaundice, cyanosis, ecchymosis, erythema, and its relationship to disease processes)?	
	What are methods of assessing skin color changes (comparing variations and similarities between different ethnic groups)?	
	Are there conditions of hypopigmentation and hyperpigmentation (e.g., vitiligo, mongolian spots, albinism, discoloration caused by trauma)? Why would these be more striking in some ethnic groups?	
	Are there any skin conditions more prevalent in a distinct ethnic group (e.g., keloids in Blacks)?	
	Is there any correlation between oral and skin pigmentation and their variations among distinct racial groups when doing assessment of oral cavity (e.g., leukoedema is normal occurrence in Blacks)?	
	What are variations in hair texture and color among racially different groups? Ask patient about preferred hair care methods or any racial/cultural restrictions (e.g., not washing "hot-combed" hair while in clinical setting, not cutting very long hair of Raza/Latina patients).	

Continued

TABLE 3-1   Bloch's Ethnic/Cultural Assessment Guide   (cont'd)

Data categories	Guideline questions/instructions	Data collected
Biological/physiological (cont'd)		
	Are there any variations in skin care methods (e.g., using Vaseline on Black skin)?	
Diseases more prevalent among ethnic/cultural group	Are there any specific diseases or conditions that are more prevalent for a specific ethnic/cultural group (e.g., hypertension, sickle cell anemia, G6-PD, lactose intolerance)?	
	Does patient have any socioenvironmental diseases common among ethnic/cultural groups (e.g., lead paint poisoning, poor nutrition, overcrowding [prone to tuberculosis], alcoholism resulting from psychological despair and alienation from dominant society, rat bites, poor sanitation)?	
Diseases ethnic/cultural group has increased resistance to	Are there any diseases that patient has increased resistance to because of racial/cultural background (e.g., skin cancer in Blacks)?	

LIST OF EMIC CARE/CARING CONSTRUCTS DERIVED FROM LEININGER'S CULTURE CARE THEORY RESEARCH (1960-91)

These *emic* (within the culture) care/caring constructs were identified in approximately 54 cultures through ethnonursing qualitative research methods from 1960 to 1991. The cultural informants identified four or five dominant care constructs with their key meanings and action modes. None of the cultures identified more than eight major constructs. The professional nurses *etic* (or outsider's views) of care are not included in this list. The findings reveal a wide diversity in the *emic* culture care meanings and action modes. All foreign care/caring terms were documented and translated into English. This is only a small glimpse of the total care research findings.

Care and/or Caring Meanings and Action Modes:

1. Acceptance
2. Accommodating
3. Accountability
4. Action (ing) for/about/with
5. Adapting to
6. Affection for
7. Alleviation (pain/suffering)
8. Anticipation (ing)
9. Assist (ing) others
10. Attention to/toward
11. Attitude toward
12. Being nonassertive
13. Being aware of others
14. Being authentic (real)
15. Being clean
16. Being genuine
17. Being involved
18. Being kind/pleasant
19. Being orderly
20. Being present
21. Being watchful
22. Bribing
23. Care (caring)
24. *Caritas* (charity)
25. Cleanliness
26. Closeness to

From *Culture care diversity and universality: A theory of nursing,* p.368, by M. Leininger, 1991, New York: National League for Nursing.

automation. Variations from these values can be frustrating if they are perceived to result from disregard for the dominant culture values; however, it should be understood that not all persons want to be cured at any expense. Some persons may opt to die with their bodies intact rather than to endure potentially lifesaving surgeries. Others may not value self-care and will expect family members and nurses to do all care. Still others may arrive late for appointments because time is not a critical element to their lifestyle.

If used, nursing diagnoses require cautious application so as not to reflect an ethnocentric assessment. Categories such as "noncompliant" or "ineffective coping" are often not appropriately applied when dealing with clients whose behaviors differ from the nurses. Goal setting requires an appreciation of the client's values, wishes, and needs, and goals need to be validated with the client.

Interventions from the generic and professional sectors are applied as deemed appropriate by the nurse and by the client's emic view. **Cultural care preservation** is used when the client's familiar mode of action is an effective alternative and needs not be changed. When aspects of the clients's generic care pattern and the professional care pattern are complementary, **cultural care accommodation** would be the appropriate mode of action in retaining cultural norms. When the client's usual pattern is detrimental, then **cultural care repatterning** is warranted; however, any proposed changes must be meaningful to clients and when possible should be determined by the client with nursing support. Nurse-client intervention may be selected from the professional care system, but the cultural relevance must be validated with the client to assure **culturally congruent care** that is meaningful in the context of the client's culture.

The following cases demonstrate the frustrations, errors, and detrimental results that stem from the lack of cultural awareness and sensitivity. In each instance, refer to the Sunrise model in Figure 3-2 and the acculturation health care assessment enabler (tool) (Figure 3-3). You may begin to assess at any stage of the model starting with cues from each case. What pitfalls can you identify in each case? How would you act differently to provide culture-congruent care?

■ CASE STUDY 2

A young family immigrated to a North American city from India. One of the daughters experienced many childhood illnesses and required frequent prolonged hospitalizations. On one occasion when the mother arrived at the hospital to visit her daughter, she was called into a meeting with a familiar physician who informed her that before her arrival an interdisciplinary meeting had been held, and it had been alleged that she had abused her daughter. Children's aid workers had been notified and had attended the meeting. The team had planned to confront the mother and take the necessary steps to report her and to remove the child from her care. Fortunately there was a *chance* meeting with the physician who was then told of the evidence found and the team's plan. The physician informed the team that the "bruises" found on the child's lower body were in fact Mongolian Spots, a common variation in the skin of non-Caucasian babies. The team meeting was adjourned with no plans to offer an explanation or apology to the mother. Had the physician not been familiar with the skin variation, the mother was to have been notified of the conclusion reached by the team without assessment. The mother reported that she felt wrongly judged, victimized, and humiliated by the experience and remains hurt and mistrustful some 20 years later.

■ CASE STUDY 3

A Vietnamese man took his young son to the emergency department of a North American city. His family had used the generic (or folk) practice of *CaoGio,* or rubbing out the wind, as treatment for the child's illness at home (Calhoun, 1986). The treatment is done by rubbing the skin with the fingers or a coin dipped in a mentholated salve, leaving dark lines on the skin. Because there was no improvement in the child's condition, the parents took the next customary step of action, which was to transfer the child from the folk to the professional domain of health care. In the emer-gency department, the staff noticed the marks, concluded that the child had been abused, and called in the police. The young father was not proficient in English and could not explain the situation to the satisfaction of the authorities who were unfamiliar with *Cao-Gio.* He was treated with suspicion and transferred to the police department where he hanged himself due to the irreparable shame he suffered. Had action been reserved until further data could be gathered or a translator obtained, this tragedy could have been prevented.

■ CASE STUDY 4

A young Chinese woman visited a family physician in a North American city for a routine physical examination. She was informed that she was anemic based on her hemoglobin concentrations. The physician suggested inadequate nutrition as the likely reason. She received a prescription for therapeutic doses of iron tablets, which she took without question for a prolonged period. Some 10 years later the woman visited a family physician in her new location of residence. She was again told of her low hemoglobin concentration, but this time the physician suggested that she undergo further laboratory studies to identify the source of the problem. It was found that the woman had a Thalassaemia trait and was cautioned against the use of large doses of iron. This condition was never suggested or investigated by the first physician, which left the woman at risk for hepatotoxicity from high doses of iron.

■ CASE STUDY 5

A middle-aged man was readmitted to a critical care unit with end-stage hepatic failure and gastrointestinal bleeding caused by prolonged use of alcohol. He was cared for by a nurse who commented within his earshot that she didn't know why "we" should bother saving him since he had been admitted several times before and once recuperated would "head for the near-est bar." Furthermore she stated that she had no patience with his wife whom he had reportedly beaten for many years and whom she believed had "simply put up with it," and who now kept a constant vigil at his bedside. The nurse performed all necessary physical and technical activities but did not converse with the client or his wife.

These examples illustrate the perils of inadequate assessments and the importance for all nurses to develop cultural sensitivity and educate themselves in transcultural nursing to prevent inappropriate treatments. While it would be impossible for all caregivers to know all aspects of cultural care specific to all cultures, it is important that nurses become knowledgeable about the specific cultural groups who reside in their local region and, in addition, to develop skill in the application of general principles for addressing the influence of culture in unfamiliar communities.

CULTURE AND NURSING EDUCATION, ADMINISTRATION, AND RESEARCH

As the population of the continent becomes more diverse, principles of transcultural nursing cannot effectively be applied from a purely academic framework as a client care matter. If culture is considered only in reference to the nurse-client relationship, nurses then become relegated to the position of observer rather than partici-pant in the helping-caring relationship. Cultural care is not authentic in such instances. Nurse educators, administrators, researchers, and students are likely to represent the values and norms of many generations and a multiplicity of ethnic, racial, social, political, and economic cultures. The inclusion of culture is essential to all aspects of nursing, from basic education to advanced practice.

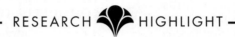

RESEARCH HIGHLIGHT

Are Nursing Students Multiculturally Competent?

The purpose of this study was to investigate undergraduate nursing students' multicultural competencies in working with culturally diverse clients. A total of 120 undergraduate nursing students (112 females, 8 males) between the ages of 18 and 43 ($\overline{X}$ 19.93), attending a developmental psychology course at a large midwestern university, consented to participate. They were from suburban, urban, and rural areas throughout the midwest and were reported to be representative of the student population enrolled in the college of nursing in terms of gender, ethnicity (98% Caucasian), and prior work experience. A total of 67% lacked experience in the nursing field, while the remaining 33% were equally divided in having worked with a minority client within the last 3 months or greater than 3 months ago.

The students' perceptions of their multicultural competency in four areas (skills, knowledge, awareness, and relationships) was measured by the Multicultural Counseling Inventory (MCI). This instrument developed by Sodowsky et al. (in press) consisted of 40 items on a four-point Likert scale with a reported internal consistency reliability of the four areas (subscales) as .83, .79, .83, and .71, respectively. For this sample, the subscale values were .81, .74, .76, and .69, respectively. Previous intersubscale correlations ranged from r = .52 to r = .23, while the results from this sample yielded values that ranged from r = .52 to r = .17. These values approximate correlations found during instrument development and suggest that the inventory is measuring related but different constructs. Further refinement of the scale is required.

The demographic information (questionnaire) sought specifically for this exploratory study included ethnic background, age, gender, academic class standing, field of study, and work experience. These variables were used to investigate differences in regard to self-reported multicultural competencies. Students did not differ significantly across self-reported variables of age or class standing, but they did differ in relation to work experience. Students who have had some work experience had significantly more self-perceived multicultural skills and knowledge but not more multicultural awareness or relationships than students who have had no work experience. This finding is further explored by the authors in their provision of possible explanations for its occurrence, but further research is acknowledged along with suggestions for future investigations.

None of the participants had completed a course or seminar addressing multicultural issues in nursing. The manner in which multicultural issues are incorporated within the nursing curriculum remains a question for educators. Because experience in the field may have had an impact on multicultural skills and knowledge, consideration might be given to the introduction of issues after students have had exposure to the clinical area.

Pope-Davis, D.B., Eliason, M.J., & Ottavi, T.M. (1994). Are nursing students multiculturally competent? An exploratory investigation. *Journal of Nursing Education, 33*(1): 31-33.

Nurse educators in the academic and practice settings can apply principles of cultural sensitivity and cultural knowledge to address differing learning styles among nurses and students.

Leininger (1978) provides educational curricula for seminar, undergraduate, and graduate nursing courses. Tuck and Harris (1988) described a comprehensive model for integrating transcultural concepts into nursing education. Nurse educators who develop cultural sensitivity and competence are able to support nurses and students from diverse backgrounds in giving care to clients from diverse backgrounds.

Nurse administrators have a multifaceted role in the arena of transcultural nursing. Culturally sensitive administrators recognize that iniquities that pervade society at large are also represented in the nursing profession. The mechanisms that promote discord between client and caregiver can also promote discord among staff members because ethnocentrism, stereotyping, and cultural imposition are not limited to nurse-client relationships.

Nursing administrators who are knowledgeable about the impact of cultural values can recognize and work deliberately to address culturally based conflicts and to promote cultural sensitivity and knowledge among staff. Administrators can also support professional advancement regardless of the nurse's cultural background as a measure to remove some of the existing cultural barriers and promote increasingly diverse representation among the administration and leadership in nursing agencies (Malone, 1993). Administrators can also collaborate with educators to promote the preparation of culturally sensitive preceptors (Williams & Rogers, 1993).

The study of culture is becoming an increasingly essential part of nursing research as well. Culturally sensitive research is conducted with consideration to differing value systems as supported by Henderson et al. (1992), Kleinman et al. (1978), Kluckhohn (1953), Leininger (1978), and Tripp-Reimer et al. (1984). Researchers who apply principles of cultural sensitivity and transcultural nursing are more likely to recognize their own beliefs and to avoid ethnocentrism and inappropriate generalization of findings (Henderson et al. 1992).

Nursing research can be conducted to demonstrate the inappropriateness of federal census and statistical hyphenated categories of aggregates. These "pigeonhole" categories are deficient in correctly identifying the cultures of North America's population. Moreover, they are inaccurate and thus are inappropriate for application in the provision of health care.

THE LEADING EDGE OF TRANSCULTURAL COMMUNITY HEALTH NURSING

With ever advancing technology and increasing speed of travel, we can be across the globe in a matter of hours. Through satellite transmission, communication in the form of news items is now instantaneous. From our North American standpoint we can no longer look at these events as being external to our lives. A societal shift toward holism and social responsibility results in a more rapid and widespread assistance of persecuted or needy persons than in the past. The influx of refugees continues as victims of upheaval seek safety and relative freedom. While newcomers may live in groups or enclaves when they first arrive, the North American values of individual rights and freedom make it possible for members of diverse groups to reside anywhere on the continent, either with aggregates or alone.

Nurses can keep abreast of the changing international political, economic, and social environments, which have implications for shifting the cultural profile of the continent. By anticipating changes in cultural population distribution, community health nurses can learn about the incoming cultures and can prepare proactive strategies to support the health of their clientele. Community health nursing agencies can include culturally relevant contexts to all aspects of operations. Very often this is written in the agency's mission statement but is overlooked in operational activities. Client assessments, care plans, visiting arrangements, staff schedules, management style, strategic plans, and quality programs are all examples of matters that can be conducted in a culturally relevant context.

Chapter Highlights

- Culture determines all learned responses to life situations, including health beliefs, practices, and care patterns.

- With increasing cultural diversity in Canada and the United States, there is interaction among a multiplicity of persons and communities holding diverse values.

- Nurses' and clients' values and beliefs interplay in the nurse-client relationship.

- There is as much diversity within cultures as among cultures; accordingly, identification or labelling by broad categories should be avoided since clients' cultural identity may span many groups. Such broad categories tend to lead to the application of a "cookbook" approach to care.

- The development of cultural sensitivity can assist the nurses to bracket their own values in deference to the clients' health values.

- Stereotyping, ethnocentrism, and cultural imposition impede the nurse-client relationship and diminish the effectiveness of care rendered.

- Culturally sensitive care can be rendered with the aid of a variety of cultural assessment enablers (tools) as listed in this chapter.

- Leininger's theory of culture care diversity and universality, and Bloch's ethnic/cultural assessment guide provide two comprehensive frameworks to facilitate culturally congruent care.

- Culture care is most effective when assessments and actions focus on the *emic* perspective.

- Nursing care of clients will only be partially effective if administration, education, and research do not occur within a framework of culture.

 CRITICAL THINKING EXERCISE

A nurse in a pediatric clinic where most of the clients are Latino becomes frustrated when they speak Spanish in her presence. She feels excluded from the conversations and uncomfortable with her role in the clinic. The nurse makes an effort to learn Spanish and begins to understand the conversations. As the weeks go by, her discomfort goes away and she begins to function with ease in the clinic.

1. What was the most effective thing the nurse did to decrease her frustration?
2. According to Bennett, what stage of development has the nurse reached in terms of cultural sensitivity?

REFERENCES

Anderson, J.M. (1987). The cultural context of caring. *Canadian Critical Care Nurse Journal, 4*(4), 7-13.

Bennett, M.J. (1986). A developmental approach to training for intercultural sensitivity. *International Journal of Intercultural Relations, 10,* 179-196.

Bloch, B. (1983). Bloch's assessment guide for ethnic cultural variations. In M. Orque, B. Bloch, & L. Monroe, (Eds.), *Ethnic nursing care: A multicultural approach.* St. Louis: Mosby.

Brink, P. (1976). *Transcultural nursing: A book of readings.* Englewoods Cliffs, NJ: Prentice-Hall.

Calhoun, M.A. (1986). Providing health care to Vietnamese in America: What practitioners need to know. *Home Healthcare Nurse 4*(5), 14-22.

Chen-Louie, T. (1983). Nursing care of Chinese-American patients. In M. Orque, B. Bloch, & L. Monroe, (Eds.), *Ethnic nursing care: A multicultural approach.* St. Louis: Mosby.

Fong, C.M. (1985). Ethnicity and nursing practice. *Topics in Clinical Nursing, 7*(3), 1-10.

Graison, B., O'Leary, L., & Wagner, J. (1984). Cultural assessment: How well do we know our patients? *Journal of Nephrology Nursing, 1*(3).

Hatton, D.C. (1992). Information transmission in bilingual, bicultural contexts. *Journal of Community Health Nursing, 9*(1), 53-59.

Henderson, D.J., Sampselle, C., Mayes, F., & Oakley, D. (1992). Toward culturally sensitive research in a multicultural society. *Health Care For Women International, 13*, 339-350.

Kavanagh, K.H., & Kennedy, P.H. (1992). *Promoting cultural diversity: Strategies for health care professionals.* Newbury Park, California: Sage Publications.

Kleinman, A., Eisenberg, L., & Good, B. (1978). Culture, illness and care. *Annals of Internal Medicine, 88*, 251-258.

Kluckhohn, F.R. (1953). Dominant and variant value orientations. In Kluckhohn, C.K., & Murray, H.A., (Eds.), *Personality in nature and society.* (pp. 342-377). New York: Knopf.

Leininger, M. (1988). Leininger's theory of nursing: Cultural care diversity and universality. *Nursing Science Quarterly, 1*(4), 152-160.

Leininger, M. (1978). *Transcultural nursing: Concepts, theories, and practices.* New York: Wiley.

Leininger, M. (1991). Becoming aware of types of health practitioners and cultural imposition. *Journal of Transcultural Nursing, 2*(2), 32-39.

Leininger, M. (1991). *Culture care diversity & universality: A theory of nursing.* New York: NLN.

Malone, B.L. (1993). Caring for culturally diverse racial groups: An administrative matter. *Nursing Administration Quarterly, 17*(2), 21-29.

Mead, M., & Metráux, R. (1959). *The Study of cultures at a distance.* Chicago: University of Chicago Press.

Murphy, K., & Clark, J.M. (1993). Nurses' experiences of caring for ethnic-minority clients. *Journal of Advanced Nursing, 18*, 442-450.

Orque, M.S., Bloch, B., & Monroe, L.S. (Eds.). (1983). *Ethnic nursing care: A multicultural approach.* St. Louis: Mosby.

Pederson, P. (Ed.). (1988). *A handbook for developing multicultural awareness.* Alexandria, Va: American Association for Counselling and Development.

Roberson, M.H.B. (1987). Home remedies: A cultural study. *Home Healthcare Nurse, 5*(1), 35-40.

Rosenbaum, J.N. (1991). A cultural assessment guide: Learning cultural sensitivity. *The Canadian Nurse, 87*(4), 32-33.

Sands, R.F., & Hale, S.L. (1988). Enhancing cultural sensitivity in clinical practice. *Journal of National Black Nurses Association, 2*(1), 54-63.

Tripp-Reimer, T., Brink, P., & Saunders, J. (1984). Cultural assessment: Content and process. *Nursing Outlook, 32*(2), 78-82.

Tuck, I., & Harris, L.H. (1988). Teaching students transcultural concepts. *Nurse Educator, 13*(3), 36-39.

Williams, J., & Rogers, S. (1993). The multicultural workplace: Preparing preceptors. *Journal of Continuing Education in Nursing, 24*(3), 101-104.

4 HEALTH CARE DELIVERY SYSTEMS

Joan M. Cookfair ◆ Katherine Jones

A system can be defined as a complex of interacting elements.

Ludwig Van Bertalanffy

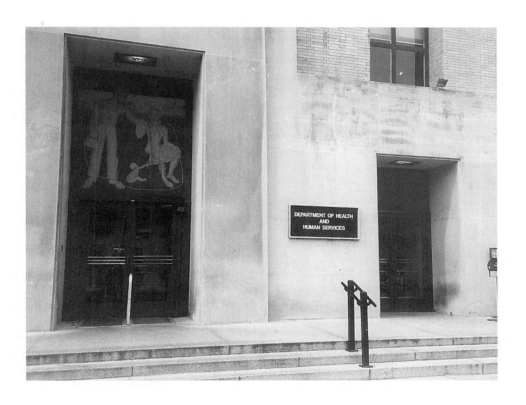

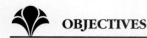 **OBJECTIVES**

At the conclusion of this chapter, the student will be able to:

1. Define the key terms listed.
2. Discuss the predisposing factors that influence the development of a formal health care delivery system.
3. Describe the major differences in health care between developed and undeveloped countries.
4. Compare and contrast and discuss the health care delivery systems in the selected countries.
5. Compare and contrast the national health care systems of selected countries.
6. Discuss the pros and cons of the Clinton Health Care Reform proposal.
7. Describe the functions and purposes of the World Health Organization.

KEY TERMS

Diagnosis-related groupings
Health care delivery system
Health maintenance organizations

Hospital insurance and the Diagnosis Services Act
Medicaid
Medicare

Medical Care Act
National health insurance system
Omnibus Budget Reconciliation Act

A **health care delivery system** is "all of the societal services and activities designed to protect or restore the health of individuals, families, groups, or communities" (Banta, 1986, p. 18).

Predisposing factors that influence the development of a formal health care system are related to the economy of a country, the level of education in a country, and the social structure. The extent to which the system will be used and who will use it depends on access, the supply and distribution of health care personnel, and affordability. Under a national insurance system, eligibility to demand service is based on the criteria of belonging to that system. In a market-oriented society, individuals are eligible to receive services if they are willing and able to pay for them. Access and affordability of insurance programs are enabling factors. The extent to which groups of people use health services relates also to percep-

tions. The recognition that a disorder may constitute a threat of morbidity may motivate an individual to seek health services. Some cultures are more likely to seek preventive health care than others. This might be called perceived morbidity. Figure 4-1 demonstrates a model of relationships relating to the development and use of health service systems (Anderson, Bice, Kohn, & Purola, 1976).

In developed countries, services are organized and financed in a systematic way. In underdeveloped countries, although there may appear to be no system, there may be a fairly complex subsystem provided by family and folk health practitioners. This system of traditions may be adaptive or it may not. Nurses who work with persons from underdeveloped countries need to acquire a fine-tuned sensitivity to traditional cultural practices (see Chapter 3).

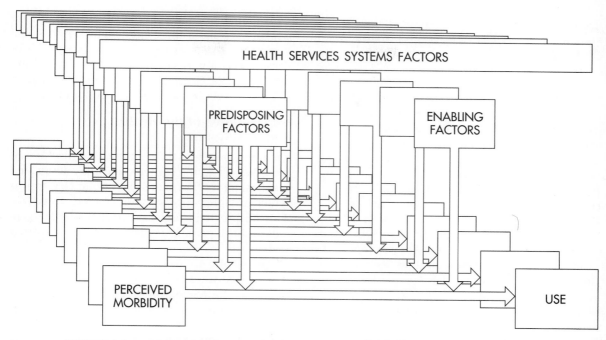

FIGURE 4-1 Model of relationships between systems and individual-level independent variables, using health services as the dependent variable.

THE UNITED STATES HEALTH CARE SYSTEM

The health care delivery system developed by the United States reflects the commitment the country has to a market economy and the rights of the individual. It has evolved into a loosely connected bureaucratic structure that is costly and inefficient, the history of which can be traced through various laws passed by Congress as far back as 1798.

Legislation Affecting the Health Care System

The official entry of the federal government into the health care delivery system began in 1798, when an act of Congress established the Marine Hospital for the relief of sick and disabled seamen. The evolution of the role of the federal government can be traced through the laws passed by Congress over the past 200 years.

Federal involvement in health care was expanded in 1935 when the Social Security Act made provisions for old-age and survivors' assistance, child health care, and aid to crippled children. The Hill-Burton Act of 1946 provided money for upgrading and equipping public and private health institutions. In 1964 the Nurse Training Act provided direct support for students and schools of nursing. Medicaid was enacted in 1965 to provide health care to certain low-socioeconomic groups. Medicare provided care for those over 65. Between 1961 and 1968, Congress passed 138 laws influencing health care delivery. The Comprehensive Health Services amendment of 1966 created health planning agencies to coordinate health services. The Occupational Safety and Health Act was enacted by the Ninety-first Congress and signed into law by President Nixon on December 29, 1970. In 1972 state labor departments began actively enforcing the Act, and every employee in the country came under the jurisdiction of the Occupational Safety and Health Administration (OSHA), which charged employers with the responsibility of furnishing their employees with safe working conditions in a site free from recognized hazards that cause or are likely to cause death or serious physical harm (Hogan & Hogan, 1977).

The Health Maintenance Act (1973) authorized grant funding and loans to stimulate funding of health maintenance organizations. The National Health Planning and Resources Act (1974) promoted collaborative efforts among local, state, and federal agencies. By 1979 a network of 205 health service agencies had been designated by state governments and approved by the Department of Health, Education and Welfare (Hawkins & Higgins, 1982) (renamed the Department of Health and Human Services in 1979). These agencies functioned until 1987, when the Health Planning and Resources Act was repealed.

In 1982 the **Omnibus Budget Reconciliation Act** was enacted, which created large cuts in domestic programs (Jonas, 1986). The legislation reduced the allowable income for persons to qualify for Aid to Families with Dependent Children (AFDC). Furthermore, families ineligible for this aid were no longer automatically eligible for Medicaid.

In 1983 the Tax Equity and Fiscal Responsibility Act (TEFRA) established a cost-per-case basis for hospital payment and placed a ceiling on the rate of increase in hospital revenues that would be supported by the Medicare program. It mandated the prospective payment system for Medicare patients.

In 1983 amendments to the Social Security Act defined a set, preestablished payment fee for types of cases defined by **diagnosis-related groupings** (DRGs). These groupings are divided into 23 major diagnostic categories, which are subdivided into 470 diagnostic groups. Each group is medically oriented, and the entire prospective payment system is based on a medical model.

In January of 1989 the Medicare Catastrophic Coverage Act expanded the scope of Medicare benefits to include an unlimited hospital stay for covered services and 150 days in a skilled nursing facility. Hospice and psychiatric benefits also were increased.

Table 4-1 outlines the history of federal legislation affecting the health care delivery system.

Local, state, and federal governments have contributed to the evolution of the health care delivery system in the United States. Professional associations, such as the American Nurses' Association, the American Medical Association, and the American Hospital Association, continue to influence and contribute to its development.

Components of the Health Services System

Each component of the multitiered health services system in the United States has designated responsibilities. There are many voluntary groups which complement the system (see Chapter 26). This chapter will focus on official public agencies and the private sector within the organized system.

The public sector

The federal government. The federal government has the responsibility for the following aspects of health care: providing direct care for certain groups such as Native Americans, military personnel, and veterans; and safeguarding the public health by regulating quarantines and immigration laws and the marketing of food, drugs, and products used in medical care. The government also prevents environmental hazards; gives grants-in-aid to states, local areas, and individuals; and supports research (Hawkins & Higgins, 1982). The most important federal agency involved with health care is the Department of Health and Human Services, which is responsible for the administration of Social Security, social welfare, and related programs. Health functions such as mental health, health resources, the National Institutes of Health (NIH), Centers for Disease Control and Prevention (CDC), and the Food and Drug Administration (FDA) are administered by the U.S. Public Health Service, which in turn works through several branches (Figure 4-2) (Clark, 1992).

A number of other agencies supervise the quality of health care in the United States. The Drug Enforcement Agency is responsible for dealing with all aspects of alcohol and drug abuse. The Health Services Administration oversees the financing of federal grants to state agencies, and the Centers for Disease Control and Prevention has the responsibility for surveillance and prevention of disease. The Food and Drug

TABLE 4-1 Federal legislation affecting the health care system

Date	Legislation
1798	Bill to create the United States Marine Hospital (Marine Hospital Service) for sick and disabled seamen
1849	Indian Health Affairs assigned to Department of Interior
1906	Pure Food and Drugs Act
1912	Creation of Children's Bureau; Marine Hospital Service renamed Public Health Service
1922	Bill to provide monies for child health care and establish child and maternity centers
1935	Social Security Act
1944	Public Health Service Act extended to all National Institutes of Health; authority to award research grants to nonfederal establishments
1946	Hill-Burton legislation, which authorized federal assistance in the construction of hospitals and health centers, improved beds per population ratios, especially in rural areas; National Mental Health Act — National Institute of Mental Health created
1949	Establishment of a common system of ten regional offices of the Federal Security Agency (later to become the nucleus of the Department of Health, Education and Welfare)
1953	Establishment of the Department of Health, Education and Welfare (DHEW) as a cabinet-status agency
1956	Authorization of the National Health Survey, a continuing interview and clinical appraisal of the health of Americans; Vocational Rehabilitation Act amendments; Housing and Urban Development Act; establishment of the National Library of Medicine
1958	Amendments to the 1906 Food, Drug, and Cosmetic Act requiring manufacturers of new food additives to submit evidence to the Food and Drug Administration (FDA) that a product's safety had been tested and established before marketing
1962	Organization of a Special Staff on Aging, later to become the Administration of Aging
1964	Nurse Training Act, aiding construction of new schools for nursing students and support for curriculum development; Economic Opportunity Act, creating the Office of Economic Opportunity (OEO)
1965	Medicare: medical health insurance for citizens 65 and older; Medicaid: medical assistance program for the indigent; Regional Medical Programs Act: regional cooperation in health care planning
1968	Vocational rehabilitation amendments extending appropriations for grants to states for services, innovation projects, and training
1970	Migrant health amendments, extending health services for migrant and other seasonal agricultural workers; creation of the Environmental Protection Agency (EPA), National Institute on Alcohol Abuse and Alcoholism, and the National Institute on Drug Abuse; Occupational Safety and Health Act (OSHA) (administered principally by the Department of Labor) to regulate and correct health hazards of the workplace
1971	National Cancer Act; Nurse Training Act: capitation grants to schools, support for advanced education; first federal law to reduce hazard of lead poisoning in children
1972	Social Security Act amendments: creating Professional Standards Review Organization (PSRO); further defined benefits under Medicaid and Medicare; important new benefits, including dialysis
1973	Health Maintenance Organization (HMO) Act: model for development of HMOs and funds for demonstration projects
1974	National Health Planning and Resources Act
1976	National Health Consumer and Health Promotion Act; establishment of the Office of Health Information
1979	Nurse Training amendments; bill to create Department of Education (cabinet level) and to rename Health, Education and Welfare, the Department of Health and Human Services
1982	Omnibus Budget Reconciliation Act, which reduced the allowable income for families with dependent children to obtain aid
1983	Tax Equity and Fiscal Responsibility Act, which mandated prospective payment for Medicare patients; amendments to the Social Security Act defined a set of preestablished payment fees for types of cases divided into 23 diagnostic-related groupings
1986	Diagnosis-related groups (DRG system) is introduced for hospital patients covered by Medicare

Modified from *Nursing and the American health care delivery system* (pp. 59-63) (ed. 3) by J. Hawkins & L. Higgins, 1989, New York: Tiresias Press.

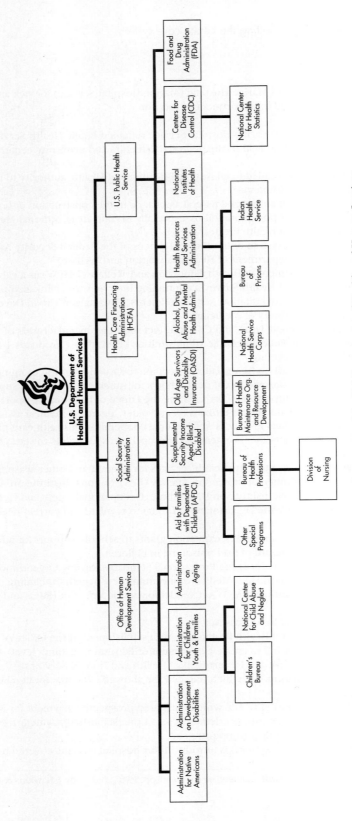

FIGURE 4-2 Partial organizational structure of the U.S. Department of Health and Human Services.

Administration is authorized to monitor the safety and effectiveness of new drugs. The Health Resource Administration is concerned with such needs as adequate personnel for health care and hospital construction. The National Institutes of Health grant monies for research to universities and other centers for research.

State governments. Many state agencies are involved in the health care delivery system, with major responsibilities in the following areas (Hawkins & Higgins, 1982):

1. Control of licensure, vital statistics, medical laboratories, fire and sanitation regulations, and enforcement of OSHA regulations.

2. Enforcement of third-party reimbursement, especially Medicaid.

3. Policy influence on communicable disease control, data collection, and assessment.

4. Delivery of services, maternal and child care, public health nursing, keeping vital records, clinic services, etc.

A sample organizational chart of a State Department of Health is depicted in Figure 4-3 (Clark, 1992, p. 40).

Local health departments. Local health departments focus on local regional needs. They usually provide immunization against infectious disease, direct environmental surveillance, and sponsor programs for maternal and infant child care. Figure 4-4 depicts a sample organizational chart of a local health department (Clark, 1992, p. 43).

The private sector

Physicians. Physicians in private practice provide care on a fee-for-service basis. They are paid directly by the patient or by third-party insurance. In private practice, physicians are largely responsible for setting fee levels.

Private hospitals. In the United States there are more than 6000 proprietary, for-profit hospitals and convalescent homes. They cater to upper-income and middle-income clients who have insurance. Unless there is an emergency situation, they may refer those unable to pay to a county, state, or federally funded hospital. Physicians may wield considerable power in privately run institutions because the hospitals depend on the physicians' good will to obtain clients.

Outpatient services. Most private hospitals offer care to ambulatory clients. Some give this service through emergency rooms rather than through hospital-based outpatient clinics. There

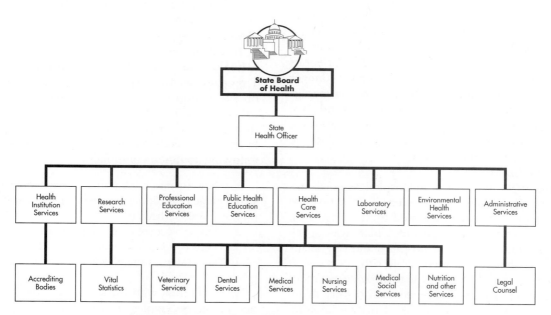

FIGURE 4-3 Typical organizational structure of a state health department.

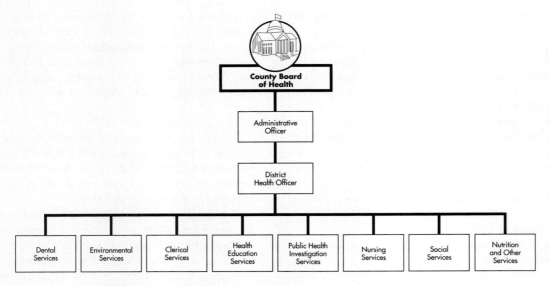

FIGURE 4-4 Typical organizational structure of a local health department.

has been a trend to provide more ambulatory services; for example, one-day surgery and satellite community clinics are available through many private hospitals.

Financing of Health Care

Medicaid and Medicare

Medicaid and **Medicare** benefits became available in 1965. Those persons eligible for Medicare benefits fit into two categories: (1) persons 65 years of age and older who are eligible for Social Security benefits; (2) disabled persons younger than 65 years who meet certain criteria for disability under Social Security regulations and have been disabled for more than 24 months (Stewart, 1979). A comparison of Medicaid and Medicare benefits is shown in Table 4-2.

Blue Cross

In the 1930s, the American Hospital Association's bill to allow subscribers to enroll in a hospital prepayment plan was adopted by the New York State legislature. This payment plan was developed from the need for hospitals and physicians to be guaranteed an income after the depression of the 1930s. It was meant to provide payment for services for eligible persons who were financially able to enroll in a group plan. Blue Cross insurance, which initially was allied with the Amer-

ican Hospital Association, formally separated from the Association in 1972.

Blue Shield

Blue Shield also was created in the 1930s. Initially associated with the American Medical Association, it is now a separate entity. Blue Cross and Blue Shield insurance is purchased through group plans in the workplace or privately by individual persons who can afford it.

Health maintenance organizations

A **health maintenance organization** (HMO) is a prepaid health cooperative with an emphasis on prevention and health maintenance. Individual persons enroll in an organization (often through the workplace) that meets most of their health care needs. All HMOs, however, have the following common components:

1. They assume contractual responsibility for a stated range of health care services, including inhospital and ambulatory care.

2. They serve a voluntary population.

3. There is a fixed annual or monthly payment.

4. The HMO assumes some financial risk or gain.

5. In contrast with physicians in private practice, physicians employed by HMOs receive a fixed salary.

TABLE 4-2 Comparison of Medicare and Medicaid benefits

	Medicaid (Title XIX)	Medicare (Title XVIII)
Description	Medical welfare for the disabled, the elderly, and families in need	Federal health insurance for the aged (65 yr and older)
Administration	Administered by welfare bureaus; federal, state, and local	Administered by Social Security Administration
Financing	Cost sharing: federal, state, and local	Financed by Social Security tax (Part B monthly premium payments)
Eligibility	Left to state's means test (some 9 million below poverty level ineligible)	Virtually all (more than 90%) persons 65 yr and older
Services provided	Services delineated	Services delineated
Provider restrictions	Choice of provider physicians who accept Medicaid	Free choice of provider physicians

Modified from *Nursing and the American health care delivery system* (p. 106) (ed. 3). J. Hawkins & L. Higgins, 1989, New York: Tiresias Press.

Independent insurance plans

Some profit-making insurance companies, such as Aetna and Metropolitan Life, sell supplemental major medical and cash payment policies that help defray costs not covered by other insurance policies. Prudential and the American Association of Retired Persons, for example, have developed a long-term care health care package for older citizens whose primary coverage is through Medicare only (Hays, 1989).

Evaluation of the Current System

Problems

Many Americans believe that all persons have a right to equal access to health care; however, there is a marked decline in access for those who are unable to pay. This lack is emphasized by the fact that Medicaid payments are based on a medical diagnosis of an illness. Thus, preventive health care is seldom available to the indigent. This is a fact that is not likely to change under the present system. Increasing the level of charity care will not solve the problem unless it includes health promotion and prevention in the community. Health care costs have risen rapidly over the past several years and are expected to continue to do so. The projection for the year 2000 alone is that health care expenditures in the United States will reach $1.5 trillion, which is 15% of the gross national product (GNP). In

1986, the health care resource allocation for each person in the United States was approximately $1837. Of these funds 60% were from private sources (either out-of-pocket or private health insurance). Local, state, and federal governmental expenditures, most of which were for Medicare (Title XVIII) or Medicaid (Title XIX) benefits, comprised the remaining 40%.

The response of providers, consumers, and legislators has been one of intense concern for the high price of health care, which sometimes has resulted in a preoccupation with cost almost to the exclusion of all else. It appears that the major issues of health care are balancing cost, quality, and equity.

Possible solutions

The implementation of the Clinton Health Security Act may be the answer. The proposal seeks to reorganize within the present structure to create a new national framework. The goal is to make health coverage "seamless," so health care benefits will have no lifetime limits. There will also be the assurance that it can never be taken away. The Act seeks to control rising costs, reduce paperwork, and make everyone responsible for care. In addition, it will seek to maintain consumer choice and improve the quality of care.

The plan would empower each state to set up health alliances that contract with health plans and bargain on behalf of consumers and employers. It would seek to cut down on paperwork and outlaw insurance practices that hurt small businesses. Malpractice reform would seek to reduce unnecessary tests and procedures. The plan is that coverage would go into effect state-by-state beginning in 1995 and be fully implemented by 1997.

THE CANADIAN HEALTH CARE SYSTEM

The Canadian health care system is a modified **national health insurance system.** A high number of health care professionals per capita and an extensive network of health care institutions and official voluntary community health agencies provide a broad spectrum of secondary and tertiary care, and preventive services. With the adoption of a comprehensive, tax-supported insurance program for hospital services in 1957 and for medical care in 1966, virtually all Canadians, regardless of age, health status, or financial means, have access to hospital and medical care on a prepaid basis, thus avoiding expensive hospital or medical bills.

While the **Medical Care Act** (1968) and the **Hospital Insurance and Diagnostic Services Act** (1961) removed financial barriers for consumers, they entrenched the most expensive means of service delivery. Federal-provincial cost sharing was and still is allowed for those services provided by physicians. Although other health care professionals are allowed to bill provincial insurance plans in some provinces, the cost of such services is, for the most part, still not incorporated into the system. Because the federal government had no direct jurisdiction in health care, both the hospital and medical insurance programs were cooperative and voluntary. To qualify for federal-provincial cost sharing, the provincial programs had only to meet certain terms of reference, which are listed as follows:

1. Universal coverage on uniform terms and conditions that do not impede reasonable access to insured persons
2. Portability of benefits from province to province
3. Insurance for all medically necessary services

4. A publicly administered nonprofit program (Vayda & Deber, 1986, p. 193).

Not only did the federal-provincial cost sharing stimulate all the provinces to act quickly to introduce their health insurance programs, but it also served as a means of redistributing income between the wealthier and poorer provinces. The 50% federal share was distributed as follows: each province was paid 25% of the per capita costs it incurred for hospital inpatient services plus 25% of the national average per capita cost multiplied by the province's population. As a result, the wealthier provinces that spent more received less than 50% of their costs. The federal government had no control over amounts expended by the provinces and received no political credit for its contributions. In 1977, Bill C-37 (Federal-Provincial Fiscal Arrangements and Established Programs Financing Act) reduced the direct federal contribution for health care to 25% of total 1975-1976 expenditures and tied any subsequent increase in federal transfer payments to the GNP. To compensate, federal income and corporate taxes were decreased to create "tax room" for the provinces which could (and did) then raise their tax rates to balance the federal reductions without increasing total taxation levels. As a result, the provinces had greater fiscal responsibility.

As early as 1969, both federally and provincially, concerns were being expressed about the escalating costs of health care. The 1969 federal Task Force on the Costs of Health Service concluded that increased costs could only be dealt with by reduced standards of care, increased taxes, premiums and/or deterrent fees, or more efficient operation of the system. While health care expenditures continued to range between 7% and 8% of the GNP, and economists and politicians hailed this as an example of successful containment, service providers (both physicians and hospitals) charged that the system was underfunded and began to seek private money through user fees, extra billing (charging over and above amounts publicly funded), and private insurance. Confrontations increased, work stoppages occurred, and many hospitals went from line to global budgets where rates of increase were often less than inflation. Hospitals protested these inadequate increases and were often successful in obtaining additional money to cover budgetary deficits.

The Lalonde Report (1975) of the Federal Department of National Health and Welfare stressed the importance of health promotion, lifestyle modification, and greater individual responsibility for health instead of increased provision of medical services. This report was discounted by many providers as a government justification for reduced spending for medical services. Many provinces commissioned similar studies, which reached the same conclusions. In 1979, within this climate of confrontation and charges of underfunding and diversion of health care dollars to other programs, the federal government asked Justice Emmett Hall to examine the universal health insurance program recommended in his 1964 Royal Commission Report. As a result of his review and the 1972 Hastings Report and the Lalonde Report, the federal government published a position paper on the preservation of Universal Medicare in 1983 and legislated the Canada Health Act (Bill C-3) in 1984. Active and successful lobbying by other health care service providers such as the Canadian Nurses Association caused the Act to refer to health care practitioners with the appropriate phraseology attached to allow provincial governments to determine and authorize which professional groups could provide insured services. The Ontario government, for example, has enacted the Regulated Health Professions Act (Bill 100, 1992), which recognizes 23 independent practitioners. Table 4-3 describes some of the laws that have affected the system.

Although many physicians continue to function as independent entrepreneurs within a publicly funded system, their power and influence has been considerably eroded. Most provinces still allow the physicians to act as gatekeepers determining access to the health care delivery system; however, the trend is changing. Hospitals are downsizing and in some cases closing. Others are having to rationalize their services and expenses. Competition is intense for new high-tech

TABLE 4-3 Laws that have affected the Canadian system

Date	Legislation
1957	Comprehensive tax-supported insurance for hospital services
1961	Hospital services and diagnostic services
1968	Medical Act
1977	Bill C-37, Federal Provincial Fiscal Arrangements and Financing Act
1984	Canada Health Act, Bill C-3
1992	Regulated Health Professionals Act, Bill 100

diagnostic capabilities such as computerized axial tomography (CAT) scanners and magnetic resonance imaging (MRI), but provincial governments have been supporting increased regionalization and collaboration with corresponding reductions in duplication of services.

Hospitals in close geographic proximity no longer provide all the same or similar services. The recent amalgamation of the Toronto Western and General Hospitals is an excellent example whereby patients with certain health care problems are treated at the Western branch and others at the General branch. In smaller communities, duplications in expensive emergency room and coronary and intensive care units have been reconciled. Ambulance and airlift transport provide opportunities for transfer of more acutely ill patients to highly specialized centers for treatment with minimal delays once the patient is stabilized. Canada spends less per capita to provide universal accessibility to necessary medical services and health promotion and illness prevention programs, such as immunization, than the United States. Some of the more advanced research technologies, such as in vitro fertilization, are no longer considered essential medical services and caps or restrictions have been placed on the implementation of such programs as a means of cost containment.

Problems and Solutions

Abuses of the system still occur and the media continue to draw attention to the defects as opposed to the aspects that are working. In some cases, bed shortages and lack of staff are cited for delays in obtaining needed surgery such as coronary bypasses and organ transplants. At the same time, health promotion and prevention programs directed at eliminating the need for such surgery are largely ignored. Cost containment measures have been criticized for reducing the perceived quality of health care. However, Canadians are now being reoriented towards appropriate use of health care delivery facilities and cost containment issues. Canadians who walk into emergency departments for nonemergency problems such as enduring toothaches or the need for prescription renewals are being redirected to medical walk-in clinics or community health centers for more appropriate follow-up of presenting health problems.

Although seniors over the age of 65 who receive Canada Pension Plan or Old Age Security benefits may obtain their prescription medications for a minimal fee or no charge, some of the newer, more expensive proprietary drugs are no longer covered without some cost to the consumer. Private insurance and drug benefit plans may cover the cost of such drugs, particularly for those individuals who, following retirement, continue to participate in plans offered by their previous employers. Not all employers offer such supplementary benefit plans, but the trend is on the rise.

Individuals who would find self-insurance or private health insurance plans prohibitively expensive are able to take advantage of less expensive group plans through their employers. Such plans cover benefits not universally accessible, such as eye examinations and eyeglasses, dental care, prescription drugs, and services of other health care professionals such as chiropractors, naturopaths, private duty nurses or nursing assistants, and prosthetic or assistive devices that may be only partially covered by provincial insurance programs.

With the deepening recession and more reductions in federal transfer payments, most provinces are becoming more creative in educating the public regarding appropriate use of health care services. Community Health Centres have been one means of coping with the coordi-

nation of service delivery, with multidisciplinary teams addressing wellness, health promotion, prevention, and social issues as opposed to primarily treatment and curative functions. Community-based programs receive grants and incentives, and the hospital is seen less significantly as the center for health care delivery. Hospitalizations and hospital stays have been markedly reduced in most areas of the country, except perhaps in the more remote northern areas where a community hospital may be serving a very diverse and geographically dispersed population.

Within this context, the role of the nurse is steadily expanding in many areas of community health nursing because funding is more consistently provided to the lowest cost level of qualified health care provider. Also, more clients are discharged earlier and therefore, possibly sicker, from the hospital or they are maintained in the community with adequate supports.

Nursing's Contribution to System Development

In spite of the fact that Canada is a market economy, there has always been an altruistic commitment to assist the poor and unfortunate. Nurses have contributed significantly to the development of the valuing of concern and care for all people. Public health nurses as employees of official agencies became more involved with health promotion aspects, education, monitoring of high risk populations, and school health and immunization programs. Voluntary agencies such as the VON and the St. Elizabeth Visiting Nurses Association took over more aspects of the direct caregiving curative, and palliative roles. More recently, the change in approach to public health nursing to provide health promotion and program planning has resulted in a perceived loss of direct client contact. Nurses from voluntary agencies provide most of the direct client care and visiting aspects under the auspices of provincial home care and private insurance programs. Entrepreneurial nurses have also developed their own businesses to provide services and programs not covered by universal accessibility to health care.

In underserviced and isolated areas, the role of the public health nurse is not as clearly differ-

Factors That Influence the Nurse Practitioner's Performance

The purpose of the following descriptive study was reflected in the following two questions: (1) "What nurse practitioner employment setting(s) has most helped and most hindered your performance of the nurse practitioner role? (2) What factors within the nurse practitioner work setting have helped and hindered your role performance?" Ninety-one of 200 randomly selected nurse practitioners certified by the Commonwealth of Pennsylvania, between the ages of 27 and 65 years ($\bar{X}$ 40 ± 8), replied to a mailed survey that requested demographic information in addition to responses to the aforementioned questions. A criterion for participation was the "prior or active" involvement as a practitioner in "providing direct patient care." All nurse practitioner specialties "(adult, family, pediatrics, neonatal, gerontology, and obstetrics and gynecology)" were represented.

The average work experience of the respondents as nurses, most of whom were women (93%) and master's prepared (64%), was 9 years, and as nurse practitioners, 6 years. Thirty-eight percent of nurse practitioners had worked in 1 setting, 43% had worked in 2 settings, and the remainder had worked in 3 or more settings. A wide variety of health care settings, categorized as inpatient, acute or long term (31%), outpatient primary care or community clinics (51%), and "other (emergency rooms; student, employee, occupational health; physician private practice and home care)" were identified. While both inpatient and outpatient set-tings were identified by 13 of 50 respondents (some provided multiple responses) who had worked in more than one position as hindering practice, there was no one setting that was consistently identified as "not being conducive to nurse practitioner practice." Nine settings were identified by 30 respondents (some provided multiple responses) as positively contributing to their role, and 17 of the 30 stipulated that "outpatient clinic settings were well suited for (their) practice." The number one specialty area was "family planning/reproductive health ($n = 7$)." Many factors (some of them situation-specific) either hindered or helped practice, but "the presence or absence of support from either coworkers or superiors (physicians, nurse practitioners, nurses, administration, and other staff members) was the overwhelming factor influencing nurse practitioner role performance." A finding which was described as incidental was "most master's-prepared nurse practitioners changed jobs more frequently than did non–master's-prepared nurse practitioners." Two main implications of this study were that "nurse practitioners need to identify settings that are appropriate for their practice and seek employment in these settings, and support systems are an area where they need to focus their attention. Although the characteristics of the sample were fairly consistent with the national sample," the response rate (46%) from one state and an absence of reasons for choices (survey) were limitations identified in the study.

From Hupcey J.E. (1993). Factors and work settings that may influence nurse practitioner practice. *Nursing Outlook, 41*(4), 181-185.

entiated because nurse practitioners perform the roles of public health nurses, visiting nurses, midwives, and physician's assistants.

Political Structure

Canada is a loose confederation of ten provinces and two territories (one third will be created by the division of the Northwest Territory in 1997 to provide for the self-rule by aboriginal peoples in that area). The British North America of 1867, which established Canada, set up the organizational structure for the nation and divided powers between the federal government in Ottawa and the provincial governments. The Act assigned all matters of national concern plus those activities likely to be most costly to the federal government, which had the broadest tax base. Ottawa was given jurisdiction over such items as railways, canals, coinage, and, in the health field, quarantine, marine hospitals, and health services for native peoples and the armed forces. The provinces were given authority for local concerns which at the time were considered unlikely to be costly, including roads, education, and the establishment of hospitals, asylums, and charities. The shared responsibilities between the federal government and the provinces cause stresses and difficulties but Canadians remain dedicated to a policy of health for all. They have adopted a framework for health promotion based on the International Conference on Health Promotion convened in Ottawa in November 1986 (Epp, 1986).

THE NORWEGIAN HEALTH CARE SYSTEM

Norway has universal health care, with the central government controlling the entire organization. Hospitals are government owned, and regulation of the quality of care rests with the government. Medical coverage is extended to everyone, although there is a policy of cost sharing for those who can pay. Poor people pay nothing for medical care, and dental care is free to all children.

The rate of physicians to the population is approximately the same as it is in the United States, but more physicians work in primary care and fewer in specialty areas (Roemer, 1977).

HEALTH CARE IN THE UNITED KINGDOM

The United Kingdom is composed of England, Wales, Scotland, and Northern Ireland. The National Health Service was implemented in 1948. The goal was to make medical care available to every citizen, regardless of income. The federal government controls financing and the regulation of care. The country is divided into regions, which fund such services as community health clinics. The regional services are then broken down into district offices. All medical care is provided through the public sector. In 1989, Margaret Thatcher stated that The National Health Service would continue to be available to all regardless of income, and it would be financed mainly through general taxation. "There has recently been a move to introduce more market elements into the National Health Service with the idea that it may increase competition and efficiency. The idea that health care should be avail-

able to all continues to form policy (Culyer and Mead, 1992).

THE WORLD HEALTH ORGANIZATION

The most extensive health service system in the world is the World Health Organization (WHO). Now in its forty-sixth year, it is made up of 147 member countries. The headquarters are in Geneva, Switzerland, and there are six regional offices: one in Africa, two in the United States, one in Copenhagen, one in Alexandria, one in New Delhi, and one in Manila. These offices service South America, Europe, India, Egypt, and Southeast Asia. The organization accumulates statistics about the state of the world's health. It also provides, on request, teams of consultants to assist with real or potential health problems and in times of disaster. In 1977, the World Health Assembly decided that the main social target of governments and WHO in the coming decade should be the attainment of a level of health that will permit all citizens of the world to lead socially and economically productive lives by the year 2000. Table 4-4 depicts a history of WHO and its international cooperation in public health.

The executive board of WHO is composed of 31 individuals who are technically qualified in the field of health, each one designated by a Member State elected to do so by the World Health Assembly. Member states are elected for 3-year terms, and the individuals they designate act in their personal capacity. The executive board meets at least twice a year; the main meeting is normally in January, with a second shorter meeting in May, immediately following the health assembly. The main functions of the executive board are to give effect to the decisions and policies of the health assembly, to advise it, and generally to facilitate its work.

The secretariat is staffed by some 4500 health and other experts in both professional and general service categories, working at headquarters, in the six regional offices and in countries. The secretariat is headed by the director-general, who is appointed by the World Health Assembly on the nomination of the executive board. The director-general is assisted by one deputy director-general and five assistant directors-general.

TABLE 4-4 History of WHO and international cooperation in public life

Date	Event	Date	Event	Date	Event
1830	Cholera overruns Europe		clude provisions against smallpox and typhus.		Sanitary Regulations adopted by the Fourth World Health Assembly, replacing the previous International Sanitary Conventions.
1851	First International Sanitary Conference is held in Paris to produce an international sanitary convention, but fails.	1935	International Sanitary Convention for aerial navigation comes into force.		
1892	International Sanitary Convention, restricted to cholera, is adopted.	1938	Last International Sanitary Conference held in Paris. Conseil Sanitaire, Maritime et Quarantinaire at Alexandria is handed over to Egypt. (The WHO Regional Office for the Eastern Mediterranean is its lineal descendant.)	1969	These are renamed the International Health Regulations, excluding louse-borne typhus and relapsing fever, and leaving only cholera, plague, smallpox, and yellow fever.
1897	Another international convention dealing with preventive measures against plague is adopted.				
1902	International Sanitary Bureau, later re-named Pan American Sanitary Bureau, and then Pan American Sanitary Organization, is set up in Washington, D.C. This is the forerunner of today's Pan American Health Organization (PAHO), which also serves as WHO's Regional Office for the Americas.	1945	United Nations Conference on International Organization in San Francisco unanimously approves a proposal by Brazil and China to establish a new, autonomous, international health organization.	1973	Report from the executive board concludes that there is widespread dissatisfaction with health services. Radical changes are needed. The Twenty-sixth Wold Health Assembly decides that WHO should collaborate with, rather than assist, its member states in developing practical guidelines for national health care systems.
1907	L'Office International d'Hygiène Publique (OIHP) is established in Paris, with a permanent secretariat and a permanent committee of senior public health officials of member governments.	1946	International Health Conference in New York approves the Constitution of the World Health Organization (WHO).		
		1947	WHO Interim Commission organizes assistance to Egypt to combat cholera epidemic.	1974	WHO launches an Expanded Programme on Immunization to protect children from poliomyelitis, measles, diphtheria, whooping cough, tetanus, and tuberculosis.
1919	League of Nations is created and is charged, among other tasks, with taking steps in matters of international concern for the prevention and control of disease. The Health Organization of the League of Nations is set up in Geneva, in parallel with the OIHP.	1948	WHO Constitution comes into force on 7 April (now marked as World Health Day each year), when the 26th of the 61 member states who signed it ratified its signature. Later, the First World Health Assembly is held in Geneva with delegations from 55 governments that by then were members.	1977	Thirtieth World Health Assembly sets as target: that the level of health to be attained by the turn of the century should be that which will permit all people to lead socially and economically productive lives. Health for All by the Year 2000.
1926	International Sanitary Convention is revised to in-	1951	Test of new International	1978	Joint WHO/UNICEF (United Nations Chil-

Continued

TABLE 4-4   History of WHO and international cooperation in public life   cont'd

Date	Event	Date	Event	Date	Event
	dren's Fund) International Conference in Alma-Ata, USSR, adopts a Declaration on Primary Health Care as the key to attaining the goal of Health for All by the Year 2000.	1979	ment and peace. A Global Commission certifies the worldwide eradication of smallpox, the last known natural case having occurred in 1977.	1987	rate with WHO. United Nations General Assembly expresses concern over the spread of the AIDS pandemic. The Global Programme on AIDS is launched within WHO.
1979	United Nations General Assembly, as well as the Thirty-second World Health Assembly, reaffirms that health is a powerful lever for socioeconomic develop-	1981	Global Strategy for Health for All by the Year 2000 is adopted, and is endorsed by the United Nations General Assembly, which urges other concerned international organizations to collabo-	1988	Fortieth Anniversary of WHO is celebrated. Forty-first World Health Assembly resolves that poliomyelitis will be eradicated by the year 2000.

From *Facts about Who* (pp 1-3) by The World Health Organization, 1990, Geneva: Author.

Past directors-general have been Dr. Brock Chisholm, Canada (1948-1953); Dr. Marcolino G. Candau, Brazil (1953-1973); and Dr. Halfdan Mahler, Denmark (1973-1988).

The present Director-General is Dr. Hiroshi Nakajima, of Japan, who assumed the post in July of 1988. Dr. Nakajima, a specialist in neuropsycho-pharmacology, joined WHO in 1973 and served as WHO Regional Director for the Western Pacific for 9 years, beginning in 1979.

In 1978 the Joint WHO/UNICEF International Conference on Primary Health Care adopted the Declaration of Alma-Ata. In 1981 the World Health Assembly—the annual meeting of delegates from all member states, usually held in Geneva—unanimously adopted a Global Strategy for Health for All by the Year 2000 (WHO, 1990, p. 2).

The emphasis placed on primary health care includes the development of health care systems that are adaptable to various local programs and that include measures for health promotion, disease prevention, diagnosis, therapy, and rehabilitation. Strategies to be encouraged are those involving specific measures to be taken by individuals and families in their homes. International support of national action through information exchange, research and development, technical support, training, and assisting with the coordination between the health sector and other sectors, is spelled out. WHO maintains that:

Primary health care is essential health care based on practical, scientifically sound, and socially acceptable methods and technology made universally accessible to individuals and families in the community through their full participation and at a cost that the community and country can afford to maintain, at every stage of their development in the spirit of self-reliance and self-determination. It forms an integral part both of the country's health system, of which it is the central function and main focus, and of the overall social and economic development of the community. It is the first level of contact of individuals, the family, and the community with the national health system, bringing health care as close as possible to where people live and work, and constitutes the first element of a continuing health care process.

Primary health care rests on the following eight elements:

- Education concerning prevailing health problems and the methods of preventing and controlling them;
- Promotion of food supply and proper nutrition;
- An adequate supply of safe water and basic sanitation;

- Maternal and child health care, including family planning;
- Immunization against the major infectious diseases;
- Prevention and control of locally endemic diseases;
- Appropriate treatment of common diseases and injuries;
- Provision of essential drugs.

Following the adoption in 1981 of the Global Strategy for Health for All, it became evident that national health systems needed to be reoriented and reorganized if the goal was to be achieved and the eight elements of primary health care to be provided. The main areas of concern have been equitable resource allocation, community involvement, and intersectoral collaboration, which require good planning and bold decisions to change existing patterns (WHO, 1990, p. 3).

HEALTH SERVICE ISSUES IN UNDERDEVELOPED NATIONS
Somalia

Somalia is one of the world's least developed countries. The per capita income is $200 per year. Women are confined to purely domestic roles, and they are subject to restrictive Islamic laws. Infibulation (stitching up of the labia majora) and clitoridectomy (female circumcision), are common practices. A young nurse, educated in Belgium, decided to work for a while in Somalia. Her assignment was in an OB/GYN ward in a small hospital in Mogadishu. Her dismay at the problems encountered by the women of Somalia because of these practices was profound. There were repeated infections and pain throughout life. Most women needed multiple episiotomies to deliver a child. If help was not available, some could not deliver. The nurse related that the women taught her much about acceptance and courage, but that it was a difficult personal experience. For 2 years afterward she could not speak of it. She ultimately chose to become a nurse educator for the Agency for International Development. She has trained more than 2000 people in midwifery in many different countries (Vansintejan, 1989). The need for the education of women and improvement in the health of women and children in poor countries such as Somalia is urgent.

It is incumbent on the world community to assist underdeveloped countries to improve health services, not just for humanitarian reasons, but because of the increased risk of the spread of infectious diseases. According to statistics from the World Health Organization, tuberculosis has once again become a global threat. Tuberculosis has a deadly link with AIDS. Both diseases are prevalent throughout Africa (Nakajima, 1993).

Peru

Peru is a very poor country that is considered to be in transition. There has never been central control or equity in the availability of health care. People in the countryside are treated by "curanderos," who are traditional healers. In January of 1991, an outbreak of cholera resulted in such a devastating loss of human life that a cholera control command was established. The ministry of health of Peru obtained technical help from the Pan American Health Organization, and the start of a system of organized care for the poor, and for the rich, began to become a reality. The government has begun surveillance of infectious disease, and has implemented programs to improve sanitation (Loyola & Hevia, 1993).

WHO works closely with other organizations within the United Nations system. It is a constitutional requirement that WHO should "establish and maintain effective collaboration with the United Nations . . . and provide health services and facilities." UNICEF has been one of the closest partners; in 1989 WHO and UNICEF jointly launched an initiative for mothers and children called "Facts for Life" (WHO, 1990, p. 4).

WHO also maintains close working relationships with bilateral agencies, intergovernmental, and nongovernmental organizations (NGOs). At present, some 160 NGOs are in official relations with WHO.

In addition, leading health-related institutions around the world are officially designated as WHO Collaborating Centres. There are now over 1000 such centers (WHO, 1990, p. 4).

The address and phone number of the World Health Organization and the addresses and phone numbers of the regional offices can be found in the box on page 82.

REGIONAL OFFICES OF THE WORLD HEALTH ORGANIZATION

World Health Organization
CH-1211 Geneva 27, Switzerland
Tel: (022) 791 21 11 Fax: (022) 791 07 46
Telex: **UNISANTE GENEVA** 415416

Africa
WHO, Regional Office for Africa
P.O. Box 6
Brazzaville, Congo
Tel: (242) 83 38 60 Fax: (242) 83 18 79
Telex: **UNISANTE BRAZZAVILLE** 5217/5364

Americas
WHO, Regional Office for the Americas
Pan American Sanitary Bureau
525 23rd Street, N.W.
Washington, DC, 20037, United States of America
Tel: (202) 861 32 00 Fax: (202) 223 59 71
Telex: **OFSANPAN WASHINGTON** 248338

Southeast Asia
WHO, Regional Office for South-East Asia
World Health House, Indraprastha Estate
Mahatma Gandhi Road
New Delhi 110002, India
Tel: (91) 331 78 04 Fax: (91 11) 331 86 07
Telex: **WHO NEW DELHI** 3165095

Europe
WHO, Regional Office for Europe
8, Scherfigsvej, DK-2100 Copenhagen 0
Denmark
Tel: (4531) 29 01 11 Fax: (45) 31 18 11 20
Telex: **UNISANTE COPENHAGEN** 15348

Eastern Mediterranean
WHO, Regional Office for the Eastern Mediterranean
P.O. Box 1517
Alexandria 21511, Egypt
Tel: (203) 483 0097 Fax: (203) 483 8916
Telex: **UNISANTE ALEXANDRIA** 54028

Western Pacific
WHO, Regional Office for the Western Pacific
P.O. Box 2932
1099 Manila, Philippines
Tel: (632) 521 84 21 Fax: (632) 52 11 036
Telex: **UNISANTE MANILA** 27652

WHO liaison office with the United Nations
2, United Nations Plaza
DC-2 Building, Rooms 0956 to 0976
New York, NY 10017
United States of America
Tel: (212) 963 60 05 Fax: (212) 223 29 20
Telex: **UNISANTE NEW YORK** 234292

Chapter Highlights

- A health care delivery system is "all of the societal services designed to protect or restore the health of individuals, families, groups, or communities" (Banta, 1986, p. 18). A health care delivery system is influenced by economy, education, and social structure.

- Since the 1798 bill to create the U.S. Marine Hospital Service for sick and disabled seamen, the federal government has taken an active role in providing direct care for certain groups such as native Americans, military personnel, and veterans, as well as regulating quarantines, immigration laws, and the marketing of food and drugs and preventing environmental hazards.

- In the United States, state health departments control licensure, collect vital statistics, enforce third-party payment, influence communicable disease control, and deliver selected types of service.

- Local health departments in each state provide immunizations against infectious disease, perform environmental surveillance, and sponsor programs for maternal and infant child care.

- Financing the health care in the public sector has been regulated through legislation (Medicare and Medicaid) that focuses primarily on indigent and elderly populations and is medically oriented.

- The private sector is composed of physicians in private practice, private hospitals, and private outpatient services. Financing for the private sector is available through Blue Cross and Blue Shield, health maintenance organizations, and other independent insurance plans.

- The Clinton proposal seeks to lower the cost of health care and provide access to health care for all United States citizens.

- Canada provides health care to all its citizens. This is provided by cost-sharing through the federal government and the provinces.

- Underdeveloped countries suffer from lack of organized health services. There are frequently subsystems in these countries. Care is provided by families and folk healers.

- The World Health Organization has 147 member countries. It advocates health for all citizens of the world by the year 2000. It advocates a system of primary health care for all countries to accomplish this goal.

 CRITICAL THINKING EXERCISE

A small town in India reported four cases of pneumonic plague. Plague is spread by infected fleas on rodents and by infected individuals through droplet infection. The level of education in the town is not high. There is very little money and no formal health care delivery system. Health care workers may be hampered by the fact that many of the people are Hindu and do not believe in destroying any kind of life, even the rats that are spreading the plague.

1. As a member of a health team sent to assist them, how would you proceed?
2. Considering the predisposing factors and the perceived morbidity of the group, what is a realistic approach?

REFERENCES

Anderson, D.O., Bice, T.W., Kohn, R., & Purola, T. (1976). *Theoretical orientation. Health care: An international study.* New York: Oxford University Press.

Banta, D. (1986). What is health care? In S. Jonas (Ed.), *Health care delivery in the United States* (3rd ed.) (p. 18). New York: Springer.

Baumgart, A., & Larsen, J. (1988). *Canadian nursing faces the future.* Toronto: Mosby.

Begin, M. (1983). *Preserving national Medicare.* Ottawa: Ministry of National Health and Welfare.

Bertalanffy, L.V. (1968). *General systems theory.* New York: George Braziller.

Canadian Nurses' Association. (1984). *Brief to the House of Commons standing committee on health, welfare, and social affairs in response to the Canada Health Act.* Ottawa, Canada.

Clark, M.J. (1992). *Nursing in the community.* Norwalk, CT: Appleton Lange.

Culyer, A.J., & Meads, A. (1992). The United Kingdom: Effective, efficient, equitable? *Journal of Health Politics, Policy and Law, 17*(4), 668-686.

Epp, J. (1986). *Achieving health for all: A framework for health promotion.* Ottawa: Ministry of National Health and Welfare.

Government of Canada. (1984). *Canada Health Act.* Ottawa: Queen's Printer.

Government of Ontario. (1992). Bill 100.

Hawkins, J., & Higgins, L. (1982). *Nursing care and the American health care delivery system.* New York: Tiresias Press.

Hays, A. (1989). Paying for long-term care. *Geriatric Nursing (London), 10*(1), 20.

Hogan, R.B., & Hogan, R.B. (1977). *Occupational Safety and Health Act.* New York: Matthew Bender.

Jonas, S. (1986). *Health care delivery in the United States.* New York: Springer.

Lalonde, M. (1975). *A new perspective on the health of Canadians.* Ottawa, Canada: National Health and Welfare.

Legislative update. (1988). *Health Care Financing Review, 10*(2), 131.

Loyola, L., & Hevia, P. (1993, July-August). Keeping cholera at bay. *World Health, 4.* Geneva, Switzerland, Public World Health.

Nakajima, H. (1993, May-June). The state of the world's health. *World Health, 3.* Geneva, Switzerland, Public World Health.

Roemer, M. (1977). *International health perspectives, an introduction in five volumes.* New York: Springer.

Roemer, M. (1982). *An introduction to the U.S. health care system.* New York: Springer.

Shah, C. (1987). *An introduction to Canadian health and the health care system* (2nd ed.). Toronto: University of Toronto, Department of Preventive Medicine and Biostatistics.

Stewart, J. (1979). *Home health care.* St. Louis: Mosby.

Vansintejan, G. (1989). Midwifery, an international career. *Journal of Nurse-Midwifery, 34*(6), 355-358.

Vayda, J., & Deber, J. (1986). *The Canadian health care system: An overview.* Toronto, Canada: Department of Health Administration, University of Toronto.

World Health Organization. (1990). *Facts about WHO.*

5

NURSING THEORY AND NURSING PROCESS IN THE COMMUNITY

Carol Batra

The knowledge base of nursing resides in the schools of thought espoused through nursing theories and frameworks. . . . It is nursing's unique contribution to the health care system.

Rosemary Rizzo Parse

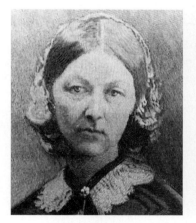

Florence Nightingale

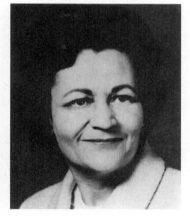

Imogene King

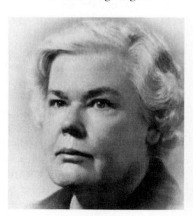

Dorothea E. Orem

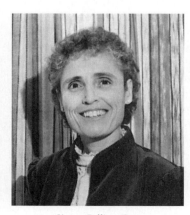

Sister Callista Roy

OBJECTIVES

At the conclusion of this chapter, the student will be able to:

1. Apply the steps of the nursing process to the community setting.
2. Compare the relationship of the nursing process to the Standards of Clinical Nursing Practice and the Standards of Community Health Nursing Practice.
3. Use the North American Nursing Diagnoses Association (NANDA) nursing diagnosis taxonomy and the Omaha Visiting Nurse Association Problem Classification Scheme to specify nursing diagnoses for a community.
4. Use the Iowa Nursing Intervention Classification (NIC) for nursing interventions specific to a community.
5. Use the nursing frameworks of King, Nightingale, Orem, and Roy to structure the nursing process for a community setting.

KEY TERMS

Assessment
Diagnosis
Dorothea Orem
Evaluation
Florence Nightingale
Imogene King
Implementation
North American nursing diagnosis association (NANDA)

Nursing frameworks
Nursing intervention classification (NIC)
Nursing process
Omaha problem classification scheme

Plan
Sr. Callista Roy
Standards of clinical nursing practice
Standards of community health nursing practice

Theory-based practice is becoming commonplace in nursing (Huch, 1988). In Canada, professional nursing associations are mandating theory-based nursing as a standard of practice (Canadian Nurses' Association, 1980). Canadian public health departments are introducing nursing models to be consistent with the provincial licensing body requirement of a conceptual model for public health nursing practice (Beynon & Laschinger, 1993). Laschinger and Duff (1991) found that nurses believed that theory-based practice helped them collect useful data and plan comprehensive care.

Nursing practice is implemented from a frame of reference. Reilly (1975) helps us to understand

this idea when she says that we all have a private image or concept of nursing practice. In turn, this private image influences our interpretation of data, our decisions, and our actions. Conceptual models of nursing are the formal presentations of some nurses' private images of nursing. These models may be considered world views or these nurses' views of the world of nursing, particularly the nature of the relationships between people and their environments (Fawcett, 1984).

The way the nurse approaches a person, a family, or a community reflects the nurse's world view. The knowledge and beliefs of the nurse are manifest in the way the nurse talks and listens to a person, what the nurse is most concerned about, and how the nurse moves with the flow of the situation (Parse, 1992). When the nurse is guided by a particular nursing framework, conceptual model, or nursing theory, the nurse performs the nursing process by using the language, concepts, categories, and world view of that nursing theorist's framework.

Nurse leaders (Barrett, 1993; Parse, 1990, 1992; Reed, 1993) have stressed that nursing actions must be based on the unique body of nursing knowledge. The nursing frameworks, conceptual models, or nursing theories constitute this unique body of nursing knowledge and nursing's unique contribution to health care.

Both the American Public Health Association (1980) and the American Nurses' Association (1980) have called for a synthesis of public health and nursing knowledge. To achieve this synthesis, it is appropriate for nursing frameworks to guide the use of the nursing process in nursing practice for clients, whether they are individuals, families, aggregates, or communities (Hanchett, 1990).

This chapter discusses each of the phases of the nursing process as applied to the community setting and to the standards of community health nursing practice. The North American Nursing Diagnoses Association (NANDA) nursing diagnosis taxonomy, Omaha Visiting Nurse Association Problem Classification Scheme, and the Iowa Nursing Intervention Classification (NIC) are described for use by community nurses. Four **nursing frameworks,** each of which contributes a useful world view to community health nurses, are presented as a structure for the nursing process. These perspectives include the following: King's open systems and theory of goal attainment, Nightingale's environmental model, Orem's self-care model, and Roy's adaptation model. Neuman's systems model is discussed in Chapter 2. Leininger's cultural assessment model is discussed in Chapter 3.

The first case study in Chapter 2 is used to show how each of four nursing frameworks can be applied to the five-phase nursing process in a community. Both the NANDA and Omaha Visiting Nurse Association Problem Classification Schemes are used to determine nursing diag-

noses, and the Iowa NIC is used to propose some nursing implementations.

NURSING PROCESS AND THE STANDARDS OF COMMUNITY HEALTH NURSING PRACTICE

Two driving forces in nursing practice in the 1990s have been the emphases both on quality and on cost containment. If nurses are to survive the competitive challenge in the next decade, they must provide a quality service that clients value. The **nursing process** provides a tool for the nurse to continually evaluate and improve the quality of nursing care (Murray & Atkinson, 1994).

In 1991 the American Nurses' Association published the Standards of Clinical Nursing Practice, which define the responsibilities of nurses in all clinical settings. The Standards specify the nurse's responsibility to the public. They hold the nurse accountable for the use of the nursing process. Table 5-1 shows the relationship of the **standards of clinical nursing practice** to each phase of the nursing process.

In 1986, the American Nurses' Association also developed **standards of community health nursing practice** for the specialty area of community health. For each standard, the Association established (1) structural criteria to judge the environment and resources to meet the standard; (2) process criteria to describe the activities of the nurse to meet the standard; and (3) outcome criteria to describe the expected outcome of the nurse's action. These standards help the nurse to apply the nursing process to the community setting, with respect to the individual, family, and community (see Chapter 1, p. 16).

ASSESSMENT

Definition: An organized and systematic process of collecting data from a variety of sources to analyze the health status of the client. *Activities:* Collect data through interviews, histories, examinations, records and reports, surveys; document data (subjective, objective).

Community health nurses need to collect data from a wide variety of sources. They may be collecting data on an individual client; for example,

TABLE 5-1 Relationship of the nursing process to the standards of clinical nursing practice

Nursing process	Standards of nursing practice
Assessment	I. The nurse collects health data.
Diagnosis	II. The nurse analyzes the assessment data in determining diagnoses.
Plan	
Outcome Identification	III. The nurse identifies expected outcomes individualized to the client.
Planning	IV. The nurse develops a plan of care that prescribes interventions to attain expected outcomes.
Implementation	V. The nurse implements the interventions identified in the plan of care.
Evaluation	VI. The nurse evaluates the client's progress toward attainment of outcomes.

Adapted from American Nurses' Association. (1991). *Standards of Clinical Nursing Practice.* Kansas City, MO: Author.

a newborn infant who has just returned home from the hospital and is having difficulties. The nurse will complete a physical examination of the infant. Through interviews with the mother, the nurse will obtain the infant's health history. The nurse may contact the newborn nursery in the hospital to compare records obtained there with current data on the infant.

School nurses may conduct surveys of the families of children in the school to obtain data on the morning dietary habits of the children. This information may be sought to determine the need for a school breakfast program for needy or latchkey children.

Nurses who work in community clinics may use epidemiologic reports on the incidence of particular communicable diseases in that community. This information may be needed to plan an immunization program at a community clinic.

Hamilton (1983) points out that if the community is viewed as a spatial unit, demographic data will be assessed through the use of maps, census bureau reports, and morbidity and mortality statistics. If the community is viewed as a way of life that emphasizes a cultural dimension, the nurse will obtain lists of civic groups, observe neighborhoods, and examine census reports on ethnicity. If the community is considered to be a place to live, then opinion polls, oral and written community histories, crime rates, employment figures, and housing and work conditions need to be assessed. To assess the social forces at work in the community, the nurse would obtain personal reports of conflicts and cooperation among groups in the community; community agency directories; city, county, state, and federal budgets; voting records; and newspaper articles.

Community health nurses use a wide variety of records for documenting assessment data on the client. Automated documentation systems provide computerized assessments of clients. Throughout this text, assessment categories are provided according to the topic under discussion. Later in this chapter, assessment formats in each of four different nursing theoretical frameworks will be demonstrated.

DIAGNOSIS

Definition: A clinical judgment about individual, family, or community responses to actual and potential health problems or life processes. Nursing diagnoses provide the basis for selection of nursing interventions to achieve outcomes for which the nurse is accountable (NANDA, 1990). *Activities:* Classify assessment data, interpret assessment data, identify significant data by comparing with standards/norms, recognizing patterns or trends, comparing with norms and models. Validate the accuracy of the data interpretation with client or significant others, with health professionals, and/or with reference sources, document the diagnostic statement, the use of a taxonomy and two-part statement (Iyer, Taptich, & Bernocchi-Losey, 1991).

Hamilton (1983) has identified that community nursing diagnoses are different from nursing diagnoses of individuals. Community diagnoses are generated from the state of the community as a physical, sociocultural, experiential entity; relational statements imply interventions that may institute a change in the present community. The implied direct client is the community, and the indirect client is the individual. Hamilton suggests that there may be a difference between nursing care of individuals in the community, nursing care of individuals influenced by the community, and nursing care of the community directly.

Neufield and Harrison (1990) identify the difficulties in verifying nursing diagnoses of aggregates or groups in the community. Several groups may have the same health concern; for example, children in a day-care center, their parents, and the staff in the center. The nurse will have to decide which client aggregate to select for the nursing diagnosis. Access to the client group, potential for success, motivation of the group, funding resources available, and the skills of the nurse in working with the different groups are all factors to take into consideration to make this determination.

Zink (1994) reviewed nursing diagnosis documentation in home care settings. She points out that many documentation systems developed in community and home care settings use nursing diagnoses for their organizational base. The problem-oriented record system has been blended with nursing diagnosis to strengthen the concept of the nursing process. One nursing diagnosis system has incorporated a standardized procedure for recording nursing assessments. This system relates nursing theory to third-party reimbursement requirements. Nurses can document patient care faster and monitor the quality and cost of care with this system.

Iyer, Taptich, and Bernocchi-Losey (1991) identify the first step in the diagnostic process as data processing, whereby the nurse classifies the assessment data. Assessment tools provide specific categories to facilitate this process. Such categories as body systems, functional health patterns, historical data, and significant symptoms may be used. The assessment data are then interpreted. Significant data are identified, compared with standards or norms, and interpreted as patterns or trends. In data-processing, the nurse verifies the accuracy of the data interpretation by interviewing the client or significant others, other professionals, and looking at reference sources. The outcome of the diagnostic process is the diagnostic statement. These statements may be made using a number of different diagnostic classification systems.

THE NORTH AMERICAN NURSING DIAGNOSIS SYSTEM (NANDA)

The **NANDA** system of diagnosis was adopted by the American Nurses' Association in 1988 as the official system of diagnosis for the United States. The box on page 90 shows a sample of a NANDA-approved nursing diagnosis that a community health nurse may encounter. The box on page 91 consists of a listing of the NANDA-approved nursing diagnoses.

PROBLEM CLASSIFICATION SCHEME, VISITING NURSE ASSOCIATION, OMAHA, NEBRASKA

The Visiting Nurse Association (VNA) of Omaha, Nebraska, has developed a classification system useful and relevant for a community-focused practice. Entitled the **Omaha Problem Classification Scheme** (Martin, 1989), the list contains 40 client-focused problems or signs and symptoms that are in one of four domains: environmental, psychosocial, physiological, and health-related behaviors (see box, page 93). These problems, particularly the environmental problems, form the basis of nursing diagnosis statements in the community. At times in the community setting there may be many related factors, or there may be unknown related factors. Figure 5-1 (see p. 99), suggests some examples of related factors. Table 5-2 (see p. 99), contains some examples of community nursing diagnosis statements using the Omaha Problem Classification Scheme.

GUIDELINES FOR WRITING COMMUNITY NURSING DIAGNOSIS STATEMENTS

Iyer, Taptich, and Bernocchi-Losey (1991) provide the following 10 important guidelines for writing nursing diagnosis statements:

1. Write the diagnosis in terms of the client response rather than the nursing need.

2. Use "related to" rather than "due to" or "caused by" to connect the two parts of the statement.

3. Write the diagnosis in legally advisable terms.

4. Write the diagnosis without value judgments.

5. Avoid reversing the parts of the statement.

6. Avoid using single symptoms in the first part of the statement.

7. The two parts of the statement should not mean the same thing.

8. Express the related factor in terms that can be changed.

9. Do not include medical diagnoses in the nursing diagnosis statement.

10. State the diagnosis clearly and concisely.

PLAN

Definition: Development of strategies to reinforce healthy client responses or to prevent, minimize, or correct unhealthy client responses identified in the nursing diagnosis (Iyer, Taptich, & Bergnocchi-Losey, 1991). *Activities:* Establish priorities, develop outcomes, develop nursing interventions, write nursing orders, document the plan.

There may be many nursing diagnoses identified for the client's care. The nurse needs a way to prioritize those that should be pursued first. Iyer, Taptich, and Bergnocchi-Losey (1991) use a refined hierarchy of Maslow's model of needs as a basis for prioritization. The nurse would focus on nursing diagnoses that involve the needs of the most basic survival level before focusing on higher-order needs.

Once the nurse and the client have agreed on the priority needs, the next step in planning is to develop outcomes. Outcomes refer to goals or behavioral objectives. They define how the nurse and the client will know that the response identified in the first part of the diagnostic statement has been prevented, modified, or corrected. Outcomes are related to client responses and identify alternative healthy responses that are desirable. They are always client-centered and start with, "The client will be able to. . . ." Client outcomes should be clear and concise and should be stated in measurable and observable behaviors. Outcomes should be realistic and have time limits, and should be determined together by the

SAMPLE OF NANDA APPROVED NURSING DIAGNOSES (1990)

Diagnosis name:

Parental role conflict (1988)

Definition:

The state in which a parent experiences role confusion and conflict in response to crisis

Defining characteristics

Major:

Parent(s) expresses concerns/feelings of inadequacy to provide for child's physical and emotional needs during hospitalization or in the home

Demonstrated disruption in caretaking routines

Parent(s) express(es) concerns about changes in parental role, family functioning, family communication, family health

Minor:

Expresses concern about perceived loss of control over decisions relating to the child

Reluctant to participate in usual caretaking activities even with encouragement and support

Verbalizes, demonstrates feelings of guilt, anger, fear, anxiety, and/or frustrations about effect of child's illness on family process

Related factors:

Separation from child as a result of chronic illness

Intimidation with invasive or restrictive modalities (e.g. isolation, intubation), specialized care centers, policies

Home care of a child with special needs (e.g., apnea monitoring, postural drainage, hyperalimentation)

Change in marital status

Interruptions of family life as a result of home care regimen (treatments, caregivers, lack of respite)

NANDA-APPROVED NURSING DIAGNOSTIC CATEGORIES

Pattern 1: exchanging

Altered nutrition: More than body requirements
Altered nutrition: Less than body requirements
Altered nutrition: Potential for more than body requirements
Potential for infection
Potential altered body temperature
Hypothermia
Hyperthermia
Ineffective thermoregulation
Dysreflexia
Constipation
Perceived constipation
Colonic constipation
Diarrhea
Bowel incontinence
Altered patterns of urinary elimination
Stress incontinence
Reflex incontinence
Urge incontinence
Functional incontinence
Total incontinence
Urinary retention
Altered (specify type) tissue perfusion (renal, cerebral, cardiopulmonary, gastrointestinal, peripheral)
Fluid volume excess
Fluid volume deficit (1)
Fluid volume deficit (2)
Potential fluid volume deficit
Decreased cardiac output
Impaired gas exchange
Ineffective airway clearance
Ineffective breathing pattern
Potential for injury
Potential for suffocation
Potential for poisoning
Potential for trauma
Potential for aspiration
Potential for disuse syndrome
Impaired tissue integrity
Altered oral mucous membrane
Impaired skin integrity
Potential impaired skin integrity

Pattern 2: communicating

Impaired verbal communication

Pattern 3: relating

Impaired social interaction
Social isolation

Altered role performance
Altered parenting
Potential altered parenting
Sexual dysfunction
Altered family processes
Parental role conflict
Altered sexuality patterns

Pattern 4: valuing

Spiritual distress (distress of the human spirit)

Pattern 5: choosing

Ineffective individual coping
Impaired adjustment
Defensive coping
Ineffective denial
Ineffective family coping: disabling
Ineffective family coping: compromised
Family coping: potential for growth
Noncompliance (specify)
Decisional conflict (specify)
Health seeking behaviors (specify)

Pattern 6: moving

Impaired physical mobility
Activity intolerance
Fatigue
Potential activity intolerance
Sleep pattern disturbance
Diversional activity deficit
Impaired home maintenance management
Altered health maintenance
Feeding self care deficit
Impaired swallowing
Ineffective breastfeeding
Bathing/hygiene self care deficit
Dressing/grooming self care deficit
Toileting self care deficit
Altered growth and development

Pattern 7: perceiving

Body image disturbance
Self esteem disturbance
Chronic low self esteem
Situational low self esteem
Personal identity disturbance
Sensory/perceptual alterations (specify) (visual, auditory, kinesthetic, gustatory, tactile, olfactory)
Unilateral neglect
Hopelessness
Powerlessness

Continued

nurse and the client, family, aggregate, or community.

The next stage of planning is to develop nursing interventions. Nursing interventions need to be individualized to the family, group, or the community. The nurse must assure a safe environment, use principles of teaching and learning, and involve the use of appropriate and available resources (Iyer, Taptich, & Bernocchi-Losey, 1991). Nursing interventions include specific strategies to assist clients to achieve outcomes.

Jones (1993) describes outcomes analysis as a means of achieving desired client outcomes in the most cost-effective manner. Sources of data for the measurement of outcomes include discharge data, medical records, and large public or private data bases. Outcomes are the end result of care, or a measurable change in the health status of a client. Traditionally, outcomes of care have focused on hospital-based care. Alternative measures of outcomes relate to quality of life, such as the client's health status, functional status, improved mobility, return to work or normal activities, and client satisfaction with services received and with providers delivering care. These measures are particularly relevant to nurses and their care plans.

The trend in outcomes measurement is toward measuring outcomes across the continuum of care, or across defined episodes of care that transcend organizational boundaries. This devel-opment is consistent with the introduction of case management programs that include critical pathways with pre-hospitalization, inpatient, outpatient, and home-care events. Additionally, outcomes such as reduced pain and improved mobility are particularly appropriate for such home care services as hospice (Jones, 1993).

Hegyvary (1991) proposed four categories of outcomes assessment to accommodate the multiple perspectives of providers, consumers, and purchasers. Clinical outcomes determine client responses to medical and nursing interventions. Functional outcomes measure maintenance or improvement of physical functioning. Financial measures indicate outcomes that demonstrate the most efficient use of resources. Finally, perceptual outcomes provide indicators of client satisfaction with outcomes, care received, and providers.

Documentation of the planning stage is found on a client record. The nursing care plan is completed by the nurse, is kept current, and contains the nursing diagnosis, client outcomes, and nursing orders. Care plans are found in the client's record and may be taken with the nurse during the home visit or in the clinic for updating. Documentation of the future will evolve into a very different format, as the need for legal, financial, and ethical verification increases. Nursing information systems will incorporate assessment data, nursing decisions, and a transaction log (Turley, 1992).

Text continued on page 98.

PROBLEM CLASSIFICATION SCHEME, VISITING NURSE ASSOCIATION, OMAHA, NE

Domain I. environmental

Refers to the material resources and physical surroundings of the home, neighborhood, and broader community.

01. *Income:*
Health promotion
Potential deficit
Deficit
   01. Low/no income
   02. Uninsured medical expenses
   03. Inadequate money management
   04. Able to buy only necessities
   05. Difficulty buying necessities
   06. Other

02. *Sanitation:*
Potential deficit
Deficit
   01. Soiled living area
   02. Inadequate food storage/disposal
   03. Insects/rodents
   04. Foul odor
   05. Inadequate water supply
   06. Inadequate sewage disposal
   07. Inadequate laundry facilities
   08. Allergens
   09. Infectious/contaminating agents
   10. Other

03. *Residence:*
Health promotion
Potential deficit
Deficit
   01. Structurally unsound
   02. Inadequate heating/cooling
   03. Steep stairs
   04. Inadequate/obstructed exits/entries
   05. Cluttered living space
   06. Unsafe storage of dangerous objects/substances
   07. Unsafe mats/throw rugs
   08. Inadequate safety devices
   09. Presence of lead-based paint
   10. Unsafe gas/electrical appliances
   11. Inadequate/crowded living space
   12. Homeless
   13. Other

04. *Neighborhood/workplace safety:*
Health promotion
Potential deficit
Deficit
   01. High crime rate
   02. High pollution level
   03. Uncontrolled animals
   04. Physical hazards
   05. Unsafe play area
   06. Other

05. *Other*
   01. Other

Domain II. psychosocial

Refers to patterns of behavior, communications, relationships, and development.

06. *Communication with community resources:*
Health promotion
Potential impairment
Impairment
   01. Unfamiliar with options/procedures for obtaining services
   02. Difficulty understanding roles/regulations of service providers
   03. Unable to communicate concerns to service provider
   04. Dissatisfaction with services provider
   05. Language barrier
   06. Inadequate/unavailable resources
   07. Other

07. *Social contact:*
Health promotion
Potential impairment
Impairment
   01. Limited social contact
   02. Uses health care provider for social contact
   03. Minimal outside stimulation/leisure time activities
   04. Other

08. *Role change:*
Health promotion
Potential impairment
Impairment
   01. Involuntary reversal of traditional male/female roles
   02. Involuntary reversal of dependent/independent roles
   03. Assumes new role
   04. Loses previous role
   05. Other

Continued

PROBLEM CLASSIFICATION SCHEME, VISITING NURSE ASSOCIATION, OMAHA, NE cont'd

09. *Interpersonal relationship:*
Health promotion
Potential impairment
Impairment
01. Difficulty establishing/maintaining relationships
02. Minimal shared activities
03. Incongruent values/goals
04. Inadequate interpersonal communication skills
05. Prolonged, unrelieved tension
06. Inappropriate suspicion/manipulation/compulsion/aggression
07. Other

10. *Spiritual distress:*
Health promotion
Potential
Actual
01. Expresses spiritual concerns
02. Disrupted spiritual rituals
03. Disrupted spiritual trust
04. Conflicting spiritual beliefs and medical regimen
05. Other

11. *Grief:*
Health promotion
Potential impairment
Impairment
01. Fails to recognize normal grief responses
02. Difficulty coping with grief responses
03. Difficulty expressing grief responses
04. Conflicting stages of grief process among family/individual
05. Other

12. *Emotional stability:*
Health promotion
Potential impairment
Impairment
01. Sadness/hopelessness/worthlessness
02. Apprehension/undefined fear
03. Loss of interest/involvement in activities/self-care
04. Narrowed perceptual focus
05. Scattering of attention
06. Flat affect
07. Irritable/agitated
08. Purposeless activity
09. Difficulty managing stress

10. Somatic complaints/chronic fatigue
11. Expresses wish to die/attempts suicide
12. Other

13. *Human sexuality:*
Health promotion
Potential impairment
Impairment
01. Difficulty recognizing consequences of sexual behavior
02. Difficulty expressing intimacy
03. Sexual identity confusion
04. Sexual value confusion
05. Dissatisfied with sexual relationships
06. Other

14. *Caretaking/parenting:*
Health promotion
Potential impairment
Impairment
01. Difficulty providing physical care/safety
02. Difficulty providing emotional nurturance
03. Difficulty providing cognitive learning experiences and activities
04. Difficulty providing preventive and therapeutic health care
05. Expectations incongruent with stage of growth and development
06. Dissatisfaction/difficulty with responsibilities
07. Neglectful
08. Abusive
09. Other

15. *Neglected child/adult:*
Health promotion
Potential
Actual
01. Lacks adequate physical care
02. Lacks emotional nurturance/support
03. Lacks appropriate stimulation/cognitive experiences
04. Inappropriately left alone
05. Lacks necessary supervision
06. Inadequate/delayed medical care
07. Other

16. *Abused child/adult:*
Health promotion
Potential
Actual
01. Harsh/excessive discipline

PROBLEM CLASSIFICATION SCHEME, VISITING NURSE ASSOCIATION, OMAHA, NE cont'd

02. Welts/bruises/burns
03. Questionable explanation of injury
04. Attacked verbally
05. Fearful/hypervigilant behavior
06. Violent environment
07. Consistent negative messages
08. Assaulted sexually
09. Other

17. *Growth and development:*
Health promotion
Potential impairment
Impairment
01. Abnormal results of development screening tests
02. Abnormal weight/height/head circumference in relation to growth curve/age
03. Age-inappropriate behavior
04. Inadequate achievement/maintenance of developmental tasks
05. Other

18. *Other*
01. Other

Domain III. physiological

Refers to the functional status of processes that maintain life.

19. *Hearing:*
Health promotion
Potential impairment
Impairment
01. Difficulty hearing normal speech tones
02. Absent/abnormal response to sound
03. Abnormal results of hearing screening test
04. Other

20. *Vision:*
Health promotion
Potential impairment
Impairment
01. Difficulty seeing small print/calibrations
02. Difficulty seeing distant objects
03. Difficulty seeing close objects
04. Absent/abnormal response to visual stimuli
05. Abnormal results of vision screening test
06. Squinting/blinking/tearing/blurring
07. Difficulty differentiating colors
08. Other

21. *Speech and language:*
Health promotion
Potential impairment
Impairment
01. Absent/abnormal ability to speak
02. Absent/abnormal ability to understand
03. Lacks alternative communication skills
04. Inappropriate sentence structure
05. Limited enunciation/clarity
06. Inappropriate word usage
07. Other

22. *Dentition:*
Health promotion
Potential impairment
Impairment
01. Abnormalities of teeth
02. Sore/swollen/bleeding gums
03. Ill-fitting dentures
04. Malocclusion
05. Other

23. *Cognition:*
Health promotion
Potential impairment
Impairment
01. Diminished judgment
02. Disoriented to time/place/person
03. Limited recall of recent events
04. Limited recall of long past events
05. Minimal calculating/sequencing skills
06. Limited concentration
07. Minimal reasoning/abstract thinking ability
08. Impulsivity
09. Repetitious language/behavior
10. Other

24. *Pain:*
Health promotion
Potential
Actual
01. Expresses discomfort/pain
02. Elevated pulse/respirations/blood pressure
03. Compensated movement/guarding
04. Restless behavior
05. Facial grimaces
06. Pallor/perspiration
07. Other

25. *Consciousness:*
Health promotion
Potential impairment

Continued

PROBLEM CLASSIFICATION SCHEME, VISITING NURSE ASSOCIATION, OMAHA, NE   cont'd

Impairment
01. Lethargic
02. Stuporous
03. Unresponsive
04. Comatose
05. Other

26. *Integument:*
Health promotion
Potential impairment
Impairment
01. Lesion
02. Rash
03. Excessively dry
04. Excessively oily
05. Inflammation
06. Pruritus
07. Drainage
08. Ecchymosis
09. Hypertrophy of nails
10. Other

27. *Neuromusculoskeletal function:*
Health promotion
Potential impairment
Impairment
01. Limited range of motion
02. Decreased muscle strength
03. Decreased coordination/balance

28. *Respiration:*
Health promotion
Potential impairment
Impairment
01. Abnormal breath patterns
02. Unable to breathe independently
03. Cough
04. Unable to cough/expectorate independently
05. Cyanosis
06. Abnormal sputum
07. Noisy respirations
08. Rhinorrhea
09. Abnormal breath sounds
10. Other

29. *Circulation:*
Health promotion
Potential impairment
Impairment
01. Edema
02. Cramping/pain of extremities
03. Decreased pulses

04. Discoloration of skin/cyanosis
05. Temperature change in affected area
06. Varicosities
07. Syncopal episodes
08. Abnormal blood pressure reading
09. Pulse deficit
10. Irregular heart rate
11. Excessively rapid heart rate
12. Excessively slow heart rate
13. Anginal pain
14. Abnormal heart sounds/murmurs
15. Other

30. *Digestion-hydration:*
Health promotion
Potential impairment
Impairment
01. Nausea/vomiting
02. Difficulty/inability to chew/swallow/digest
03. Indigestion
04. Reflux
05. Anorexia
06. Anemia
07. Ascites
08. Jaundice/liver enlargement
09. Decreased skin turgor
10. Cracked lips/dry mouth
11. Electrolyte imbalance
12. Other

31. *Bowel function:*
Health promotion
Potential impairment
Impairment
01. Abnormal frequency/consistency of stool
02. Painful defecation
03. Decreased bowel sounds
04. Blood in stools
05. Abnormal color
06. Cramping/abdominal discomfort
07. Incontinent of stool
08. Other

32. *Genitourinary function:*
Health promotion
Potential impairment
Impairment
01. Incontinent of urine
02. Urgency/frequency
03. Burning/painful urination

PROBLEM CLASSIFICATION SCHEME, VISITING NURSE ASSOCIATION, OMAHA, NE cont'd

04. Difficulty emptying bladder
05. Abnormal urinary frequency/amount
06. Hematuria
07. Abnormal discharge
08. Abnormal menstrual pattern
09. Abnormal lumps/swelling/tenderness of male/female reproductive organs
10. Dyspareunia
11. Other

33. *Antepartum/postpartum:*
Health promotion
Potential impairment
Impairment
01. Difficulty coping with body changes
02. Inappropriate exercise/rest/diet/habits
03. Discomforts
04. Complications
05. Fears delivery procedure
06. Difficulty breastfeeding
07. Other

34. *Other*
01. Other

Domain IV. health-related behaviors

Refers to activities that maintain or promote wellness; promote recovery; or maximize rehabilitation.

35. *Nutrition:*
Health promotion
Potential impairment
Impairment
01. Weighs 10 percent more than average
02. Weighs 10 percent less than average
03. Lacks established standards for daily calorie/fluid intake
04. Exceeds established standards for daily calorie/fluid intake
05. Unbalanced diet
06. Improper feeding schedule for age
07. Nonadherence to prescribed diet
08. Other

36. *Sleep and rest patterns:*
Health promotion
Potential impairment
Impairment
01. Sleep/rest pattern disrupts family
02. Frequently wakes during night
03. Somnambulism
04. Insomnia

05. Nightmares
06. Insufficient sleep/rest for age/physical condition
07. Other

37. *Physical activity:*
Health promotion
Potential impairment
Impairment
01. Sedentary life style
02. Inadequate/inconsistent exercise routine
03. Inappropriate type/amount of exercise for age/physical condition
04. Other

38. *Personal hygiene:*
Health promotion
Potential impairment
Impairment
01. Inadequate laundering of clothing
02. Inadequate bathing
03. Body odor
04. Inadequate shampooing/combing of hair
05. Inadequate brushing/flossing/mouth care
06. Other

39. *Substance misuse:*
Health promotion
Potential
Actual
01. Abuses over-the-counter/street drugs
02. Abuses alcohol
03. Smokes
04. Difficulty performing normal routines
05. Reflex disturbances
06. Behavior change
07. Other

40. *Family planning:*
Health promotion
Potential impairment
Impairment
01. Inappropriate/insufficient knowledge of family planning methods
02. Inaccurate/inconsistent use of family planning methods
03. Dissatisfied with present family planning method
04. Other

41. *Medical/dental supervision:*
Health promotion
Potential impairment

Continued

PROBLEM CLASSIFICATION SCHEME, VISITING NURSE ASSOCIATION, OMAHA, NE cont'd

Impairment
01. Fails to obtain routine medical/dental evaluation
02. Fails to seek care for symptoms requiring medical/dental evaluation
03. Fails to return as requested to physician/dentist
04. Inability to coordinate multiple appointments/regimens
05. Inconsistent source of medical/dental care
06. Inadequate prescribed medical/dental regimen
07. Other

42. *Prescribed medication:*
Health promotion
Potential impairment
Impairment
01. Deviates from prescribed dosage
02. Demonstrates side effects
03. Inadequate system for taking medication
04. Improper storage of medication

05. Fails to obtain refills appropriately
06. Fails to obtain immunizations
07. Other

43. *Technical procedures:*
Health promotion
Potential impairment
Impairment
01. Unable to demonstrate/relate procedure accurately
02. Does not follow/demonstrate principles of safe/aseptic techniques
03. Procedure requires nursing skill
04. Unable/unwilling to perform procedure without assistance
05. Unable/unwilling to operate special equipment
06. Other person(s) unable/unavailable to assist
07. Other

44. *Other*
01. Other

From *Nursing diagnosis: A case study approach.* pp. 391-401 by J.H. Carlson, C.A. Craft, A.D. McGuire, & S. Popkess-Vawter, 1991, Philadelphia: WB Saunders. Reprinted by permission.

Dolan (1990) has compiled community and home health care plans. She states that they are for hands-on nursing care for patients in the home setting. The care plans are organized by clinical care plans, general care plans, and community-based care plans. The box on page 100 demonstrates a sample.

The clinical care plans are divided by systems: cardiovascular, respiratory, neurologic, gastrointestinal, integumentary, musculoskeletal, endocrine, reproductive, renal and urinary, and psychological problems. Under each system, Dolan has selected a variety of diseases for which she lists a description, health history and physical findings, diagnostic studies, and several nursing diagnoses from the NANDA classification, with suggested interventions and rationales.

The general care plans cover such topics as pain, ineffective coping, grief, sleep disorders, sexuality, intermittent intravenous (IV) therapy, malnutrition, and total parenteral nutrition. Fi-

nally, the community-based care plans include such topics as sexually transmitted diseases, AIDS, teenage pregnancy, postpartum period, lyme disease, substance abuse, smoking cessation, and hospice care. The box on page 90 shows, as an example, the NANDA diagnosis of parental role conflict. The box on page 100 portrays a related example from Dolan's general care plans for the nursing diagnosis of ineffective family coping: compromised, related to inadequate resources.

IMPLEMENTATION

Definition: The carrying out of the plan of care by the client and nurse to assist the client to achieve the desired outcomes. *Activities:* Perform interventions, collaborate with health team, make ongoing assessment, update and revise plan, document responses.

Nursing interventions should be consistent with the plan of care. They should be based on

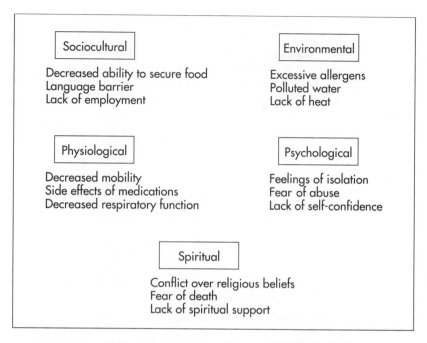

FIGURE 5-1   Examples of related factors for nursing diagnosis statements.

nursing knowledge and designed specifically for each client situation. A safe and therapeutic environment is always the foremost consideration. As indicated in the plan, the nurse uses client-teaching strategies and facilitates the involvement of appropriate resources on the client's behalf. The nurse collaborates with other health team members and community agencies. It is the nurse's responsibility to be aware of what resources are available for the client. In the community setting, the nurse must undergo much investigating and learning to find out what is available.

At all times the nurse is reassessing the client. Possible complications or changes in priorities need to be identified with the client. Nursing knowledge, assessment, and interviewing skills are all critical throughout the implementation stage.

IOWA INTERVENTION PROJECT: NURSING INTERVENTION CLASSIFICATION (NIC)

The Iowa Intervention Project was completed in 1992. It was created to assist nurses in documenting nursing care given and to facilitate the

development of nursing knowledge through the evaluation of patient outcomes (McCloskey & Bulechek, 1992). From the Project, a **Nursing Intervention Classification (NIC)** was established (see box on page 103). This classification system may be used for documenting nursing care in the community setting. Many of the categories are highly appropriate for client care in

TABLE 5-2   Examples of nursing diagnosis statements using the Omaha problem classification scheme

Client response		Related factors
Unable to breathe independently (28.04)	related to	excessive allergens
Abdominal discomfort (31.06)	related to	polluted water
Pain in extremities (29.02)	related to	lack of heat

the home setting, for groups, or for communities as a whole. Intervention categories such as abuse protection, area restriction, communication enhancement, coping enhancement, and environmental management for safety or violence prevention are a few relevant examples. The case study samples within the nursing theoretical frameworks in the next section of this chapter use many of the NIC categories of nursing interventions. This classification:

1. creates a standardized language for nurses to describe their behaviors when delivering nursing treatments.

2. expands nurses' knowledge about the similarities and differences among diagnoses, treatments, and outcomes.

3. explores possibilities of current and future nursing and health care information systems.

4. can be used to teach decision making to nursing students.

SAMPLE OF DOLAN'S HOME HEALTH CARE PLAN FOR INEFFECTIVE FAMILY COPING

Description and time focus

Ineffective coping is an impairment of adaptive behaviors and problem-solving abilities to meet life's demands and roles. A serious illness or injury, such as cerebrovascular accident or amputation, usually forces the patient and family to make difficult adjustments in life-style and role performance. This clinical plan focuses on the patient who is having difficulty coping with these adjustments. The nurse may determine that the patient's environment is conducive to effective coping only to discover that he exhibits poor coping techniques. Nursing care centers on helping the patient identify factors that impede effective coping, take positive steps to make the patient's life as comfortable as possible, establish reliable support systems, and adapt successfully to life-style changes effected by the patient's illness.

■ Typical home health care length of service for a patient with impaired coping skills: depends on the underlying disease

■ Typical visit frequency: depends on the underlying disease

Health history findings

In a health history interview, the patient may report many of these findings:
- Severe anxiety
- Erratic or unstable attitudes and emotional responses
- Illness in the family
- Role changes in the family
- Loss of self-control
- Insomnia

Physical findings

In a physical examination, the nurse may detect many of these findings:

Cardiovascular
- High blood pressure
- Tachycardia
- Dysrhythmia

Respiratory
- Hyperventilation

Neurologic
- Restlessness
- Lethargy
- Insomnia

Gastrointestinal
- Vomiting
- Diarrhea
- Stress ulcer
- GI bleeding
- Constipation

Integumentary
- Diaphoresis
- Rash

Musculoskeletal
- Muscle tension
- Pain

Diagnostic studies

Studies vary according to the disease. For detailed information, see "Diagnostic Studies" in the applicable care plan.

SAMPLE OF DOLAN'S HOME HEALTH CARE PLAN
FOR INEFFECTIVE FAMILY COPING   cont'd

Nursing diagnosis:

Ineffective family coping: compromised, related to inadequate resources

Goal:

To promote effective family coping by coordinating available resources

Interventions

1. Assess the patient's relationship with each family member. Identify those on whom the patient relies most often for support and guidance, particularly the primary caregiver.

2. Assess the family's financial ability to meet the patient's medical needs. Refer them to a social worker for financial counseling, if necessary, and give them a comprehensive list of community resources that can assist with other needs.

Rationales

1. Assessing family relationships helps the nurse employ members effectively in caring for the patient. Usually, one member emerges as the primary caregiver, and the nurse must work closely with this person to enhance the patient's health.

2. The family's financial status may influence decisions they must make about health care. A social worker can help them explore private- and community-funding options. Other community resources — such as support groups, mental health clinics, religious organizations, libraries, and Meals On Wheels — can provide emotional support, information on the patient's disease, and assistance with transportation, medical equipment, or homemaking needs.

Associated care plans

- Developmental disabilities
- Grief and grieving
- Hospice care
- Pain
- Sex and sexuality

Networking of services

- Meals On Wheels
- Mental health organizations
- Religious organizations
- Libraries

Care team involved

- Nurse
- Doctor
- Patient and family
- Social worker
- Recreational therapist

Implications for home care

- Functional features of the home
- Telephone (communication)

Patient education tools

- List of necessary medical equipment
- Literature on each prescribed medication, particularly mood-altering medications
- Audiocassettes or videocassettes on relaxation techniques, self-improvement, and (of permitted) moderate exercises

Discharge plan from home health care

Before discharge from home health care, the patient should:

- Know the method of administration, dosage, action, and adverse effects of each prescribed medication, especially mood-altering medications
- Understand dietary requirements
- Know personal stressors and methods to minimize or eliminate them
- Know how to reach care team members or community resources if necessary
- Post telephone numbers for the doctor and home health agency by the phone for follow-up care, if necessary
- Understand the problems that may occur in sexual functioning
- Develop effective coping skills
- Feel that he has control over many aspects of his life.

From *Community and home health care plans.* pp. 257-259 by M.B. Dolan, 1990, Springhouse, PA: Springhouse. Reprinted by permission.

5. can be used to determine the costs of services nurses provide for the creation of a reimbursement system for nurses.

6. can assist nursing administrators to plan more effectively for staff and equipment needs.

7. provides the language to communicate the unique function of nursing.

8. helps demonstrate the impact that nurses have on the system of health care delivery.

The box on page 106 shows an example of caregiver support, which is one of the interventions. Each intervention is defined and lists specific nursing activities for the intervention.

EVALUATION

Definition: A systematic, continuous process of comparing the client's responses with outcomes defined by the plan of care. *Activities:* Gather client data on health status, compare data with outcomes, revise plan of care.

The nurse is continually in the evaluation phase at every step of the nursing process. During assessment, the nurse is evaluating which client responses are significant. During diagnosis, the nurse evaluates the most appropriate diagnosis for the particular client. During planning, the nurse evaluates the potential effectiveness of proposed nursing interventions. During the implementation phase, the nurse observes the client's responses and evaluates the appropriateness of the planned interventions. In the evaluation phase, the nurse is focusing on the client's responses in light of the client outcomes that are sought.

In addition to evaluation of care for specific clients, families, aggregates, or communities, nurses are involved in quality assurance or continued quality improvement (CQI), which is a planned and systematic evaluation of care given to a group of clients. Chapter 11 will explore in depth this aspect of evaluation.

NURSING PROCESS FRAMEWORKS

The remainder of this chapter will examine the use of the nursing process within the frameworks of King, Nightingale, Orem, and Roy. For each theorist, the nursing process will be applied to the first case study outlined in chapter 2, which utilized Betty Neuman's theoretical nursing framework and her concept of the nursing process.

King's Open Systems and Theory of Goal Attainment

King's theory for nursing has been used with the nursing process in three ways. **Imogene King** (1992) compared the nursing process as method with the nursing process as theory. The assessment phase incorporates King's concepts of perception, communication, and interaction of the nurse and the client. The planning phase makes use of King's concepts of decision making about goals and agreement on ways to attain these goals. For implementation, King states that transactions are made. The evaluation phase determines if the goals have been attained.

King (1981) operationalized the nursing process components through the Goal-Oriented Nursing Record (GONR). Fawcett (1984) adapted King's GONR to include a data base, problem list, goal list, plan, and progress notes (see box on page 107). The terminology and structure of this record are very similar to the problem-oriented record system that was used for many years in public health departments (King, 1983).

Hanchett (1988) used all the subconcepts of the personal, interpersonal, and social systems of King's theory to structure a community health assessment. George (1985) used King's theory in a similar fashion to structure the assessment of the individual client.

The first case study presented in Chapter 2, which was written in Neuman's systems framework, will be used to demonstrate a combination of the above approaches for using King's theory for nursing to structure the nursing process in the community setting (Table 5-3). NANDA nursing diagnoses are identified and the Iowa NIC is used to specify nursing implementations.

Nightingale's Environmental Model

Nightingale's (1969) *Notes on Nursing* were written in 1860. **Florence Nightingale's** concepts are more relevant today than ever in terms

NURSING INTERVENTIONS CLASSIFICATION (NIC)
OF THE IOWA INTERVENTION PROJECT

Abuse Protection

Acid-Base Management

Acid-Base Management:
  Metabolic Acidosis

Acid-Base Management:
  Metabolic Alkalosis

Acid-Base Management:
  Respiratory Acidosis

Acid-Base Management:
  Respiratory Alkalosis

Acid-Base Monitoring

Active Listening

Activity Therapy

Admission Care

Airway Insertion and Stabilization

Airway Management

Airway Suctioning

Allergy Management

Amputation Care

Analgesic Administration

Anesthesia Administration

Anger Control Assistance

Animal Assisted Therapy

Anticipatory Guidance

Anxiety Reduction

Area Restriction

Art Therapy

Artificial Airway Management

Aspiration Precautions

Assertiveness Training

Attachment Promotion

Autogenic Training

Bathing

Bed Rest Care

Behavior Management

Behavior Modification

Bibliotherapy

Biofeedback

Birthing

Bleeding Precautions

Bleeding Reduction

Bleeding Reduction: Gastrointestinal

Bleeding Reduction: Nasal

Bleeding Reduction: Wound

Blood Products Administration

Body Image Enhancement

Body Mechanics Promotion

Bottle Feeding

Bowel Incontinence Care

Bowel Irrigation

Bowel Management

Bowel Training

Calming Technique

Cardiac Care

Cardiac Care: Acute

Cardiac Care: Rehabilitative

Cardiac Precautions

Caregiver Support

Cast Care: Maintenance

Cast Care: Wet

Cerebral Edema Management

Cesarean Section Care

Chemotherapy Management

Chest Physiotherapy

Childbirth Preparation

Circulatory Care

Circulatory Precautions

Code Management

Cognitive Restructuring

Cognitive Stimulation

Communication Enhancement

Communication Enhancement:
  Hearing Deficit

Communication Enhancement:
  Visual Deficit

Confusion Management

Constipation/Impaction Management

Contact Lens Care

Coping Enhancement

Cough Enhancement

Counseling

Crisis Intervention

Culture Brokerage

Cutaneous Stimulation

Decision-Making Support

Delirium Management

Diarrhea Management

Diet Staging

Discharge Planning

Distraction

Dressing

Dying Care

Dysreflexia Management

Dysrhythmia Management

Ear Care

Eating Disorders Management

Electrolyte Management

Electrolyte Management:
  Hypercalcemia

Electrolyte Management:
  Hyperkalemia

Electrolyte Management:
  Hypermagnesemia

Electrolyte Management:
  Hypernatremia

Electrolyte Management:
  Hyperphosphatemia

Electrolyte Management:
  Hypocalcemia

Electrolyte Management:
  Hypokalemia

Electrolyte Management:
  Hypomagnesemia

Electrolyte Management:
  Hyponatremia

Electrolyte Management:
  Hypophosphatemia

Electrolyte Monitoring

Embolus Care: Peripheral

Embolus Care: Pulmonary

Embolus Precautions

Emergency Care

Emotional Support

Energy Management

Enteral Tube Feeding

Environmental Management

Environmental Management:
  Attachment Process

Environmental Management:
  Comfort

Environmental Management: Safety

Environmental Management:
  Violence Prevention

Epidural Analgesia Administration

Exercise Promotion

Exercise Therapy: Ambulation

Exercise Therapy: Balance

Exercise Therapy: Joint Mobility

Exercise Therapy: Muscle Control

Eye Care

Fall Prevention

Family Integrity Promotion

Continued

NURSING INTERVENTIONS CLASSIFICATION (NIC)
OF THE IOWA INTERVENTION PROJECT   cont'd

Family Integrity Promotion: Childbearing Family
Family Involvement
Family Mobilization
Family Planning: Contraception
Family Planning: Infertility
Family Planning: Unplanned Pregnancy
Family Process Maintenance
Family Support
Family Therapy
Feeding
Fetal Monitoring
Fever Treatment
First Aid
Flatulence Reduction
Fluid/Electrolyte Management
Fluid Management
Fluid Monitoring
Fluid Resuscitation
Foot Care
Gastrointestinal Intubation
Genetic Counseling
Grief Work Facilitation
Guilt Work Facilitation
Hair Care
Hallucination Management
Health Screening
Health System Guidance
Heat Exposure Treatment
Heat/Cold Application
Hemodialysis Therapy
Hemodynamic Regulation
Hemorrhage Control
Home Maintenance Assistance
Hope Instillation
Humor
Hyperglycemia Management
Hypervolemia Management
Hypnosis
Hypoglycemia Management
Hypothermia Treatment
Hypovolemia Management
Immunization/Vaccination Administration
Incision Site Care
Infant Care
Infection Control

Infection Protection
Intracranial Pressure (ICP) Monitoring
Intrapartal Care
Intravenous (IV) Insertion
Intravenous (IV) Therapy
Invasive Hemodynamic Monitoring
Lactation Management
Lactation Suppression
Learning Facilitation
Learning Readiness Enhancement
Limit Setting
Mechanical Ventilation
Mechanical Ventilatory Weaning
Medication Administration
Medication Administration: Enteral
Medication Administration: Interpleural
Medication Administration: Oral
Medication Administration: Parenteral
Medication Administration: Topical
Medication Management
Meditation
Memory Training
Milieu Therapy
Music Therapy
Mutual Goal Setting
Nail Care
Neurologic Monitoring
Newborn Care
Newborn Monitoring
Nonnutritive Sucking
Nutrition Management
Nutrition Therapy
Nutritional Counseling
Nutritional Monitoring
Oral Health Maintenance
Oral Health Promotion
Oral Health Restoration
Ostomy Care
Oxygen Therapy
Pain Management
Parent Education: Adolescent
Parent Education: Childbearing Family

Parent Education: Childrearing Family
Patient Contracting
Patient Controlled Analgesia (PCA) Assistance
Patient Rights Protection
Perineal Care
Peripheral Sensation Management
Peripherally Inserted Central (PIC) Catheter Care
Peritoneal Dialysis Therapy
Physical Restraint
Play Therapy
Positioning
Positioning: Neurologic
Positioning: Wheelchair
Postmortem Care
Postpartal Care
Pregnancy Termination Care
Prenatal Care
Preparatory Sensory Information
Presence
Pressure Management
Pressure Ulcer Care
Pressure Ulcer Prevention
Progressive Muscle Relaxation
Prosthesis Care
Radiation Therapy Management
Rape-Trauma Treatment
Reality Orientation
Recreation Therapy
Referral
Reminiscence Therapy
Respiratory Monitoring
Respite Care
Resuscitation
Risk Identification
Risk Identification: Childbearing Family
Role Enhancement
Seclusion
Security Enhancement
Seizure Management
Seizure Precautions
Self-Awareness Enhancement
Self-Care Assistance
Self-Care Assistance: Bathing/Hygiene

NURSING INTERVENTIONS CLASSIFICATION (NIC)
OF THE IOWA INTERVENTION PROJECT   cont'd

Self-Care Assistance: Dressing/
  Grooming
Self-Care Assistance: Feeding
Self-Care Assistance: Toileting
Self-Esteem Enhancement
Self-Modification Assistance
Self-Responsibility Facilitation
Sexual Counseling
Shock Management
Shock Management: Cardiac
Shock Management: Vasogenic
Shock Management: Volume
Shock Prevention
Sibling Support
Simple Guided Imagery
Simple Massage
Simple Relaxation Therapy
Skin Care: Topical Treatments
Skin Surveillance
Sleep Enhancement
Smoking Cessation Assistance
Socialization Enhancement
Specimen Management
Spiritual Support
Splinting
Subarachnoid Hemorrhage
  Precautions
Substance Use Prevention
Substance Use Treatment
Substance Use Treatment: Alcohol
  Withdrawal

Substance Use Treatment: Drug
  Withdrawal
Substance Use Treatment: Over-
  dose
Suicide Prevention
Support Group
Support System Enhancement
Surgical Assistance: Circulating
Surgical Assistance: Scrubbing
Surgical Preparation
Surveillance
Surveillance: Safety
Sustenance Support
Suturing
Swallowing Therapy
Teaching: Disease Process
Teaching: Group
Teaching: Individual
Teaching: Infant Care
Teaching: Preoperative
Teaching: Prescribed
  Activity/Exercise
Teaching: Prescribed Diet
Teaching: Prescribed Medication
Teaching: Procedure/Treatment
Teaching: Psychomotor Skill
Teaching: Safe Sex
Technology Management
Temperature Regulation
Therapeutic Touch
Therapy Group

Total Parenteral Nutrition (TPN)
  Administration
Touch
Traction Care
Transcutaneous Electrical Nerve
  Stimulation (TENS)
Transport
Triage
Truth Telling
Tube Care
Tube Care: Chest
Tube Care: Gastrointestinal
Tube Care: Urinary
Tube Care: Ventriculostomy/Lum-
  bar Drain
Urinary Catheterization
Urinary Catheterization: Intermit-
  tent
Urinary Elimination Management
Urinary Incontinence Care
Urinary Retention Care
Values Clarification
Ventilation Assistance
Visitation Facilitation
Vital Signs Monitoring
Weight Gain Assistance
Weight Management
Weight Reduction Assistance
Wound Care
Wound Care: Closed Drainage
Wound Irrigation

From *Iowa intervention project: Nursing interventions classification (NIC)* by J.C. McCloskey & G.M. Bulechek, 1992, pp. xx-xxiv. St. Louis: Mosby.

of the health of a community. The concepts, which focus on the health of houses, specifically, noise, variety, light, and cleanliness have become especially meaningful in the 1990s. Many communities struggle with toxic waste, polluted water, polluted air, high industrial noise levels, and radon gas.

Table 5-4 demonstrates the use of Nightingale's concepts to structure the nursing process in the community setting. The Omaha Visiting Nurse Association Problem Classification Scheme

is used for the nursing diagnoses. The Iowa NIC is used for the nursing implementations in the case study.

Orem's Self Care Model

Dorothea Orem's self-care model has been evolving since 1971, with the most recent revision in 1995. Many authors have used Orem's model with the nursing process for the individual client (Fawcett, 1984; Stanton, 1985). Higgs and Gustafson (1985) have taken Orem's major

SAMPLE OF A NURSING INTERVENTIONS CLASSIFICATION (NIC) OF THE IOWA INTERVENTION PROJECT

Caregiver support

Definition:

Provision of the necessary information, advocacy, and support to facilitate primary patient care by someone other than a health care professional.

Activities:

Determine caregiver's level of knowledge

Determine caregiver's acceptance of role

Accept expressions of negative emotion

Explore with the caregiver his/her strengths and weaknesses

Acknowledge dependency of patient on caregiver as appropriate

Encourage caregiver to assume responsibility as appropriate

Encourage the acceptance of interdependency among family members

Monitor family interaction problems related to care of patient

Provide information about patient's condition in accordance with patient preferences

Teach caregiver the patient's therapy in accordance with patient preferences

Provide for follow-up health caregiver assistance through phone calls and/or community nurse care

Monitor for indicators of stress

Teach caregiver stress management techniques

Educate caregiver about the grieving process

Support caregiver through grieving process

Encourage caregiver participation in support groups

Teach caregiver health care maintenance strategies to sustain own physical and mental health

Foster caregiver social networking

Identify sources of respite care

Inform caregiver of health care and community resources

Teach caregiver strategies to access and maximize health care and community resources

Act for caregiver if overburdening becomes apparent

Notify emergency services agency/personnel about the patient's stay at home, health status, and technologies in use with consent of patient and family.

From *Iowa intervention project: Nursing interventions classification (NIC)* by J.C. McCloskey & G.M. Bulechek, 1992, p. 161. St. Louis: Mosby.

concepts; that is, universal, developmental, and health deviation requisites, and applied them to the nursing process in the community setting with different, but related, subconcepts. Hanchett (1988, 1990) has provided the most closely aligned application of Orem's original framework to the nursing process in the community setting.

Using the same case study as in previous tables, Table 5-5 demonstrates the use of Orem's model with the nursing process, with definitions applied specifically to the community setting. The NANDA taxonomy is used for the community nursing diagnoses, and the Iowa NIC system

is used for the nursing implementations for the community case study application.

Roy's Adaptation Model

Sr. Callista Roy has been developing her model since the early 1970s, first as a framework for a curriculum to teach assessment to student nurses, and then in the 1980s as a world view of the person as an adaptive system. Roy has completed extensive research studies on selected concepts in her model (1988), as well as specified six steps in the nursing process within her framework (Roy, 1984).

Roy's adaptation framework and her specifica-

Text continued on p. 115.

FAWCETT'S MODIFICATION OF KING'S GOAL-ORIENTED NURSING RECORD (GONR)

I. Data base

A. Composed of all information gathered about a person on entry into the health care system
   1. Nursing history and health assessment
   2. Physician history and physical examination
   3. Results of laboratory tests and x-ray examinations
   4. Information from such sources as family and social workers

B. Classification of patient
   1. According to severity of illness
   2. According to ability to perform activities of daily living

II. Problem list

A. List of nursing problems
B. Purposes
   1. Provides a consistent approach that may be used by many nurses to implement a plan of nursing care
   2. Serves as a guide for continuous assessment of subjective and objective signs and symptoms of a disturbance or interference in client's ability to function in usual roles
   3. Serves as a guide to identify a nursing diagnosis and to plan for the patient's immediate nursing care
   4. Provides an approach for coordination of nursing problems with medical and allied professionals' problem lists

III. Goal list

A. List of nursing goals
B. Purposes
   1. Provides a consistent and systematic approach to help individuals move toward a healthy state
   2. Serves as a guide to nurses in monitoring the disturbances and interferences in patients and to be alert for any new patient information
   3. Provides a means for nurses and clients to interact, to share information, to set mutual goals, to explore means, and to agree on means to achieve goals

4. Provides for continuity of care
5. Serves to focus attention on clients' participation in decisions about their care
6. Provides for growth and learning for both nurse and client through the interaction required to set goals

IV. Plan

A. Plan is based on assessment of the problem
B. Format for assessment (SOAP)
   1. Subjective data
      a. How does the client perceive the problem?
      b. How does the client feel about the problem?
   2. Objective data
      a. Physical examination
      b. Laboratory test results
      c. X-ray findings
      d. Activities of daily living
      e. Other pertinent objective data
   3. Assessment of the problem
      a. Identify problem
      b. Monitor changes in problem status
   4. Plan
      a. Nursing diagnosis
      b. Means agreed upon to resolve the problem and to attain goals
      c. May include client education as an integral component

V. Progress notes

A. Narrative notes
   1. Concise summary of client's progress
   2. Written when flow sheets indicate changes in the client
B. Flow sheets
   1. Used to record routine information
   2. Used for continuous or repetitive recording of specific information
   3. Used to record daily routine care
   4. Used to record cumulative data
C. Final summary or discharge notes
   1. Discussion of each problem
   2. Statement of each goal
   3. Statement regarding attainment of goal
   4. Identification of future goals

From *Analysis and evaluation of conceptual models of nursing*, pp. 98-99 by J. Fawcett, 1984, Philadelphia: Davis. Reprinted by permission.

TABLE 5-3   Nursing process in the community setting from a King framework

Nursing process in King's framework	Definitions	Case study application
Community assessment		
Personal systems		
Perception	Community's perceptions of: • health and health needs • barriers to health • health care resources • meaning of persons, objects, events	Playground and corner near day care center is a drug drop Lack of police surveillance Concerned about food pantry visitors to neighborhood
Self	Self-esteem of groups in community may be reflected by high-risk behavior	High incidence of crime Dogs for protection Cats control rats
Growth and development	Developmental levels of infants, children, adolescents, adults in community	11% were under 5 yrs old 23% were 5-14 yrs old 11% were 15-19 yrs old 49% were 20-64 yrs old 6% were 65-74 yrs old 25% infant deaths Neonatal death 3.9 times higher Postneonatal death 3.6 times higher
Body image	Social significance of body image in a particular culture	21% Caucasian 33% African-American 5% Native American 36% Hispanic 4% Other
Space	Spaces used in community Quality of play space, living space, work space	Few trees and flowers Crowded living quarters Houses run down Fences broken Yards untended Playgrounds had broken equipment Many dogs and cats in streets
Time	Experiences of people waiting	City fire department slow to answer calls Snow removal slow
Interpersonal systems		
Human interactions	Quality of interactions Limitations of prejudice Density of ethnic or economic groups	36% Hispanic and Spanish-speaking; language 33% African-American 5329 people in 4 square miles Houses crowded
Communication	Accessibility and openness of communication channels Telephone services Social support	Stable population Children kept in own yards because of drug sites in neighborhood playgrounds Groups of men in front of stores, on corners are verbally abusive

TABLE 5-3   Nursing process in the community setting from a King framework   cont'd

Nursing process in King's framework	Definitions	Case study application
Interpersonal systems Cont'd		
Transactions	Between individuals Between individuals and families Between individuals and community groups How are goals achieved in the community?	Concerns and complaints but no voiced plans change them: • food pantry visitors • drug drop sites • lack of police surveillance • high crime rates • slow city services
Role	Roles in the community Local influentials	780 households headed by women
Stress	Sources of stress in home and work environments	Low income 50% earned under $5000 26% adults unemployed High incidence of crime
Social systems		
Organization	Type of government Informal organization — the grapevine, racism, sexism, agism	Governed by the city Local officials said Native Americans refused census because they belonged to the Indian nation
Authority	Individuals and groups with authority in community: • newspapers • interviews	Local councilman aware of problems, but no plans to respond
Power	Media influences Political parties, legislators Lobbyists, voting behavior Proposed solutions to problems	Local newspaper Local councilman aware of problems, but no plans to respond Fewer than half adults finished high school
Status	Socioeconomic status of community from census Relative size and condition of buildings Physical facilities' condition: • schools • churches • hospitals • malls • sports centers	Low income urban area Many on public assistance Most working in clerical, service jobs Houses run down Playgrounds not usable with broken equipment One private physician Neighborhood food pantry Available by bus: • county hospital • ambulatory clinic • library, city college
Decision making	Community decision making evident at meetings, in documents	No attempt by local authorities to impound roaming dogs

Continued

TABLE 5-3 Nursing process in the community setting from a King framework   cont'd

Nursing process in King's framework	Definitions	Case study application
Social systems Cont'd		Local councilman aware of needs, no plans to respond
Community diagnoses	Disturbances, problems, concerns about which patients seek help	Fear related to lack of police surveillance, high crime rate, slow fire department assistance Potential for violence related to high unemployment and low income Unilateral neglect related to high infant mortality rates
Community plans	Setting goals with clients and making decisions with them on how to reach goals	Organize community meetings with police, fire departments, and local councilman to improve their responses Identify reasons for high unemployment Identify reasons for infant mortality rate
Community implementation	Activities that seek to meet the goals	Family involvement by meeting with mothers through the schools and day-care centers to organize for change, and mutually identify reasons for problems Mutual goal setting by using local newspaper to generate interest
Community evaluation	Attainment of client goals Effectiveness of nursing care	Were mothers interested in meeting to seek changes?

TABLE 5-4   Nursing process in the community setting from a Nightingale framework

Nursing process in Nightingale's framework	Definitions	Case study application
Community assessment		
Ventilation	Fresh air without impurities #1 in importance	Low-income urban area Living quarters close together
Light	Living arrangements structured so that light is everywhere #2 in importance	Run-down houses in need of repair Boarded or heavily-shaded windows
Warmth	Warm environment to prevent chilling	Harsh winters, deep snow, cold and damp spring and fall Run-down houses in need of repair
Effluvia (smells)	Foul odors Highly noxious and dangerous emanations from ill persons	Large numbers of dogs and cats roaming the streets; cats needed to control the rats
Pure water	Clean water without impurities	City water
Efficient drainage	Removal of wastes from houses in a safe way	City waste removal City snow removal slower in winter than in local neighborhoods
Cleanliness	Clean, sanitary houses inside and outside	Crowded houses in need of repair; untended yards; broken fences
Petty management	How to manage what needs to be done when homeowners are not home	Lack of police surveillance; high crime rate; city fire department slow to answer calls for assistance Language barrier: Spanish-speaking residents No police attempt to enforce leash law for loose dogs
Noise	Disturbing noises in the living area	Low-income urban area bordered by a main street to downtown Many roaming cats and dogs Groups of men on street corners and in front of stores were verbally abusive to passersby
Variety	Beautiful objects, brilliant color, bright-colored flowers	Few trees and flowers Playgrounds not usable because of broken equipment Fences broken, yards untended
Diet	Cooking, choice of diet, choice of dining times	Low income, half of families earn under $5000 annually
Bed and bedding	Clean bedding	Low income, half of families earn under $5000 annually
Cleanliness of rooms and walls	Dust-free; clean carpets and walls	Low-income urban area Crowded, run-down houses in need of repair Fences broken, yards untended, broken equipment in playground Snow removal delayed

Continued

TABLE 5-4   Nursing process in the community setting from a Nightingale framework   cont'd

Nursing process in Nightingale's framework	Definitions	Case study application
Community assessment Cont'd		
Shattering hopes	Hearing good news without false hopes	Local community newspaper Local councilman aware of needs but no plan to respond Neonatal deaths 3.9 times and postneonatal deaths 3.6 times higher than surrounding county (25.4 deaths/1000)
Community diagnoses	What is lacking in environment to restore health	Neighborhood safety deficit related to high crime rate and unsafe play area Sanitation deficit related to rats, loose dogs and cats Residence deficit related to crowded living space, run-down houses in need of repair, broken fences, untended yards
Community plans	Identify area of environment needing modification	Improve police surveillance for crimes Legislation to get rid of rats and enforce control of cats and dogs Investigate reasons for lack of repairs to houses
Community implementation	Carry out actions to change the environment to provide conditions to improve health	Environmental management for violence prevention through meetings with police department and community residents Environmental management for safety through meetings with SPCA and police department on leash law, loose animals, and rodent control Environmental management for comfort through meetings with landlords and residents about house repairs
Community evaluation	How effective were the actions to create changes in the environment to improve health?	Were changes planned to decrease the crime rate? Were actions taken to decrease the numbers of loose dogs, cats, rats in the neighborhood? Were plans made to repair houses, fences, yards?

TABLE 5-5 Nursing process in the community setting from an Orem framework

Nursing process in Orem's framework	Definitions	Case study application
Community assessment		
Universal requisites		
Sufficient intake of air	Index of air pollution	Few trees and flowers
	Temperature and weather factors	Urban area bordered by a main street to downtown shopping
		Harsh winters, cold and damp spring and fall
Sufficient intake of water	Degree of water pollution	City water
	Availability of water	
Sufficient intake of food	Growing, selling, preparing food	Low-income urban area
	Eligibility for food supplement programs	Half of families earned under $5000, many on public assistance
	Location and costs of supermarket items	780 households headed by women
		Neighborhood food pantry
	Influence of climate and soil on farming	Hispanic, African-American, Native American cultures
	Cultural meaning of food	
Care for eliminative processes and excrements	Plumbing facilities	Houses need repairs
	Sewage disposal	City sewage disposal
	Cleanliness of neighborhood	Many dogs, cats, rats roaming the streets
Balance between activity and rest	Work and recreation availability	Half of residents over 25 yrs of age had no high school education
	Child care availability	26% over 16 yrs unemployed
		Most in clerical/service jobs; 16% in lower-level management
		Playgrounds not usable because of broken equipment
		Drug drop in playground and near day-care facilities
		Yards untended
		Lack of police surveillance, many crimes
Balance between solitude and social interaction	Finding, creating, and maintaining space and time for both	Urban area near main street to downtown
		Houses crowded
	Available child care and support groups	Groups of men on corners
		High crime rate
		Drug drop near day-care facilities, in playground
Prevention of hazards to human life, functioning, and well being	Safe driving, prevention of accidents or hazards	Broken equipment and fences
		Houses run down and need repair
	Availability of emergency services	Drug drops in child areas
		Lack of police protection
		Fire department slow to respond
		Snow removal slow
Promotion of human functioning and development	Desire to be normal	Local councilman aware of needs but no plans to respond
	Environment for community development	

Continued

TABLE 5-5   Nursing process in the community setting from an Orem framework   cont'd

Nursing process in Orem's framework	Definitions	Case study application
Developmental requisites		
Conditions to support life and promote development	Neonatal, child, adult statistics Pregnancy rates	Neonatal deaths 3.9 times and postneonatal deaths 3.6 times higher than local counties
Provision of care to overcome conditions affecting development	Educational deprivation, social problems, violence, losses, oppressive living conditions	High crime rates, crowded and run-down houses Less than half of residents over 25 yrs of age have any high school education 780 households headed by women Many on public assistance
Health deviation requisites		
Seeking medical care for exposure to risks	Disaster plans Exposure to toxicities	Drug drops in area High crime rates One physician in area
Attending to effects and results of pathologic conditions	Morbidity and mortality data Availability of physicians, emergency care	Neonatal deaths 3.9 times and postneonatal deaths 3.6 times higher than local areas (25.4/1000) One physician in area By bus, large county hospital
Carrying out diagnostic, therapeutic, and rehabilitative measures	Availability of pharmacies, outpatient departments, nurses, hospitals, physicians	By bus, large county hospital, ambulatory care clinic
Attending to discomforting effects of medical care measures	Self-help groups Pharmacists Nurses Patient education	By bus, ambulatory care clinic
Modifying the self-concept to accept health state and need for health care	Support groups Counseling Patient education	By bus, ambulatory care clinic, public library
Learning to live with effects of pathology and of medical, diagnostic, and treatment measures in lifestyle promoting development	Self-help groups Counseling Social and recreational activities; sheltered workshops	By bus, hospital, ambulatory care clinic, library, city college Local newspaper
Community diagnoses		
	Self-care deficits in above requisites	Potential for injury related to self-care deficits in police, fire, snow removal services Fear related to high crime rate and local drug drops Knowledge deficit in prenatal and infant care related to unknown etiology

TABLE 5-5 Nursing process in the community setting from an Orem framework   cont'd

Nursing process in Orem's framework	Definitions	Case study application
Community plans		
	Increase self-care capability	Organize grass roots political activism to improve city services
	Decrease self-care demands	
	Provide dependent care	Support families in setting up neighborhood watch programs
		Provide prenatal care, family planning, infant care classes
Community implementation		
	Acting or doing for the community	Security enhancement by acting for families by joint meetings with city officials on services
	Providing support	
	Guiding clients	Providing support groups for families in efforts to set up programs for a safer environment
	Teaching clients	
	Providing a developmental environment	Teaching prenatal care, infant care, family planning to women in their homes
Community evaluation		
	Is community attempting self-care?	Is community working with nurse to meet with city officials?
	Is community accepting care and assistance from nurse?	Is community willing to organize safety programs being initiated by the nurse?
	Is nurse supporting, teaching, guiding the community?	Are families receptive to nurse's teaching to decrease infant mortality rates? Are rates declining?

tion of the nursing process have been applied by several authors to describe the nursing process with the individual (Fawcett, 1984; Galbreath, 1985; Stanton, 1985; Andrews & Roy, 1986). Roy (1983) demonstrated how to use her model and nursing process framework with the family as client, as did Hanson (1984), and Martz (1990).

Roy's model has been applied to the community as client by Higgs and Gustafson (1985), using community functions, stimuli, and adaptive responses. Hanchett (1988, 1990) described Roy's nursing process in terms of community health nursing, exclusively using Roy's concepts with Hanson's (1984) application of them to the family.

Table 5-6 demonstrates the use of Roy's model with the nursing process, including definitions useful for the community setting. The concepts are derived from Roy's (1983) application of her concepts for the individual to a family situation, from Hanson's assessment of the family in Roy's (1984) text, and from Hanchett's (1988) use of Roy's framework in the community setting. The Omaha Visiting Nurse Association Problem Classification Scheme is used for the nursing diagnosis, and the Iowa NIC is used for the implementation.

TABLE 5-6   Nursing process in the community setting from a Roy framework

Nursing process in Roy's framework	Definitions	Case study application
Community assessment		
First level assessment		
Survival (physiologic mode)		
Physical maintenance of members		
Food	Availability	Low-income urban area
	Quality, cost	Many on public assistance
		Neighborhood food pantry
Clothing	Availability	On main street to downtown shopping
	Affordability	Half of families earn income of under $5000 annually
Shelter	Adequacy	Houses crowded, run down, in need of repair
	Affordability	Winters harsh, deep snow, spring and fall cold and damp
		Few trees and flowers
Allocation of resources for health care needs		
Emergency care	Responsiveness	Lack of police surveillance
	Access	Fire department slow to answer calls
Medical care	Access	One physician in area
		Large county hospital by bus
		Ambulatory care clinic by bus
Dental care	Access	Large county hospital by bus
Preventive care	Access	Ambulatory care clinic by bus
Allocation of space and equipment for:		
Rest	Solitude	High crime rate, drug drops
		Yards untended, broken fences
		780 households headed by women
Exercise	Recreational resources	Playground is a drug drop, also not usable because of broken equipment; low income urban area bordered by two other low-income areas, one middle-income area, main street
Aloneness and togetherness	Support systems	Drug drop near day-care center
Growth (self-concept mode)		
Solidarity and social integration	Families in the community	780 households headed by women; 17% newcomers in 5 years; multi-ethnic groups
Understanding and companionship	Support systems	Groups of men on corners verbally abusive to passersby
		Most residents over 16 yrs of age in clerical or service jobs; 16% in lower-level management

TABLE 5-6 Nursing process in the community setting from a Roy framework   cont'd

Nursing process in Roy's framework	Definitions	Case study application
First level assessment Cont'd		
Moral-ethical values	Cultural values	36% Hispanic
		33% African-American
		21% Caucasian
		4.5% Native American
Time orientation	Future and present orientation	17% newcomers in past 5 years
		45% under 20 years old
Conflict management	How are problems resolved?	Children kept in yards because of fears of drug drops
		Local councilman aware of problems, but no plans to respond
Continuity (role function mode)		
Decision-making	Who has power?	Local councilman; no response
Communication	Clarity	Language barrier; many Spanish-speaking persons
	Appropriateness	
		Groups of men on corners verbally abusive
Roles	Clarity	Concerns about lack of fire, police, snow removal service
	Tolerance for changes	
Division of responsibility	How are community tasks achieved?	Local councilman unresponsive
Transactional patterns (interdependence mode)		
Interactions of groups	How do groups intermingle?	Children kept in own yards because of drug drops
		Groups of men on corners
		Drug drops in playground, near day-care center
Support systems	What are community supports?	Hispanic, African-American, Native American cultures
Significant others	Who are community resources?	Local councilman; not responsive
Member control (physiological mode, role function mode)		
Behaviors in formal/ informal systems	Families, schools, churches	Fewer than half of residents over 25 yrs of age have any high school education
	Values	Library, city college by bus
		780 households headed by women
		High crime rates
		High infant mortality rates
Social control by agencies	Police department	Lack of police surveillance
	Public health department	Fire department slow to answer calls
	Planning commission	Snow removal slow
		Local councilman has no plans to respond to known needs

Continued

TABLE 5-6   Nursing process in the community setting from a Roy framework   cont'd

Nursing process in Roy's framework	Definitions	Case study application
Second level assessment		
Focal stimuli	Groups' needs Changes within and among groups Changes in environment	Concerned about lack of police surveillance and high crime rate; slow fire department and snow removal response
Contextual stimuli	Support Nurturance Socialization	High infant mortality rate Low income, half of families earn under $5000 annually Half of residents over 25 years of age have no high school education 780 households headed by women; fears for child safety with drug drops
Residual stimuli	Previous experiences	17% newcomers in last 5 years Hispanic, African-American, Native American groups
Community diagnosis		
	Adaptive or ineffective responses	Deficit in neighborhood safety related to high crime rate, lack of police surveillance, slow fire department and snow removal responses
Community plans		
	Increase adaptive responses for survival, continuity, growth	Identify community leaders to mobilize action to increase community safety for family survival
Community implementation		
	Management of the three stimuli	Focal stimulus: safety Environmental management: Safety by identifying leaders, helping to plan meetings of residents to correct police, fire, snow removal deficits; to work with public officials and organize informal actions to improve safety
Community evaluation		
	Are coping mechanisms enabling community to adapt effectively to stimuli?	Are community leaders identified and making efforts to organize residents for action?

Chapter Highlights

- The nursing process is a means for the community health nurse to be accountable to the American Nurses' Association Standards of Clinical Nursing Practice and the American Nurses' Association Standards of Community Health Nursing Practice.

- Nursing assessments are structured by some form of data collection in the community.

- Nursing diagnoses are written according to specific guidelines and may be based on the NANDA system of nursing diagnosis, or the Omaha Visiting Nurse Association Problem Classification Scheme.

- Nursing plans are stated in terms of client outcomes and may include nursing orders.

- Nursing implementations may be based on the Iowa NIC scheme.

- Evaluation of nursing care is conducted for the client and for a group of clients, which ensures continuous quality improvement.

- King's framework directs community assessment of personal, interpersonal, and social systems; and mutual agreement of problems and goals and on means to achieve those goals.

- Nightingale's framework directs assessment of the physical aspects of the environment and interventions on the environment to enable the community to restore its health.

- Orem's framework enables assessment of the universal, developmental, and health deviation requisites of a community; and to establish its self-care deficits and nursing implementations through five helping methods.

- Roy's framework provides for first level assessment of the four modes, second level assessment of the focal, contextual, and residual stimuli; and to identify adaptive or ineffective responses that will be the basis of the nurse's management of the three stimuli.

 CRITICAL THINKING EXERCISE

A community health nurse receives a referral to do a health assessment on a person newly diagnosed as having Alzheimer's disease. The referral simply states "teaching and counseling." A visit to the home reveals a 72-year-old client who is forgetful and sometimes emotionally labile. He is able to take care of his physical needs with verbal prompting, but sometimes thinks he is in his boyhood home. His primary caretaker is his 68-year-old wife.

During the interview, she seems very apprehensive, especially about her ability to handle their finances. She asks for help with this. She cries often and says she understands that their life as a couple will be going through many changes.

1. Using nursing process, arrive at a nursing diagnosis for this family.
2. Using King's conceptual framework as a guide, develop a plan of care that will move the family toward maintenance of present family processes. Include sub-goals, rationales for interventions, and outcome assessment criteria.

REFERENCES

American Nurses' Association. (1980). *Nursing: A social policy statement.* Kansas City, MO: Author.

American Nurses' Association. (1986). *Standards of community health nursing practice.* Kansas City, MO: Author.

American Public Health Association. (1980). *The definition and role of public health nursing in the delivery of health care.* Washington, D.C.: Author.

Andrews, H.A., & Roy, C. (1986). *Essentials of the Roy adaptation model.* Norwalk, CT: Appleton-Century-Crofts.

Barrett, E.A.M. (1993, Fall). Nursing centers without nursing frameworks: What's wrong with this picture? *Nursing Science Quarterly, 6*(3), 115-117.

Bellack, J.P., & Edlund, B.J. (1992). *Nursing assessment and nursing diagnosis* (2nd ed.). Boston: Jones and Bartlett.

Beynon, C., & Laschinger, H.K. (1993, September). Theory-based practice: Attitudes of nursing managers before and after educational sessions. *Public Health Nursing, 10*(3), 183-188.

Canadian Nurses' Association. (1980). *A definition of nursing practice.* Ottawa: Author.

Carlson, J.H., Craft, C.A., McGuire, A.D., & Popkess-Vawter, S. (1991). *Nursing diagnosis: A case study approach.* Philadelphia: WB Saunders.

Carroll-Johnson, R.M. (Ed.). (1991). *Classification of nursing diagnoses: Proceedings of the ninth conference.* Philadelphia: JB Lippincott.

Cross, J.R. (1985). Betty Neuman. In George, J.B. (Ed.), *Nursing theories: The base for professional nursing practice* (2nd ed.) (pp. 258-286). Englewood Cliffs, NJ: Prentice-Hall.

Dolan, M.B. (1990). *Community and home health care plans.* Springhouse, PA: Springhouse.

Fawcett, J. (1984). *Analysis and evaluation of conceptual models of nursing.* Philadelphia: Davis.

Galbreath, J.G. (1985). Sister Callista Roy. In George, J.B. (Ed.), *Nursing theories: The base for professional nursing practice* (2nd ed.) (pp. 300-318). Englewood Cliffs, NJ: Prentice-Hall.

George, J.B. (1985). Imogene M. King. In George, J.B. (Ed.), *Nursing theories: The base for professional nursing practice* (2nd ed.) (pp. 235-257). Englewood Cliffs, NJ: Prentice-Hall.

Hamilton, P. (1983, April). Community nursing diagnosis. *Advances in Nursing Science, 5*(3), 21-36.

Hanchett, E.S. (1988). *Nursing frameworks and community as client: Bridging the gap.* Norwalk, CT: Appleton & Lange.

Hanchett, E.S. (1990, Summer). Nursing models and community as client. *Nursing Science Quarterly, 3*(2), 67-72.

Hanson, J. (1984). The family. In Roy, C. (Ed.), *Introduction to nursing: An adaptation model* (2nd ed.) (pp. 519-533). Englewood Cliffs, NJ: Prentice-Hall.

Hegyvary, S.T. (1991). Issues in outcomes research. *Journal of Nursing Quality Assurance, 5*(2), 1-6.

Higgs, Z.R., & Gustafson, D.D. (1985). *Community as client: Assessment and diagnosis.* Philadelphia: Davis.

Huch, M.H. (1988, February). Theory-based practice: Structuring nursing care. *Nursing Science Quarterly, 1*(1), 6-7.

Iyer, P.W., Taptich, B., & Bernocchi-Losey, D. (1991). *Nursing process and nursing diagnosis* (2nd ed.). Philadelphia: WB Saunders.

Jones, K.R. (1993, May-June). Outcomes analysis: Methods and issues. *Nursing Economics, 11*(3), 145-152.

King, I.M. (1981). *A theory for nursing: Systems, concepts, process.* New York: Wiley.

King, I.M. (1983). King's theory of nursing. In Clements, I.W., & Roberts, F.B. (Eds.), *Family health: A theoretical approach to nursing care* (pp. 177-188). New York: Wiley.

King, I.M. (1992, Spring). King's theory of goal attainment. *Nursing Science Quarterly, 5*(1), 19-26.

Laschinger, H.K., & Duff, V. (1991). Practicing nurses' attitudes toward nursing-theory based practice. *Canadian Journal of Nursing Administration, 1*(1), 16-19.

Martin, K.S. (1989). Omaha System. In American Nurses' Association. *ANA classification systems for describing nursing practice.* Kansas City, MO: Author.

Martz, C.M. (1990). Nursing process of the family client: Application of Friedman's and Roy's models. In Christensen, P.J., and Kenney, J.W. (Eds.), *Nursing process: Application of conceptual models* (3rd ed.) (pp. 305-331). St. Louis: Mosby.

McCloskey, J.C., & Bulechek, G.M. (1992). *Iowa intervention project: Nursing interventions classification (NIC).* St. Louis: Mosby.

Murray, M.E., & Atkinson, L.D. (1994). *Understanding the nursing process: The next generation* (5th ed.). New York: McGraw-Hill.

Neufeld, A., & Harrison, M.J. (1990, December). The development of nursing diagnoses for aggregates and groups. *Public Health Nursing, 7*(4), 251-255.

Nightingale, F. (1969). *Notes on nursing: What it is, and what it is not.* New York: Dover.

Orem, D.E. (1995). *Nursing: Concepts of practice* (5th ed.). St. Louis: Mosby.

Parse, R.R. (1990, Summer). Nursing theory-based practice: A challenge for the 90s. *Nursing Science Quarterly, 5*(4), 53.

Parse, R.R. (1992, Winter). The performing art of nursing. *Nursing Science Quarterly, 5*(4), 147.

Reed, K.S. (1993, Summer). Adapting the Neuman systems model for family nursing. *Nursing Science Quarterly, 6*(2), 93-97.

Reilly, C.E. (1975). Why a conceptual framework? *Nursing Outlook, 23,* 566-569.

Roy, C. (1983). Roy adaptation model. In Clements, I.W., & Roberts, F.B. (Eds.), *Family health: A theoretical approach to nursing care* (pp. 255-278). New York: Wiley.

Roy, C. (1984). *Introduction to nursing: An adaptation model* (2nd ed.). Englewood Cliffs, NJ: Prentice-Hall.

Roy, C. (1988, February). An explication of the philosophical assumptions of the Roy adaptation model. *Nursing Science Quarterly, 1*(1), 26-34.

Stanton, M. (1985). Nursing theories and the nursing process. In George, J.B. (Ed.), *Nursing theories: The base for professional nursing practice* (2nd ed.) (pp. 319-337). Englewood Cliffs, NJ: Prentice-Hall.

Not in Alma
by barcode or title

Torres, G. (1985). Florence Nightingale. In George, J.B. (Ed.), *Nursing theories: The base for professional nursing practice* (2nd ed.) (pp. 34-49). Englewood Cliffs, NJ: Prentice-Hall.

Turley, J.P. (1992, July-August). A framework for the transition from nursing records to a nursing information system. *Nursing Outlook, 40*(4), 177-181.

Zink, M.R. (1994). Nursing diagnosis in home care: Audit tool development. *Journal of Community Health Nursing, 11*(1), 51-58.

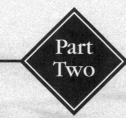

Part
Two

Strategies and Tools for Health Promotion

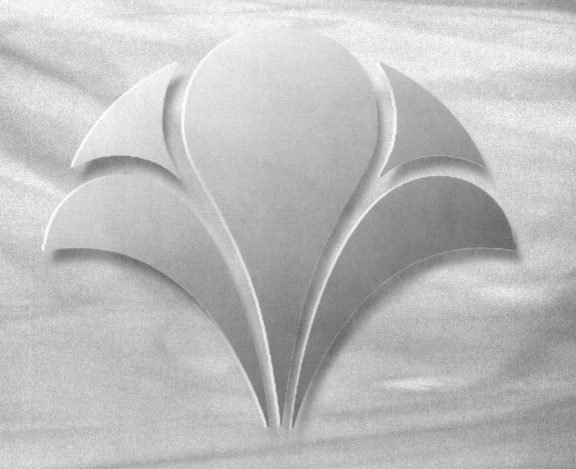

Promoting health and wellness is an integral part of the role of the nurse in the community. Part II describes several strategies and tools that may be used to accomplish this.

Chapter 6 describes the epidemiologic process and includes research methods that can be used to study patterns and trends in human populations. Included is a model of the natural history of disease in humans. Other epidemiologic concepts that can be used by the nurse to predict and prevent disease and disability are presented as well.

Chapter 7 presents a number of conceptual models that will assist the nurse when assessing the health states of individuals and families. It also provides a holistic perspective of nursing care and includes some alternative techniques that might be considered when providing that care.

Teaching strategies and an overview of the teaching/learning process are discussed in Chapter 8.

Chapter 9 provides information about leadership, control, planning, and organization in health care. This information is invaluable when attempting to bring about change or plan methods of case management.

Chapter 10 outlines the importance of group process and describes types of groups that can be organized in the community to promote wellness and teach disease prevention.

Chapter 11 deals with various models of quality that can be used in the evaluative process. Cost containment and consumer advocacy are discussed as is total quality management.

6

EPIDEMIOLOGY IN COMMUNITY HEALTH NURSING

Diane L. Cookfair ◆ Joan M. Cookfair

Any modification of the conditions of life as they exist in a community . . . requires something more than a knowledge of specific organisms of disease. It equally requires a knowledge of the community, of the psychology of the people, their social organization, the conditions and events of their everyday life. It requires that the knowledge of fundamental causes of disease be fitted together with the knowledge of people into a practical epidemiology, directly applicable to prevention.

Wade Hampton Frost

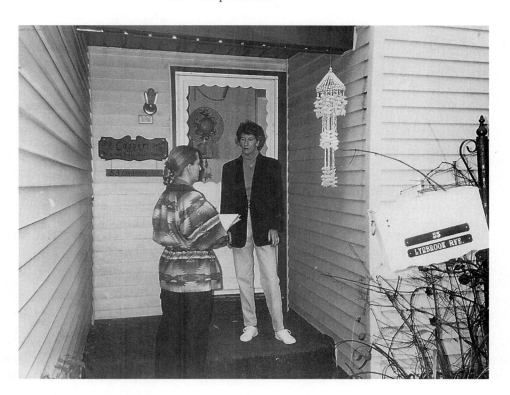

OBJECTIVES

At the conclusion of this chapter, the student will be able to:

1. Define the key terms used.
2. Describe the historical evolution of epidemiology.
3. Describe key epidemiologic concepts.
4. Describe measures of disease frequency.
5. Describe measures of association.
6. Describe key statistical concepts.
7. Identify methods of study used in epidemiologic research.
8. Describe sources of data used in epidemiologic research.
9. Describe the application of epidemiology to community health nursing.

KEY TERMS

Analytic study
Case-control study
Causal relationships
Cohort study
Cross-sectional study
Descriptive study
Epidemiologic triangle
Epidemiology

Experimental study
Incidence rate
Mode of transmission
Morbidity
Mortality
Natural history of disease
Observational study
Prevalence rate

Primary prevention
Relative risk
Reservoirs of infection
Secondary prevention
Sensitivity
Specificity
Tertiary prevention

Epidemiology is a science that studies the occurrence of disease in human populations (Ahlbom & Norell, 1990). Epidemiologists identify differences in disease distribution among population groups and investigate the determinants of these differences. Information concerning patterns of disease occurrence and factors that place individuals at increased risk of developing disease are used for the purpose of preventing disease and maintaining and promoting health. Epidemiologists study *groups* of individuals.

Epidemiologists are concerned with both the measurement of disease frequency and the measurement of environmental exposures, host fac-

tors, and other risk factors that may be associated with disease occurrence. Epidemiologic studies may be either observational or experimental in nature. Observational studies include both descriptive and analytic studies. Descriptive studies examine differences in disease distribution among different population groups (person), assess variations in disease occurrence by geographic location (place), and record variations in disease occurrence over time. Analytic studies test specific hypotheses regarding the etiology (the cause or causes) or the prevention of disease. They are used to identify the factors that account for differences in disease distribution by person, place, and time; for example, factors that place an individual at high risk of developing a disease.

Experimental studies test the effectiveness of specific interventions designed to prevent disease (prophylactic trials) or to treat existing disease (therapeutic trials). Experimental studies may also be conducted to determine the sensitivity and specificity of a new screening test.

HISTORICAL EVOLUTION OF EPIDEMIOLOGY

The epidemiologic method is based on the premise that disease does not occur by chance alone. This type of reasoning can be seen as early as the fifth century BC in Hippocrates' book, *Airs, Waters and Places.* In his book, Hippocrates specified that for proper medical investigation one must take into account the seasons, the water supply, the orientation of the city and its topography, and the customs and occupations of the population under observation. Hippocrates' work clearly suggests that environmental factors influence patterns of disease occurrence.

Centuries before the development of the germ theory, this type of reasoning led to the practice of isolating persons with contagious diseases. During the fourteenth century, bubonic plague, or "Black Death," as it was called, swept over Europe killing between one third and two thirds of the inhabitants in Europe's largest cities (Tuchman, 1978). The plague was almost always fatal. Often the dead remained unburied because no one remained to bury them. It was not surprising, therefore, that people were frightened and often reacted violently against the mere mention of the word plague. Quarantine procedures were strictly enforced by many European cities. In Milan, Archbishop Giovanni Visconti ordered the first three homes in which the plague was discovered to be permanently walled up, enclosing both the living and the dead together (Tuchman, 1978). A less drastic version of this type of quarantine was practiced in London during the epidemic of the sixteenth century (Smith, 1941). At that time town officials shut up the houses where the plague was found, confining well persons in the home with the sick and posting watchers at the door to prevent escape.

Despite these early observations concerning the spread of disease, it was not until the late 1800s that the germ theory received widespread acceptance. However, the development of germ theory was preceded by the concept that disease does not occur randomly. This led physicians and researchers to look for patterns in **mortality** (death) and **morbidity** (illness). Parish clerks and village priests kept records, called bills of mortality, about deaths that occurred in London and Hampshire. In the seventeenth century John Graunt, a pioneer in the field of epidemiology, began to look carefully at these statistics and to draw inferences from them. He examined differences in urban and rural mortality and also differences in mortality caused by both acute and chronic disease. His work, *Natural and Political Observations,* published in 1692, presented a strong case for the accurate recording of vital statistics to provide a database for research (Lilienfeld, 1980).

Another pioneer in the field of epidemiology was Dr. William Farr, who was in charge of the General Registrar's office established in England in 1837. Farr compiled statistical data about morbidity and mortality and made epidemiologic inferences about the effect of inadequate sanitation and overcrowding on the spread of disease. Farr is credited with developing the first modern vital statistics system (Farr, 1975). In the 1850s, Florence Nightingale patterned her reports to superiors on the health conditions of the military during the Crimean War after Farr's work, presenting detailed statistics and their implications. On the basis of these reports she acquired funding to implement changes that significantly reduced the mortality rate of British troops in hospitals (Cohen, 1984). Nightingale continued to use an epidemiologic model in her early work to demonstrate the role of environment in health and its relevance to disease patterns (Stanhope & Lancaster, 1992).

In the 1850s John Snow, a contemporary of William Farr's, conducted a classic series of epidemiologic studies concerning the transmission of cholera in London (Snow, 1936). He compared the incidence (number of cases) of cholera reported in various households according to their source of drinking water. His results clearly indicated that the cholera rates of houses supplied by the Southwork and Vauxhall Company were between eight and nine times higher than those households whose water was not supplied by that company. Snow had isolated an indirect cause (drinking water), and improved sanitation of the water supply reduced the incidence of cholera long before the direct cause of cholera was known. In fact, this logical ordering of events and empirical reasoning used to identify the source of cholera occurred many years before Pasteur formulated the germ theory of disease and Koch discovered the bacillus that caused cholera *(Vibrio cholerae)* (Lilienfeld, 1980).

Another important contribution to the development of modern epidemiology was made in the United States by Joseph Goldberger in the early twentieth century (Lilienfeld, 1980). Pellagra is a nutritional disorder caused by severe niacin deficiency, characterized by changes in the mucous membrane, cutaneous lesions, and central nervous system and gastrointestinal symptoms (Berkow, 1992). Before Goldberger's work, pellagra was thought to be an infectious disease. Cases were regularly reported throughout the United States, especially in institutional settings. Goldberger's initial studies were based on his own observations. He studied residents in asylums and orphanages, comparing diet among groups with a high incidence of pellagra, and groups with a low incidence of pellagra (Goldberger, 1964). The striking results of these observational studies led Goldberger to conduct a series of experimental studies. In one experiment pellagra was induced in prison farm volunteers (Goldberger, 1964). One group of prisoners was fed the type of diet that had been associated with a high incidence of pellagra in Goldberger's earlier observational studies. The control group was fed a less restricted diet. Further comparative studies were conducted in orphanages, where children placed on supplemental "preventive" diets were compared with control groups of children who received the institution's normal diet (Goldberger, 1923). Goldberger's work led to the virtual elimination of pellagra in the United States and other industrialized nations.

As effective treatments and methods of preventing acute infectious diseases were developed, epidemiology began to increase its focus on chronic disease. New methodologies began to be developed to address the more complex problems posed by the study of chronic disease, where exposure to a causal agent may take place decades before disease develops, and "cause" may be multifactorial in nature, as with cancer (Rothman, 1986). With the recognition that multiple factors frequently interact to "cause" disease, a new approach to disease control was taken, and increased emphasis was placed on developing interventions that could reduce the risk of developing disease.

KEY BIOLOGIC AND EPIDEMIOLOGIC CONCEPTS
Primary, Secondary, and Tertiary Prevention

Earlier chapters in this book refer to the concept of primary, secondary, and tertiary prevention. **Primary prevention** is the prevention of disease by altering susceptibility or reducing exposure of susceptible individuals. It is accomplished by health promotion (teaching and advocacy) or specific protection (immunizations and altered environment).

Secondary prevention is the early detection and treatment of disease by such techniques as case finding and screening. Early detection not only leads to early treatment, which may benefit the individual with the disease, but also helps to prevent the spread of communicable disease, which represents primary prevention for healthy, susceptible individuals. **Tertiary prevention** is the alleviation of disability that results from disease and the attempt to restore effective functioning. It can be achieved by means of rehabilitation or palliative methods if rehabilitation is not possible.

Natural History of Disease

Epidemiologic methods may be used to learn more about the **natural history of disease.** Information on the natural history of disease is helpful in planning studies concerning disease etiology and is essential for the development of effective interventions to prevent and treat disease.

THE NATURAL HISTORY OF DISEASE IN MAN

Time Period:	PREPATHOGENESIS	PERIOD OF PATHOGENESIS	
Stage:	Prior to Development of Disease	Presymptomatic → Early Clinical Disease →	Advanced Clinical Disease

Level of Prevention:
 	
Activities:
	Primary Prevention
	
	• Health Promotion
	
	  a. Health Education
	  b. Counseling
	
	• Specific Protection
	
	  a. Immunizations
	  b. Prevent exposure to carcinogens and other agents which cause disease
	  c. Protect against occupational hazards and accidents
		Secondary Prevention
		
		• Early Case Finding:
		
		  a. Individuals
		  b. Families
		  c. Community (Screening Programs)
		
		• Early Treatment
		
		  a. Cure or prevent progression of disease
		  b. Prevent spread of disease (represents primary prevention for unaffected individuals)
		  c. Prevent complications and sequelae
			Tertiary Prevention
			
			• Limit Disability
			
			  a. Arrest or slow disease process
			  b. Prevent death if possible
			  c. Provide supportive care
			
			• Rehabilitation
			
			  a. Retraining
			  b. Occupational Therapy
			  c. Physical Therapy

FIGURE 6-1 Adapted from *Preventive medicine for the doctor in his community: An epidemiologic approach* (3rd Ed.) (1965) by Leavell, H.R., & Clark, E.G. New York: McGraw-Hill.

Leavell and Clark (1965) developed a model that outlines the natural history of disease in human beings (Figure 6-1). The prepathogenetic period is the time before the development of disease, or before pathogenesis. The pathogenetic period involves a presymptomatic stage followed by the development of recognizable clinical disease with specific signs and symptoms.

During the prepathogenetic period, interactions may occur between the host, agent, and environment that increase an individual's susceptibility to disease. For example, smoking increases an individual's risk of contracting lung disease. Health education before the event (smoking) may prevent an individual from smoking and thus minimize the risk of a lung disease such as emphysema (primary prevention). If during early pathogenesis a smoker with a chronic cough can be encouraged to prevent further sequelae by quitting smoking, disease progression still may be altered (secondary prevention). Should a pathologic condition such as emphysema develop, rehabilitation or limitation of disability still is possible if the smoker is encouraged to cease smoking and make maximum use of remaining capabilities (tertiary prevention).

Agent, Host, and Environment

The epidemiologic triangle. For infectious diseases and many chronic diseases a specific factor or agent must be present to cause disease. An agent does not cause disease unless (1) it connects with a susceptible host, and (2) the host is susceptible to the agent when the contact is made. These two factors, a causative agent and a susceptible host, along with a third factor, a conducive environment, make up the **epidemiologic triangle.**

The triangle model assumes all three factors are important in predicting patterns of disease occurrence. For example, in Philadelphia during the summer of 1976 there were 24 deaths and more than 200 persons became seriously ill as a result of an outbreak of *Legionella pneumophila* (Lattimer, 1981; Fraser, 1977). This epidemic affected participants of an American Legion convention who had all stayed in the same hotel. The *agent* in this case was an airborne bacteria; outbreaks such as this one have been traced to

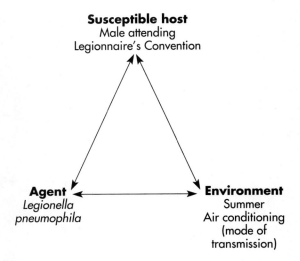

FIGURE 6-2   The epidemiological triangle applied to the 1976 outbreak of Legionnaires' disease.

air-conditioning systems (environment). Susceptible *hosts* frequently have depressed immunity. Elimination of any one of the factors (host, agent, or environment) could have prevented the outbreak of Legionnaires' disease. If the men had not attended the convention, they would not have become ill. If the agent had not been present, illness would not have occurred. If the air conditioning system had not been operating, the disease would not have been transmitted (Figure 6-2).

The wheel model. The wheel model of human-environmental interactions (Figure 6-3) is another model used to visualize this type of phenomenon (Mausner, 1974). The hub of the wheel is the host, which has a unique genetic core. The surrounding environment is biological, social, or physical. The size of the wheel's components depends on the disease in question. For a hereditary disease such as Tay-Sachs disease, the genetic core is prominent. In a disease such as AIDS, the host's immune state and the social and biological environments (hubs) are more prominent.

Reservoirs of Infection

Reservoirs of infection are defined as living organisms or inanimate objects (soil, for example) that harbor an infectious agent (Mausner, 1985). Some reservoirs are specific to some infectious

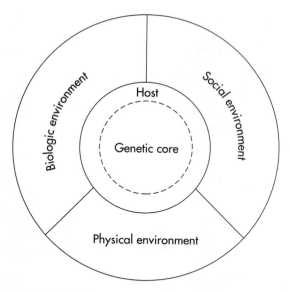

FIGURE 6-3 The wheel model of human-environmental interactions. From *Epidemiology* (2nd ed.) by J. Mausner (1974). Philadelphia: WB Saunders Co.

agents. Most viral and bacterial diseases are transmitted from one human being to another. Bovine tuberculosis, rabies, and brucellosis are known as zoonoses. Zoonoses are infectious diseases that are transmissible from vertebrate animals to humans.

Mode of Transmission

Any mechanism whereby an infectious agent is spread through the environment to members of a population is called the **mode of transmission.** It can be either direct or indirect. An example of direct transmission is the transfer of the human immunodeficiency virus (HIV) through the body fluid of one person to that of another. By contrast, indirect transmission can occur without human contact. For example, *E. coli* organisms may be transmitted in contaminated water, and Rickettsie are transmitted by a tick. As described earlier, *L. pneumophila* is transmitted via air.

Immunity

The concept of resistance to infectious disease is related to the concept of immunity. Artificial active immunity to a specific disease can be ac-

quired by immunizing susceptible individuals with live attenuated toxins. For example, childhood disease such as mumps, rubella, diphtheria, and pertussis can be prevented through immunization. Temporary artificial passive immunity by gamma globulin administration can protect persons exposed to a disease, such as Hepatitis A. Active natural immunity to some diseases is acquired by having the disease; for example, varicella (chicken pox). For a limited period after birth, passive natural immunity to certain diseases the mother may have had is transferred to the child across the placental barrier during the last trimester of pregnancy. Herd immunity refers to the resistance of a group or population to the invasion or spread of an infectious agent.

MEASURES OF DISEASE FREQUENCY

To study the distribution of disease in a population group, an epidemiologist must be able to describe how common the disease is in the population that is being studied. A rate describes the number of events (in this instance cases of disease or death) that occur in a population of a certain size during a specific period. A rate is given as a fraction, where the numerator is the number of events (cases or deaths) during a specific period, and the denominator is the number of people at risk of the event during that period.

$$\text{Rate} = \frac{\text{Number of cases or deaths in a period}}{\text{Population at risk in same period}}$$

Rates are used to describe the frequency of illness (morbidity) from specific causes and the frequency of death (mortality) from specific causes.

The two most common measures of disease frequency are incidence rate and prevalence rate. **Incidence rate** measures the number of *new* cases of a disease that develop in a population during a given period. **Prevalence rate** measures all cases (old cases plus new cases) that exist in a population during a given period. Because the prevalence rate describes all existing cases, it depends on two factors: the incidence of the disease and the duration of the disease. For an acute disease of short duration, such as measles, incidence and prevalence will be similar. For a lifelong chronic disease, such as multiple sclerosis, which generally strikes young and middle-age adults, incidence will be much lower than prevalence for any given year.

Measures of disease mortality include the crude mortality rate, specific mortality rates (age, sex, race, and cause-specific), and the case fatality rate (Morton, 1990). The crude mortality rate measures the number of overall deaths in a community per 1000 population in a 1-year period. Case-specific mortality rates measure death resulting from a specific cause (*i.e.,* lung cancer) that occur in a community per 1000 population in a 1-year time period. Because cause of death and frequency of death differ so much by age, it is also common to see number of deaths described in terms of age-specific mortality rates. For instance, the incidence of mortality from pertussis is rare after a child is 2 years of age, and pertussis is seldom serious in older children. Therefore, an age-specific rate is a more appropriate way of describing mortality caused by per-

tussis in young children than a crude mortality rate.

The case fatality rate is used to describe the probability of death in a *diagnosed* case (Morton, 1990). It describes the relationship between incidence of a disease and mortality from that disease. The case fatality rate for a disease such as multiple sclerosis is lower than the case fatality rate for a disease such as lung cancer.

Case fatality rate

$$= \frac{\text{No. of deaths caused by the disease during 1 year}}{\text{No. of cases of the disease occurring in the same year}}$$

When studying acute disease outbreaks (epidemics), the attack rate is used to describe the proportion of a population that contracts a disease out of all those at risk of contracting the disease during a given period. Other rates that are important in describing the general health or level of wellness in a community include birth

TABLE 6-1 Formulas of commonly used rates

Rates		Population size
Age-specific death rate =	$\dfrac{\text{No. of deaths among persons in a given age group in 1 year}}{\text{Average (mid-year) population in the age group specified}}$	per 1000
Birth rate =	$\dfrac{\text{No. of live births}}{\text{Estimated mid-year population}}$	per 1000
Cause-specific mortality rate =	$\dfrac{\text{No. of deaths from specific cause during 1 year}}{\text{Average population at risk mid-year}}$	per 100,000
Crude death rate =	$\dfrac{\text{No. of overall deaths during 1 year}}{\text{Average mid-year population at risk}}$	per 1000
Incidence rate =	$\dfrac{\text{No. of new cases of specified illness during a specific time interval}}{\text{Estimated mid-interval population at risk}}$	per 1000
Infant mortality rate =	$\dfrac{\text{No. of deaths under 1 year of age during 1 year}}{\text{No. of live births in same year}}$	per 1000 live births
Maternal mortality rate =	$\dfrac{\text{No. of deaths from puerperal causes during 1 year}}{\text{No. of women giving birth during same year}}$	per 100,000
Neonatal mortality rate =	$\dfrac{\text{No. of deaths of infants under 28 days of age in 1 year}}{\text{No. of live births in same year}}$	per 100,000 live births
Prevalence rate =	$\dfrac{\text{No. of old and new cases of specified illness during a specified time interval}}{\text{Estimated mid-interval population at risk}}$	per 1000

rate, fertility rate, maternal mortality rate, neonatal mortality rate, and infant mortality rate. Table 6-1 provides formulas for these and other rates that are described in this chapter.

SOURCES OF DATA

There are several sources of data routinely collected on disease occurrence. Local, state, and federal health departments regularly conduct disease surveillance activities; both incidence and mortality rate data are generated as part of these activities.

Vital records, including birth certificates, marriage certificates, and death certificates are filed for every individual. Each state maintains death certificates for every person who dies in that state. Death certificates contain information on date, place, and cause of death, along with the date of birth, the age at death, usual occupation, and next-of-kin information for the deceased. Several public health agencies require disease notification and registration for a number of communicable diseases and certain chronic diseases such as cancer. Morbidity surveys such as the National Health Survey are another important source of information.

Data on special populations such as the Armed Forces, participants in medical care, or insurance plans are also used. Data on both disease occurrence and risk factors for disease occurrence may be generated from hospital records, medical records, school records, and occupational records. Descriptive surveys and interviews also may be conducted to provide data on risk factors and, less frequently, disease occurrence. Sometimes laboratory data generated as part of an earlier study may be available; other times biologic measurements are made using blood or other samples collected specifically for a particular study. In an experimental trial, participants may routinely undergo physical examinations at regular intervals throughout the study to monitor health status.

METHODS USED IN EPIDEMIOLOGIC RESEARCH
Observational Studies

There are two major types of study design used in epidemiologic research; one is observational, the other experimental. Figure 6-4 provides an outline of the various study designs used in epidemiologic research. In an **observational study,** data are generated through "observations" of study participants. Observational studies may be either descriptive or analytic.

Descriptive studies. In a **descriptive study,** an epidemiologist studies patterns of disease occurrence by person, place, or time to develop hypotheses concerning disease etiology. Important clues may be derived by looking at differences in disease incidence or mortality by geographic location, ethnicity, race, sex, age, or socioeconomic status. Clustering of disease cases by time and place may be significant. Trends in mortality or incidence rates over time are also of interest.

In an *ecologic* study the investigator compares aggregate data for entire populations; for example, lung cancer rates for the population of urban counties with high air pollution levels might be compared with lung cancer rates for rural counties with low air pollution levels (Shy & Struba, 1982). The problem with this type of study is that the researcher is looking at averaged data for an entire group or community. One cannot be sure whether those persons with the disease are actually the persons who were exposed to the risk factor of interest. The two groups being compared may be different in other ways, leading the investigator to draw the wrong conclusion about any association he or she observes. For example, in the study of lung cancer mentioned above, perhaps the difference in group rates is a result of the supposition that urban residents are more likely to smoke cigarettes than rural inhabitants and not because of differences in air pollution. For these reasons, it is also important to conduct analytic studies before assuming that any associations or patterns seen in a descriptive study are causal in nature.

Analytic studies. An **analytic study** is focused on a specific hypothesis regarding disease etiology. In laboratory studies the investigator may conduct experiments in which disease is induced in animals by exposing them to the agent suspected of carrying the disease. For both ethical and practical reasons, this method is *not* used to determine the cause of disease in human populations, except in a few very rare instances in-

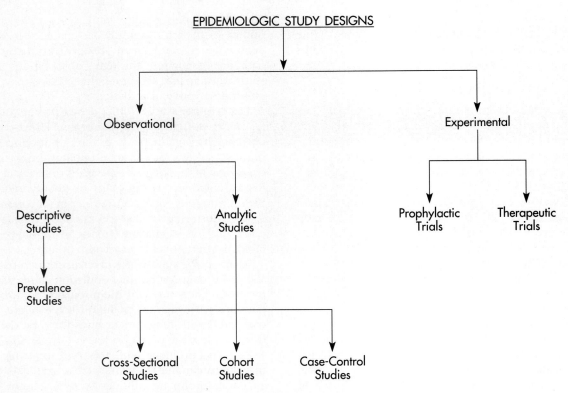

FIGURE 6-4 Various study designs used in epidemiologic research.

volving volunteers. Data are generated through observation rather than direct intervention and experimental manipulation of study participants. There are three types of analytic study designs used by epidemiologists to *test* hypotheses regarding disease etiology: the cross-sectional study, the case-control study, and the cohort study.

Cross-sectional studies. In a **cross-sectional study,** the risk factor and disease outcome of interest are assessed at the same point. For example, the researcher may study a group of textile workers to determine whether workers exposed to Fiber X are more likely to have lung disease than workers with jobs that do not involve exposure to Fiber X. The problem with cross-sectional studies is that the workers are studied at only one point. The investigator cannot always be sure that exposure preceded disease. Perhaps a worker had lung disease before being exposed to Fiber X. Furthermore, it is possible that lung disease actually develops more fre-

quently in workers exposed to Fiber X than other workers. However, once lung disease develops in the workers, they are no longer able to do the heavy work required by their job and are transferred to less physically demanding desk jobs where there is no exposure to Fiber X. In this case, the investigator might see no difference in the proportion of currently exposed workers with lung disease and the proportion of currently unexposed workers with lung disease even though Fiber X actually causes lung disease. For these reasons, the cross-sectional design is not used as commonly as the case-control or cohort approach.

Cohort studies. In a **cohort study,** the investigator starts by determining the exposure status of a cohort (group) of individuals. The cohort is then followed *prospectively* (forward) to determine their disease experience over time. The incidence of disease in exposed cohort members is then compared with the incidence of disease in nonexposed cohort members. Studies of chronic diseases such as cancer are often difficult to conduct in this fashion because there may be many years between exposure to a carcinogenic agent and the subsequent development of cancer. Sometimes it is possible to conduct a historical cohort study. For example, if a factory has the original employment records of all workers going back to 1950, an investigator could take the cohort of workers hired between 1950 and 1960, classify them as to their occupational exposures using plant records from that time, and then follow them to the present to determine which workers contracted or died from the disease in question. When a cohort study is not feasible, either because of the number of years it would take to complete or because the disease being studied is relatively rare, an alternative is to conduct a case-control study.

Case-control studies. The **case-control study** is *retrospective* in nature. The investigator begins with a group of people who have already contracted the disease under study (cases), and compares them with a group of people who do not have the disease (controls). Controls are generally selected so as to be similar to cases with regard to other factors that affect disease risk, such as age, race, and sex. This is called matching. Past exposure to the suspected risk factor is then determined for both cases and controls.

Experimental Studies

In an **experimental study** there is a deliberate *intervention* by the investigator. Study participants are randomly assigned to an intervention group by the investigator at the beginning of the study. The effects of the intervention may then be determined by comparing subsequent disease experience in the different intervention groups. Preventive trials evaluate whether an intervention successfully prevents the development of disease; therapeutic trials test the effectiveness of interventions designed to treat existing disease.

STATISTICAL CONCEPTS

Once epidemiologic data are collected, they are analyzed, and the results of these analyses are then interpreted. To understand and apply the epidemiologic literature, it is important for the community health nurse to understand related statistical concepts he or she may encounter during review of the literature.

Measures of Association

The *correlation coefficient* (r) measures the strength of association between two variables. It ranges from −1.0 to 1.0; zero indicates no association. A positive value for r indicates that the two variables are positively correlated. That is, as one variable increases so does the other. A negative value for r indicates that the two variables are inversely correlated. That is, as one variable increases, the other decreases. For example, if researchers looked at the height and weight of 100 school children, and found that the two variables had a correlation coefficient of −10.8, they could conclude that there is a strong, positive correlation between height and weight. If they found a correlation coefficient of −0.5, they would conclude that there is a moderate inverse correlation between the variables; in other words, as height goes up, weight goes down, and vice versa. A correlation coefficient measures only whether two variables are associated. It can not be used to infer cause and effect.

The **relative risk** measures the strength of association between a specific factor or exposure, and risk of disease.

$$\text{Relative risk} = \frac{\text{Incidence rate among exposed individuals}}{\text{Incidence rate among nonexposed individuals}}$$

Basically, it describes the risk of the exposed group relative to the risk of the unexposed group. A relative risk (RR) of 2.0 means that exposed individuals are twice as likely to contract a disease as unexposed individuals. In case-control studies, risk is reported using the odds ratio (OR), which is interpreted in a similar fashion to relative risk. Keep in mind that relative risk estimates indicate the *probability* of contracting disease, given exposure. Not everyone who is exposed to the suspected risk factor necessarily contracts the disease; not everyone who has a disease has been exposed to the suspected risk factor.

Attributable risk is a measure of the *absolute* amount of risk or incidence of disease that can be attributed to exposure. The attributable risk is equal to the incidence rate in the exposed population *minus* the incidence rate in the unexposed population.

Screening Tests

Screening programs are an important part of disease prevention. To be effective, a screening test must be acceptable to the persons who will be screened (Valanis, 1992). It must also be relatively inexpensive, since it will be administered to large groups of individuals, and it must be simple and safe to administer. The test must be able to detect disease at an early enough stage so that prompt treatment will be effective in altering disease outcome, and an effective treatment must be available. If there is no effective treatment for the disease in question, one must seriously consider whether it is ethical to screen for that disease at all. Finally, the disease of interest must be sufficiently serious to warrant the cost involved in administering the screening program.

Screening tests are frequently used in the secondary prevention of disease. To determine the usefulness of a screening test, one must know the sensitivity, specificity, and predictive value of the test. **Sensitivity** measures the probability that a person with a disease will be classified as having the disease. **Specificity** measures the probability that a person who is free of disease will be classified as disease-free.

Sensitivity

$$= \frac{\text{Number of diseased people with positive test results}}{\text{Number of people with disease}}$$

Specificity

$$= \frac{\text{Number of disease-free people with negative test results}}{\text{Number of disease-free people}}$$

A screening test can have high sensitivity without having high specificity, and vice versa. For example, the hemoccult test screens for the presence of blood in human feces. It is used as a screening test for colon cancer. Most individuals with colon cancer will have positive hemoccult test results (Greegor, 1971, 1972). Therefore, the test is highly *sensitive*. However, there are many other diseases that may lead to the presence of blood in the feces. Therefore, the hemoccult test is not very *specific* as a test for colon cancer. Sigmoidoscopy, which involves a direct examination of the sigmoid colon with a colonoscope, is far more specific and has high sensitivity as well. However, it is invasive and relatively expensive and therefore not practical as a screening test for a large population group. The hemoccult test is relatively noninvasive, easy to administer, and inexpensive. Therefore, despite its low specificity, it is widely used. Persons with positive test results are then referred for more specific testing.

The other statistic commonly reported for a screening test is the predictive value. The predictive value indicates what proportion of people with positive test results actually have the disease in question.

Predictive Value

$$= \frac{\text{Number of diseased people with positive test results}}{\substack{\text{Number of people with positive test results} \\ \text{(true positive plus false positive)}}}$$

Other Measures

In experimental trials the researcher is generally interested in the magnitude (size) of the difference between groups. There are specific statistical tests that are used to determine whether any differences observed are statistically significant. For continuous outcome data such as blood pressure, the researcher might report the difference in *mean* (average) blood pressure levels for the group treated with drug Z (treatment group) and the group not treated with drug Z (placebo group).

The researcher may also look at differences in the proportion of patients who die of a disease in one group versus another. For example, suppose the researcher is asked to evaluate the effectiveness of a new chemotherapeutic agent for the treatment of pancreatic cancer. He or she might compare the proportion of patients in the treatment group who have died after 6 months and the proportion of patients in the placebo group who have died after 6 months. It is important to note that in a clinical trial both the placebo group and the treatment group always receive the best available medically established treatment for their disease. The treatment group *also* receives the experimental drug under evaluation.

Statistical Significance

When a researcher tests the statistical significance of an association between two or more variables, the hypothesis to be tested is always given as the *null hypothesis.* For tests that involve the comparison of two groups, the null hypothesis states that there is no difference between the two groups with regard to the variable of interest (*e.g.,* a risk factor or experimental intervention) (Morton, 1990). In a case-control study concerning the association between cigarette smoking and lung cancer, the null hypothesis would be that there is no association between cigarette smoking and lung cancer in the cases and controls being studied. If the investigator found a statistically significant association between the two variables (*i.e.,* lung cancer and cigarette smoking), the null hypothesis of no association would be *rejected.*

Sometimes a difference between groups is nothing more than a chance finding, the result of random variation. The *p*-value indicates the likelihood that a difference between groups or an association between two variables, such as a risk factor and disease, can be accounted for by chance alone. When an investigator reports that a result is statistically significant at the $p < 0.05$ level, it means there is only a 5% possibility of rejecting the null hypothesis when it should not be rejected. Another way of saying this is that there is a 95% probability that an association is real, rather than a chance finding.

The *p*-value is important in determining the statistical significance of a finding. However, it is important to keep in mind that a difference between groups may be nonsignificant and still be real, especially if the sample size is small. Also, when a study has a very large sample size, small differences between groups may be *statistically* significant without being *clinically* significant.

CAUSALITY

Detecting **causal relationships** may be the key to interrupting a chain of events that can lead to disease or disability. However, when interpreting the results of a single epidemiologic study, a researcher *cannot* automatically assume that an association between risk factor and disease is causal. It may actually be an artifact caused by a chance occurrence or bias in the study methods. Measurement error and bias arising from the selection of study participants are examples of bias that can lead to spurious relationships. It is also possible that an association may be real but noncausal in nature. A noncausal relationship may result when the disease causes the risk factor (rather than the other way around), or when the disease and the exposure are both related to a third variable. In this case the risk factor associated with the disease in a study could just be an indirect measure of another exposure variable that the investigator has not considered. Before a causal association can be established, other possible risk factors that could explain the finding must be eliminated. There must be sufficient evidence that the risk factor of interest increases or decreases the likelihood that a disease event may occur. To achieve validity, studies must be repeated in unrelated population groups.

The 1964 Surgeon General's report regarding smoking and health outcomes established five criteria that must be fulfilled to establish a causal relationship (U.S. Department of Health, Education, and Welfare,* 1964):

1. Temporality: Exposure precedes disease.
2. Strength of association:
    a. The larger the risk ratio, the greater the likelihood that the risk factor affects the disease outcome.
    b. Dose-response gradient: With increasing levels of exposure to the risk factor, a corresponding increase in the occurrence of disease is found.
3. Specificity: It must be possible to predict the occurrence of one variable (*e.g.,* exposure) in relation to the extent or occurrence of another (*e.g.,* disease outcome).
4. Consistency: The association found in one study must persist in other studies with other populations and/or different designs.
5. Biological plausibility: There must be a reasonable biological explanation for the occurrence of an event, one that coincides with current knowledge about the factor and the disease or disability.

* The Department of Health, Education, and Welfare is now the Department of Health and Human Services.

This list was expanded to include three additional criteria by Sir A. Bradford Hill in his landmark presidential address on association and causation (Hill, 1965). The additional criteria discussed by Hill include:

6. Biological coherence: Agreement of results with findings of experimental research and clinical observations.
7. Effect of intervention: Removal of the putative cause results in a significant reduction in disease incidence.
8. Analogy: Drugs or chemicals that are structural analogs of a harmful agent may also induce similar harmful effects (considered a weak criterion).

Hill notes that some of the eight criteria summarized above are stronger than others, and that it is not necessary to fulfill all of these criteria to establish causality.

The 1980 surgeon general's report entitled *The Health Consequences of Smoking for Women* provides an example of how these criteria may be applied to determine whether there is a causal association between a risk factor and a disease outcome (U.S. Department of Health, Education, and Welfare, 1980). A review of various research findings concerning maternal smoking during pregnancy and low birth-weight infants revealed the following:

• Temporality: Many investigators have documented that women who smoke during pregnancy are more likely to deliver low birth-weight infants than women who do not smoke during pregnancy. Exposure, which occurs during pregnancy while the fetus is developing, precedes event (low birth-weight infant).
• Strength of association: The results of many studies about the relationship between smoking and birth weight are reviewed in the surgeon general's report; they show a strong association between maternal cigarette smoking and delivery of infants of lower birth weight. Infants born to mothers who smoke were reported to be two times more likely to have a birth weight under 2500 grams than infants born to women who do not smoke. There also is a dose-response relation-ship: the more cigarettes a woman smokes, the greater the reduction in birth weight.

• Biological plausibility: Available evidence shows that cigarette smokers' infants tend to be smaller for gestational age rather than gestationally premature.
• Specificity: Infants of smokers have lower birth weights than do infants of nonsmokers. When a variety of other factors (*e.g.,* age, parity, previous pregnancy history, and prenatal visits) that are also known or suspected to exert an influence on birth weight have been controlled for, cigarette smoking is still shown to be related to low birth weight.
• Consistency: The association between maternal smoking and low birth weight has been shown in many countries among different cultures and in different geographical settings. Results have been replicated in many different populations by a variety of investigators using different types of study design.
• Biologic coherence: The infants of smokers experience an accelerated growth rate during the first 6 months after delivery compared with infants of nonsmokers. Data from experiments in animals have documented that exposure to various constituents of cigarette smoking (*e.g.,* nicotine) may result in the delivery of low birth-weight offspring.
• Effect of intervention: If a woman gives up smoking by her fourth month of gestation, risk of delivering a low birth-weight infant is similar to that of a nonsmoker.

Based on this assessment, a causal association between smoking and low birth weight was established, and appropriate warning labels are now carried on packages of cigarettes (see also U.S. Department of Health, Education, and Welfare, 1979).

INVESTIGATING A NEW DISEASE

To carry out effective disease prevention activities at the primary, secondary, and tertiary levels, it is first necessary to know something about the natural history of a disease; high risk groups must be identified, and risk factors associated with the disease of interest must be determined. When a clinical report concerning a new or unusual complex of symptoms first appears in the medical literature, it is just the beginning of a long and complicated process. To provide the information necessary to plan appropriate disease prevention and control activities, epidemiologists and other public health professionals must investigate this new disease or condition in a systematic manner. The box below provides a brief overview of the various steps that must be carried out when investigating a new disease or syndrome. Of particular importance is the establishment of a working case definition, which can then be used by different researchers investigating the new disease or syndrome. This helps to ensure that researchers are all studying the same condition, and provides a starting point for the investigations that are to be conducted. Frequently the initial case definition is refined once more information is available on the natural history and etiology of the condition (Valanis, 1992).

APPLICATIONS OF EPIDEMIOLOGIC CONCEPTS TO COMMUNITY HEALTH NURSING

The community health nurse can participate in the epidemiologic process in a number of ways. He or she may work as part of a research team, conducting interviews or collecting other types of data, or becoming involved in monitoring the health status of individuals taking part in a preventive or therapeutic trial. The community health nurse working in a health agency can also use data on disease frequency in planning the allocation of health agency resources within a community. Most importantly, the community health nurse can apply epidemiologic concepts and use study results to plan and conduct disease prevention activities at the primary, secondary, and tertiary levels. The information generated by epidemiologic studies may be used during a case study assessment to help determine which individuals in a family or community are at high risk of contracting a disease or disability. On a community level, epidemiologic data and concepts may be used to identify high risk groups within the community and to develop health education and promotion programs appropriate for these groups of individuals. The case study provided is an example of one way in which community health nurses may apply epidemiologic information and concepts in their work.

INVESTIGATING A NEW DISEASE

- Establish case definition
- Conduct active case finding
- Determine incidence, prevalence of disease
- Revise case definition
- Determine risk factors associated with disease
- Conduct therapeutic and/or prophylactic trials
- Implement disease control activities (primary, secondary, tertiary prevention) at the community level

---

■ CASE STUDY

Nurse Smith works for the Elmwood County health department. She has been placed in charge of developing new guidelines on AIDS prevention for community health nurses who work for the county. These guidelines must provide information on prevention activities at the primary, secondary, and tertiary levels. As part of her background research, Ms. Smith reviews the epidemiologic literature concerning the distribution and etiology of AIDS; she also researches the most current information available concerning the natural history of AIDS, and investigates AIDS prevention programs currently in place at other county health departments. During this process she determines the incidence and prevalence of HIV-positive and AIDS cases in the United States, and reviews available information on incidence and prevalence of AIDS for her own state and county. She collects the latest information concerning the manner in which HIV is transmitted and methods of preventing its transmission. Nurse Smith identifies groups of individuals who are at high

TABLE 6-2   Prepathogenesis and pathogenesis of acquired immunodeficiency syndrome (AIDS)

Prepathogenesis:	Period of pathogenesis:		
Primary prevention Health promotion Specific protection*	**Secondary prevention** Early diagnosis and treatment: HIV positive (latent stage)	**Tertiary prevention** Limitation of disability: onset of clinical symptoms of AIDS	Rehabilitation/palliative: onset of opportunistic infections known as disease indicators

1. Encourage education of children as early as possible about the manner in which HIV is transferred
2. Screen all blood products for presence of HIV
3. Educate IV drug users about danger of sharing needles
4. Teach safer sexual practices:
  a. avoid sexual practices that injure mucosal tissue
  b. limit partners
  c. use condoms
  d. consider abstinence
5. Educate health care workers to use universal precautions recommended by the CDC
6. Teach HIV positive individuals how to avoid passing infection, including:
  a. teach/use good hand washing
  b. teach/use needle precaution
  c. teach/use universal precautions
  d. use gloves during contact with body fluids
  e. use bleach such as Clorox for spills and clothes washing, etc.
	Men:
	1. Avoid infections
	2. Have regular checkups
	3. Avoid passing infection (see Primary Prevention)
	4. Get adequate rest, nutrition, exercise
	5. Maintain full employment, confidentiality
	Women (in addition to above):
	1. Avoid pregnancy
	2. If pregnant, request a cesarean section
	3. Do not breast-feed
	Child:
	1. Encourage medical supervision
	2. Avoid infection
	3. Maintain quality of life
	4. Check status of parents
		1. Encourage compliance with medical regimen
		2. Make patient aware of side effects
		3. Encourage employment as long as possible
		4. Provide counseling for client and family
		5. Take appropriate precautions to prevent opportunistic infection
			1. Counsel patients and family
			2. Maintain medical regimen
			3. Maintain quality of life by maintaining nutrition and limiting discomfort
			4. Assist patient/family in obtaining social sevices and financial assistance

*Specific protection: prevent HIV exposure of susceptible HIV-negative individuals (no vaccine available).
AIDS, Acquired immunodeficiency syndrome; HIV, human immunodeficiency virus; IV, intravenous.
Modified from *The natural history of disease in man.* (p. 21) by H.R. Leavell & E.G. Clark, 1965, New York: McGraw Hill.

risk of becoming infected with HIV, and she evaluates high-risk behaviors for HIV transmission among these groups.

After completing her background research, Ms. Smith develops guidelines for primary, secondary, and tertiary prevention activities using the Leavell and Clark model of the natural history of disease in hu-

mans as a framework. This allows her to organize her recommendations in such a way that they may be applied according to the clinical status (stage of disease) of the individual client seen by the community health nurse. The guidelines developed by Nurse Smith are summarized in Table 6-2.

Chapter Highlights

- Epidemiology is a science that studies the occurrence of disease in human populations.

- The science of epidemiology has evolved over a long period. Pioneers in the field of epidemiology include John Graunt, William Farr, John Snow, and Joseph Goldberger.

- Important biologic concepts include the natural history of disease, mode of transmission, reservoirs of infection, and immunity.

- Important epidemiologic concepts include the epidemiologic triangle, the three levels of prevention, and causality.

- The incidence rate and the prevalence rate are important measures of disease frequency (morbidity, mortality).

- Observational study designs used by epidemiologists include ecologic studies, cross-sectional studies, case-control studies, and cohort studies.

- Experimental studies include preventive trials and therapeutic trials. Experimental studies involve a specific intervention.

- Important measures of association include the correlation coefficient, relative risk, attributable risk, and the odds ratio.

- An association between a risk factor and a disease may be spurious, noncausal, or causal. Certain criteria must be met before a causal relationship may be established.

- Community health nurses can apply epidemiologic concepts and principles to their practice.

 ## CRITICAL THINKING EXERCISE

The health consequence of smoking for women described in the surgeon general's report in 1980 indicated a causal relationship between smoking and low birth weight.

1. What kind of research determined causality?
2. Describe primary, secondary, and tertiary prevention that will prevent low birth weight in the children of mothers who smoke.

REFERENCES

Ahlbom, A. & Norell, S. (1990). *Introduction to modern epidemiology* (2nd ed.). Chestnut Hill, MA: Epidemiology Resources, Inc.

Benenson, A.S. (1990). *Control of communicable diseases in man* (15th ed.). Washington, D.C.: American Public Health Association.

Berkow, R. & Fletcher, A.J. (Eds.) (1992). *The Merck manual of diagnosis and therapy* (16th ed.). Rahway, N.J.: Merck & Co., Inc.

Cohen, I. (1984). Florence Nightingale. *Scientific American 20*(3), 128, 133.

Farr, W. (1975). *Vital statistics: A memorial volume of selections from the reports and writings of William Farr.* Metsusen, N.J.: New York Academy of Medicine.

Fraser, D.W., Tsai, T.R., Orenstein, W., Parkin, W.E., Beecham, H.J., Sharrer, R.G., Harris, J., Mallisons, G.F., Martin, S.M., McDade, J.E., Shepard, C.C., Brachman, P.S., & the Field Investigation Team (1977). Legionnaires' disease: Description of an epidemic of pneumonia. *New England Journal of Medicine 297*:1189-97.

Frost, W.H. (1923). The importance of epidemiology as a function of health departments. *Medical Officer 29*:113-114.

Frost, W.H. (Ed.). (1936). *Snow on cholera.* New York: The Commonwealth Fund.

Goldberger, J. & Wheeler, G.A. (1964). The experimental production of pellagra in human subjects by means of diet. In Terrace, M. (Ed.). *Goldberger on Pellagra.* Baton Rouge: Louisiana State University Press.

Goldberger, J., Waring, C.H., & Tanner, W.F. (1923). Pellagra prevention by diet among institution inmates. *Public Health Reports 38*:2361-2368.

Greegor, D.H. (1971). Occult blood testing for detection of asymptomatic colon cancer. *Cancer 28*:131-134.

Greegor, D.H. (1972). A progress report: Detection of colorectal cancer using guaic slides. *Cancer 22*:360-363.

Hill, A.B.H. (1965). The environment and disease: Association or causation? *Proceedings of the Royal Society of Medicine 58*:295-300.

Hippocrates. (1939 Translation). *The genuine works of Hippocrates translated from the Greek by Francis Adam.* Baltimore: Williams & Wilkins.

Lattimer, G. & Ormbsbee, R.A. (1981). *Legionnaires' disease.* New York: Marcel Dekker, Inc.

Leavell, H.R. & Clark, E.G. (1965). *Preventive medicine for the doctor in his community: An epidemiologic approach* (3rd ed.). New York: McGraw-Hill.

Lilienfeld, A. & Lilienfeld, D. (1980). *Foundations of epidemiology.* New York: Oxford University Press.

Lilienfeld, A.M. (1983). Wade Hampton Frost: Contributions to epidemiology and public health. *American Journal of Epidemiology 117*:379-383.

Mausner, J.S. & Bahn, A.K. (1985). *Epidemiology, An introductory text* (2nd ed.). Philadelphia: WB Saunders Co.

Morton, R.F., Hebel, J.R. & McCarter, R.J. (1990). *A study guide to epidemiology and biostatistics* (3rd ed.). Rockville, MD: Aspen Publishers, Inc.

Rothman, K.J. (1986). *Modern epidemiology.* Boston: Little, Brown & Co.

Shy, C.M., & Struba, R.J. (1982). In D. Schottenfeld & F. Fraumene (Eds.), *Air and water pollution in cancer, epidemiology, and prevention* (Ch. 19). Philadelphia: WB Saunders.

Smith, G. (1941). *Plague on us.* London: Oxford University Press.

Snow, J. (1936). *On the mode of communication of cholera* (2nd ed.). Reprinted in: Frost, W.H., (Ed.) (1936). *Snow on cholera.* New York: The Commonwealth Fund.

Stanhope, M. & Lancaster, J. (1992). *Community health nursing.* St. Louis: Mosby.

Tuchman, B.W. (1978). *A distant mirror.* New York: Alfred A. Knopf.

U.S. Department of Health, Education, and Welfare (1964). *Smoking and health: Report of the Advisory Committee to the Surgeon General of the Public Health Service.* Public Health Service Publication No. 1103, Washington, D.C.: U.S. Government Printing Office.

U.S. Department of Health, Education, and Welfare, Public Health Service, Office on Smoking Health (1979). *Smoking and health: A report of the Surgeon General.* DHEW Publication No. (PHS) 79-50066. Washington, D.C.: U.S. Government Printing Office.

U.S. Department of Health and Human Services, Public Health Service, Office on Smoking and Health (1980). *The health consequences of smoking for women: A report of the surgeon general.* Washington, D.C.: U.S. Government Printing Office.

Valanis, B. (1992). *Epidemiology in nursing and health care* (2nd ed.). Norwalk, CT: Appleton & Lange.

Health and Wellness in the Community

Carole A. Gutt

There will either be an increase in wellness or a depressed, deprived, depleted and short-lived society which will not be recognizable. We can't continue to survive living the way we do, physically, economically, and environmentally. Since there are too many survivors among us, wellness must and will prevail.

Donald B. Ardell

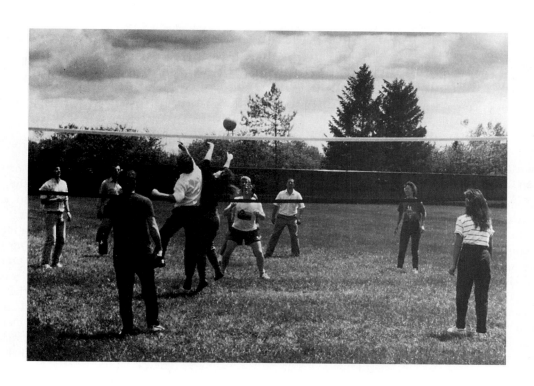

OBJECTIVES

At the conclusion of this chapter, the student will be able to:

1. Define the key terms listed.
2. Describe the historical development of the wellness movement in the United States.
3. Identify individuals who have contributed to the development of the wellness movement.
4. Differentiate among wellness, disease prevention, health education, medical self-care, health promotion, and holistic health.
5. Describe selected wellness models that can be applied to community health nursing.
6. Integrate concepts of teaching/learning with selected wellness models.
7. Discuss the components of wellness.
8. Describe alternative treatment modalities in holistic care.
9. Discuss the role of the community health nurse in wellness education.

KEY TERMS

Alternative or complementary treatment modalities
Disease prevention
Environmental sensitivity
Health
Health behavior contract

Health belief model
Health education
Health promotion
Holistic health
Inner harmony
Lifestyle assessment questionnaire

Medical self-care
Nutrition
Physical fitness
Self-efficacy model
Wellness

HISTORICAL DEVELOPMENT OF THE WELLNESS MOVEMENT

The Roman philosopher Seneca said more than 1900 years ago, "Man does not die, he kills himself." The growing public awareness of wellness as a concept is related to several contributing factors and movements that occurred in the late 1970s. These trends came together as a force and shaped the climate and nature of the wellness movement.

Until the late 1970s the approach to health was curative rather than preventive. At that time several landmark publications brought to the public's attention the need to emphasize preventive aspects of health. In 1975 several prominent American foundations pooled their resources

and published a two-volume collection of works that reflected growing concern with the status quo of the health care delivery system at that time and the need for sweeping reforms to include wellness concepts and changes in lifestyle. These works were John Knowles's *Doing Better and Feeling Worse* (1977) and *Future Directions in Health Care. Dietary Goals,* a report issued by the Senate Select Committee on Nutrition and Human Needs (1977), showed a direct link between diet and disease and called for major adjustments in American dietary patterns, including marked decreases in consumption of meat, dairy products, sugar, and salt.

In 1979 the American Hospital Association (AHA) issued a policy statement entitled "Hospitals' Responsibility for Health Promotion." As a result, several American hospitals established health promotion and wellness programs. These programs became a routine extension of hospital-based care in the 1980s; however, at the time of the AHA report the concept was relatively unknown and innovative.

Perhaps the most well-known and significant report in terms of impact was the 1979 document entitled *Healthy People* issued by the secretary of the Department of Health, Education, and Welfare (now the Department of Health and Human Services). *Healthy People* stressed that many of the illnesses prevalent in our society could be avoided by a change in lifestyle and environment. A shift from high-technology, medical-model, and acute hospital-based care was urged, with emphasis on health promotion and disease prevention.

A major contributing factor in the development of the wellness movement of the 1970s was the cost crisis that occurred in health care. Americans suddenly found that medical bills were soaring to unheard-of heights. There were annual increases in health care spending both at the federal governmental level in terms of the percentage of the gross national product being consumed for health care and personal individual expenses. Large corporations and businesses found that employees' medical costs, coupled with rising inflation rates, were cutting into their profit margins, necessitating increased costs to their customers. Financial motivation proved to be a powerful impetus for companies to look at ways to improve the health of their employees before they became ill. Direct benefits to companies were measurable in terms of reduced absenteeism and turnover and improved employee morale. Cures are costly, and sustaining chronic illnesses with resulting disability proved overwhelming for many companies. Wellness measures with lifestyle-related interventions were cost effective and easy to design and implement not only in the workplace but also in school and community settings.

Blue Shield of Northern California initiated what was perhaps the first practical application of these concepts when it issued the "Stay Well Plan" in 1978. Employees of the Mendocino school district were the target population of the plan. They were offered classes on a variety of topics related to health and self-care. They also were offered financial incentives if they used less than $500 of medical care benefits in 1 year. The district saved considerable monies in insurance premiums, and Blue Shield was able to decrease its premium rates as a result of the program.

Consumer consciousness came to play a vital role in the development of the wellness movement. The media became increasingly involved with dissemination of health information to the public. At the same time the public began to emphasize its desire to care for its own minor medical needs. American consumers wanted to take an active part in the control of their own health needs rather than having those needs dictated by health professionals. This public interest in self-treatment has been referred to as the "third wave of health" by some prominent health educators. Coupled with a growing consumer consciousness was a heightened mind-body awareness resulting from political, ideological, and sociological changes that occurred in this country after the Vietnam War. The "baby boom" generation had reached young adulthood and placed an awesome burden on the health care delivery system. This segment of the population, which began to approach middle age in the 1980s, is beginning to fall prey to many of the lifestyle-related diseases first noted in the 1970s. For example, individuals who have been sedentary and obese as young adults will be at greater risk of contracting heart disease as they age. The influence of Eastern philosophies and psychological theories of self-actualization also was evident as consumers of health care began to seek holistic alternatives to the scientific models of care to which they had been accustomed.

During this same time frame, several other shifts were occurring in society. The women's movement became a strong political and personal force in this country. Its proponents urged women to question their medical care and assume personal responsibility for their own health needs. Ecologists also began to give loud public voice to concerns related to environmental effects on health. Physical fitness became almost an obsession with large segments of the American population. This was due in part to published results of studies on the growing incidence of coronary heart disease in this country. Americans were urged to jog, do aerobics, and eat natural, healthful foods. The quality of life was seen as something that the health consumer could and should control. Researchers began to supply health care deliverers with findings relevant to the impact of improved lifestyles on health and the quality of life. The 1970 Framingham study on risk factors and heart disease formed the baseline for many of our current health hazard appraisal instruments. Also in 1970, the surgeon general's report on smoking and health provided the first definitive link between smoking and various diseases of both a chronic and lethal nature. Several organizations played a key role in the wellness movement, including the President's Council on Physical Fitness and Sports, the Society for Prospective Medicine, the American Federation of Fitness Directors in Business, and chapters of the Young Men's Christian Association throughout the country. It is important to note that none of these factors operated in isolation. It was the dovetailing and meshing of the various forces that produced the wellness/health movement of today (Ardell, 1985).

PROMINENT INDIVIDUALS IN THE WELLNESS/HEALTH MOVEMENT

Halpert L. Dunn was perhaps the most notable visionary in the early wellness movement. In 1961 he published his landmark work entitled *High-Level Wellness,* the first publication to signifi-cantly influence health professionals and introduce them to the total concept of wellness. Dunn stressed the need for mind/body/spirit connections and their importance to total well-being. He repeatedly stressed the need for valued purposes in life and the necessity of personal satisfaction in the maintenance of a healthy state. Health, according to Dunn, was much more than nonillness, which was the traditional view of health until this time.

Belloc and Breslow (1972) studied the effect of health care skills on life expectancy and quality of life. Their results showed that individuals who observed six to seven basic practices could expect to live longer lives. These practices included moderate use of alcohol or abstinence, daily breakfast, three regular meals daily, moderate weight, non-smoking, 7 to 8 hours of sleep daily, and moderate exercise twice weekly.

John Travis, one of Dunn's earliest followers, developed a health/wellness model (1977) that compared traditional views of health to a self-responsibility model. The illness-wellness continuum is used frequently by wellness-oriented practitioners (Figure 7-1). At one end of the continuum is the treatment model, which moves along the continuum and stops at a neutral point in the middle. At this point there is no discernible illness or wellness. The model for self-responsibility goes beyond this point and encompasses education, growth, and self-actualization, with the achievement of high-level wellness at the other end of the continuum. Travis' *The Wellness Workbook for Helping Professionals,* pub-

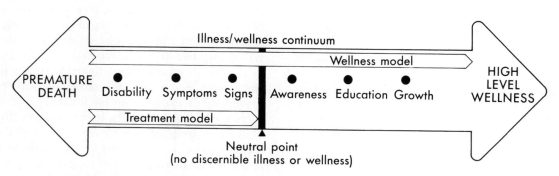

FIGURE 7-1 Travis' illness/wellness continuum. (*From* The wellness workbook *by J.W. Travis & R.S. Ryan, 1981, Berkeley, CA: Ten Speed Press. Copyright 1981 by Ten Speed Press. Reprinted by permission.*)

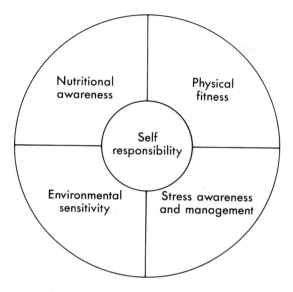

FIGURE 7-2 Ardell's wellness model. (*From* 14 Days to a wellness lifestyle *by D. Ardell, 1982, San Rafael, CA: New World Library. Copyright 1982 by New World Library. Reprinted by permission.*)

lished in 1977 and updated in 1981, still is used extensively today in wellness courses throughout the country.

Another book, Donald Ardell's *High-Level Wellness: An Alternative to Doctors, Drugs and Disease* also was published in 1977. This work provided a framework and an ethic that were to guide most future programs in wellness. Ardell outlined five dimensions of wellness that need to be considered by practitioners in the development of wellness approaches and programs: self-responsibility, nutritional awareness, stress management, physical fitness, and environmental sensitivity. Self-responsibility is depicted as the center of the other dimensions. It is crucial to the development and implementation of well-related behaviors in the other four spheres (Figure 7-2).

William Hettler, while serving as the head of the student health service at the University of Wisconsin during the 1970s, developed the first student-led wellness model. This model is used extensively in colleges and universities throughout the country. His efforts led to the inception of the annual wellness festivals held at Stevens

Point, Wisconsin, which were instrumental in dissemination of wellness-promoting activities nationwide (Ardell, 1985).

Certainly numerous other individuals contributed to the development of the wellness movement as it has come to be called, but the individuals named here defined the foundations and key concepts of wellness.

TERMS USED IN THE WELLNESS MOVEMENT

Students who read on the topic of wellness might easily become confused by the vast spectrum of terminology that describes wellness and its related concepts. Very often these terms are used interchangeably, which increases the general confusion.

Health itself has been defined in a variety of ways and from differing perspectives. The first definition of health to deviate from a purely biological orientation was that issued by the World Health Organization in 1947. It defined health as "a state of complete physical, mental, and social well-being and not merely the absence of disease or infirmity." The importance of this definition was its inclusion of psychosocial considerations. Halpert Dunn's definition of health is considered conclusive: "health is an integrated method of functioning which is oriented toward maximizing the potential of which the individual is capable, within the environment where he is functioning" (Dunn, 1961, p. 5). Donald Ardell integrated concepts of health, wellness, and prevention and defined what he called high-level wellness as "a lifestyle-focused approach designed for the purpose of pursuing the highest level of health within one's capability. A wellness lifestyle is dynamic or everchanging as the individual evolves throughout life. It is an integrated lifestyle in that it incorporates some approach or aspect of each wellness dimension" (Ardell, 1977, p. 65).

Rene Dubos, philosopher and microbiologist, defined health from an ecological perspective as an expression of fitness to the environment, that is, as a state of adaptedness. It is the condition of the whole person engaged in effective and fruitful interaction with the physical and social environment. Health then represents freedom from physical and mental discomfort (Dubos, 1965). The well-known social critic, Ivan Illich, defined health as "the intensity with which individuals cope with their internal states and their environmental conditions" (1977, p. 271).

Recently, health promotion has come to be viewed from a feminist perspective that challenges individual self-determination in health-related choices and lifestyles. This feminist conception of health promotion proposes that demographics and social structure, *not* self-choice, determine the ability of individuals to engage in responsible health behaviors. According to Hartsock (1983), one's personal identity, role assignment, and opportunities in life are largely influenced by factors such as sex, skin color, age, income, and place of origin. For example, media promotion of smoking might have a stronger influence on women and African Americans who seek greater upward mobility and liberation in today's society than on other groups within that same society. This outlook on health has great implications for nursing practice. In the future, "nurses need to turn their attention to the conditions that control, influence, and produce health or illness in human beings" (Chooparian, 1986, p. 53).

People in a low income bracket can become more actively involved in their own health promotion through developing social movements such as the American Health Decisions. Grassroots level participation in health care education on current issues and problems offers a social process for groups who by virtue of social strictures feel powerless to become more directly involved in health care policy decisions. Nursing's role would be one of active encouragement of such groups in these decision-making processes (Williams, 1991, pp. 271-276).

Social change and other political activities such as community organizing, coalition building, and health policy may need to be coupled with personal change concepts to lead to a new view on health promotion for future nurses (Williams, 1989, pp. 20-23).

Several nursing theorists also have presented views on health. Neuman, Parse, and Pender are considered to be among the foremost health theorists in nursing. These three theorists view the individual holistically and perceive health as a process that reflects person-environment relationships. Persons are seen not as passive receivers of health care or respondents to their environments but rather as self-determining beings in continuous interaction with their environment, with resultant positive and negative consequences. Pender defines health as "the actualization of the person's potential through goal-directed behavior, competent self-care and satisfying relationships with others while adjustments are made as needed to maintain structural integrity and harmony within the environment" (Pender, 1987, p. 27). The following terms are seen frequently in wellness-related literature and are defined here for clarity. "Alternative" or "Complementary" Treatment Modalities are based on the theory that a balance of human/universal energy dynamics or the interlocking and influence of mind and body on each other is necessary for wellness (Rapacz, 1993). Holistic care by nurses can include the practices of acupuncture, relaxation techniques, massage therapy, aromatherapy, polarity, therapeutic touch, and imagery. All of these involve an exchange or a synergistic interaction of mind and body.

Disease prevention encompasses those activities that contain or actually prevent the spread of disease. It includes primary, secondary, and tertiary levels of prevention.

Health promotion refers to a wide variety of activities, including risk-reduction classes (*e.g.,* weight loss and smoking cessation clinics), testing, health hazard assessments, jogging and other fitness activities, and physical examination. Health-promotion activities are examples of primary prevention (Ardell, 1985).

Health education focuses on risk reduction and alleviation of problems through retraining of attitudes and behavior. It assists persons with medical concerns and problems to function and cope more effectively.

Holistic health emphasizes the mind-body connection in health and illness, personal responsibility, and a balanced lifestyle. In this approach, fitness, stress management, and nutrition, along with other aspects of optimal functioning, are integrated into a total approach. Nondrug, nonsurgical interventions for the treatment of illness conditions are stressed in holistic health.

Medical self-care stresses personal responsibility for health by teaching appropriate levels of self-sufficiency with self-monitoring of blood pressure, diet, exercise, and routine health-related procedures such as breast and pelvic examinations.

Wellness is defined as "an integrated method of functioning which is oriented toward maximizing the potential of which the individual is capable. It requires that the individual maintain a continuum of balance and purposeful direction within the environment where he is functioning" (Dunn, 1977, pp. 5-6). It includes a conscious and deliberate approach to an advanced state of physical, psychological, and spiritual health and is a dynamic, fluctuating state of being.

In addition to basic definitions of wellness-related terms as they are used in nursing literature, it is important to understand the various approaches to wellness. These approaches often are referred to as *conceptual frameworks* or *models*. These terms mean that a viewpoint or structure is presented by an expert in the field of wellness, which provides a way of viewing wellness or understanding how best to present the concepts to the client.

MODELS OF WELLNESS
Health Belief Model

A frequently used model in the development of wellness programs is the **health belief model** developed by Rosenstock (Becker, Haefner, Kasl, Kirscht, Maiman, & Rosenstock, 1977). This model attempts to explain why and under what conditions persons take action to prevent, detect, or comply with treatment. The model asserts that the decision to undertake preventive health measures is influenced by an individual's perception of personal susceptibility to a particular condition and the severity of consequences if that condition develops. Motivation to take action to promote health or to prevent disease is based on how strongly the individual believes that the following statements apply to him or her (Becker, 1974):

1. I am personally susceptible to the disease.
2. The illness would affect my life in a significant way.
3. Taking action would reduce my susceptibility or, if the illness occurred, would reduce its severity.
4. Taking action would not require me to endure significant financial strain, inconvenience, pain, or embarrassment.
5. Disease can be present even in the absence of apparent illness or symptoms.

Together these perceptions produce a readiness that will result in the desired behavior when there is an appropriate cue to action, a lack of barriers, and belief of the usefulness of the action. Consider the wellness behavior of breast self-examination. A woman's estimated probability that she will encounter breast cancer constitutes perceived susceptibility. Given an appropriate cue (exposure to the media) and the lack of significant barriers (fear, embarrassment, or a lack of knowledge), a woman would find the value of breast self-examination enhanced by the recognition that she is susceptible to breast cancer, by her perception of the severity of the negative aspects of breast cancer, and by the belief that performing breast self-examination is useful. According to the health belief model the woman who is most likely to carry out the behavior of breast self-examination in the prescribed way will be one who believes that she is especially vulnerable to breast cancer (Calnan & Rutter, 1986).

Rosenstock's model includes two variables, a psychological state of readiness to take action and the extent to which a particular action is believed to be beneficial. Rosenstock defined the state of readiness as the person's perceived susceptibility to a condition and the perceived seriousness of that condition (Figure 7-3). Previous research has established a relationship between perceived susceptibility and preventive health behaviors.

The health belief model was tested by Larson et al. (1979) by studying the relationship of certain health beliefs and values to the influenza vaccination and the effect of a postcard reminder concerning vaccination dates. The persons who followed up and received the vaccine believed

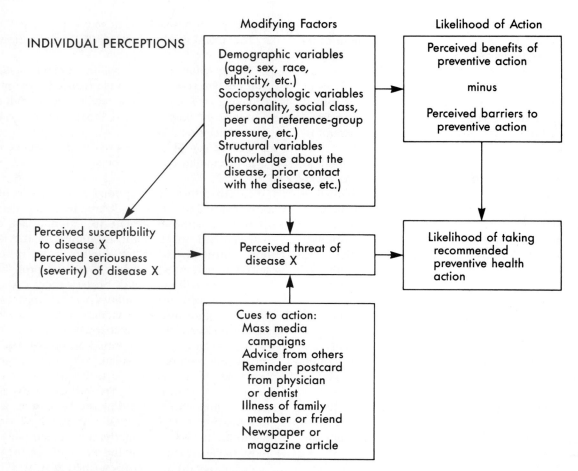

FIGURE 7-3   Rosenstock's health belief model. *(From Selected psychosocial models and correlates of individual health-related behaviors by M.D. Becker, D.P. Haefner, S.V. Kasl, J.P. Kirscht, L.A. Maiman, & I.M. Rosenstock, 1977, Medical Care, 15(5) (suppl.), p. 27. Copyright 1977 by J.B. Lippincott Company. Reprinted by permission.)*

vaccination to be more efficacious than did those who remained unvaccinated. In addition, those individuals who were not vaccinated were less satisfied with their medical care in general; they also considered the vaccine to be more expensive than did those who were vaccinated. The study indicated that persons who perceive the benefits of a preventive behavior as outweighing the barriers usually have a higher health value orientation and thus undertake the preventive behavior (Larson, Bergman, Herdricht, Alvin, & Schneeweiss, 1979).

Evaluation of a model encompassing many health-promoting variables was conducted on a sample of 589 individuals enrolled in a health promotion program.

Findings indicated that those individuals practicing healthier lifestyles demonstrated perception of health as high-level wellness, an internal locus of control, and competence in handling life situations (Pender, Walker, Sechrist, & Frank-Stromborg, 1990).

The Self-Efficacy Model

Recent work in the field of wellness has suggested that the health belief model would be enhanced by the addition of concepts from the **self-efficacy model** (Desmond & Price, 1988).

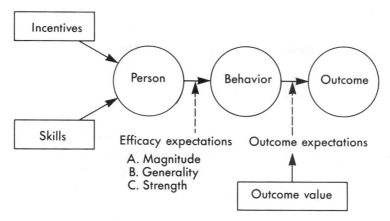

FIGURE 7-4 The self-efficacy model. *(Modified from Self-efficacy and weight control by S.M. Desmond & J.H. Price, 1988, Health Education, 19(1), 13 [Modified from A. Bandura, 1977, Psychological Review, 84(2), p. 191.])*

Bandura's theory of self-efficacy looks at whether an individual will initiate a healthy behavior and how long that person will maintain that behavior and/or strive to achieve it (Bandura, 1977). Use of the perceived self-efficacy model is an effective vehicle for bringing about desired behavior changes in a specific area of lifestyle (Figure 7-4). A person's belief regarding (1) ability to perform a specific health-related behavior, and (2) the probability that the performed behavior will lead to the anticipated outcome directly affect its performance or lack of it.

Consider the case of Jack M., who decides it would be healthy to embark on an exercise regimen. Jack's physician suggests that he attend aerobic classes three times a week. Although Jack knows that his work schedule prohibits attendance at such a class three times a week on a consistent basis, he agrees to try to meet this goal. During the first week Jack regularly attended the classes. His second week's attendance drops to twice a week. The classes are rigorous and tiring, and Jack has difficulty keeping up with the fast tempo. The only perceivable outcomes at this point are increased stress from trying to meet the proposed attendance schedule and sore, aching muscles. By the end of 1 month Jack no longer is attending the classes and has decided that maybe he really does not need to exercise after all. Thus this client's *efficacy expec-*

tations (i.e., what he hopes to achieve—in this case improved health) were incongruent with his outcome expectations (sore muscles and stress).

Efficacy expectations vary in magnitude, generality, and strength, which, combined, affect performance. *Magnitude* refers to the difficulty level of the involved tasks and the person's belief regarding ability to perform them. The individual's perception of whether the expected behavior relates to only one specific situation or to a variety of situations is referred to as *generality* of self-efficacy. *Strength* of efficacy expectation relates to the individual's resoluteness of belief in the ability to perform the health-related behavior. Sources of efficacy expectations include the way the individual accomplishes the performed task, observance of successful performance of the task by others, verbal persuasion to convince the individual that he or she can perform the behavior, and emotional arousal to convince the client of his or her ability to complete the task (Desmond & Price, 1988).

Consider again Jack's situation regarding the need for an exercise program. Taking into account his rigorous work schedule and lack of conditioning at the time, the occupational health nurse at his work setting suggests that Jack begin his exercise program by walking for 15 minutes daily during his lunch hour for a 2-week period.

She also suggests that Jack walk with another person in the company who has been involved in a walking program for 1 month. Jack begins walking and achieves success. His co-worker encourages him and stresses how much better he feels since embarking on the walking program. Jack then decides he would like to engage in some other type of exercise program to develop and tone other body muscle groups.

The nurse suggests stopping at a local gymnasium twice a week, one of the days to be a weekend day when Jack would have no work commitments. This particular facility designs individual exercise programs after assessing preexercise tone levels, age, and ability to work with weights and toning machines. It opens early in the morning and Jack schedules his weekday visits on Wednesdays at 7 AM, which is a lighter day for him in terms of workload. The nurse and Jack discuss specific benefits he wishes to see from his exercise program and how certain he is that he can carry out his new goals. Jack finds that his lunchtime walking program and the twice-weekly individually tailored program at the local gym meet his needs for an exercise regimen. He also feels that he is able to accomplish his goals, and he continues to receive encouragement and support from the occupational nurse, his walking partner, and the staff members of the exercise facility he has chosen. Jack's efficacy expectations and outcome expectations are congruent this time, and he is successful in maintaining his exercise program over a specified period of time.

A study done to examine factors affecting the participation of a cohort of labor class individuals in a wellness worksite program found self-efficacy to be the most distinguishing characteristic for the participating individuals. The participating group saw fewer barriers and more benefits from involvement in the worksite program. Their nonparticipating counterparts saw factors such as age, fitness level, work schedules, and personal responsibilities as deterrents to improving health status (Alexy, 1991, pp. 37-40).

Self Reliance

Spiritual well-being is not often a consideration in the development and implementation of wellness programs, which tend to concentrate on the physical domains. Recent programs developed by the Boulder County YMCA in Colorado and the University of Maryland, College Park, used Carl Jung's model definition of spirituality as "self-reliance." Self-reliance then encompasses awareness, inner faith, self-worth, humility, patience, acceptance, and self-confidence. A breakdown in one's personal beliefs can lead to a spiritual crisis and impediments to wellness. Through workshops, classes and lectures involving stress-management techniques, value clarification, and confidence building, spiritual well-being is enhanced, leading to improved overall wellness. This model has been incorporated into many substance abuse and weight control programs with success (Seaward, 1989).

Contracting

The **health behavior contract** is another useful approach for achieving behavior changes in the wellness area. A health behavior contract is a formal written agreement between the nurse and the client, which is designed to systematically change a behavior within the client's lifestyle (Figure 7-5). Important components of behavior contracts include short- and long-term goals, measurable behaviors, planning for steps needed to achieve the goal, and consideration of positive and negative factors that may affect goal achievement. A self-care contract should provide rewards and punishments and indicate a target date for reevaluation of goal achievement. Behavior contracts have been shown to improve goal-setting abilities and awareness of behavior cues. Clients also can be assisted to substitute positive health practices for negative ones (Kittleson & Hageman-Rigney, 1988). Health-behavior contracts stress self-responsibility and the need to take control of one's health and lifestyle management.

Social Support

Most wellness models include some reference to the importance of social support for achievement of wellness behavioral changes. Effective models contain two components: a direct support component and a modeling component. Supportiveness is the degree to which respondents perceive others in their environment as ac-

---

NURSE-CLIENT CONTRACT/AGREEMENT

Statement of health goal: _____ Nutritional planning for weight control _____

I _____ Jean Jones _____ promise to _____ Maintain a dietary _____
       (Client)

_____ intake log of all foods eaten daily _____
       (Client responsibility)

for a period of _____ one week _____ , whereupon,

_____ Cheryl Jenkins _____ will provide _____ a copy of _____
       (Nurse)

_____ Ann Smith's book, Nutrition and Weight Control _____
       (Nurse responsibility)

on _____ Friday, January 7, 1989 _____ to me.
       (Date)

If I do not fulfill the terms of this contract in total, I
understand that the designated reward will be withheld.

Signed: _____
       (Client)

_____
       (Date)

_____
       (Nurse)

_____

FIGURE 7-5 Nurse-client contract/agreement.

tively supporting or helping them in their efforts to change health-related behaviors. Modeling refers to the degree of personal involvement of significant others in the individual's health-related efforts. Research findings suggest that change is affected both by social supports that help the person stay motivated and by the modeling of positive health-related behaviors on the part of others in that person's environment (Robbins & Slavin, 1988).

A study conducted on a program implemented to reduce cardiovascular disease risks of employees at three different plant sites used four different intervention models. Identified risk factors addressed were cigarette smoking, obesity, and high blood pressure. Sustained health improvement and greater cost effectiveness was achieved through the models that incorporated health education, personal outreach, ongoing counseling, and social organization within the site (Erfurt, 1991, pp. 440-448). Therefore, it is suggested that a health-support index be used in conjunction with education and counseling when designing a wellness program to assess the degree of support individuals receive from their environments.

Individuals of course rarely function in isolation in our society; they are viewed instead as part of a system. Thus the "Heart Smart" cardiovascular health program (Johnson, Nicklas, Arbeit, Franklin, & Berenson, 1988) has developed a family health-promotion model that incorporates and relates many of the aforementioned models and concepts to the family setting. The program seeks to modify cardiovascular risk factors in parents and children through alterations in behavior in the areas of diet, exercise, and stress management. Major components of the maintenance program are intrafamily and interfamily social support, personal self-management, and reinforcement of the cardiovascular health program.

Contact with program participants was maintained by telephone, mail, or personal contact over a 5-year period. Designers of the program sought to help families maintain changes in the previously cited areas for the purpose of improving cardiovascular health. Based on the success of such groups as Weight Watchers and Alcoholics Anonymous, Heart Smart's family health promotion program enlisted participants to carry the message to new members, to share their experiences, and to offer support personally or by

---

The "Heart Smart" Family Health Promotion Maintenance Data Collection Timeline

Weekly
24-hour food records (self-monitored)
Exercise log (self-monitored)
Behavioral records (self-monitored)

Monthly
Grocery receipts (self-monitored)
Weight

Quarterly
Blood pressure
Group 24-hour dietary recalls

Semiannually
Risk factor screening (including venipuncture and urine collection)

Annually
Paper-and-pencil questionnaires

FIGURE 7-6 Data collection time line. (*From A comprehensive model for maintenance of family health behaviors: The heart smart family health promotion program" by C. Johnson et al., 1988,* Family and Community Health, *11(1), p. 6, with permission of Aspen Publishers, Inc, copyright 1988.*)

telephone contact. Personal self-management was achieved by teaching adults and children to become in essence their own counselors. The participants kept eating behavior and exercise logs and were responsible for self-observation and monitoring. Clients were taught stimulus control principles and were urged to reward themselves for weekly self-monitoring. Self-evaluation was based on comparison of behavioral records and individual goals. Self-reinforcement was provided through reciprocal contracts and rewards during the maintenance phase. The overall effectiveness of the Heart Smart maintenance model was monitored by physiological assessments and self-reported behaviors. Figure 7-6 shows an example of a data collection timeline used in the program.

The MATCH Model

The models presented thus far have viewed wellness and health promotion from a personal and family perspective. A great deal of controversy surrounds the area of focus for health/wellness educational efforts. A multilevel intervention approach has been proposed (Simons-Morton, D.G., Simons-Morton, B.G., Parcel, G.S., & Bunker, J.F., 1988), which is useful in influencing both personal preventive services and community preventive services. The multilevel approaches toward community health (MATCH) model conceptualizes intervention directed at individual, organizational, and governmental levels (Figure 7-7). Individual health is affected through personal behaviors, whereas organizations affect the health of their members through policies and practices. A government affects its electorate's health by public action and legislation. Thus community health intervention can consist of "(1) influencing individuals to reduce personal risk factors for disease and (2) influencing organizations and governments to reduce environmental risk factors for disease and to facilitate positive influences on personal behaviors and physiology" (Simons-Morton et al., 1988, p. 27).

Phase I of the MATCH model consists of the selection of health goals for the target population. The target population is in this instance those persons whose health is of concern. It can be an individual client, a group, or an identified

community. Appropriate health goals are selected for the target population.

In Phase II appropriate interventions are planned to achieve the health goals in the target population through environmental and personal change. An example of intervention at the individual level is reduction in the personal disease risk factors of individual participants. Organizational-level objectives include changes in or establishment of organizational policies or programs, and government-level objectives include changes in or establishment of local, state, or federal governmental policies, programs, and legislation.

Individual target populations are family groups as well as the individual members themselves. Organizational-level target populations include decision makers and persons of influence in the targeted organization. Governmental-level target populations include leaders and persons of power and influence in the targeted governmental entity.

Phase III involves several steps. These include development and implementation of the interventions selected in Phase II, development and testing of needed materials, hiring of additional personnel, scheduling meeting or class sites, and conducting interventions. Phase IV evaluates the achievement of health goals and intervention objectives from Phases I and II.

Consider the example of coronary artery disease. To decrease the prevalence and severity of this health problem in the community, nurses who use the MATCH model might consider influencing the process at all three levels (Simons-Morton et al., 1988, pp. 31-32), as follows:

. . . *individuals* to eat foods that are low in fat and salt, to do aerobic exercise on a regular basis, and to not smoke, *organizations* to provide low-fat and low-salt selections for food purchase, to establish exercise facilities, and to implement smoking restriction policies, and *governments* to fund research on dietary practices to lower CHD [coronary heart disease] risk, to provide food commodities that meet dietary recommendations to lower CHD risk, to initiate community education campaigns, and to pass ordinances, laws, and regulations restricting smoking in public places.

This model is unique in that it involves health and education professionals, as well as others, in

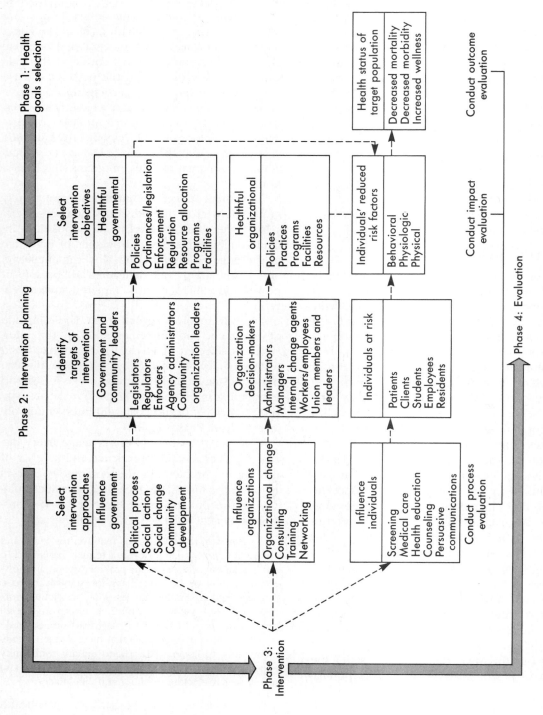

FIGURE 7-7 The MATCH model for community health intervention. *(From Influencing personal and environmental conditions for community health: a multi-level intervention model by D.G. Simons-Morton, B.G. Simons-Morton, G.S. Parcel, & J.F. Bunker; August 1988,* Family and Community Health, *11(2), p. 29. Copyright 1988 by Aspen Publishers, Inc. Reprinted by permission.)*

intervention efforts to improve the health of the population. Laypersons, institutions, and political action groups all can make a significant contribution.

The Community Wellness Program

Rural health has become a focus for health care reform in the United States. Health hazards from new farming technology involving chemicals, the closing of rural hospitals, AIDS, teenage pregnancy and abortion, and the increased incidence of chronic illness have combined to create a rural population that is sicker, older, and underinsured. A group empowerment model used by county cooperative extension service agents in Georgia entitled the Community Wellness Program has achieved a positive influence on rural health problems. It involves several phases including assessment of specific community health needs with interventions designed to meet those needs, community-based program planning, community empowerment, and a community-wide support system. The Community Wellness Program begins with a single resource level involv-

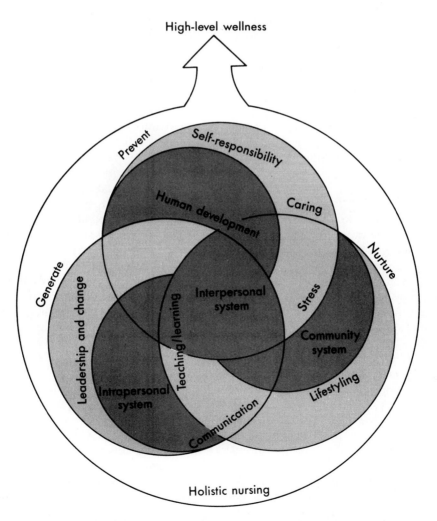

FIGURE 7-8 The holistic nursing model. *(From* Holistic Nursing *(p. 24) by B. Blattner, 1981, Englewood Cliffs, NJ: Prentice-Hall. Copyright 1981 by Prentice-Hall. Reprinted by permission.)*

ing programs the county extension agent can implement alone such as stress management for teachers. The second level is the multiple resources level, which requires the involvement and cooperation of other health professionals or agencies; for example, a cholesterol screening program for a local business.

The third stage is community-wide resources. Here more complex programs such as community-wide health fairs that require organizational involvement in collaboration and coordination are initiated. The last level of the community wellness process involves formation of task force resources to address mechanisms for improving overall education, health care, employment, or transportation issues (e.g., a Community Wellness-Council).

Community participation for initiation, innovation, and support of programs helps link ideas with resources and ultimately leads citizens to individual and collective empowerment. Total involvement by persons within the rural community is needed to determine needs, plan approaches, and undertake solutions (Jenkins, 1991).

The Holistic Nursing Perspective

Another wellness model reflects the holistic nursing perspective (Blattner, 1981). This model (Figure 7-8) has many interlocking circles, half-circles, and eclipses that show the relationships and connectedness of the systems and their relationship to the holistic nursing process. Central to the figure are three circles that represent nurturant, generative, and preventive nursing interventions. The nine areas that require processing to achieve wellness are self-responsibility, caring, stress, lifestyle, human development, problem solving, communication, teaching-learning and leadership, and change. Superimposed on these areas are the intrapersonal, interpersonal, and community systems. Intrapersonal encompasses the nurse/client relationship, interpersonal involves groups such as families, and community denotes organizations or persons with common interests. High-level wellness is achieved through the nine life processes within these three systems.

ASSESSMENT OF WELLNESS BEHAVIORS

Nurses first must understand their own wellness practices and philosophies if they are to be effective teachers and models of wellness. Self-assessment of lifestyle beliefs and behaviors is a good starting point. Several tools for wellness lifestyle assessment have been developed that require only a short time for completion (Figure 7-9). Complete the questionnaire and determine your own "wellness score." What deficits and strengths did you find? How might this affect your ability to effectively teach wellness concepts to your clients?

Completion of a **lifestyle assessment questionnaire** by clients enables them to look objectively at their wellness practices and assess positive as well as negative areas. For total accuracy of responses the client should be allowed to complete the questionnaire without interference. Clients generally find this exercise interesting and often revealing. It is important to recognize that a client's ability to incorporate wellness concepts into personal beliefs and behaviors is governed by many factors, including a positive self-concept and attitude, a holistic perspective on health, cultural beliefs, and self-discipline. The ability to make wellness choices depends in part on the client's flexibility and capacity for change.

Individual marketing plans must be designed and tailored to diverse needs of the main target groups on the age continuum. These would include preschool and school-age children, homemakers, unskilled, semi-skilled, and skilled laborers, professionals and business executives, the unemployable, and the elderly (Goldman, Adamson, Raymond, & Shore, 1989).

Values

Values play a key role in wellness choices because they affect motivation, thought, affect, and behavior. For a value to be internalized as a wellness behavior, the client must choose the value freely from among several alternatives. The outcomes of the various alternatives must have been considered in a deliberate fashion. The selected value must be prized or cherished and made known to others. Clients then must be willing to act upon the value and incorporate it into

Text continues on p. 162.

SELF-TEST FOR HEALTH STYLE

Directions

This is not a pass-fail test. Its purpose is simply to tell you how well you are doing in staying healthy. The behaviors covered in the test are recommended for most Americans. Some of them may not apply to persons with certain chronic diseases or handicaps. Such persons may require special instructions from their physician or other health professional.

The test has six sections: smoking, alochol and drugs, nutrition, exercise and fitness, stress control, and safety. Complete one section at a time by circling the number corresponding to the answer that best describes your behavior (2 for "Almost always", 1 for "Sometimes", and 0 for "Almost never"). Then add the numbers you have circled to determine your score for that section. Write the score on the line provided at the end of each section. The highest score you can get for each section is 10.

Smoking	Almost always	Sometimes	Almost never
If you never smoke, enter a score of 10 for this section and go to the next section.			
1. I avoid smoking cigarettes.	2	1	0
2. I smoke only low-tar and nicotine cigarettes, or I smoke a pipe or cigars.	2	1	0

Smoking score: _____

Alcohol and drugs	Almost always	Sometimes	Almost never
1. I avoid drinking alcoholic beverages, or I drink no more than one or two drinks a day.	4	1	0
2. I avoid using alcohol or other drugs (especially illegal drugs) as a way of handling stressful situations or the problems in my life.	2	1	0
3. I am careful not to drink alcohol when taking certain medicines (for example, medicine for sleeping, pain, colds, and allergies) or when pregnant.	2	1	0
4. I read and follow the label directions when using prescribed and over-the-counter drugs.	2	1	0

Alcohol and drugs score: _____

Eating habits	Almost always	Sometimes	Almost never
1. I eat a variety of foods each day, such as fruits and vegetables, whole grain breads and cereals, lean meats, dairy products, dry peas and beans, and nuts and seeds.	4	1	0
2. I limit the amount of fat, saturated fat, and cholesterol I eat (including fat on meats, eggs, butter, cream, shortenings, and organ meats, such as liver).	2	1	0
3. I limit the amount of salt I eat by cooking with only small amounts, not adding salt at the table, and avoiding salty snacks.	2	1	0
4. I avoid eating too much sugar (especially frequent snacks of sticky candy or soft drinks).	2	1	0

Eating habits score: _____

FIGURE 7-9 Self-test for health style. *(From U.S. Department of Health and Human Services, Office of Health Information, Health Promotion, and Physical Fitness and Sports Medicine. Washington, DC: U.S. Government Printing Office.)*

Continued

Exercise / fitness	Almost always	Sometimes	Almost never
1. I maintain a desired weight, avoiding overweight and underweight.	3	1	0
2. I do vigorous exercises for 15-30 minutes at least three times a week (examples: running, swimming, brisk walking).	3	1	0
3. I do exercises that enhance my muscle tone for 15-30 minutes at least three times a week (examples: yoga and calisthenics).	2	1	0
4. I use part of my leisure time participating in individual, family, or team activities (such as gardening, bowling, golf, and baseball) that increase my level of fitness.	2	1	0

Exercise / fitness score: _____

Stress control	Almost always	Sometimes	Almost never
1. I have a job or do other work that I enjoy.	2	1	0
2. I find it easy to relax and express my feelings freely.	2	1	0
3. I recognize early, and prepare for, events or situations likely to be stressful for me.	2	1	0
4. I have close friends, relatives, or others whom I can talk to about personal matters and call on for help when needed.	2	1	0
5. I participate in group activities (such as church and community organizational activites) or hobbies that I enjoy.	2	1	0

Stress control score: _____

Safety	Almost always	Sometimes	Almost never
1. I wear a seat belt while riding in a car.	2	1	0
2. I avoid driving while under the influence of alcohol and other drugs.	2	1	0
3. I obey traffic rules and the speed limit when driving.	2	1	0
4. I am careful when using potentially harmful products or substances (such as household cleaners, poisons, and electrical devices).	2	1	0
5. I avoid smoking in bed.	2	1	0

Safety score: _____

FIGURE 7-9, cont'd.

Your healthstyle scores

After you have figured your scores for each of the six sections, circle the number in each column that matches your score for that section of the test.

Smoking	Alcohol and drugs	Eating habits	Exercise fitness	Stress control	Safety
10	10	10	10	10	10
9	9	9	9	9	9
8	8	8	8	8	8
7	7	7	7	7	7
6	6	6	6	6	6
5	5	5	5	5	5
4	4	4	4	4	4
3	3	3	3	3	3
2	2	2	2	2	2
1	1	1	1	1	1
0	0	0	0	0	0

Remember, there is no total score for this test. Consider each section separately. You are trying to identify aspects of your lifestyle that you can improve in order to be healthier and to reduce the risk of illness. So let's see what your scores reveal.

Scores of 9 and 10: Excellent! Your answers show that you are aware of the importance of this area to your health. More importantly, you are putting your knowledge to work for you by practicing good health habits. As long as you continue to do so, this area should not pose a serious health risk. It's likely that you are setting an example for your family and friends to follow. Since you got a very high score on this part of the test, you may want to consider other areas where your scores indicate room for improvement.

Scores 6 to 8: Your health practices in this area are good, but there is room for improvement. Look again at the items you answered with a "Sometimes" or "Almost never." What changes can you make to improve your score? Even a small change can often help you achieve better health.

Scores of 3 to 5: Your health risks are showing! Would you like more information about the risks you are facing and about why it is important for you to change these behaviors? Perhaps you need help in deciding how to make successfully the changes you desire. In either case, help is available.

Scores 0 to 2: Obviously, you were concerned enough about your health to take the test, but your answers show that you may be taking serious and unnecessary risks with your health. Perhaps you are not aware of the risks and what to do about them. You can easily get the information and help you need to improve, if you wish. The next step is up to you.

FIGURE 7-9, cont'd.

lifestyle practices. Consider the nurse who counsels the hypertensive client about the hazards of smoking but smokes two packs of cigarettes per day. An inconsistent message is given to the client, which indicates that the nurse advocates choosing the value of nonsmoking but does not prize it or act upon it. Individuals who have determined what is important in their lives (choosing a value) tend to make responsible decisions regarding their lifestyle (acting upon the value). Nurses who work with clients cannot prescribe wellness activities and choices for a client but must maintain an open, supportive, and nonjudgmental attitude. Nurses should serve as catalysts to help clients move toward self-responsibility in a wellness lifestyle (Gutt, 1983).

Motivation

Motivation is a crucial element in understanding why a client will accept and practice a wellness behavior. Clients first must become aware of things as they are, then as they might be. Strategies for bridging the gap must be devised, and the client must believe in his or her ability to carry out the strategies. This incorporates both the self-efficacy model and the health belief model. The client's social support and locus of control also must be considered in motivation assessment. Social support can be material or psychological support. It can include the expectations that the support group places on the client. The locus of control can be internal or external. Internally controlled individuals believe that their actions control outcomes in their lives. Externally controlled individuals believe that their outcomes are determined by others (Blattner, 1981).

Empowering potential is a recent motivational term used to explain initiation and maintenance of health behaviors. Individual motivation for health change is seen as "a continuous process of growth and development which facilitates the emergence of new and positive health patterns" (Fleury, 1991, p. 289). Individuals undergo a threefold process of readiness appraisal, change, and change integration. Imaging and social support systems are key elements within the empowerment process (Fleury, 1991).

Numerous strategies can be used by the nurse

in working with clients to achieve wellness goals (Dossey, Keegan, Guzzetta, & Kolkmeier, 1988). The client's health beliefs (positive or negative) and social support (adequate or absent) are assessed, and the client is placed in one of four categories. Specific teaching strategies are then chosen to implement wellness learning and behaviors depending on the category in which the client falls. Not all strategies are useful in each of the categories, which may account for a client's lack of adherence to a wellness program. Figure 7-10 presents a diagrammatic interpretation of these categories and strategies that the nurse can use in wellness education.

ALTERNATIVE OR COMPLEMENTARY TREATMENT MODALITIES

Nonwestern cultures have traditionally employed **alternative or complementary treatment modalities** in their healing practices. These include acupuncture, reflexology, and herbalism, among others. Positive and negative aspects of energy, or what the Chinese refer to as the *Yin* and *Yang,* interact both in the individual and in the supersystem of the universe to create bodily and universal harmony. Disruption of any of the key elements that balance humans and nature (fire, earth, metal, wood, and water) can lead to illness. Alternative or complementary therapies are seen as a means to achieve harmony of energy, for example, the *Yin* and *Yang,* and to return the body to a state of wellness or holism (Kleiman, 1980; Liu, 1988).

The holistic concept of practice has led to the holistic care movement in nursing itself. Nurses are increasingly using alternative treatment modalities as a means of incorporating traditional nursing values with concrete interventions. Techniques such as massage can be used as an adjunct to traditional bedside care or in independent nursing practice.

Massage techniques involve the use of the fingers, hands, and other body parts by the nurse for manipulation of the soft tissues (connective and muscular tissues). Benefits include improved circulation and skin condition, neurological, and psychological benefits (Schubert, 1989). *Aromatherapy* is often used in conjunction with massage and uses essential oils of flowers and

	Positive Beliefs and Attitudes	Negative Beliefs and Attitudes
Adequate supports	**Category 1** Teaching strategies Structured to facilitate affective, cognitive, psycho-motor learning. Discuss important points first and repeat. Present clearly and concisely in logical categories. Aim printed material at learner reading level. If denying, give basic survival information. If client focuses on the problem, give him detailed information.	**Category 2** Teaching strategies Focus on consciousness-raising techniques. Use nurse/client discussions to explore feelings. Form self-help groups with clients having similar problems. Use values clarification. Use behavior modification techniques by identifying a list of rewards ahead of time and giving temporary artificial rewards for healthy behavior. Identify cues for healthy and unhealthy behaviors. Keep a log or diary for several days to identify cues.
Inadequate supports	**Category 3** Teaching strategies Increase social support and cognitive strengthening. Provide family and friends with important information and encourage involvement with therapy regime discussions and value clarification sessions. Use assertiveness training, relaxation and imagery. If clients have external locus of control, involve them with community agencies and self-help groups. If clients have internal locus of control, use problem-solving and goal-setting approaches.	**Category 4** Teaching strategies Use foot-in-the-door strategies and aim for the minimal behavior change needed to accomplish the goal with a positive result. Provide simple regimens with basic goal-setting. Give rewards and reinforcements for healthy behaviors. Break goals into subsets moving from simple to complex. Use written versus verbal contracts.

FIGURE 7-10 Integrated health belief and social support model. (*Modified from* Holistic nursing: A handbook for practice, p. 140, by B. Dossey, I. Keegan, C.E. Guzetta, & I.G. Kolkmeier, 1988, Rockville, MD:Aspen. Copyright 1988 by Aspen Publishers, Inc. Reprinted by permission.)

fruits to effect healing. *Acupuncture* uses fine needles to alter body physiology and change body energy balance. The needles are inserted along pathways that closely follow the nervous system of the body and is used to treat a variety of disorders (McGregor, 1989). *Therapeutic touch* is a modality introduced by Dolores Krieger in 1972 and is a combination of several ancient healing practices. Therapeutic touch involves energy transfer to facilitate the client's own healing, relaxation, or pain amelioration responses (Krieger, 1990) by the therapeutic laying-on of hands of the practitioner. Imagery and relaxation techniques will be discussed in detail in the section on inner harmony.

Nurses practicing holistic care modalities must undergo appropriate training, investigate the legal and insurance implications, and seek policy development for the practice setting involved. Consent of client, family, or caregiver is imperative. Appropriate consultation with relevant health team practitioners is necessary. Authorization must be obtained if therapies are conducted in an agency context or setting. Documentation should be carried out each time a treatment is given in any setting (Rankin-Box, 1991). There are many additional modes of therapy that are being used by nurses in holistic care, and the popularity of these is increasing as nursing struggles to form its unique professional identity.

Consideration of client value systems, locus of control, social support, and motivation is necessary for the successful development and implementation of individual or group wellness programs.

WELLNESS COMPONENTS
Physical Fitness

Today's sedentary lifestyle, with its dependency on high technology, is a deterrent to active use of the body and the total self in either the workplace or home setting. The wellness movement stressed a total body-mind integration, and as a result, many Americans began to exercise on a regular basis. Several benefits were noted. Among them were increased longevity and prevention of several lifestyle-related diseases such as diabetes, obesity, and coronary heart disease. Other benefits, more noticeable on a daily basis, included better sleep habits, decreased stress, improved posture and energy, and a general sense of well-being.

Physical fitness programs include several types of movement. Aerobic exercise targets the heart, blood vessels, and lungs; it is achieved through such activity as dancing, swimming, jogging, cycling, rowing, and aerobic walking. It is important to engage in this type of exercise at least three times a week. (Figure 7-11 illustrates two types of exercise that are beneficial and in-

expensive.) The exercise activity should include a 5-minute warm-up period, sustained exercise for at least 20 to 30 minutes, and a cool-down period of 5 minutes. To achieve maximum benefit from aerobic exercise, participants must attain and maintain what is known as the *target heart rate* (THR). To calculate the THR, the person's age is subtracted from 220. This number is then called the maximum heart rate (MHR) and is multiplied by 60% to 85%, depending on age and general condition. Older or extremely sedentary persons would use the 60% figure to calculate their THR. Younger, reasonably fit persons would multiply by 75%. Individuals who already participate in a regular, vigorous exercise plan would use 85% of the MHR to calculate their target rate. For example, consider Mary M., aged 62 years, a recently retired office worker who feels she would like to go to Jazzercise sessions at the YWCA with her friend Judy now that she has more leisure time. *Mary had not before participated in any type of exercise program.* The following calculation provides Mary's THR:

$$
\begin{array}{ll}
220 & \\
\underline{-62} & \text{(Mary's age)} \\
= 158 & \text{(MHR)} \\
\underline{\times 65\%} & \text{(appropriate for Mary's age and condition} \\
= 102.70, \text{ or } 103 & \text{(Mary's THR)}
\end{array}
$$

The pulse rate must be checked frequently during the exercise session to be sure that the THR is being sustained for the entire half-hour period.

Yoga and stretching exercises can be used to improve flexibility and to enhance a regular exercise regimen. These types of exercises should be done slowly and gradually to achieve maximum range of motion.

Exercises to increase muscle strength and endurance are termed *isotonic and isokinetic.* Calisthenics and weightlifting programs frequently involve this type of exercise.

Isometric exercise produces a contraction of muscle groupings, with little or no joint movement. Unlike aerobic exercise, it does not affect the heart and lungs.

Nurses frequently are asked to counsel clients about wellness exercise programs. Clients should be advised to learn what types of programs are available in their areas. Consultation with a physi-

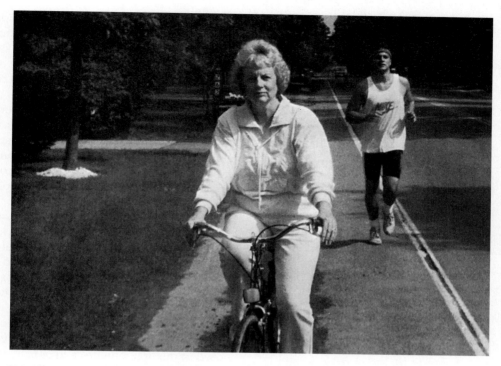

FIGURE 7-11 Exercise activities can be varied to suit the age and fitness levels of the individual. Note the middle-aged adult riding the bicycle, while in the background a young adult is seen jogging for fitness.

cian or exercise physiologist is advised if the client is older than 35 years of age or has a handicapping or chronic condition. Age 35 generally is used as a parameter for the middle-adulthood grouping. Clients must be assisted to establish long- and short-term goals and a specific schedule and timetable for the exercise program. It is important to evaluate any type of exercise program monthly to determine results, problems, and client satisfaction. The saying "no pain—no gain" is untrue; exercise should be enjoyable as well as beneficial. The client who feels pain while exercising should proceed with caution because injuries can result.

Fitness programs now are part of many nursery school activities and senior citizen programs. Fitness for everyone is the goal. Looking good should include not only the external manifestations of fitness, such as slimness and muscle development, but also the condition of the internal organs, particularly the cardiovascular system.

More specific information on physical fitness can be found in any comprehensive wellness or health education text.

Nutrition

Good **nutrition** management is an essential component of a wellness lifestyle and therefore an inherent element of any wellness program, individual or group. It is necessary for individuals to nurture the body through dietary intake; however, recent discoveries in the field of nutrition indicate that caloric consumption cannot be the only guiding factor in dietary selection. It has been found that the amounts of salt, sugar, fiber, and saturated fats that an individual consumes relate directly to the prevention or the incidence of several diseases. These include diabetes, cancer, ulcers, heart disease, hypertension, and stroke. Knowledge of basic dietary principles to maintain ideal body weight and to assist in the maintenance of a prudent diet can be the key to

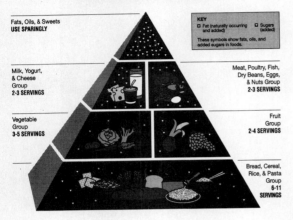

Food Guide Pyramid
A Guide to Daily Food Choices

FIGURE 7-12   The Food Guide Pyramid. The Food Guide Pyramid emphasizes foods from the five major food groups shown in the three lower sections of the pyramid. Each of these food groups provides some, but not all, of the nutrients you need. No one of these major food groups is more important than another — for good health, you need them all.

improved energy, better health, and longer life span.

In the U.S. government publication *Dietary Goals for the United States* (1977) a Senate subcommittee looked at the issue of nutrition and its links to health and established seven basic dietary goals for the remainder of this century. These include eating a variety of foods, maintaining healthy weight, and choosing a diet low in fat, saturated fat, and cholesterol with a high intake of vegetables, fruits, and grain products. Sugars, salt (sodium), and alcohol are to be used in moderation. Fat intake in particular should be limited to 30% of the total caloric intake with saturated fats being limited to 10% of the total.

The Food Guide Pyramid (Figure 7-12) emphasizes five basic food groups and the amounts necessary from each to provide adequate nutrients for a healthful diet.

The American public is inundated with an ever-changing array of dietary do's and don'ts. One term frequently heard in everyday "wellness chatter" is RDA or recommended daily allowances. These are essential nutrients considered necessary for human well-being. It is impor-

tant for nurses to be aware that there is no international standardization of RDAs. Thus incorporation of the recommended average daily amounts in the diet should actually be averaged so that the average intake occurs over a three-day period.

Diets geared toward health promotion should consider individual client factors such as height, weight, age, growth and development, gender, exercise, and lifestyle. Client risk factors, physiological condition, and preexisting medical conditions must also be attended to in the dietary plan (Herron, 1991).

Clients must receive health teaching regarding the need to eat foods that are as free as possible from excessive processing and chemical contamination. They should be encouraged to exclude foods from the diet that contain excessive additives, toxins, chemicals, and preservatives. Consumers must become label conscious, carefully screening lists of ingredients and recognizing misleading statements. The food we eat is exposed to multiple processes to enhance the shelf life of the product and at times its appearance. Clients need to be made aware of the hazards of food irradiation, meat and poultry supplementation, and chemical additives and preservatives. Irradiation causes depletion of vitamins A, C, E, and B complex and creates radioactive trace chemicals in the treated food. Some sources suggest that these elements may over time have carcinogenic properties. Hormones and antibiotics are given to farm animals and poultry to increase size and weight and therefore market value. The long-range effects of these procedures is unknown. Chemical additives are found in many foods to enhance color and taste. Again, the long-range effects of many of these dyes and flavor enhancers over time is unclear. Nurses need to be aware of these issues and be prepared to act as client advocates if necessary (Dossey, Keegan, Guzzetta, & Kolkmeier, 1988).

An important wellness consideration in the nutrition component is that of weight. Although Americans are eating more, they are not necessarily eating better. A successful weight-control program views psychological factors, environmental concerns, and genetics in assessing the client's weight gain. Additional factors in assessment are family history of obesity, situational factors that trigger eating, and psychological components of eating patterns. A dietary log that tracks what is eaten daily and weekly, as well as the circumstances, helps clients analyze factors relevant to their eating patterns. Caution is needed to avoid diets in which fewer than 1000 calories are allowed, which are deficient in essential vitamins or minerals, or which actually may contain hidden sources of fat. Fad diets come and go, and most are not only ineffective for sustained weight loss but may, in fact, be harmful to health. The greatest success in achieving and maintaining weight loss occurs through a combination of a nutritionally balanced food plan and behavior-modification techniques in a self-help setting. The importance of support groups, be they friends, co-workers, or family cannot be overemphasized in long-term maintenance of weight loss (Swinford & Webster, 1989).

All weight-loss programs should incorporate exercise if they are to be effective. Here it is important to assess the client's age, fitness level, and existing health state to ensure that too rigorous an exercise program is not chosen. For some individuals, exercises to tone tissue and muscle may be accomplished through isometrics or low-impact aerobics without posing any hazards to health.

Clients can be referred to nutrition counselors, weight-loss support groups, and a variety of literature sources for additional information regarding nutritional and dietary concerns as they relate to wellness.

Inner Harmony

The ability to feel, think, and act well depends in great part on the ability to partake in the banquet of life. In contemporary society individuals are continually subjected to time, role, and social stressors that can affect the best-planned physical wellness program. The loss of family interaction and support, friends with whom to share positive and negative events, and the ability to laugh and enjoy takes its toll over time. The inability to cope with stressors in one's personal and extrapersonal environment often leads to symptoms of anxiety and stress.

Stress can manifest itself in a variety of do-

mains. Clients may complain of insomnia, fatigue, irritability, anger, depression, hyperactivity, lack of concentration, forgetfulness, changes in eating habits, frequent tears, and impulsive behaviors. Physical symptoms abound and can include headaches, diarrhea, tics, backache, teeth grinding, shortness of breath, heart pounding, and vertigo.

The Social Readjustment Rating Scale (Figure 7-13), which is an assessment tool to evaluate the statistical probability of contracting an illness, is based on stressors or change experienced by clients during the previous year. It is important to note that happy or joyful events such as a new job or a wedding are changes that also are accompanied by a certain degree of stress. Individual scores are totaled, and ranges provide guidelines for the probability of illness occurring in the next 2 years. Quite often, clients are amazed at their scores and unaware of the cumulative effect of the many changes in their lives.

Coping strategies to produce relaxation and to assist in stress management must begin with awareness of stress, identification of specific stressors or stressful situations, and an evaluation of usual coping methods. Lifestyle behaviors must be scrutinized to ensure that adequate rest, nutrition, and physical activity are part of the daily routine. A regular exercise program is helpful in relieving stress and anxiety. Clients who participate in such activity on a regular basis state that missing the activity makes a definite difference in their attitude and coping in stressful situations.

A variety of other techniques and exercises are available to aid in achievement of **inner harmony.**

Progressive relaxation is a simple technique that can be done anywhere and at any time, particularly when one feels tension mounting. Through a combination of deep breathing and alternate tensing and relaxation of body muscle groups, clients can be taught to rid themselves of excess stress. A comfortable position is assumed, and muscle groups are first contracted, held, and then relaxed, progressing from the toes up through the neck and face muscles. Soothing music can be used in accompaniment to the exercise. Participants usually find the exercise helpful

Social Readjustment Rating Scale

Rank	Event	Value	Score
1	Death of a spouse	100	_____
2	Divorce	73	_____
3	Marital separation	65	_____
4	Jail term	63	_____
5	Death of a close family member	63	_____
6	Personal injury or illness	53	_____
7	Marriage	50	_____
8	Fired from work	47	_____
9	Marital reconciliation	45	_____
10	Retirement	45	_____
11	Change in family member's health	44	_____
12	Pregnancy	40	_____
13	Sex difficulties	39	_____
14	Addition to family	39	_____
15	Business readjustment	39	_____
16	Change in financial status	38	_____
17	Death of a close friend	37	_____
18	Change to different line of work	36	_____
19	Change in number of marital arguments	35	_____
20	Mortgage or loan over $10,000	31	_____
21	Foreclosure of mortgage or loan	30	_____
22	Change in work responsibilities	29	_____
23	Son or daughter leaving home	29	_____
24	Trouble with in-laws	29	_____
25	Outstanding personal achievement	28	_____
26	Spouse begins or stops work	26	_____
27	Starting or finishing school	26	_____
28	Change in living conditions	25	_____
29	Revision of personal habits	24	_____
30	Trouble with boss	23	_____
31	Change in work hours, conditions	20	_____
32	Change in residence	20	_____
33	Change in schools	20	_____
34	Change in recreational habits	19	_____
35	Change in church activities	19	_____
36	Change in social activities	18	_____
37	Mortgage or loan under $10,000	17	_____
38	Change in sleeping habits	16	_____
39	Change in number of family gatherings	15	_____
40	Change in eating habits	15	_____
41	Vacation	13	_____
42	Christmas season	12	_____
43	Minor violation of the law	11	_____

Score of less than 150: 37% chance of illness during the next 2 years.

Score of 150-300: 51% chance of illness during the next 2 years.

Score of more than 300: 80% chance of illness during the next 2 years.

FIGURE 7-13 The Social Readjustment Rating Scale. *(From Social Readjustment Rating Scale by T.H. Holmes & R.H. Rabe, 1967,* Journal of Psychosomatic Research, *11, p. 213. Copyright 1967 by Pergamon Press, Ltd. Reprinted by permission.)*

as an escape valve for excess tension.

Biofeedback is a technique that provides ongoing input to the client about internal physiological responses (generally believed to be good indicators of stress) such as pulse, temperature, blood pressure, and muscle tension. This is accompanied by placing a type of electronic monitoring device on the client and providing a meter reading of tension levels. With practice, clients can learn to monitor and control their specific body responses when they are under stress.

Meditation is useful to many clients in the achievement or maintenance of a non-stressful state. It involves assuming a comfortable, relaxed position, freeing the body of extraneous thoughts, and concentrating on the inner mind and spirit through low, soft repetition of a mantra or chant. Words used as mantras are such resonant phrases as *om* and *lum.* A 10- to 15-minute period is needed to free the body of excess pressures and to achieve a true meditative state.

Hypnosis has of late come into prominence as a useful tool in specific client management areas such as smoking cessation and pain control. Self-hypnosis has been found helpful in increasing the ability to cope with stressors. One way clients can use self-hypnosis is through audiotapes specifically geared to their individual relaxation or lifestyle intervention needs.

Imagery, also known as visualization, is an excellent coping strategy for dealing with stress. Memories, dreams, or fantasies experienced by clients can be used to focus the client's experience. Relaxing or soothing music can be used as a background to the imagery exercise. Clients assume a comfortable position, engage in deep breathing to relax, and imagine a place or time that holds positive or beautiful memories, for example, a favorite beach. They then are asked to visualize the sounds, sights, and smells associated with that experience; for example, a beach would include hearing the waves, tasting the sea spray, and smelling the sea breezes. The exercise is carried out for a 10- to 15-minute period, with a gradual awakening or return to the real world. Imagery "minibreaks," which often are useful to defuse a stressful workday and to assist in coping, can be practiced for a 3- to 5-minute period if more time is not available.

Humor is gaining prominence as an inexpensive and accessible way to deal with tension. It has long been said that "laughter is the best medicine." Muscle tension decreases after laughter. The cardiovascular system also shows positive effects from laughter. Humor makes everything look better and often opens new avenues of communication. Nurses can use positive humor in client/nurse situations and in their own stressful work climates. Clients undergoing chemotherapy, with its accompanying hair loss, have used laughter at their own appearance during support group sessions to diminish their stress levels during treatment (Swinford & Webster, 1989).

Environmental Sensitivity

Environmental sensitivity is an integral dimension of wellness. Historically, nurses played key roles in environmental consciousness and improvement of living conditions for their clients/patients. Today this role again is becoming increasingly important, with concerns about chemical contamination, air pollution, and radiation noted daily in the media. Human beings are in constant interaction with their environment, both immediate and global, yet have little ability to control the myriad of negative factors that exist in that environment.

A person's immediate environment usually consists of home and workplace. In the workplace prolonged exposure to noise levels above 75 decibels has been shown to cause hearing loss and cardiovascular changes. Inharmonic sound (random, unstructured noise), although it may not be excessively loud, can cause restlessness and irritability. These exposures over time take their toll on the human body systems. Noise problems are seen not only in factory settings but in office environments where typewriters, telephones, and office machinery all become cumulative culprits.

Air pollution occurs through contamination from vehicles and machines, as well as cigarette smoke. Sidestream smoke from breathing air contaminated by family members' or co-workers' smoke has been found to be as hazardous to health as actual mainstream smoking. Kidney disease, respiratory diseases, and cancer have been linked to air pollution and pose a grave environ-

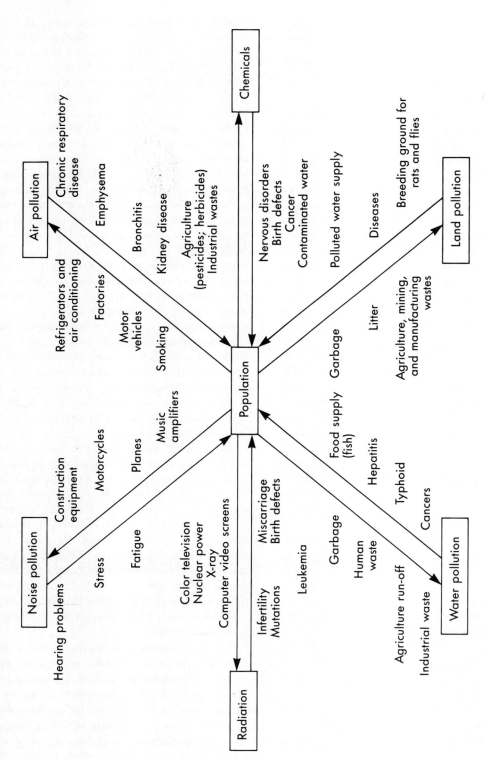

FIGURE 7-14 Environmental hazards. (*From Ecominnea; A strategy for teaching environmental health by K.L. Rotter, 1989, 17(4) pp. 26-27. Copyright 1989 by Association for the Advancement of Health Education. Reprinted by permission.*)

mental concern. Automobile exhaust fumes and by-products of industrial manufacturing contribute greatly to the "dust domes" seen in many major cities. Work environments also have proved hazardous. Prolonged exposure to workplace chemicals, asbestos, and trace fibers used for insulation have fostered the "sick building syndrome." When workers employed in these settings began to complain of symptoms of malaise, headaches, rash, and upper respiratory irritation, investigation showed links to workplace pollutants (Dossey, Keegan, Guzzetta, & Kolkmeier, 1988).

Throughout the nation there are waste dumps, in which toxic substances of a carcinogenic nature are stockpiled, and many citizen ad-

vocacy groups have begun to lobby actively for their removal. An example of one such waste site is the now infamous Love Canal area in Niagara Falls, New York, which had served as a waste dump for the many chemical companies located in that city. Chapter 27 contains a detailed discussion of the problems related to toxic waste dumps and the role of the nurse in helping families living in such areas.

Nurses, as professional health care workers, must act as advocates for clients in issues relevant to environmental concerns. This role includes informing clients about these hazards and urging self-responsibility in monitoring environmental health. Figure 7-14 presents a complete overview of the many sources of risk to clients

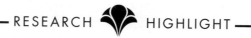

RESEARCH HIGHLIGHT

Humor and the Older Adult

An equal distribution of 60 older adults (36 women and 24 men) from three settings (private residence, senior citizen housing, and long-term care facility), categorized in two age groups (10 over 80 years, $\overline{X}$ 93, and 10 between 65 and 80 years, $\overline{X}$ 74), were selected to explore how they viewed humor. Responses from semistructured audiotaped interviews were analyzed to investigate the influence of place of residence, age, gender, functional ability, perceived health status (3-point scale from poor to good) and regard for and use of humor (4-point scale from poor to good). Field notes were used to document individual nonverbal behaviors and other contextual information. Transcriptions, category codes, and category indicators were reviewed by an experienced researcher and the established intercoder reliability was .97. Validity of the findings was confirmed by six older adults who reviewed the data analysis and found it to be consistent with their experience.

The following six functional categories evolved from participants' descriptions of humor: connectedness, relaxation, restoration, freedom, joy, and per-

spective. Comical everyday experiences and antics of children and pets were preferred sources of humor. While gentle humor was viewed as appropriate, humor that ridiculed or excluded an individual was seen as inappropriate. Profanities and sexist language were considered inappropriate by women, but men indicated that the use of humor that included such language depended upon the situation. This was the only reported gender difference. In addition, receptivity to humor (ability to take in and appreciate) varied according to age, place of residence, and level of health and functional ability but not gender.

Descriptions of the ways in which humor may be incorporated into the lives of older adults were provided along with the suggested use of the findings as a guide to the development of instruments to ascertain the needs for humor of individuals in light of their attitudes and practices. Instruments could be used by nurses to identify and to evaluate therapeutic strategies for intervention based on humor preferences and receptivity.

Herth, K.A. (1993). Humor and the older adult. *Applied Nursing Research, 6*(4), 146-153.

Chapter Highlights

- Several landmark publications alerted the public to the need for preventive health care, including *Dietary Goals, Hospitals' Responsibility for Health Promotion, Healthy People, Doing Better and Feeling Worse,* and *Future Directions in Health Care.*

- The rapidly rising costs of health care in the 1970s motivated employers and insurance companies to find ways to cut costs through prevention of illness and disability.

- Individuals who contributed to the wellness movement include Halpert L. Dunn, John Travis, Donald Ardell, and William Hettler.

- *Health* has been defined in a variety of ways. Recent definitions incorporate concepts of well-being and psychosocial aspects, as well as absence of disease.

- The concept of wellness refers to maximizing an individual's ability to function. It is a dynamic, fluctuating state of being.

- According to Rosenstock's health belief model, an individual's decision to perform a health action is determined by perceptions of susceptibility to an illness, severity of the illness, and personal threat of the illness.

- The self-efficacy model is a useful tool for bringing about desired behavioral changes in a specific area of lifestyle. The more likely a behavior is perceived as leading to a desired outcome, the more likely it is to be performed.

- A contract between the nurse and client stresses the need for the individual to take responsibility for health and lifestyle management.

- The multilevel approaches toward community health (MATCH) model is useful in implementing changes at the levels of individual, community, and government.

- Blattner's wellness model is based on the holistic nursing perspective and the processes needed to achieve wellness.

- Self-assessment of lifestyle beliefs and behaviors enables clients to assess their positive and negative health behaviors.

- Nurses cannot prescribe wellness activities for a client but should serve as catalysts to help clients move toward self-responsibility.

- Regular exercise is beneficial in helping to prevent many chronic diseases, as well as in promoting a general sense of well-being.

- Aerobic exercise raises the heart rate and benefits the heart, blood vessels, and lungs.

- Good nutrition is an integral component of health promotion.

- Contemporary society contains many stresses that can be manifested in a variety of physical symptoms. Effective stress management strategies are necessary to achieve high-level wellness.

- Strategies to produce relaxation and improve stress include progressive relaxation, biofeedback, meditation, hypnosis, imagery (or visualization), and humor.

- Environmental hazards that can negatively affect health include air pollution, chemicals, noise pollution, and toxic waste.

- Community health nurses can play a key role in health promotion. To do so, they must develop skills in information dissemination, communication, and advocacy.

CRITICAL THINKING EXERCISE

A nurse employed by a college conducts a survey concerning the overall wellness in a college community. The survey reveals that 70% of the students and faculty are overweight, and 40% smoke more than 20 cigarettes a day. The results of the survey prompt the college board to ask the nurse to set up a plan that will teach the students about nutrition and cessation of smoking. Realizing that the problem is complex, the nurse decides to design a plan based on the MATCH model.

Phase I: Goals

(a) The college community will develop an awareness of the health benefits of prudent eating habits and exercise.

(b) The college community will understand the health threat caused by primary and secondary smoke.

(c) Smoking cessation programs will become available to the college community.

Using the MATCH model, plan Phases II, III, and IV of the program.

REFERENCES

Alexy, B.B. (1991). Factors associated with participation or nonparticipation in a workplace wellness center. *Research, Nursing and Health, 14*(1), 33-40.

American Hospital Association, Center for Promotion, *Hospital's responsibility for health promotion.* Chicago, IL: Author.

Ardell, D.B. (1977). *High level wellness: An alternative to doctors, drugs and disease.* Emmaus, PA: Rodale Press.

Ardell, D.B. (1982). *14 days to a wellness lifestyle.* Mill Valley, CA: Whatever Publishing.

Ardell, D.B. (1985). The history and future of wellness. *Health Values, 9,* 37-56.

Bandura, A. (1977). Self-efficacy: Toward a unifying theory of behavioral change. *Psychological Review, 84*(2), 191-215.

Becker, M.H. (Ed.). (1974). *The health belief model and personal health behavior.* Thorofare, NJ: Charles B. Black.

Becker, M.H., Haefrer, D.P., Kasl, S.V., Kirscht, J.P., Maiman, L.A., & Rosenstock, I.M. (1977). Selected psychosocial models and correlates of individual health-related behaviors. *Medical Care, 15*(5) (suppl.), 27-30.

Belloc, N.B., & Breslow, L. (1972). Relationship of physical health status and health practices. *Preventive Medicine, 1,* 409-421.

Blattner, B. (1981). *Holistic nursing.* Englewood Cliffs, NJ: Prentice-Hall.

Blue Cross Association. (1977). The Rockefeller Foundation and the Health Policy Program at the University of California (San Francisco): *The proceedings of the conference on future directions in health care: the dimensions of medicine,* Chicago, IL: Author.

Calnan, M., & Rutler, D.R. (1986). Do health beliefs predict health behavior? An analysis of breast self-examination. *Social Science Medicine, 22*(6), 673-678.

Chooparian, T. (1986). Reconceptualizing the environment. In P. Maccia (Ed.) *New approaches to theory development* (pp. 39-54). New York: National League for Nursing.

Desmond, S.M., & Price, J.H. (1988). Self-efficacy and weight control, *Health Education,* February/March, *19*(1), 12-21.

Dossey, B., Keegan, L., Guzzetta, C.E., & Kolkmeier, L.G. (1988). *Holistic nursing: A handbook for practice.* Rockville, MD: Aspen Publishers.

Dubos, R. (1965). *Man adapting.* New Haven, CT: Yale University Press.

Dunn, H.L. (1961). *High level wellness.* Arlington, VA: R.W. Beatty.

Erfurt, J.C., Foote, A., & Heirich, M.A. (1991). Worksite wellness programs: Incremental comparison of screening and referral alone, health education, follow-up counseling, and plant organization. *American Journal of Health Promotion,* July-August 5(6), 438-448.

Fleury, J.D. (1991). Empowering potential: A theory of wellness motivation. *Nursing Research,* September-October, *40*(5), 286-291.

Goldman, R.L., Adamson, T.E., Raymond, G.L., & Schore, J.E. (1989). It is time to move from health maintenance to health promotion. *Journal of Hospital Marketing, 3*(2), 115-119.

Gutt, C. (1983). *Wellness discovery curriculum and instructor guide.* Buffalo, NY: Greater Buffalo Chapter American Red Cross.

Hartsock, N. (1983). The feminist standpoint: Developing the ground for a specifically feminist historical materialism. In S. Harding & M. Hintikka (Eds). *Discovering reality: Feminist perspectives on epistemology, metaphysics, methodology, and philosophy of science,* (pp. 283-310). Boston: D. Reidel Publishing Co.

Herron, D. (1991). Strategies for promoting a healthy dietary intake. *The Nursing Clinics of North America,* December, *26*(4), 875-884.

Illich, I. (1977). *Medical nemesis.* New York: Bantam Books.

Institute of Medicine. (1978). *Perspectives of health promotion and disease prevention in the U.S.* Washington, DC: National Academy of Sciences.

Jenkins, S. (1991). Community wellness: A group empowerment model for rural America. *Journal of Health Care for the Poor and Underserved,* Spring, *1*(4), 388-404.

Johnson, C., Nicklas, T., Arbeit, M., Franklin, F., & Berenson, G. (1988). A comprehensive model for maintenance of family health behaviors: The "Heart Smart" family health promotion program. *Family & Community Health,* May, *11*(1), 1-7.

Kittleson, M.J., & Hageman-Rigney, B. (1988). Wellness and behavior contracting. *Health Education,* April/May, *19*(2), 8-11.

Kleiman, A. (1980). *Patient and healers in the context of culture.* Berkeley, CA: University of California Press.

Knowles, J.H. (Ed.). (1977). *Doing better and feeling worse.* New York: Norton.

Krieger, D. (1990). Therapeutic touch: Two decades of research, teaching and clinical practice. *NSNA/Imprint,* September-October, 83-88.

Larson, E.B., Bergaman, J., Herdricht, F., Alvin, B.L., & Schneeweiss, R. (1982). Do postcard reminders improve influenza compliance? Prospective trial of different postcard cues. *Medical Care,* June, *20*(6), 639-648.

Liu, Y. (1988). *The essential book of traditional Chinese medicine.* New York: Columbia University Press.

Maglacas, A. (1988). Health for all: Nursing's role. *Nursing Outlook,* March/April, 66-71.

McGregor, B. (1989). The step beyond. *The Lamp,* April, 17-19.

National Heart, Lung, and Blood Institute. (1970). *National cooperative pooling project.* Bethesda, MD: Author.

Neuman, B.N. (1989). *The Neuman Systems model* (2nd ed.). Norwalk, CT: Appleton & Lange.

Orem, D. (1985). *Nursing: Concepts of practice* (3rd ed.) New York: McGraw-Hill.

Parse, R.R. (1981). *Man-living health: a theory of nursing.* New York: John Wiley, 25-36.

Pender, N.J. (1987). *Health promotion in nursing practice* (2nd ed.). East Norwalk, CT: Appleton-Century-Crofts.

Pender, N.J., Walker, S.N., Sechrist, K.R., & Frank-Stromborg, M. (1990). Predicting health-promoting lifestyles in the workplace. *Nursing Research,* November-December, *39*(6), 326-332.

Public Health Service. (1981). *Health style: A self-test.* U.S. Department of Health and Human Services, Office of Disease Prevention and Health Information, Health Promotion, Physical Fitness and Sports Medicine. (Publication No. 81010877). Washington, DC: U.S. Government Printing Office.

Public Health Service. (1979). *Healthy people: The surgeon general's report on health promotion and disease prevention* (DHHS Publication No. 79-55071). Washington, DC: U.S. Government Printing Office.

Rankin-Box, D. (1991). Proceed with caution. *Nursing Times,* November, *87*(45), 34-35.

Rapacz, K. (1993). Alternative treatment modalities. *Search,* Summer, *16*(2), 9.

Redeker, N. (1988). Health beliefs and adherence in chronic illness. *Image,* 20, 31-34.

Robbins, S., & Slavin, L. (1988). A measure of social support for health-related behavior change. *Health Education,* June/July, *19*(3), 36-39.

Rosenstock, I.M. (1966). Why people use health services. *Milbank Memorial Fund Quarterly,* July, *44,* 94-127.

Schubert, M. (1989). Massage-perspectives in nursing. *The Lamp,* April, 20-21.

Seaward, B,L. (1989). Giving wellness a spiritual workout. *Health Progress,* April, *70*(3), 50-52.

Senate Select Committee on Nutrition and Human Needs. (1977). *Dietary goals for the United States.* (Publication No. 052-070-03913-2). Washington, DC: U.S. Government Printing Office.

Simons-Morton, D.G., Simons-Morton, B.G., Parcel, G.S., & Bunker, J.F. (1988). Influencing personal and environmental conditions for community health: A multi-level intervention model. *Family & Community Health,* August *11*(2), 29.

Swinford, P., & Webster, J. (1989). *Promoting wellness: A nurse's handbook,* Rockville, MD: Aspen Publishers.

Travis, J.W. (1977). *The wellness workbook for helping professionals.* Mill Valley, CA: Wellness Associates.

Travis, J.W., & Ryan, R.S. (1981). *The Wellness Workbook.* Berkeley, CA: Ten Speed Press.

Williams, D.M. (1989). Political theory and individualistic health promotion. *Advances in Nursing Science, 12*(1), 14-25.

Williams, D.M. (1991). Policy at the grassroots: Community-based participation in health care policy. *Journal of Professional Nursing,* September-October 7(5), 271-276.

Williamson, J., & Danaher, K. (1978): *Self-care in health,* London: Croom Helm.

World Health Organization: Constitution of the World Health Organization, *Chronicles of WHO,* 1-2, 1947.

8

HEALTH TEACHING IN THE COMMUNITY

Janet E. Jackson ◆ Elizabeth Johnson Blankenship

Things are experienced but not in such a way that they are composed into an experience if there is distraction and dispersion in what we observe and what we think.

John Dewey

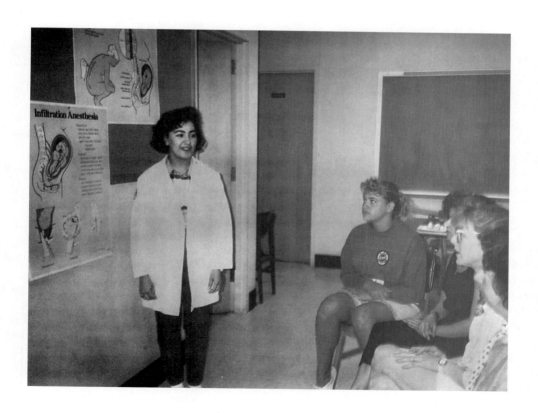

OBJECTIVES

At the conclusion of this chapter, the student will be able to:

1. Define the key terms listed.
2. Discuss the differences between teaching and learning.
3. Review the development of client teaching throughout the history of nursing.
4. Discuss the legal implications of health teaching in the community.
5. Identify principles of health teaching.
6. Relate the teaching/learning process to the nursing process.
7. Identify the areas of assessment related to health teaching.
8. Discuss the use of various teaching methods and audiovisual materials.
9. Identify guidelines that assist in the implementation of the teaching plan.
10. Recognize common barriers, problems, and mistakes.
11. Explore methods of evaluating the teaching plan and the teacher.

KEY TERMS

Affective domain
Assessment
Client education
Cognitive domain
Compliance
Educational need

Expected outcome
Extrinsic motivation
Goal
Intrinsic motivation
Learning
Objective

PRECEDE model
Psychomotor domain
Readiness to learn
Teaching/learning process
Teaching situation

According to the American Nurses' Association (ANA) and the American Public Health Association (APHA), community health nursing focuses on the prevention of illness and the promotion and maintenance of health. To accomplish these goals the community health nurse directs practice in two areas. The first area is the direct care given to individuals, families, and groups within a community. The second area is the concern for the health of the total population and the community health problems and issues that affect individuals, families, and groups. In both areas of practice the community health nurse uses nursing interventions that involve client education, counseling, advocacy, and the management of care. To effect these interventions the nurse must possess knowledge of concepts such as family-centered care, principles of teaching/learning, and assessment skills. The community health nurse takes on many roles, such as communicator, educator, and community advocate (Peters, 1989).

HISTORICAL BACKGROUND

In considering the role of health educator it is important to look at the historical background and legal issues related to health teaching. The value placed on health, the right to health care, and the right to know how to attain better health care all have become very important to the consumer.

This need for knowledge regarding one's health is not new to nurses. Nurses have been providing health teaching to their clients as early as the mid-nineteenth century. The public health nurses and the visiting nurses both in England and in the United States who were caring for clients in their homes recognized the great need for health teaching. In 1918 the National League of Nursing specified the need to include preventive care and health teaching in nursing curricula. The incorporation of teaching/learning principles is found in almost all nursing curricula.

Whether the client is an individual, a family, or a group, education is a basic community health nursing intervention. In the past several years the demand for health education in the community has greatly increased and will continue to do so as changes occur in our health delivery systems. Consumers of health care actively seek health ed-

ucation in many areas to maintain and improve their health. In addition, the rapidly growing field of home health care has been included in the realm of community health nursing and greatly increases the need for client education.

Historically and currently, community health nursing focuses on health promotion and disease prevention, whereas home care nursing focuses on individuals who are experiencing disease or infirmity (Humphrey, 1988). The nurse who is involved in home care is able to gain access to families that often are in great need of health education concerning care for an ill family member. A survey of 35 home health agencies indicated that 83% reported seeing clients whose conditions were more acute and less stable than in the past, including some clients discharged directly home from intensive care units (Hardy, 1989). The acuity of the home care client has increased dramatically. All these factors point to the increasing need for client education. The community health nurse may be teaching classes on nutrition to

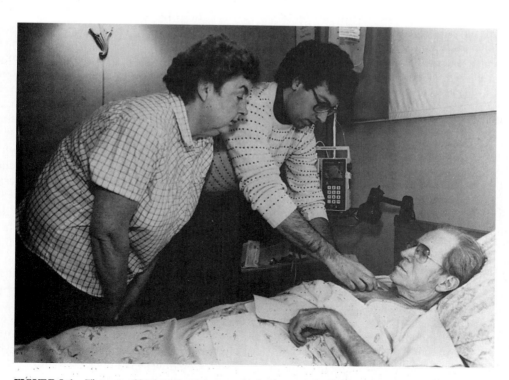

FIGURE 8-1 The use of high-tech equipment in the home has increased the need for client teaching. *(By permission of Visiting Nurses' Association of Buffalo, NY.)*

teenaged mothers or teaching a spouse how to manage technologically sophisticated equipment in the home (Figure 8-1). Whatever the setting, the nurse is not only asked but expected to provide client teaching as part of daily practice.

Client education may be provided at the primary, secondary, or tertiary level of prevention. Education programs often encompass all three levels. For example, a class related to cardiovascular disease might include clients who are trying to avoid heart disease by learning about risk factors (primary prevention), clients who have angina and are trying to change their lifestyles (secondary prevention), and clients who have had a myocardial infarction and are trying to achieve optimal health (tertiary prevention).

It becomes evident that the role of educator is a dominant one for community health nurses; education is an integral component of practice. The nurse must therefore become familiar with the teaching/learning process, which is the only way to ensure effective teaching. The following discussion of health teaching and the teaching/learning process encompasses the traditional setting of community health nursing and also the area of home care. Within these areas the community health nurse has the opportunity and challenge to meet the needs of clients through health teaching (Peters, 1989).

LEGAL ISSUES IN HEALTH TEACHING

With the development of nurse practice acts, nurses now are held accountable for their practice by law. The purpose of the practice acts is to protect the lay public from incompetent practitioners by means of establishing licensing procedures and defining the practice of nursing. Some state practice acts are ambiguous, but many are highly specific and include health teaching as a component of nursing practice.

Helen Creighton, a leading authority on legal issues in nursing, has identified a list of legal issues in home care. These include adequately prepared nurses, a thoroughly documented assessment, appropriate nursing judgment related to the assessment, use of appropriate terminology in documentation, complete documentation of all activities, adequate supervision of staff, and the inclusion of client education. She also indi-

cates that nurses in the home cannot assume that teaching was carried out in the hospital; often the information from the hospital must be reinforced or retaught.

The American Hospital Association prepared a document entitled "A Patient's Bill of Rights" in 1975. The goal of this document was to ensure high-quality care. Although written for the hospital, these rights apply equally to care in the client's home. The document establishes that clients have a right to knowledge concerning their condition, the health care delivery system, the immediate environment, and skills needed to care for self-care.

TEACHING/LEARNING THEORIES

The literature abounds with descriptions of theories and definitions of teaching and learning. Some define teaching as a process that facilitates learning, which results when a behavioral change occurs (Chatham & Knapp, 1982). Others define teaching as activities by which the teacher helps the student learn, as the process of facilitating learning, and as a deliberate action that is undertaken to help another person learn to do something (Narrow, 1979; Redman, 1988). **Learning** is said to have occurred when a person becomes capable of doing something he or she could not do before. To take it one step further, the person who has learned will be able to explain, discuss, demonstrate, or make something by using a set of ideas (Stanton, 1985). Rankin & Duffy (1983) describe client teaching as an act in which the nurse becomes involved in assisting clients to become active members of the health care team and to make informed choices regarding the quality of their life. It also enables clients to learn things that may help them live a longer and/or fuller life and to reach an optimal level of health.

A learning theory is "a systematic integrated outlook in regard to the nature of the process whereby people relate to their environments in such a way as to enhance their ability to use both themselves and their environment more effectively" (Bigge, 1982, p. 3). Many learning theories have been developed over the years.

Before the twentieth century most Western learning theories were based on learning as a mental discipline. Early theorists believed the learner has a substantive mind separate from the body. Different points of view developed. Some saw the mind as innately bad and in need of correction and advocated the use of strict discipline. This theory was called theistic mental discipline. Others described the mind as neutral and in need of exercise, which formed the basis of the humanistic mental discipline theory. The third was the natural unfoldment or self-actualization theory, based on the belief that the mind was good and should unfold naturally. The last of the mental discipline theories, termed apperception theory, viewed the mind as passive and neutral. It encouraged the process of new ideas associating themselves with old ones.

A new category of learning theories was developed in the twentieth century; these are classified as stimulus-response theories. The stimulus-response bond theory states that certain stimuli, with conditioning, evoke certain response patterns. In the co-reinforcement theory, desired responses depend on the learner's innate reflexive drives to accomplish the desired response after conditioning. Reinforcement theory states that the desired response will be elicited by the use of successive, systematic changes in the learner's environment to enhance the probability of desired responses.

More contemporary theories are those cognitive theories of Gestalt psychology, which emphasizes a holistic approach to learning. These theories assume that human beings are neither good nor bad, that they simply interact with their environment and that learning is related to perception. The insight theory views learning as a process in which the learner develops new insights or changes old ones. Goal insight theory is similar to insight theory but suggests that teachers assist learners in higher level insights as they begin to form and attain conceptual thought processes. The cognitive field theory states that the learner has purpose and is problem centered. The learner still is assisted to gain new insights. Today these theories are the most popular.

Learning theories provide the framework for the development of a philosophy of teaching. Theories help the nurse to sort out beliefs regarding the teaching/learning process; thus the

knowledge base increases and teaching should improve.

TYPES OF LEARNING

The nurse should become familiar with the different types or domains of learning (Bloom, 1969): (1) cognitive learning, (2) affective learning, and (3) psychomotor learning.

Cognitive Learning

The **cognitive domain** deals with "recall or recognition of knowledge and the development of intellectual abilities and skills" (Bloom, 1969, p. 7). It involves the mind and thinking processes. Six major categories comprise a hierarchical classification of behavior, with the simplest being first.

Knowledge. This is the lowest level and involves recall. Nurses often call upon this behavior. For example, the nurse teaches clients the signs and symptoms of congestive heart failure or hyperglycemia. The client who can identify the signs and symptoms of hyperglycemia has reached this level.

Comprehension. This level of learning combines remembering with understanding. Nurses want their clients to understand why it is important to possess certain health behaviors. The client who learns the signs and symptoms of hyperglycemia should understand how medication and lifestyle affect blood glucose levels. It certainly is a level the nurse would like to see the client reach.

Application. In the third level of cognitive learning, learners can take material they understand and apply it to theoretical and actual situations. The test of application is a transfer of understanding into practice. In teaching a client about a diet, application would be seen when the client displayed a food diary that reflects knowledge of a diet to help control blood-glucose levels.

Analysis. This stage requires the mastery of knowledge, comprehension, and application. To analyze, the learner must break information into parts, understand the relationships among parts, and distinguish among elements. This level of learning leads to problem solving. In community health nursing this level often is promoted as clients are encouraged to use analytical methodology. An example of this would be a person with newly diagnosed diabetes explaining the relationship among diet, insulin, activity, and blood glucose.

Synthesis. Synthesis is the ability to form elements into a unified whole. It brings all the previous levels of cognitive learning to the stage of developing a plan. Through assistance and encouragement from the nurse, the client can formulate a plan. By answering a question such as "What do you think you can do to keep your blood glucose in a normal range?" the client demonstrates synthesis.

Evaluation. The highest level of cognitive learning occurs when the learner uses appropriate criteria to judge the value of ideas, procedures, and methods. The client must compare one situation with another or judge a health behavior in relation to set standards. Through evaluation of daily blood glucose levels the client can decide if the new actions are meeting set goals. This level enables the client to examine closely the newly found health behavior, judge its adequacy, and decide if there is need for improvement.

Measuring cognitive learning is not difficult. It can be seen easily in the client's actions. It is important to recognize the client's cognitive abilities and plan the teaching accordingly. The nurse and the client's behaviors will vary depending on the client's cognitive level.

Affective Learning

The **affective domain** deals with "changes in interest, attitudes, values, and the development of appreciations, and adequate adjustment" (Bloom, 1969, p. 7). Through health teaching nurses promote healthier behavior patterns. The acceptance of these patterns may depend on how they are communicated to the client. Past reference has indicated the importance of health beliefs in relation to health teaching. Nurses can greatly influence a client's attitudes and values. They also must be aware of their own values and attitudes, which may not concur with those of the client.

Affective learning occurs on several levels as learners respond with varying degrees of involvement and commitment (Spradley, 1985). At the first level the learner is receptive. He or she listens, pays attention, and shows awareness of what is going on. At the second level the learner is responsive, showing some willingness to read or respond to what is being taught. The third level is valuing. The client finds value in the information being taught. The information is accepted, and the client may make a commitment to changing behavior. At the fourth level the client internalizes or conceptualizes an idea or value. The information that is learned is put into practice. The last level is that of adoption. The learner now takes the information learned and adopts a behavior consistent with what was taught.

It is difficult to measure affective learning. It is also difficult to change values and attitudes. However, through cognitive learning the client often will experience affective learning as well.

Psychomotor Learning

The **psychomotor domain** includes observable performance of skills that require some degree of neuromuscular coordination. The skill will vary depending on the task to be learned. The psychomotor skills taught to community health nursing clients are numerous. Bathing infants, breast self-examination, self-injection, food preparation, catheter irrigation, tracheostomy care, central line care, crutch walking, and dressing changes are a few examples.

For psychomotor learning to take place, the learner must first have the necessary ability. A client with diabetes and Parkinson's disease may not have the manual dexterity to perform insulin self-injections. Clients with limited intelligence should not be expected to learn complex skills. The learner also must have a sensory image of how to carry out a skill; that is, the client must be able to visualize a procedure to perform it in a logical sequence. A sensory image is obtained through demonstration of a task. The client also must have the opportunity to practice the skill. Through repetition of a task, the client will achieve mastery of the skill.

In addition to these theories there are two models that relate directly to health teaching.

PRECEDE Model

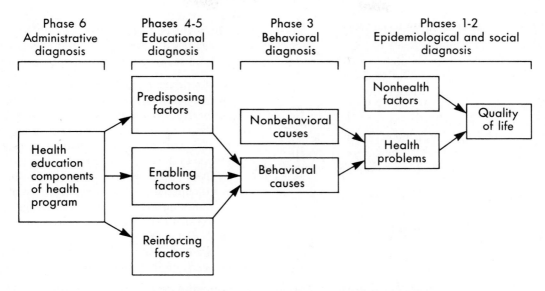

FIGURE 8-2 The PRECEDE model. *(From Health education planning: A diagnostic approach (pp 14,15) by L.W. Green, M.W. Kreuter, S.G. Deeds, & K.B. Partridge, 1980, Palo Alto, CA: Mayfield. Copyright 1980 by Mayfield Publishing Company. Reprinted by permission.)*

These are the PRECEDE model and the health belief model.

The **PRECEDE model** is a health education planning model (Green, 1980). PRECEDE stands for predisposing, reinforcing, and enabling causes in educational diagnosis and evaluation (Figure 8-2). The model indicates that certain environmental factors motivate the individual to exhibit certain health behaviors. It is based on the theory that because health and health behavior are determined by several factors, efforts to change behaviors must be multidimensional. The model works by means of a process in which the individual considers the desired outcomes and works back to the original cause. The model is applied by means of the following seven steps:

1. Consider the quality of life of the group or person involved.
2. Identify specific health problems and choose the one deserving the most attention.
3. Identify specific health-related behaviors that appear to be causing the health problem.

4. Categorize factors that have direct impact on the behavior selected:
   - Predisposing factors: attitudes, beliefs, values, and perceptions that may facilitate or hinder motivation
   - Enabling factors: barriers created by outside forces
   - Reinforcing factors: related to feedback that the learner receives from others, be it positive or negative
5. Decide which factors will be the focus of intervention.
6. Select interventions and assess problems that may arise.
7. Evaluate.

The health belief model is discussed in detail in Chapter 7.

Both these models indicate the importance of the relationship among motivation, the learning process, and **compliance.** The nurse may do an excellent job of teaching a client, but if the client was not motivated to learn or change behavior, very little is accomplished, and noncompliance may result.

PRINCIPLES OF TEACHING/LEARNING

Nurses in the community are expected to teach on a daily basis as part of their practice. To do this nurses must have a solid knowledge base, not only of theories and models of the teaching/learning process but of general principles of teaching/learning. Nurses recognize certain cues from the client that indicate a need to learn. When nurses respond to that cue, they are teaching. Teaching may be simple or complex; it may take a short time or many days to complete. Client teaching requires great involvement by both the nurse and the client (Jackson & Johnson, 1988). The nurse's knowledge of teaching/learning principles will enhance the teaching relationship established with each individual, family, or group.

The primary goal of teaching is learning. This holds true for health teaching also, but there are other goals to consider: those of promoting health, preventing illness, and coping with illness (Narrow, 1979). To reach these goals of health teaching the nurse should take into consideration the following principles (Dugas, 1972):

- Learning is more effective when it is a response to a felt need of the learner.
- Active participation on the part of the learner is essential if learning is to take place.
- Learning is made easier when the material to be learned is related to what the learner already knows.
- Learning is facilitated when the material to be learned is meaningful to the learner.
- Learning is retained longer when it is put into immediate use than when its application is delayed.
- Periodic plateaus occur in learning.
- Learning must be reinforced.
- Learning is made easier when the learner is aware of his or her progress.

Table 8-1 reiterates some of these principles but suggests the existence of superior conditions of learning and related principles of teaching.

The nurse also must look closely at the client. Whether the client is a group or an individual in the home, the person or persons who are learning often are adults. Adults bring to educational activities different self-images, experiences, and goals than do children. Knowles (1984, p. 174, 175), considered the father of adult education, offers the following guidelines in teaching adults:

- Adults prefer learning activities based on active involvement and the problems they encounter in their everyday work environment.
- Adults tend to withdraw from learning situations that are potentially humiliating and detrimental to their self-concept.
- Adults possess a large reservoir of life and work experiences and desire opportunities to capitalize on and share their knowledge.
- Adults possess a variety of individual learning styles and rates.
- Adults have many compelling and conflicting demands on their time and thought processes.

Of course the community health nurse will deal with clients other than adults. Often the client may be a child or group of children. Learning ability and appropriate teaching methods related to age are found in Table 8-2.

THE TEACHING/LEARNING PROCESS AND THE NURSING PROCESS

Community health nurses function as a primary source for health teaching. Their knowledge, opportunities for teaching, and the nature of the client-nurse relationship enable them to assume this role. In Table 8-3 different nursing theorists views are described. As nurses use their knowledge of nursing and teaching/learning principles, they should consider the following questions (Jackson & Johnson, 1988):

- What factors influence readiness to learn?
- Does the client want to learn?
- How important is it that the client learn?
- What should the client learn?
- What does the client want to learn?
- What is the best way to teach the information?
- What can you do to increase the likelihood that your client will learn what you taught?
- How can you tell when a person has learned something?

These questions can be answered by means

TABLE 8-1 Superior conditions of learning and principles of teaching

Conditions of learning	Principles of teaching
The learners feel a need to learn.	1. The teacher exposes students to new possibilities for self-fulfillment. 2. The teacher helps each student clarify his own aspirations for improved behavior. 3. The teacher helps each student diagnose the gap between his aspiration and his present level of performance. 4. The teacher helps the students identify the life problems they experience because of the gaps in their personal equipment.
The learning environment is characterized by physical comfort, mutual trust and respect, mutual helpfulness, freedom of expression, and acceptance of differences.	5. The teacher provides physical conditions that are comfortable (as to seating, smoking, temperature, ventilation, lighting, decoration) and conducive to interaction (preferably, no person sitting behind another person). 6. The teacher accepts each student as a person of worth and respects his feelings and ideas. 7. The teacher seeks to build relationships of mutual trust and helpfulness among the students by encouraging cooperative activities and refraining from inducing competitiveness and judgementalness. [sic] 8. The teacher exposes his own feelings and contributes his resources as a colearner in the spirit of mutual inquiry.
The learners perceive the goals of a learning experience to be their goals.	9. The teacher involves the students in a mutual process of formulating learning objectives in which the needs of the students, of the institution, of the teacher, of the subject matter, and of the society are taken into account.
The learners accept a share of the responsibility for planning and operating a learning experience, and therefore have a feeling of commitment toward it.	10. The teacher shares his thinking about options available in the designing of learning experiences and the selection of materials and methods and involves the students in deciding among these options jointly.
The learners participate actively in the learning process.	11. The teacher helps the students to organize themselves (project groups, learning-teaching teams, independent study, etc.) to share responsibility in the process of mutual inquiry.
The learning process is related to and makes use of the experience of the learners.	12. The teacher helps the students exploit their own experiences as resources for learning through the use of such techniques as discussion, role playing, case method, etc. 13. The teacher gears the presentation of his own resources to the levels of experience of his particular students. 14. The teacher helps the students to apply new learnings to their experience, and thus to make the learnings more meaningful and integrated.
The learners have a sense of progress toward their goals.	15. The teacher involves the students in developing mutually acceptable criteria and methods for measuring progress toward the learning objectives. 16. The teacher helps the students develop and apply procedures for self-evaluation according to these criteria.

From *The modern practice of adult education: From pedagogy to andragogy, revised and updated* (pp. 57-58) by M.S. Knowles, 1980, Engelwood Cliffs, N.J.: Prentice Hall, Inc. Reprinted by permission.

TABLE 8-2   Developmental capacities for learning

Learning capacity	Teaching methods
Infant	
Infant relies on parents for basic needs.	Keep routines (e.g., feeding, bathing) consistent.
Infant learns to trust adults when they convey love and compassion.	Hold infant firmly while smiling and speaking softly to convey sense of trust.
Infant explores environment through senses.	
Toddler	
Toddler learns to understand words and express feelings verbally.	Use play to teach procedure or activity (e.g., handling examination equipment, applying bandage to doll).
Toddler learns by associating words with objects.	Offer picture books that describe story of children in hospital or clinic.
Toddler likes to explore environment through play.	Use simple words such as *cut* instead of *laceration* to promote understanding.
Preschooler	
Vocabulary grows.	Use role playing, imitation, and play to make it fun for preschoolers to learn.
Preschooler uses language without comprehending meaning of words, especially concepts (e.g., right or left, time).	Encourage questions and offer explanations. Use simple explanations and demonstrations.
During play, child expresses feelings more through actions than words.	Encourage children to learn together through pictures and short stories of how to perform hygiene.
Preschooler asks questions and imitates adults.	
School-age child	
Child interacts with adults and peers outside immediate family.	Teach psychomotor skills needed to maintain health. (Complicated skills, such as learning to use a syringe, may take considerable practice.)
Child begins to acquire ability to relate series of events and actions to mental representations that can be expressed verbally and symbolically.	Offer opportunities to discuss health problems and answer questions.
Child is able to make judgments.	
Child matures physically.	
Play becomes more formal and imaginative.	
Child is inquisitive and asks many questions about health.	
Adolescent	
Adolescent struggles between childlike feelings of dependence and independence of adults.	Help adolescent learn about feelings and need for self-expression.
Teenager wants to be in control but, during illness, fears loss of self-concept or body image.	Use teaching as collaborative activity.
Adolescent is able to solve abstract problems.	Allow adolescents to make decisions about health and health promotion (e.g., safety, sex education, substance abuse).
Teenager learns best when immediate benefit is gained.	Use problem solving to help adolescents make choices.

TABLE 8-2 Developmental capacities for learning cont'd

Learning capacity	Teaching methods
Young or middle adult	
Adult complies with health teaching because client fears the results, is trying to gain approval, is responding to nurse's attitude, or knows it is in best interest.	Encourage participation in teaching plan by setting mutual goals.
Learning occurs when adult values information being taught.	Encourage independent learning. Offer information so that adult can understand effects of health problem.
Older adult	
Often, there is decline in visual and auditory acuity, which impairs perception of stimuli.	Teach when client is alert and rested.
Sensory alterations, mobility limitations, and physical coordination problems affect capacity to learn.	Involve adult in discussion or activity. Focus on wellness and the person's strength.
Sleep-wake cycles are more fragmented.	Use approaches that enhance sensorially impaired client's reception of stimuli.
Older adult takes pride in being independent and caring for self.	Keep teaching sessions short.
There is no decline in intelligence with age.	

From *Fundamentals of nursing* (ed. 3) by P.A. Potter & A.G. Perry, 1993, St. Louis: Mosby.
Data from *Preoperative patient education seminar presentation by S.* Woodard, 1983, Denver: Resource Applications.

of the nurse's understanding of the **teaching/ learning process.**

The nursing process is the foundation of nursing practice. It is an orderly sequence of steps that include assessment, diagnosis, planning, implementation, and evaluation. The nursing process can provide a framework in which a nurse can develop, plan, and carry out client teaching. By employing knowledge of the nursing process and teaching/learning principles, the nurse can provide client education in such a way that both the nurse and client will grow in a cooperative relationship (Jackson & Johnson, 1988). The teaching/learning process and the nursing process fit very easily together, providing an excellent framework for developing an effective teaching plan. The five steps of the nursing process and how the teaching/learning process fits into the process are described in the box on p.186. Each of the steps would be used in developing a teaching plan.

Assessment

To formulate a teaching plan a thorough educational assessment must be performed. This in-

cludes **assessment** of the need, the learner, the teaching situation, and the teacher. All these areas are vital to a complete assessment of educational needs.

The educational need. Before the assessment is begun, the resources available to provide the needed information should be examined. Table 8-4 describes sources that can be used.

The following list presents four classifications of educational needs (Atwood & Ellis, 1971):

1. A real need is one that is based on a deficiency that actually exists.

2. An educational need is one that can be met by a learning experience.

3. A real educational need indicates that specific skills, knowledge, and attitudes are required to assist the client in attaining a more desirable condition.

4. A felt need is recognized as important by the learner.

It is important to recognize educational needs because they determine the specific content to be taught. Even though clients often will identify their needs, the nurse must be able to recognize needs not perceived by the client and to ques-

TABLE 8-3   Elements of selected nursing models that are instructive for patient education

Model author	Elements of model instructive for patient education
Peplau	Nursing helps patients gain intellectual and interpersonal competencies beyond those that they have at the point of illness. Nursing is an educative instrument that facilitates the patient's ability to transform symptom-bound energy into problem-solving energy.
Henderson	Function of the nurse is to assist the individual, sick or well, in performance of activities that he or she would perform unaided if he or she had the necessary strength, will, or knowledge to do so.
Orem	When the patient's self-care agency is inadequate to meet the therapeutic self-care demand, a self-care deficit occurs. Nursing assists patients to develop self-care abilities.
Neuman	Nurses teach individuals and communities how to respond to stressors.
Allen (McGill Model)	Nursing engages the client/family in the search for healthy being by structuring appropriate learning experiences that use pertinent health information by giving the client/family opportunities to share, discuss, and test appropriate plans of action.
Watson	Nursing includes a commitment to caring as a moral ideal. Two of the ten carative factors used by nurses are the use of problem-solving techniques for decision making and the promotion of interpersonal teaching-learning.

From *The process of patient education* (ed. 7) by B.K. Redman, 1993, St. Louis: Mosby.

THE TEACHING/LEARNING PROCESS AND THE NURSING PROCESS

1. Assessment
   a. The need
   b. The learner
      • Ability to learn
      • Readiness to learn
      • Attitude and motivation
   c. The teaching situation
   d. The teacher
2. Diagnosis
   a. Identify the problem
   b. Establish a diagnosis
3. Planning
   a. Establish a plan of teaching
   b. Formulate learning objectives
   c. Develop contracts
   d. Select teaching methods and audiovisual materials
4. Implementation
   a. Carry out teaching
   b. Recognize obstacles
5. Evaluation
   a. Teaching effectiveness
   b. Teaching ability

Modified from *Patient education in home care* (p. 20) by J. Jackson & E. Johnson, 1988, Rockville, MD: Aspen Publishers, Inc., copyright 1988. Reprinted by permission.

---

tion suspect health practices. Ten areas to consider in assessing the client's educational needs are:

- normal body functions
- health problems and diagnosis
- medication prescribed
- diet
- activity limitations
- diagnostic tests
- preventive and/or health promotion activities
- community resources
- financial resources
- and future plans for the use of the health care system (Chatham & Knapp, 1982).

Often the teaching is related to the client's prescribed medical regimen. In assessing the client's educational needs in this area, the nurse

TABLE 8-4 Informational resources related to educational need

Source	Information provided
Client	Attitude toward learning
	Motivation, values, beliefs
	Interest and readiness to learn
	Medical, social, cultural, and educational background
	Activities of daily living
	Routine coping mechanisms
	Likely areas of noncompliance
	Support systems
	Comprehension level
Family or significant other	Insight into past experience
	Reinforcement of information obtained from client
Client's chart	Medical diagnosis and prognosis
	Current treatment regimen
	Client's response to treatment
	Teaching that has been done and client response
Nursing care plan	Identification of unique individual characteristics of client
	Goals of the present illness
	Daily life-style modifications
	Nursing interventions and response
Other health care professionals	New client information
	Coordination of teaching efforts
	Information already taught and client's response
Standardized teaching plans for specific diagnosis; literature regarding teaching content for specific diagnosis	Help in formulation of the teaching plan
	Provide knowledge for the teacher
	Access to available resources dealing with the content to be taught

should consider the following questions: Why is it done? Who does it? When is it done? How long does it take? What is the cost? What is the client required to do? Can the client do it?

The areas of health teaching are vast, reflecting the client's many different educational needs.

In assessing these needs, the client, family, and teachers should consider certain questions (Chatham & Knapp, 1982):

1. What should the patient know about his or her health condition(s), testing, treatments, prognosis?

2. What skills should the patient be able to perform to implement prescribed and recommended therapeutic or rehabilitative interventions?

3. What attitudes should the patient possess to adopt and integrate health-related skills and practices into his or her daily life?

4. What long-term health practices should the patient incorporate into his or her lifestyle?

5. What resources does the patient need to accomplish all the above?

Many different questions and areas are considered in the assessment of educational needs. Identification of educational needs is vital to the assessment. Once these are established, the nurse can move on to assessment of the learner.

The learner. In community health practice the learner may be a community, a group, or an individual. The individual may be a child or an adult. The learner also may be the spouse, parent, or significant other. Whoever the learner is, three areas to consider are (1) readiness to learn, (2) ability to learn, and (3) attitude and motivation.

Readiness to learn. The nurse implements a well-organized teaching plan, yet the client does not learn. The client is not ready to learn. Assessment of the client's readiness will save much time in the teaching/learning process. Client readiness greatly influences teaching effectiveness.

Readiness to learn is described as the state of being both willing and able to use health teaching (Narrow, 1979). There are two types of learner readiness: emotional readiness, which is described as motivation or willingness, and experiential readiness, which includes the client's background of experiences, skills, attitudes, and ability to learn (Redman, 1988).

Many factors influence a client's readiness to learn. Among them are comfort, energy, capability, and motivation. A client's health or lack of health also can influence readiness. A client who is anxious or in pain certainly is not ready to learn. The nurse must consider the client's physical and psychological comfort, emotions, and level of energy. The client's developmental stage also is important: "The teachable moment for adults is when the content and skills to be taught are consistent with the developmental tasks" (Stanhope & Lancaster, 1988, p. 190). Because of the multiplicity of influences on learning, it is imperative that the nurse know the client and recognize the effect of these factors on learning.

Ability to learn. The ability to learn can be easily assessed; it can be observed, tested, and measured. Ability is influenced by many factors, including age, maturation, previous learning, physical and mental health, and the environment. If the client has physical or intellectual disabilities, these must be recognized. A client who has hemiplegia cannot be expected to accomplish a psychomotor task that requires the use of both hands. Strength, coordination, dexterity, and the senses must be taken into account. Mathematics, reading, and verbal skills must be assessed. Printed material should not be used as a teaching tool if the client's reading skills are poor. (Readability of learning material is discussed later in the chapter.) Previous experience and past learning must be assessed. The client's ability provides a basis for formulating the teaching plan related to the client's needs.

Attitude and motivation. The client's attitudes toward learning and health are paramount in learning the information presented. Motivation too is a major determinant of client learning. In relation to health teaching, it is essential that the learner wants to learn and perceives the importance of the activity before actually participating (Dracup & Meleis, 1982). The health belief model and the PRECEDE model are based on the importance of both attitudes and motivation.

There are two types of motivation: intrinsic and extrinsic. **Intrinsic motivation** is defined as values, attitudes, perceptions, and/or unmet needs. **Extrinsic motivation** comes from outside forces such as family pressure, environmental factors, and/or changes in lifestyle. A client can possess an abundance of knowledge but, if motivation is lacking, rarely will comply (Cohen, 1979). Clients must recognize the need for information and be mentally and physically ready be-

fore they can be motivated (Falvo, 1985).

Motivation moves people to action. The desire to know and understand, get well, return to work, avoid complications, please others, and manage their own care are all factors that can motivate clients to learn. What motivates is unique to each client, and any motivation to learn is a valid one.

All these aspects of assessment—the need, learner readiness, ability, and motivation—are necessary components of an educational assessment. The nurse must be knowledgeable and adept in all aspects. Although the client is the most important component of assessment, a complete assessment also includes the teaching situation and the teacher.

The teaching situation. The nurse should provide an environment that is conducive to learning. Three aspects of the environment must be assessed: the physical environment, the interpersonal environment, and the external environment.

The physical environment is the actual room where teaching occurs. The room should have comfortable physical surroundings, minimal distractions, and provide a comfortable setting for both client and teacher. It would be foolish to attempt to help a mother with breast-feeding in a room where Grandma is visiting with the next-door neighbor and three children are playing. Although there are times when control over the environment is impossible, the nurse must carefully and judiciously choose where the teaching will take place whenever possible.

The interpersonal environment is one over which the nurse has control. A trusting, caring relationship, with mutual respect, should be developed. Active listening is important. A rapport must be established for teaching to be effective. The nurse must listen, make eye contact, ask for the client's opinion, avoid reading or writing while the client is talking, and check with the client for clarification of what is understood. All these actions can foster a positive interpersonal environment.

The external environment includes the resources and support that are available to the educational process, for example, available specialists or consultants, time, money and materials, administrative support, collegial support, physician support, and familial support.

The nurse may question the need for physician support, believing that she or he is capable of identifying the client's educational needs. If, however, the client is being seen in the home and the visit is eligible for Medicare reimbursement, then the nursing service must be approved or ordered by a physician. Support from all the aforementioned areas allows for a more effective learning experience.

The teacher. All too often assessment of the teacher is ignored. Teaching is an integral component of nursing practice and a responsibility of each nurse. However, is every nurse capable of teaching? Nurses must carefully examine their own beliefs concerning the teaching/learning process (Jackson & Johnson, 1988), and all nurses should work to develop better teaching skills.

Four factors are considered in assessing the ability to teach: energy, attitude, knowledge, and skill. The act of teaching takes great energy and can be very time-consuming. The nurse's attitude should be considered in relation to teaching, the client, and the subject matter. The nurse's knowledge base should be examined. Knowledge of the topic to be taught is necessary to facilitate learning. Last, the nurse should possess skills that reflect teaching/learning principles and should be knowledgeable about content. All nurses who assume the role of teacher should evaluate themselves in these areas. The nurse who supervises other nurses who teach must also evaluate their teaching ability. Once the assessment is completed, the process continues to the next step, that of establishing the diagnosis.

Diagnosis

Nursing diagnosis can be defined in various ways. It is the end of the assessment. The North American Nursing Diagnosis Association (NANDA) defines nursing as a clinical judgment about an individual, family, or community response to actual or potential health problems and life processes. Nursing diagnosis provides the basis for selection of nursing interventions to achieve outcome for which the nurse is accountable.

Although some might think that a nursing diagnosis is not relevant in developing a teaching plan, one of NANDA's diagnostic categories is that of knowledge deficit. The diagnosis of knowledge deficit can easily be used in teaching plans. The problem (knowledge deficit) and the factors that contribute to the problem (e.g., dietary management of a low-sodium diet) are identified. This diagnosis would be stated as knowledge deficit related to inability to manage a low-sodium diet. From the diagnosis a teaching plan can be developed.

Although knowledge deficit is still considered a nursing diagnosis it has been identified that a knowledge deficit does not represent a human response, alteration, or a pattern of dysfunction, but rather a related factor (Jenny, 1987).

Many other nursing diagnoses may indicate the need for client teaching by including statements where the knowledge deficit is the "related to" portion of the nursing diagnosis, such as anxiety related to knowledge deficit of tube feedings and gastrostomy care, altered health maintenance related to knowledge deficit of hypertension and prescribed medical regimen, and so on.

Planning

With the assessment completed and a diagnosis established, the nurse prepares a teaching plan in collaboration with the client. The family and client must be involved in this part of the process. The questions of what, how, where, and when must be answered.

Writing objectives. At this point learning objectives with expected outcomes should be established. The terms **goal, expected outcome,** and **objective** are often used interchangeably in nursing literature. Regardless of the terms, they are all statements of what is expected to be accomplished by a certain time. The purpose of planning is to identify a specific means to evaluate the client's response to nursing care (Hickey, 1990). It has been suggested that when writing a goal statement, the objective should be a broad statement, and the expected outcomes should be the more specific applications of the objective. An example would be: The client will demonstrate knowledge of medical regimen (objective) by verbalization of drug names, doses, times, purpose, and side effects (expected outcome) (Al-faro, 1990). These statements serve the following functions:

- To identify activities regarding content and methods to be used
- To inform the patient of what is expected
- To provide a basis for evaluation
- To promote continuity of the teaching activities when more than one discipline is involved
- To enable the setting of priorities regarding information the patient needs
- To provide a guide for patient teaching that ultimately should save time

Each of the following factors should be included in the writing of learning objectives:

- Behaviors the patient is expected to accomplish as a result of the teaching
- Objectives that are client-centered, including what the client will do
- A clear, concise statement that includes an action verb and the criterion for measurement

Objectives should be written in behavioral terms and categorized into the three domains of learning: cognitive, affective, and psychomotor. Examples of verbs related to the cognitive do-

---

Date _____

Health-care contract

Contract goal: (Specific outcome to be attained)

I, (client's name), agree to (detailed description of required behaviors, time and frequency limitations) in return for (positive reinforcements contingent upon completion of required behaviors; timing and mode of delivery of reinforcements).

I, (provider's name), agree to (detailed description of required behaviors, time and frequency limitations).

(Optional) I, (significant other's name), agree to (detailed description of required behaviors, time and frequency limitations).

(Optional) Aversive consequences: (Negative reinforcements for failure to meet minimum behavioral requirements).

(Optional) Bonuses: (Additional positive reinforcements for exceeding minimum contact requirements).

We will review the terms of this agreement, and will make any desired modifications, on (date). We hereby agree to abide by the terms of the contract described above.

Signed:(Client) _____

Signed:(Significant other, if relevant) _____

Signed:(Provider) _____

Contract effective from (Date) _____

to (Date) _____

FIGURE 8-3 Example of a client contract. (*From* Patient education and counseling *by N.K. Jany, M.H. Becker, & P.E. Hartman, 1984 5[4], p. 178. Copyright 1984 by Elsevier Scientific Publishers Ireland Ltd. Reprinted by permission.*)

main that can be used in writing objectives follow:

Knowledge: count, define, identify, list, report

Comprehension: compare, distinguish, describe, discuss, explain

Application: apply, demonstrate, practice, relate, utilize

Analysis: analyze, differentiate, distinguish, question, summarize

Synthesis: assemble, design, formulate, organize, plan

Evaluation: assess, determine, evaluate, measure, recommend

Developing contracts. The number of objectives depends on the individual needs of each client. From the assessment data the nurse and the client may set priorities related to the objectives. This is a time when a client-nurse contract may be developed. Figure 8-3 provides an example of a written contract, and Table 8-5 illustrates

TABLE 8-5 Good patient contracts: characteristics and examples

Characteristics of a good patient contract	Questions health professionals can ask to help patient set an achievable goal	Sample contract: Mr. Dixon, 47, is an obese businessman, who had a heart attack 4 months ago. His goals:	Sample contract: Ms. Waverly, 56, is a plump woman with angina pectoris, who finds she snacks constantly. Her goals:
Realistic	Does goal seem possible? Have you ever had regular exercise? Sound reasonable at this time?	Walk the dog.	Lose weight.
Measurable	How often can you do this? What will show you have done this?	Walk the dog around the lake for 30 minutes.	Lose 5 pounds.
Positive	What goals are you working toward? What are you going to do for yourself? What strengths can you build on?	I will do this following exercise . . .	I will lose weight by a. Eating three meals b. Sitting down to eat c. An evening snack of an apple or other fruit
Time-dated	When can you start this? What will you do in the next 2 weeks?	Walk the dog each night before supper for the next 2 weeks.	Lose 5 pounds by the end of the month, which is my birthday.
Written	Could I write down your ideas? Would you write down these goals we are discussing?	Will walk dog 30 minutes around a lake before supper — 2 weeks.	I'll lose 5 pounds by my birthday. 1. Eat three meals a day 2. Sit down 3. Fruit snack at bedtime
Rewardable	If you make this effort, what reward could you give yourself?	New walking shoes if I accomplish my goal.	A long-distance telephone call to my sister.
Evaluated	How can I help you evaluate your goals? Can you share your goals with anyone?	I'll come back in to see you to report progress in 2 weeks.	I'll ask my sister to work on these goals with me. I will send you a postcard the first of next month with my results.

From "Hows and why of patient contracting" by P. A. Herje, 1980, *Nurse Educator, 5,* p. 30. Copyright 1980 by J.B. Lippincott Co. Reprinted by permission.

characteristics and examples of good client contracts. A contract usually specifies what is to be learned, how long it will take to learn, how the learning will be evaluated, and possibly a reward. Contracting is believed to strengthen the involvement and responsibility of the learner and therefore increase the likelihood of effective teaching (Figure 8-4).

Selecting teaching methods and audiovisual materials. During the planning stage the nurse must choose a teaching method or methods and educational materials needed to carry out the teaching plan. The choices should coincide with the stated objectives. Consideration must be given as to whether the nurse is teaching a group or an individual and the characteristics of the learner. Table 8-6 describes various teaching methods. Teaching methods can be matched with the domains and levels of learning (Table 8-7).

When making home visits, the nurse most often will be instructing one or a few individuals, but many times in the community the nurse will be instructing larger groups. Group instruction offers many advantages. It is economical, groups of learners can be reached with one teaching plan, it offers structured time, and usually allows for planning of content in advance. Common teaching methods used with groups include role playing, lecture, discussions, demonstrations, and case studies. Groups also can benefit the learner. They provide security and the opportunity to share experiences, resources, and to learn from one another (Stanhope & Lancaster, 1988). The nurse's role in working with groups is discussed in detail in Chapter 6.

The nurse must select educational materials according to the client's needs and abilities. Audiovisual materials include printed material, films, videotapes, audiotapes, records, and slides. All materials should be viewed and evaluated before they are used. The following questions should be considered in the evaluation of audiovisual materials:

What is the readability factor (if printed material)?

Is the material incorrect or contradictory of other sources being used?

Is it beyond the level of understanding of the client?

Is the quality good?

Did the client find the audiovisual helpful?

The nurse should determine if the material actually will add to teaching effectiveness or will just take up valuable time.

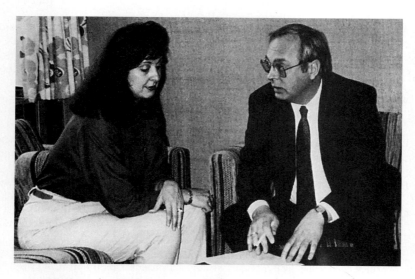

FIGURE 8-4   Nurse and client should review the contract together.

TABLE 8-6 Summary of instructional methods

Instructor-centered	Interactive	Individualized
Lecture Students are passive Efficient for lower learning levels and large classes	**Class discussion** Class size must be small May be time-consuming Encourages student involvement	**Programmed instruction** Most effective at lower learning levels Very structured Students work at own pace Students receive extensive feedback
Questioning Monitors students learning Encourages student involvement May cause anxiety for some	**Discussion groups** Class size should be small Students participate Effective for high cognitive and affective learning levels	**Modularized instruction** Can be time-consuming Very flexible formats Students work at own pace
Demonstration Illustrates an application of a skill or concept Students are passive	**Peer teaching** Requires careful planning and monitoring Utilizes differences in student expertise Encourages student involvement	**Independent projects** Most appropriate at higher learning levels Can be time-consuming Students are actively involved in learning
	Group projects Requires careful planning, including evaluation techniques Useful at higher learning levels Encourages active student participation	**Computerized instruction** May involve considerable instructor-time or expense Can be very flexible Students work at own pace Students may be involved in varying activities

Experiential learning methods				
Field or clinical Occurs in natural setting during performance Students are actively involved Management and evaluation may be difficult	**Laboratory** Requires careful planning and evaluation Students actively involved in a realistic setting	**Role playing** Effective in affective and psychomotor domains Provides "safe" experiences Active student participation	**Simulations and games** Provide practice of specific skills Produces anxiety for some students Active student participation	**Drill** Most appropriate at lower learning levels Provides active practice May not be motivating for some students

TABLE 8-7   Matching domain and level of learning to appropriate methods

Domain and level	Method
Cognitive domain	
Knowledge	Lecture, programmed instruction, drill and practice
Comprehension	Lecture, modularized instruction, programmed instruction
Application	Discussion, simulations and games, CAI,* modularized instruction, field experiences, laboratory
Analysis	Discussion, independent/group projects, simulations, field experience, role-playing, laboratory
Synthesis	Independent/group projects, field experience, role-playing, laboratory
Evaluation	Independent/group projects, field experience, laboratory
Affective domain	
Receiving	Lecture, discussion, modularized instruction, field experience
Responding	Discussion, simulations, modularized instruction, role-playing, field experience
Valuing	Discussion, independent/group projects, simulations, role-playing, field experience
Organization	Discussion, independent/group projects, field experience
Characterization by a value	Independent projects, field experience
Psychomotor domain	
Perception	Demonstration (lecture), drill and practice
Set	Demonstration (lecture), drill and practice
Guided response	Peer teaching, games, role-playing, field experience, drill and practice
Mechanism	Games, role-playing, field experience, drill and practice
Complex overt response	Games, field experience
Adaptation	Independent projects, games, field experience
Origination	Independent projects, games, field experience

From Selecting Instructional strategies by C. Weston & P. A. Cranton, 1986, *Journal of Higher Education, 57,* p. 278. Copyright 1986 by The Ohio State University Press. Reprinted with permission. All rights reserved.
*CAI: Computer-assisted instruction

If printed material is chosen, the literacy level of the client must be considered. If reading ability is not assessed, the nurse can easily embarrass the client or be unaware of why learning did not take place. The client's ability to comprehend the material is essential to client learning.

Many formulas can be used to measure readability. These include the Fry formula, the Flesch formula, and the Fog formula. These formulas are based on word and sentence length. The Fry formula can determine the level of materials from grade one through college. It must be used on passages of 300 words or more. The Flesch formula can determine the level of material be-

tween grade five through college completion. The Fog formula tests levels of material between grade four and college. Both the Flesch and the Fog are useful for short brochures and pamphlets because they can be used with only 100 words. The nurse should practice using these formulas and decide which is preferred. All printed materials should be closely evaluated and chosen according to the client's capabilities.

Implementation

The nurse who presents the plan of teaching should be knowledgeable in terms of content, and assessment of the learner's abilities should always be kept in mind. The more often the nurse takes the responsibility for teaching, the more the ability to teach and self-confidence will increase. When implementing the teaching plan, the nurse should take the following actions:

- Provide a conducive learning environment.
- Communicate the importance of learning.
- Communicate enjoyment in teaching the material.
- Express enthusiasm and concern through voice and body language.
- Take time and avoid rushing the client.
- Praise the client frequently and note progress.
- Repeat information often.
- Show flexibility, adjusting learning goals as necessary.
- Let the client share what he or she knows about the subject.
- Reinforce all information presented.
- Reward if beneficial.
- Try to allow the client to use the information learned without delay.

Obstacles to implementation. Obstacles to implementation include barriers, problems, and mistakes. These are common problems that can occur with the most organized teaching plan. Being aware of them can help when they actually are encountered in practice.

Barriers. Barriers are external problems that frequently are encountered, such as lack of administrative support, lack of time, poor resources, conflict with other disciplines, and inadequate teaching skills. Lack of administrative support can lead to almost all the other barriers listed. Administration and nursing personnel must share the same philosophy of health teaching and believe it to be beneficial and necessary. Nurses often are called on to demonstrate that health teaching is cost effective.

Lack of resources such as staff and audiovisual materials can be frustrating. Nursing staff is essential; however, audiovisual materials often are helpful but not always necessary. Both resources depend on financial assets.

Lack of time is related to inadequate staffing, high client load, and poor organization. The nurse must recognize the amount of time needed for health teaching and arrange the schedule accordingly. If staffing or high client load is the

problem, administrative personnel should be informed.

A client also may be seen by other professionals such as a physical or an occupational therapist. Thus a lack of coordination of teaching activities can occur and cause conflict. Teaching activities should be coordinated by means of team conferences when necessary.

The last barrier is that of inadequate teaching skills. The effectiveness of teaching certainly depends on how well the material is taught. The nurse is responsible for health teaching and should update and seek knowledge when needed.

Problems. Some problems the nurse may encounter relate to client situations such as a wide age range, noncompliance, and terminal illness. These problems occur in the community, in group settings, or in the home.

The client's age presents various problems. Adult learning characteristics, discussed earlier in the chapter, also apply to the elderly client. There are, however, special considerations. In teaching elderly persons, information should sometimes be presented at a slower rate. The client should be evaluated carefully for sensory deprivation related to aging. The nurse also should be alert to decreased capacity related to cerebral changes.

When the client is a child, the nurse should make the teaching plan flexible and creative, schedule short sessions, and consider the child's developmental stage and cognitive level. Incorporating play into the plan usually is helpful. Parental involvement depends on the age of the child. With a small child the parents should be included whereas with adolescents it may be best to not include them; the nurse and client must make this decision on a case-by-case basis. Adolescent knowledge must be assessed carefully inasmuch as adolescents often imply that they are knowledgeable when they are not.

Noncompliance always is a potential problem when teaching is involved. Noncompliance occurs frequently. Cohen (1979) estimated that only one third of chronically ill clients adhere to their therapeutic regimens; one third are noncompliant because they adhere to a misunderstood regimen; and one third choose to be noncompliant. The community setting may

TABLE 8-8 Common mistakes in the teaching/learning process

Assessment

This step has already been identified as one of the most important components of the teaching/learning process. Poor and ineffective assessments lead to a poor and inadequate teaching plan. Always confirm information obtained. Many times, illiterate patients end up with printed teaching material. Always reassess.

Failure to negotiate goals

One often forgets that the goals established are (or should have been) the patient's goals. The nurse may have goals, but patient goals should be given priority. Recognize when the goals need to be renegotiated. Unrealistic goals lead to noncompliance.

Territoriality and duplication

Nurses can become very possessive of their patients and may want to be the only person available to them. They also feel personally responsible for the patient's teaching. One must remember that the patient is ultimately responsible for his behavior. Duplication of information often happens when the patient goes from the hospital to home and if the home health nurse changes. This can be solved with patient care conferences and good documentation of patient teaching.

Patient overload

Too often, too much material is presented at one time. Shorter sessions are usually helpful in preventing this, and they allow the patient to synthesize and formulate questions. Be alert to the patient yawning, fidgeting, or being unable to answer questions. These may indicate overload and the need for a break in teaching.

Poor timing of patient teaching

The nurse must consider the patient's schedule, physical comfort, and stress level. Very little learning can take place if the patient is in pain or anxious about something.

Poor use of media

Never use materials that have not been reviewed. This can lead to ineffective teaching and even very embarrassing moments. Know your material. Also, never rely solely on media for teaching.

Recognition of patient's background

There are times when the nurse seems to have forgotten the information gained from the assessment. Asking a patient who has financial problems to follow an expensive dietary regimen is unreasonable. The patient's ethnic, educational, and financial background is sometimes not remembered. The nurse too often teaches from previous background.

Making assumptions

Making assumptions is very easy to do but can be detrimental to effective teaching. The following nevers should be remembered:
- Never assume that a patient understands the disease or prescribed treatment even if it has been diagnosed for some time.
- Never assume that a patient knows why a prescription drug is taken.
- Never assume because a patient is from a different socioeconomic, ethnic, or educational background that he will not be motivated or able to learn.
- Never assume that because a patient has been noncompliant in the past that he will continue to be.
- Never make assumptions!

Poor documentation

This is surely a very common mistake and a very important aspect of patient teaching, especially in home health.

From *Patient education in home care,* (pp. 43-44) by J. Jackson & E. Johnson, 1988, Rockville, MD: Aspen. Copyright 1988 by Aspen Publishers, Inc. Reprinted by permission.

contribute to noncompliance, especially in the home setting. Clients who have been compliant in the hospital often forget the regimen when they go home and return to old habits. The nurse possibly can increase client compliance by the following actions:

- Establishing a caring relationship
- Assessing the client's beliefs and values concerning health
- Encouraging the client to question what is being done
- Reinforcing the benefits of the prescribed regimen
- Praising the client frequently
- Offering realistic expectations

Mistakes. Many mistakes can occur during the teaching/learning process, the most common of which are identified in Table 8-8.

The obstacles discussed can be encountered in many areas of health teaching. Through awareness the nurse can work to prevent them and minimize disruptions in the teaching/learning process.

Evaluation

Evaluating teacher effectiveness often is the most neglected component of the teaching/learning process. The worth of teaching can be known only through evaluation of two areas: (1) teaching effectiveness and (2) teacher performance.

If learning objectives with expected outcomes were written, what the client learned can be evaluated. This can be accomplished through written tests, laboratory data, return demonstrations, compliance, and/or a follow-up questionnaire. Teacher performance can be evaluated through videotaping a teaching session or having a colleague present during teaching. Peer evaluation should be based on mutual trust and respect. The client also can evaluate the teacher through written or direct feedback.

If the teaching was deemed unsuccessful, the reasons for this are analyzed and the process begins again. It cannot be assumed that teaching was effective and that learning took place. The teaching/learning process is not complete until evaluation of the teaching and the learning based on expected outcomes.

Chapter Highlights

- Education is a basic community health nursing intervention. In the past several years the demand for health education has increased greatly.

- Teaching is a process that facilitates learning. Health teaching is an act in which a client is assisted to become an active member of the health team and to reach an optimal level of health.

- When learning occurs, there usually is a resultant change in behavior. The learner will be able to explain, discuss, demonstrate, or make something by using a new set of ideas.

- Types of learning theories include mental discipline theories, stimulus-response theories, and cognitive theories.

- The three types of learning are cognitive learning, affective learning, and psychomotor learning.

- The PRECEDE model and health belief model are useful in helping nurses to plan and carry out health teaching.

- Learning is most likely to occur when the learner perceives a need to learn, when he or she participates actively in the learning process, when the material to be learned is relevant, when it is reinforced, and when the new knowledge is put to immediate use.

- Motivation moves people to action and is paramount to learning. Intrinsic motivation comes from within the individual whereas extrinsic motivation comes from outside sources.

- The teaching/learning process can be related to the nursing process by means of the steps of assessment, diagnosis, planning, implementation, and evaluation.

- An educational assessment includes assessment of the educational need, the learner, the teaching situation, and the teacher.

- A nursing diagnosis of knowledge deficit indicates a need for client teaching.

- During the planning stage, objectives are formulated and teaching methods and materials are selected. A client contract may be developed at this time.

- The nurse carries out the teaching plan during the implementation stage.

- Obstacles to implementation of the teaching plan include external barriers, client problems, and mistakes in teaching.

- Noncompliance occurs when the client does not adhere to the medical regimen or when the client is insufficiently motivated.

- The evaluation stage includes evaluation of teaching effectiveness and teaching performance based upon objectives and expected outcomes.

 CRITICAL THINKING EXERCISE

A community health nurse receives a referral from a physician for teaching and counseling. The client is 55 years old with newly diagnosed diabetes. She is to be taught to inject her own insulin and modify her diet. An initial visit reveals an apprehensive client who has a phobia about needles. She is in complete denial about the need to modify her diet and take insulin on a planned schedule.

1. According to Bloom, what different types of learning should the nurse plan for?
2. Using the PRECEDE Model, develop a teaching plan to move the client toward self-care and keeping her diabetes under control.

REFERENCES

Alfaro, R. (1990). *Applying nursing diagnosis and nursing process: A step by step guide* (2nd ed.). Philadelphia: J.B. Lippincott.

American Hospital Association (1972). *A patient's bill of rights.* Chicago: Author.

American Nurses' Association (1980). *A conceptual model of community health nursing.* Kansas City, MO: Author.

American Public Health Association (1981). *The definition and role of public health nursing in the delivery of health care.* Washington, D.C.: Author.

Atwood, H., & Ellis, J. (1971). Concept of need: An analysis for adult education. *Adult Leadership, 19,* 210-212.

Becker, M.H. (1974). *The health belief model and personal health behaviors.* Thorofare, NJ: Charles B. Black.

Bigge, M. (1982). *Learning theories for teachers.* New York: Harper & Row.

Bloom, B.S. (ed.) (1969). *Taxonomy of educational objectives: The classification of educational goals. Handbook I: Cognitive domain.* New York and London: Longman.

Chatham, M., & Knapp, L. (1982). *Patient education handbook.* Bowie, MD: Brady.

Cohen, S. (ed.) (1979). *New directions in patient compliance.* Lexington, MA: Lexington Books.

Creighton, H. (1987). Legal implication of home health care. *Nursing Management, 18*(2), 14-17.

Dewey, J. (1958). *Art as experience.* New York: Capricorn Books, GP Putnam's Sons.

Dracup, K., & Meleis, A. (1982). Compliance: An interactionist's approach. *Nursing Research,* January/February *31*(1), 31-36.

Dugas, B. (1972). *Introduction to patient care* (2nd ed.). Philadelphia: W.B. Saunders.

Falvo, D. (1985). *Effective patient education.* Rockville, MD: Aspen.

Fitzpatrick, J., & Whall, A. (1989). *Conceptual models of nursing* (2nd ed.). Norwalk, Conn: Appleton & Lange.

Flesch, R. (1974). *The art of readable writing.* New York: Harper & Row.

Fry, E. (1968). A readability formula that saves time. *Journal of Reading, 11,* 514.

Green, L., Kreuter, M., Deeds, S., & Partridge, K. (1980). *Health education planning: A diagnostic approach.* Palo Alto, CA: Mayfield.

Gunning, R. (1952). *The Fog formula: the technique of clear writing.* New York: McGraw-Hill Book Co.

Hardy, C. (1989). Patient-centered high technology care. *Holistic Nursing Practice, 3*(2), 46-53.

Humphrey, C. (1988). The home as a setting for care. *Nursing Clinics of North America, 23,* 305-314.

Jackson, J., & Johnson, E. (1988). *Patient education in home care.* Rockville, MD: Aspen.

Jenny, J. (1987). Knowledge deficit: not a nursing diagnosis. *Image, 19*(4), 184, 185.

Knowles, M. (1978). *The adult learner: A neglected species* (2nd ed.). Houston: Gulf Publishing.

Narrow, B.W. (1979). *Patient teaching in nursing practice.* New York: John Wiley.

Peters, D. (1989). A concept of nursing discharge. *Holistic Nursing Practice, 3*(2), 18-25.

Potter, P., & Perry, A. (1993). *Fundamentals of nursing* (3rd ed.). St. Louis: Mosby.

Rankin, S., & Duffy, K. (1983). *Patient education: Issues, principles, and guidelines.* Philadelphia: J.B. Lippincott.

Redman, B.K. (1993). *The process of patient education* (7th ed.). St. Louis: Mosby.

Spradley, B.W. (1985). *Community health nursing* (2nd ed.). Boston: Little, Brown & Co.

Stanhope, M., & Lancaster, J. (1988). *Community health nursing.* St. Louis: Mosby.

Stanton, M. (1985). Patient and health education: lessons from the marketplace. *Nursing Management, 16*(4): 26-30.

Weston, C., & Cranton, P.A. (1986). Selecting instructional strategies. *Journal of Higher Education,* May/June *57*(3), Ohio State University Press.

9

MANAGEMENT CONCEPTS IN COMMUNITY HEALTH NURSING

Ruth N. Knollmueller

Adopt a new philosophy because the others no longer work.

W. Edward Deming

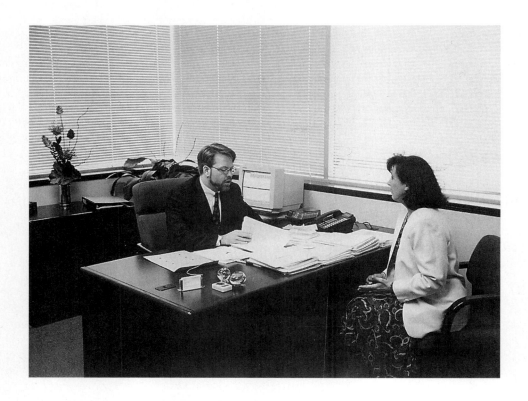

OBJECTIVES

At the conclusion of this chapter, the student will be able to:

1. Describe selected theories and concepts of management.
2. Discuss certain aspects of leadership and organizational behavior.
3. Explore significant parts of planning and organization in community health nursing practice.

KEY TERMS

Caseload management

Clinical management

Evaluation

Management models

Leadership styles

Motivation maintenance theory

Organizational management

Planning

Shared governance

Systems theory

Theory X and Theory Y

Time management

DEVELOPING MANAGEMENT THEORY

The rapid expansion of industry that took place starting in the late eighteenth century influenced thinking about management as sociologists, psychologists, and others systematically studied and wrote about this role. Theories of management were derived from time-and-motion studies, studies of hierarchy of needs among workers, and studies of human behavior and motivation among workers in the industrial setting.

Maslow's (1943) hierarchy of needs theory focused on the belief that people have needs that motivate certain behaviors (Figure 9-1). These needs are arranged in a five-step hierarchy of importance, resulting in increased motivation as basic human needs are met. The hierarchy begins with basic physiologic needs (food, water, shelter), and moves on to safety and security needs (protection from physical harm); affection and social activity needs (the need for friendship, companionship and affection, and belonging to groups); esteem and status needs (self-respect and awareness of one's importance to others); and finally, self-actualization needs (the highest level of human need, which includes full development of one's potential). Using this approach when thinking about management is helpful be-

cause the role of manager is developmental and achieved in stages. The Maslow hierarchy of needs is not a ladder on which one achieves or accomplishes goals rung by rung, but rather, captures the staging that is part of one's maturation.

McGregor (1960) described two theories of human behavior, called **Theory X** and **Theory Y.** Theory X views the worker as a person who avoids responsibility and prefers to be directed by a manager in work efforts; Theory Y views the worker as responsible and cooperative. An extremely rigid, task-oriented manager with an authoritarian style may believe in the Theory X assumptions about people. This manager usually favors one-way communication between staff and manager. This level of communication may be seen in a manager who is a stickler for following policies and procedures in an exact way and who demands an immediate response. Often these managers believe that people are basically lazy and do not want to work; people are passive, even resistive, to organizational needs and must be persuaded, rewarded, punished, and controlled; people are self-centered and not very bright; people want to be told, shown, and trained; and people lack ambi-

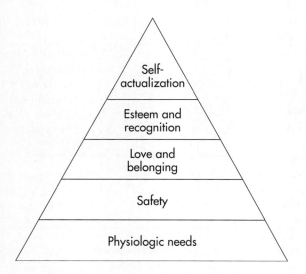

FIGURE 9-1   Maslow's hierarchy of needs.

tion and responsibility and want to be led. The style of manager who believes these Theory X assumptions will be consistent with these negative descriptors. This person will use an authoritarian form of management. Although there are situations in which the manager needs to be authoritarian, society in general, and professional employees and students in particular, now desire a more humanistic and professional approach from people in management. The increased rate of change and complexity of organizations and decision making require more sophisticated leadership skills in managers today.

Leaders who believe Theory Y assumptions tend to involve their followers more in their decision making, and two-way communication increases. Some assumptions of Theory Y are that people like to work and are not naturally passive or resistant to organizational goals; all people have potential for development and a capacity for assuming responsibility; the work itself is meaningful; and most people are capable of controlling their own work and seek responsibility. The **motivation maintenance theory** (Herzberg, Mausner, & Synderman, 1959) identifies five major "dissatisfiers": company policy and administration, supervision, salary, interpersonal relationships, and working conditions. These fac-

tors are termed *hygiene factors.* According to the motivational maintenance theory, a second group of factors, identified as "satisfiers," includes satisfying job content, task achievement, responsibility for a task, and professional achievement. These satisfiers are called *motivators* because they provide impetus to superior performance (Cookfair, 1991, p. 131).

Drucker (1954) proposed a result-oriented approach to management. This approach involves an exchange of information between the manager and the worker and setting mutual goals and an agreement on methods for achieving these goals. Drucker is best known for his "management by objectives" approach, which is based on these ideas. More recently, Drucker (1990) describes the key role of the employee as one who takes the organization's mission and moves it toward specific objectives and applications. In this case the staff member is a very active part of the organization and openly embraces the organization's purposes, whereas in more traditional settings this is left to the higher administrative level.

Management Models

The role of the manager in a community nursing agency is pivotal for achieving success in working with a group of staff and students. The manager's role is facilitative and instructive, with the goal of bringing the less experienced worker along and helping him or her to grow from a dependent level of functioning to an independent level. The process is similar to the way a community health nurse works with an individual or family. Initially, there may be dependence on the nurse, but the goal is independence.

Currently, in some **management models,** there is a strong drive toward permitting more freedom and independence among all levels of workers. Organizations seem to move from a flexible style to a bureaucratic, controlling style and back to a style of greater autonomy and independence for the individual staff member. This oscillation of styles may be a reflection of the culture of a specific organization or agency and the experience the manager brought to the community setting. Those individuals coming into an agency with modest experience in community health nursing may use a more controlling style until they feel comfortable in the management role.

Self-managing work teams (SMWT) consist of groups of employees who are given responsibility for managing and operating their own particular assigned duties. SMWTs are responsible for planning the work to be done, organizing themselves to get it done, selecting team members and assigning them to jobs, providing their own supervision (a traditional manager serves as group facilitator and does not manage), resolving team conflicts, and exercising quality control (Heneman, Schwab, Fossum & Dyer, 1989, p. 673). Considerable nurturing is necessary to make the SMWT form of management successful. Team members must be thoroughly educated, not only in technical matters but in group process skills that focus on establishing trust and respect (Figure 9-2).

SMWTs were begun in the business and industry setting and were not used as much as originally expected. Evaluations of the model are rare and productivity improvements and cost savings are claimed but not substantiated (Manz & Sims, 1987, p. 128). If health care facilities consider implementing this model, it must be kept in mind that while the potential exists to help staff members grow, it does not happen without a commitment to guide and support the SMWT both as individuals and especially as a group. This presumes that the manager assisting in developing this model is skilled in group process and is capable of being a mentor to the group (see Chapter 10).

Shared governance is a concept in management today that may have evolved from the model of participative management of the past. It is based on the premises that workers today are generally well-educated or, at least, more so than was true some years ago, and that staff deserve a voice in the decisions that affect them. In some instances, staff believe that shared governance includes decisions about salary, benefits, and patient care. Implementing shared governance has been an uneven experience in health care facili-

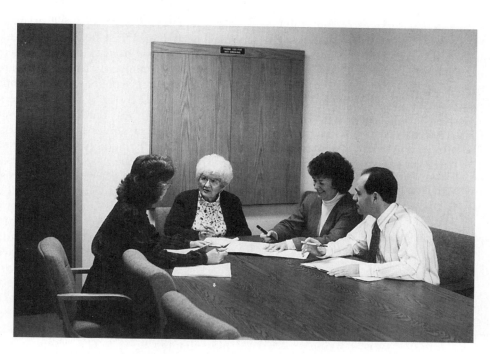

FIGURE 9-2   Team leader assigning case load to members of the team.

ties because of the mixed message that can be conveyed by the management staff and understood by the clinical staff (Szilagyi & Wallace, 1983). That is, some things are acceptable for shared governance, but directing compensation may not be one of them.

Typically, shared governance encourages staff involvement in problem solving, decision making, and team building. Its purpose is to alter the climate in the work setting so that employees can contribute to and gain more from their jobs (Szilagyi & Wallace, 1983). This process encourages staff members to identify problems, gather and analyze appropriate data, and offer some ideas toward a solution based on the findings. The concept of shared governance was developed to allow staff nurses a measure of control over their working environment in an institutional setting. Peterson and Allen (1986) describe some management assumptions that support shared governance with professional staff (see box below).

To the extent that problem solving, decision making, and team building are focused on the delivery of care, the clinical practice, and the professional aspects of the services of the community nursing agency, there is minimal tension between staff and management.

Maynard and Mehrtens (1993, p. 16) propose that the corporation in the future will shift to new models of governance, thus engendering deeper levels of trust, caring, and sharing throughout the internal corporate family. Customers will be integrated but not assimilated into corporate life. The culture of most community nursing agencies that are voluntary, nonprofit, or public agencies has traditionally been family-like. The roles of the patient and family have been highly regarded as the reasons for the existence of any community agency. In fact, historically, it was members of the community who provided the initiative (money and lay leadership) to form the corporation known as a visiting nurse association or public health nursing agency.

Leadership

Leadership, according to Bennis and Nanus (1985, p. 27), is "the marshalling of skills possessed by a majority but used by a minority; it is something that can be learned by anyone, taught to everyone, and denied to no one." Only a few people will lead nations or even lead corporations. Many, however, will lead departments or small groups and will function as leaders through a middle management role.

Hersey and Blanchard (1982, p. 84) describe leadership as a "process of influencing the activities of an individual or a group in efforts toward goal achievement in a given situation." Leadership should occur at all levels of the agency hierarchy, not just at the executive or management level. Leadership must be responsive to the job that needs to be done and to the interpersonal relationships among all of those who are part of the agency. Some would argue that being a manager does not necessarily involve leadership, and that may be so. The outcome of the quality of management that denies leadership responsibilities minimizes the potential of this key role.

To be an effective leader, one needs a variety of leadership skills. There is no one best way in which to influence people, and the style a person uses depends on the level of maturity of the group being influenced. Hersey and Blanchard (1982) describe four levels of **leadership style:** high task and low relationship behavior; high task and high relationship behavior; high relationship and low task behavior; and low relationship and low task behavior. The maturity of both the leader and the staff group influence the style of leadership that works best. A leader who uses a high relationship style is one who considers the human aspect of leadership important. Time and energy are necessary to determine the right style

---

ASSUMPTIONS OF SHARED GOVERNANCE

- People are essentially trustworthy.
- Professionals require a sense of worth.
- Each individual has a valuable contribution to make.
- Problems are best solved by those who are directly involved.
- Leadership ability at all levels of the heirarchy should be developed.
- A management labor team is necessary to accomplish clear direction.

for each person in a work group. Yet another type of leadership is a low relationship and low task behavior. In that model, workers are left alone to "do their own thing" without wanting or receiving guidance.

The appropriate leadership style of a manager today is contingent on the situation. A good leader must know how to balance autocratic (directive—based on the premise that "I am the leader, this is the law" Smith, 1980), democratic (participative—based on the premise that "we are all equal; whatever happens, happens" Smith, 1980), and laissez-faire (nondirective—based on the belief that the group is self-directing within the limits of rules and guidelines and where the leader's motto is "I am here if you need me" Smith, 1980) styles and behaviors. There are many styles that reflect varying amounts and types of two-way communication between manager and staff.

Bass and Avolio (1990), and Barker (1990, 1991) describe a new paradigm called transactional leadership and transformational leadership. The transactional leader recognizes roles and tasks required for the completion of work, and the transformational leader encourages workers to develop and perform beyond expectations. The transformational leader establishes goals and objectives with the intent of helping followers develop into leaders. Bass (1985) suggests that transformational leaders are more likely to emerge in times of growth, change, and crisis. The transactional leader works within the existing organizational culture, and the transformational leader seeks to change the culture. Transactional leadership is viewed as an essential component of effective leadership, although transformational leadership is seen as more acceptable and effective in improving outcomes because the focus is on the process of leadership rather than on a product.

Planning

Planning is an important strategy for successful management. A plan helps you to organize work, evaluate your present status during the active work phase, decide your direction, and determine the desired outcome. Developing goals and objectives constitutes a good use of time. Lack of planning, on the other hand, reveals poor use of time and energy and leads to increasing stress levels and decreasing job satisfaction. Planning is a time-consuming activity and an important management function regardless of the level of staff involved.

Thriving in your work requires you to be a good steward of your time. Planning work helps to alleviate this stress. Planning includes the ability to delegate, accommodate, and eliminate certain activities. It is easy to become tyrannized by the need to respond immediately to each of the seemingly endless series of questions that confront you when you are in a position of planning. Losing control because of inadequate planning is costly and a threat to individual and group success.

All planning involves particular steps that might be identified in the following way:

- Analyze the present situation.
- Forecast the future situation.
- Look for opportunities.
- Establish broad goals based on these opportunities.
- Reduce the broad goals to specific, time-limited tasks.
- Evaluate and revise the plans. (Table 9-1)

These steps follow the structure of the nursing process: assessment, planning, implementation, and evaluation. For example, students who wish to establish a clinical service to aged resi-

TABLE 9-1 Comparison of steps in planning for good management and the nursing process

Planning	Nursing process
Analyze the present situation	Assessment
Forecast the future situation	
Look for opportunities	
Establish broad goal based on these opportunities	Planning
Reduce the broad goals to specific, time-limited tasks	Implementation
Evaluate and revise the plans	Evaluation

dents living in an apartment complex must take an assessment of needs as related by the residents, plan program opportunities that are desired by the residents, formulate goals that can be accomplished in a limited time frame, prepare and carry out the plans, and evaluate the results through a formal evaluation tool and informal discussion with the participants.

For direct client care and student application, the steps outlined above should be structured as a clinical caseload. Students should review the visits needed for the day, estimate the frequency of visits, seek out the client or family members to carry out part or all of the treatment plan, set mutual goals for the care plan and visit requirements, and then evaluate the efficacy of that plan for further nursing intervention.

Strategic planning. Caseload planning, discussed above, has a clinical focus. Another aspect of planning is called strategic planning and usually pertains to organizational planning for selected goals in service delivery or through fiscal planning by the community agency. In strategic planning, basic goals of the agency or organization are established for specific direction and emphasis and are likely to be more long term. Strategic planning includes anticipated outcomes and a method for achieving the outcomes (Figure 9-3). For instance, it may be determined that a goal will be to provide care to high-risk newborns or to plan and implement a prevention and health promotion program for expectant parents. Through community assessment, a plan will be identified and a method of payment will be devised for the clinical services needed. If necessary, special funding will be found. The predicted outcome will be identified based on the community need and on information gained in the community assessment. This information gathering and outcome prediction are integral parts of the evaluation.

Financial planning. Planning for the use of financial resources is no longer strictly the responsibility of the Executive Director or the

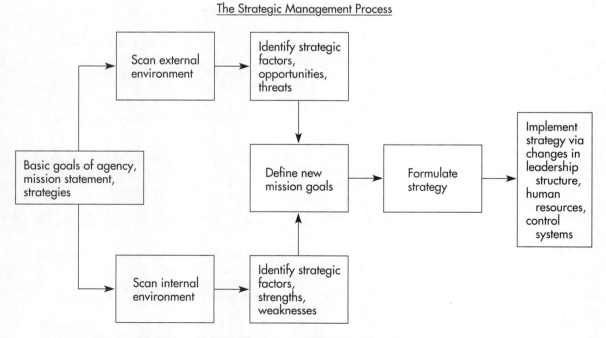

The Strategic Management Process

FIGURE 9-3   The strategic management process. *From* Management *(2nd ed) (p. 156) by R. Daft, 1991, Chicago: Holt, Rinehart, & Winston. Copyright 1991, The Dryden Press. Reprinted by permission.*

head of the agency's department of finance and business. It has become everyone's concern because the integrity of the agency often rests on its fiscal stability, which is supported by services rendered by all staff members. The most common activity pertaining to financial planning is preparation of the annual budget, which identifies costs as part of the delivery of nursing care in the community.

Budgets can be developed in line-item format or by program. The budget is based on predicted revenue that will be generated to support services, salaries, and running the office. Funding comes from a variety of sources, some of which are more predictable on a year-to-year basis, such as special grants for a certain time-limited program, or the United Way allocations or other voluntary contributions from a community drive that are divided with many community organizations. Medicaid reimbursement is mandated by each state based on an agency cost report. It may change from year to year but once it is set, it stays at that rate for the year.

Although a budget is similar to a roadmap for the agency, it is usually a dynamic tool because changes occur during the fiscal year that may have both positive and negative effects on program support. That is, a budget is not rigid, but it is a useful and essential financial planning guide for the services the community agency expects to provide. Table 9-2 shows advantages and disadvantages of budgets.

The other side of budget planning is the ability of the agency to collect data on visits and program statistics to compare the revenue generation with the actual expenses. The budget "roadmap" may be used to understand whether the predictions for the volume of service were appropriate and if the staffing was adequate to achieve the volume of activity.

Staff planning. Planning for the best balance of staffing the agency is a very important matter and should not be taken casually. In most community health nursing agencies, the largest expenses are the salaries for all employees. Salaries usually represent approximately 80% of the expense side of the budget. Typically, staff workers are both professional (nursing, therapy, social work) and nonprofessional, (commonly

TABLE 9-2 Advantages and Disadvantages of Budgets

Advantages	Disadvantages
Facilitates coordination across departments	Can be used mechanically
Translates strategic plans into department actions	Can adversely affect employee motivation because of lack of participation
Improves communication between employees	Can cause perceptions of unfairness
Improves resource allocation	Can create competition for resources and affect agency politics
Provides a tool for corrective action through reallocation	Can limit opportunities for innovation and adaptation

From Daft, R. (1991) *Management* (2nd ed.) (p. 34.) Chicago: Holt, Rinehart, & Winston. Reprinted by permission of the Dryden Press.

called support staff). Home health agencies have another employee, the home health aide, who is a vital part of the service component of the agency. As a paraprofessional doing personal care, the home health aide works under the direction and supervision of the registered nurse.

Planning for such a variety of staffing includes developing agency personnel policies, procedures, and job descriptions. This is done by the human resources, or personnel, department of an agency. State and federal regulations further demand human resource expertise in meeting Occupational Safety and Health Administration (OSHA), American Disabilities Act (ADA), and other mandates that affect the ways an agency hires and provides safety and benefits for all employees.

ORGANIZATION

Organizations use a variety of systems to explain and guide their approach to providing care as a community health nursing agency.

General Systems Theory

According to **systems theory,** a system is a set of interrelated and interdependent parts that form a complex whole, and each of those parts can be viewed as a subsystem with its own set of interrelated and independent parts (Rakich, Longest, & Darr, 1985, p. 158).

Systems are either closed or open. Closed systems are self-contained, whereas an open system is more consistent with systems concepts as applied to management because the notion that the system is constantly in a dynamic interaction with its environment is supported. (For more about open systems, see the Neuman Systems Model, which is discussed in Chapter 2.)

A systems approach emphasizes the interrelatedness, connectedness, and interdependence and interaction of organizational phenomena and dynamics (French & Bell, 1984, p. 54). Systems analysis assumes structure and stability at any given time. A systems approach encourages an analysis of events in terms of multiple causation rather than a single cause.

Viewing community health nursing practice and organization as a system provides a frame of reference for perceiving the agency as a whole with interdependent parts.

Community health nursing practice is organized primarily around nursing care, and includes health care from other providers who have assorted skills. This model forms a holistic approach to health care delivery. Care may be provided in a variety of settings, which may include visits in a home or visits in a clinic (mobile, ambulatory/hospital, neighborhood).

Organizing Community Nursing Services

Community nursing services have always provided a way to care for people in their homes. High-tech home care, with intravenous therapy, ventilators, pain control pumps, and other such equipment now common in the home, client care that requires sophisticated technology is no longer carried out exclusively in institutions, and this has made home care more challenging.

One model of care delivered at the community level is primary care, in which an advanced nurse clinician, is responsible for caring for individuals and families at a clinic or health center. Another model is the traditional approach. In this model the community is defined by geographic area and is served by a generalist community health nurse. Most community agencies in the United States and Canada use the census tracts that are formally and numerically designated by the U.S. Department of Commerce and the Canada Bureau of Statistics as the assigned areas. Census tracts are used in all areas of the country. This means that in the traditional approach model, people who live in a designated census tract are in the district assigned to the nurse. Clients are assigned to a specific district nurse according to their address within the census tract. This method of districting is very old, and its success comes from many years of experience with using it.

Organization of a staff nurse's client caseload, of an agency's services (*e.g.,* home, school, or community health aide), and of the array of community nursing program services (*e.g.,* prenatal clinic, hypertension clinic), calls for careful planning and prudent delivery of nursing care. The approach of service delivery that an agency uses is influenced by the resources available, both financial and personnel. For example, some community agencies may use a team nursing approach, in which a group of staff nurses and a physical therapist and/or medical social worker may be responsible for a geographically designated cluster of clients. There is a nonrotating team leader who assigns the care of the clients and oversees the total caseload needs. The team leader discusses with that group of clinicians the care and needs of clients and families. The team develops and carries out a plan of care as a group. Regular clinical conferencing and case review are done to ascertain the most appropriate service for each client and family. In many community nursing agencies a nurse manager fills this function.

Another approach is based on the primary care nurse, who may be a clinical nurse specialist in psychiatric-mental health nursing, a pediatric nurse practitioner, or an oncology nurse clinician. In this instance, the direct care caseload is limited to a few complex situations, and there is a plan to assign those clients to the district nurse. Most of the clinician's time is spent in clinical consultation with staff nurses or in making joint visits with staff nurses to establish a plan of care as it relates to a clinical specialty condition.

In some community nursing agencies, the use of the term primary nurse and district nurse are interchangeable. This nurse is a generalist with skills in a wide range of nursing care, including prenatal/postpartum and newborn care, care of the ill at home that requires specific treatments and assessments, and the chronically mentally ill. The generalist usually has this kind of a caseload mix and is guided by a nurse manager. In addition, the generalist nurse is supported by a clinical nurse specialist if the agency has one on staff or one is available as a consultant to staff. A faculty member with clinical credentials from an area school of nursing or an advanced nurse clinician working in the community may be hired as a clinical consultant in selected clinical specialties based on the need when the agency is not in a position to directly employ such a person.

Evaluation

Evaluation is defined as the process of determining whether a service is needed and likely to be used, whether it is conducted as planned, and whether the service actually helps people in need (Posavac & Carey, 1980, p. 6). Evaluation for the purpose of assessing whether objectives are met or planned activities are completed is referred to as formative evaluation. This type of evaluation begins with an assessment of the need for the program. Evaluation that assesses program outcomes or is a follow-up of the results of the activities is called summative evaluation (Stanhope & Lee, 1992, p. 202). For example, a program to conduct diabetes screening in a community begins with a needs assessment and a review of the initial objectives for that program once it is underway. This procedure is an example of formative evaluation. At the conclusion of the diabetes screening program, participants and referrals are measured, and the next step is determined. This is an example of summative evaluation.

Performance evaluation. As a management concept, evaluation includes both individual performance evaluation and program evaluation. The latter involves evaluating a process or a plan

or an agency structure that is working toward a reorganization for greater efficiency or a change in service focus.

Individual performance evaluation is the one form of evaluation that everyone knows about and is involved in regardless of his or her position in the agency.

The purpose of the performance evaluation is to review actual and expected performance on a given job (Knollmueller, 1986, p. 69). Too often, evaluation is a litany of criticism and finding fault with past performance. Although the past is a point from which to begin, the evaluation process should move beyond the past. An employee's performance usually varies over a long period. An evaluation of performance should give recognition and provide motivation based on the work accomplished. Another outcome of an evaluation is to encourage the staff member to improve in selected areas of the position and to provide opportunities for growth within the position. The result of this professional growth is that individuals may pursue possibilities for promotion or other responsibilities within the agency. The performance evaluation is an administrative activity that should have an educational focus. Because merit or annual salary increments are associated with performance evaluations, they are often perceived as more managerial than educational. This perception may detract from positive effects of a performance evaluation. The formal performance evaluation is the culmination of the guidance and teaching the staff member has received over a specific period of time. If the communication between supervisor and staff member or teacher and student is on target, agreement during the evaluation should be fairly consistent. If there are many differences in opinion, it is necessary to review the method of evaluation and the way goals and expectations are set.

Program evaluation. Program evaluation is a process that begins at the initial planning and continues until that program is completed. The goals of a program evaluation are to ascertain the relevance, progress, efficiency, effectiveness, and effects of program activities for the clients served (Veney & Kaluzny, 1984).

A program evaluation begins at the time the

needs assessment is conducted and reviewed. Evaluation at this stage is intended to determine if the proposed program is needed. The clients who are likely to be the recipients in the program are usually involved in this assessment. Once the program is underway, the participation of clients, the time the providers must give to the program, and funding used to implement the program are regularly monitored. Once the program has concluded, the accumulated information, such as data on participation, referrals, types of intervention, and client satisfaction, is evaluated and analyzed.

Many agencies carry out a program evaluation on at least one program each year to determine how needs are being met, whether the program is still viable, and whether changes in delivery are necessary. This should not be considered an activity that is done only for special projects or specially funded programs. The standard programs of a community nursing agency benefit from a regular and systematic review.

The typical way to evaluate a plan or a program is to review the goals and objectives that were initially established, to assess whether or not they were met and to what degree they were met, and to consider additional goals and objectives to carry the activity forward. For instance, if an agency has a program of services for at-risk pregnant women, the agency will want to know how that need has been met as viewed by the client and the clinical staff in light of the goals and objectives established for this program. Some of the questions to ask might include: Were the clients reached and given care; Were the hours and place of care acceptable; Were appointments kept; and were outcomes of these pregnancies an indication of good care? A new concept, Total Quality Management (TQM), focuses on outcomes as they are influenced by the whole agency (see Chapter 11). TQM may radically change present evaluation methods.

APPLICATION OF MANAGEMENT CONCEPTS

Students may wonder why it is necessary to begin thinking about management concepts when there is so much else to learn that is specific to nursing in general and to community health nurs-

ing, in particular during the undergraduate educational experience.

Management offers nurses opportunities to grow professionally and to develop leadership skills. It is essential that some of the basic concepts concerning development of management and leadership skills be presented during the student experience.

The next part of this chapter will discuss selected practical issues relating to the following management concepts, with special reference to student nurses: time, clinical caseloads, paraprofessionals, home visits, and managing meetings and committee work.

Time Management

Management of time is relevant in both our personal and professional lives.

Time management relates to productivity in carrying out the work assigned. The cost of delivering health care has highlighted the need to improve productivity. This is true whatever the setting of practice.

Some key concepts of productivity for the community health nurse are given in the box below. Understanding productivity entails an understanding of the expectations of the outcomes of the home visit and the standard set for what is to be achieved in the home visit (Benefield, 1988).

Management of one's time is a learned behavior although some people may be more intuitively organized than others. Attention to the amount of time needed to carry out certain tasks

---

KEY CONCEPTS OF PRODUCTIVITY

Productivity is the relationship between the use of resources and the results of that use.

Efficiency is not necessarily how fast the work is done but how well time is used.

Quality can improve at the same time the productivity increases.

Improving productivity involves all units in a community health agency.

Hands-on skills are important, but so is the nurse's ability to think creatively, solve problems, and make decisions that have an effect on the plan of care for the client.

is essential. It is evident that proper management of time is being employed when one is able to structure personal time so that the result is not only getting a particular job done but getting it done in a manner that is balanced and sensible. The way a student responds to academic work and requirements suggests how well organized and how sensitive to time management the student will be in a variety of assignments.

The goal is to complete all work in a way that avoids the rush and panic that sets in when the deadline approaches. Although there are occasions when that may happen, continuous behavior of this type must be addressed. The student must change the behavior with more appropriate planning techniques. There will always be people who believe that they do their best work in this state of panic and hurry, but in the long run it is not a valuable approach to productive use of time in community health nursing practice.

The community health nurse must be versatile, eclectic, and pragmatic. In one scenerio a nurse may have to provide for a wound and dressing treatment. If the order occurs during a hot weather spell, the nurse will have to assess and evaluate the fluid intake of this client and assess a peculiar odor that may be a precursor of an infection. In addition, in this scenario the family members responsible for the client are distracted by eviction from their house. This situation calls for a flexible practitioner who clearly understands the safe scope of clinical practice and can adapt nursing skills in ways that are useful to that client and family. That is, the nurse should attend to the wound, report the observations to the physician, and direct the family for social service assistance for the housing problem. This type of unpredictability in a clinical setting should encourage the community health nurse to carefully consider the best possible plan for provision of the needed care.

Caseload Management

Each staff nurse has an assigned caseload of primary clients. More recently, with the advent of home care agencies that provide acute nursing care to population groups with special needs such as ventilators, intravenous therapy, and the like, districting is not used as much as in the past.

However, districting is an accurate and convenient method of demarcating an area or district for home visiting by a nurse with a generalized caseload.

The caseload is usually defined as a group of clients a nurse sees in a geographic area. A typical caseload is likely to have a patient mix of both more frequent and less frequent home visits, therefore, it is difficult to give a specific number of clinical cases for each nurse.

The management of the clinical caseload often depends on the way the clinical nursing supervisor or manager assists the nurse in delegating and evaluating the clinical need of the client and family in light of the total requirements of work. Of course, daily visits are scheduled as needed, but it is up to the nurse to determine the ability of the individual or a responsible party to take over the treatment procedure. The goal is to assist the client and family or responsible party to become independent of the nurse rather than to build dependency. In community health nursing practice, the goal of independence is overtly practiced.

Besides the actual clients and their family members, **caseload management** includes coordinating care and collaborating with other providers, including family members, social service agents, clinical specialists, home health aides, physicians, and therapists in the plan of care. Making telephone calls, preparing reports, and attending case conferences with a team of providers are examples of coordination and collaboration.

Communication of facts, plans, and appropriate information is critical in providing care to clients in the home. Educating the individual and family or responsible party is also essential in regard to the scope of community health. For instance, if the nurse or student makes a home visit to perform a technical procedure for an elderly person, such as an injection of medication or care of a wound, and there are young children in the home, it is appropriate to query whether these children have received their basic immunizations and if not, to refer the family to the appropriate community resource such as a neighborhood or hospital clinic, health department, or community physician or nurse practitioner.

Clinical Management

One of the most important aspects of **clinical management** in community health nursing practice is the work of the paraprofessional. The goal of care for the community-based client and family is to become independent of clinical providers as soon as it is appropriate and possible.

Some community agencies have licensed practical or vocational nurses (LPN) on staff. These staff members legally work under the direction and supervision of a registered nurse and want and need supervision of the home visits they make. Despite the limited scope of practice of the LPN, some agencies find this level of skill useful in certain settings and for selected activities.

The role of the nurse. The key person in the clinical management of the home client is the nurse who carries out clinical responsibilities in conjunction with the family member(s) or responsible party, a physician, and perhaps other clinical providers (physical, occupational, and speech therapists; social workers; psychologists). A nurse realizes rather quickly that there are

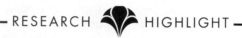

RESEARCH ✦ HIGHLIGHT

District Nurses and Caseload Management

The characteristics of recently (within 6 months) referred terminally ill or chronically physically disabled clients were compared with clients who had been followed for 5 or more years by a district nursing service to ascertain if projections for future service needs could be determined and to raise questions concerning referral and discharge policies for different teams or areas. The impetus for this study was related to the ever-increasing numbers of referrals for home care and clients' earlier discharges from the hospital at a stage when their nursing requirements were relatively high. The length of stay required examination to ensure appropriate home service delivery and effective use of what was becoming a scarce resource. Interviews were conducted to document the service of providers ($n = 619$), and to elicit randomly selected clients' ($n = 202$) perceptions of their circumstances and service provided.

The length of time clients had been seen (recent referrals and long-stay) was accompanied by the division between qualified staff (nurses) and auxiliary personnel. Thirteen clients were excluded from the analysis because there were no records of referral. In addition, examination of client characteristics was confined to qualified staff because of the rela-

tively small numbers in auxillary groups. However, both groups were considered in relation to long-stay visitation. The client composite was divided into the four teams represented in the district nursing caseloads, and proportional differences existed between recently referred and long-stay clients. Long-stay clients had chronic illnesses associated with the aging process and were visited either by qualified (nurses) or auxiliary personnel, some required injections, some were identified as younger, and others had disabling neurologic deficits.

Although physicians and delays in acquiring equipment contributed in part to the unnecessary frequency of client contact and retention, this situation was attributed in large part to the nurse's reluctance to either reduce intervention or to discharge clients from the system. Caseload mismanagement could be resolved by systematic reviews (evaluation) with adherence to schedules for maintenance of continuity simultaneous with the retention and eventual discharge of individuals who no longer required the services of the district agency. Decisions related to retention (criteria) and discharge were crucial to those awaiting services, particularly in view of the proliferation of referrals not only to this district, but to other districts as well.

From District nurses' patients-issues of caseload management by F. Badger, E. Cameron, & H. Evers, 1989, *Journal of Advanced Nursing, 14*(7), 518-527.

many players in the home care setting. It is necessary to identify the appropriate persons and to remember that the client is the central member in the configuration of "care" people.

It is important for the community health nurse to be skilled in verbal and written communication. When talking to a client, the nurse should be careful about using jargon or complex words that make understanding the discussion difficult. Written communication should describe an observation in a way that is not judgmental. Developing skill in summarizing information for purposes of reporting to other providers or third-party payors is essential, and learning to give enough data without too many words is especially useful. Sharing information with the client and other providers can assist in implementing a plan of care. Understanding the needs described by the client and family or responsible party are equally important to develop a plan of care that will successfully meet the clinical services.

The cultural background of a client and family or significant other has an effect on how any plan of care will succeed both as a partnership with that client and in keeping with the unique ethnic values and culture of that client.

In addition to providing direct hands-on clinical care for clients and families, the nurse will identify and plan to include prevention and health promotion as an integral part of the care. Sometimes prevention and health promotion will be very specific, for example, the nurse may explore whether any family member requires immunizations, or may obtain information about a therapeutic diet based on family history. At other times, prevention and health promotion will be more general, through observation of behaviors that promote or put at risk safety and life, such as smoking and seatbelt use. Creatively informing individuals about how to stay healthy will go a long way toward achieving broad goals of prevention and health promotion. Sometimes it is helpful to go over pictorial and printed materials with the client. These materials may be left in the home for future reference.

Clinical management is a broad scope of practice for the nurse and must be holistic in concept. It is a challenging and stimulating experience.

ORGANIZING THE HOME VISIT

The structure for delivering services in community health nursing lies in the home visit. Components of a home visit include planning for the visit, consideration of the most appropriate approach of the nurse in meeting the client and family, collecting the necessary supplies for the visit, and preparing for activities of the visit such as nursing care, teaching, and health counseling. Termination of a visit should include summarization of important points and a plan for the next home visit. The last steps of the home visit include recording the visit in the client's clinical file and evaluating the plan of care for the next visit.

An initial aspect of a home visit is to establish the purpose of the visit. This may consist of one or more of many activities, such as providing nursing care to an ill client, demonstrating and teaching about insulin administration to a client and family members, demonstrating and teaching about active and passive range of motion, or discussing with a mother the care of herself and her infant or providing care that is informative and supportive to the mother.

In making overall plans for the day's work, the nurse determines priorities, which are determined in part by the purpose of each visit. If the purpose is to include teaching a specific technique that a family member who works must learn, then the visit is arranged around a mutually agreeable time. The nurse must hold a broad view of the work that needs to be accomplished and then plan and execute the home visit according to the need. Planning ahead for each visit and each day is necessary to conduct current clinical consultation with other providers, and to have all of the necessary equipment, supplies for treatments, and materials for teaching.

During the first visit to an individual or family by the community health nursing agency, it is appropriate for the nurse to share some information with them about the agency. For instance, it is relevant to give information about the agency's location, how long it has been in the community, how to reach the agency by phone, and the hours of business. The first visit will probably be longer than subsequent visits. The assessment, plan, implementation, and evaluation conducted by the nurse at this time sets the tone for future visits.

Organizing careful and complete documentation of the visit takes skill that is acquired with experience. Descriptive rather than judgmental notes should be recorded. Organizing thoughts requires discipline and guidance from an experienced nurse who has developed skills that will be a model for the student.

The home visit is a vehicle for providing nursing services. It is a social and informal forum in which to accomplish serious and complex clinical interventions. A home visit requires well-organized planning to be successfully completed.

ORGANIZATIONAL MANAGEMENT

Learning basics about effective committee work may be neglected because it is perceived as easy. We have all been on committees in which the goals of the committee were difficult to accomplish. Perhaps the chairperson was not prepared for the meeting, work required to be done between meetings was not followed through by committee members, or the agenda for the meeting was not developed to help guide the discussion.

Community agencies have regularly scheduled committees, usually called standing committees, and ad hoc committees, which are designed for a special problem or issue. Students are usually not in an agency long enough or often enough to be able to participate on agency committees. However, as a part of a community health nursing clinical experience, students complete a community project of some kind. This is a good opportunity to have exposure to planning and leading meetings or to serve as a productive member of a community committee. A productive committee member is one who accepts and follows through with a particular assignment on behalf of the group, attends meetings punctually and stays for the duration, and prepares for the meeting by being informed and/or reading reports so that the work of the committee moves ahead.

Serving as the chairperson of a meeting is successful when scheduled meetings are started and ended at the agreed time and when the meeting agenda is carefully planned. Time for discussion of items is necessary and standard acceptances of fiscal and secretarial minutes must be presented and duly noted in the meeting minutes.

Perhaps the most important part of running a meeting is to learn how to develop leadership skills that strengthen the process of how one works with a group of people. An effective leader can draw the best out of others to achieve the goals of the meeting. There will be committee members who talk too much, talk too little, talk about tangential matters, or who keep the discussion focused. The leader sets goals for the meeting and often must also set limits for some group members. Having an agenda and adhering to it are critical to **organizational management.** There should be time permitted for discussion, and it is acceptable for the chairperson to establish an appropriate time limit for purposes of completing the agenda. Sometimes a content expert is invited to the meeting to further inform committee members about a particular issue. Involving as many members of the group as possible is important, and gaining a consensus for a recommendation or a solution is essential. At the conclusion of the meeting, the chairperson summarizes the primary issues, the potential alternatives, and the agreed-upon solution with a plan for follow-up, if that is appropriate. This format is useful whether one is leading a clinical case conference or discussing an agency policy.

Experience in observing people with experience as committee members or as the chairperson of a committee is a valuable opportunity for a student or new nurse. It is important to begin developing leadership skills and to continue this development over many years.

Chapter Highlights

- Application of selected management concepts and theories is useful and relevant.

- Leadership is developed at all levels of responsibility.

- A variety of approaches for implementing management concepts is possible.

- Leadership styles may vary, and it is useful to seek out new approaches.

- Planning concepts assists in greater effectiveness.

- Organizational skills are essential for effective performance, including time management, caseload management, and clinical management.

- Effective relationships with paraprofessionals are important.

- Evaluation of individual performance, of agency programs, and of organizational structure yields more effective community health nursing services.

 CRITICAL THINKING EXERCISE

A home health nurse has added several patients to a caseload that is already difficult to schedule. Realizing that the quality of care will be impossible to maintain, the nurse asks for home health aides to be placed in some of the homes. The aides will be asked to do tube feedings and some dressing changes.

1. Using Peterson and Allen's management assumptions, discuss whether you think the plan will work.
2. What leadership style do you think will work best to supervise the home health aids? Explain your answer.

REFERENCES

Barker, A.M. (1990). *Transformational leadership: A vision for the future.* Baltimore: Williams & Wilkins.

Barker, A.M. (1991). An emerging leadership paradigm. *Nursing & Health Care, 12*(4).

Bass, B.M. (1985). *Leadership and performance beyond expectations.* New York: Free Press.

Bass, B.M., & Avolio, B.J. (1990). *Transformational leadership development.* Palo Alto, California: Consulting Psychologists Press, Inc.

Benefield, L. (1988). *Home health care management.* Englewood Cliffs, New Jersey: Prentice-Hall.

Bennis, W., & Nanus, B. (1985). *Leaders: The strategies for taking charge.* New York: Harper & Row.

Cookfair, J. (1991). *Nursing Process and Practice in the Community.* St. Louis: Mosby.

Daft, R. (1991). *Management* (2nd ed.) (pp. 156, 534). Chicago: The Dryden Press.

Drucker, P. (1954). *The practice of management.* New York: Harper & Row.

Drucker, P. (1990). *Managing the non-profit organization* (pp. 5, 157). New York: Harper Collins.

French, W., & Bell, C. (1984). *Organization development: Behavioral science interventions for organization improvement.* Englewood Cliffs, New Jersey: Prentice-Hall.

Heneman, H., Schwab, D., Fossum, J., & Dyer, L. (1989). *Personnel/human resource management* (4th ed.). Homewood, Illinois: Irwin.

Hersey, R., & Blanchard, K. (1982). *Management of organizational behavior: Utilizing human resources* (4th ed.). Englewood Cliffs, New Jersey: Prentice-Hall.

Herzberg, F., Mausner, B., & Synderman, B. (1959). *The motivation to work.* New York: Wiley.

Humphrey, C.J., & Milone-Nuzzo, P. (1991). *Home care nursing: An orientation to practice.* Norwalk, Connecticut: Appleton & Lange.

Knollmueller, R.N. (1986). *The community health nursing supervisor: A handbook for community/home care managers.* New York: National League for Nursing.

Manz, C., & Sims, H. (1987). Leading workers to lead themselves: The external leadership of self-managing work teams. *Administrative Science Quarterly, 32,* 106-128.

Maslow, A. (1943). A theory of human motivation. *Psychological Review,* July, 370-396.

Maynard, H., & Mehrtens, S. (1993). *The fourth wave: business in the 21st century.* San Francisco: Barrett-Koehler.

McGregor, D. (1960). *The human side of enterprise.* New York: McGraw-Hill.

Peterson, M.E., & Allen, D.E. (1986). Shared governance: A strategy for transforming organizations. *Journal of Nursing Administration* (Part I), *15*(1).

Posavac, E.J., & Carey, R.G. (1980). *Program evaluation: methods and case studies.* Englewood Cliffs, New Jersey: Prentice Hall.

Rakich, J., Longest, B., & Darr, K. (1985). *Managing health services organizations.* Philadelphia: W.B. Saunders.

Smith, L. (1980). Finding your leadership style in groups. *American Journal of Nursing.* 80: 1301-1303.

Stanhope, M., & Lee, G. (1992). Program management. In M. Stanhope & J. Lancaster (Eds.). *Community health nursing: Process and practice for promoting health* (3rd ed.), (p. 202). St. Louis: Mosby.

Szilagyi, A.D., & Wallace, M.J. (1983). *Organizational behavior and performance.* Chicago: Scott, Foresman & Co.

Veney, J., & Kaluzny, A. (1984). *Evaluation and decision making for health service programs.* Englewood Cliffs, New Jersey: Prentice-Hall.

10

Working with Groups in the Community

Linda Janelli

A group is an open system composed of three or more people held together by a common interest or bond.

Ruth M. Tappen

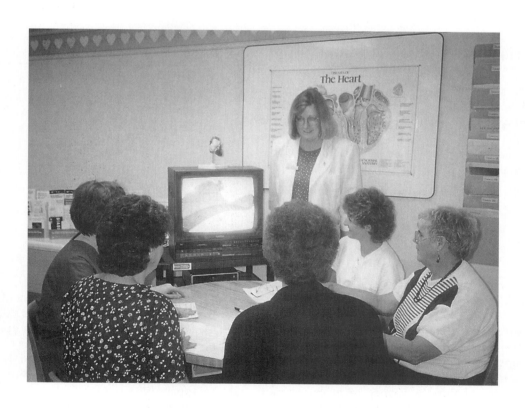

OBJECTIVES

At the conclusion of this chapter, the student will be able to:

1. Define the key terms listed.
2. Identify the three basic characteristics found in most groups.
3. Describe the five stages of group development (forming, storming, norming, performing, and adjourning) and state how they differ from one another.
4. Identify at least two task roles, two social roles, and two individual roles that could emerge from a group situation.
5. Assess those elements that can contribute to the effectiveness of a group leader.
6. Explain how Herzberg's motivational factors can affect the group process.
7. Explain the purposes of community, support, educational, and focus groups and the potential role of the community health nurse in each group.

KEY TERMS

Adjourning	Group	Power
Cohesion	Individual roles	Relationships
Community development groups	Maintenance roles	Shared leadership
Conflict	Motivational theory	Storming
Educational groups	Norming	Support groups
Focus group	Performing	Task roles
Forming		

T his chapter deals with types of groups, group development, negotiating the group process, and the use of groups to help professionals promote health. Community health nurses often have the opportunity to work with four kinds of groups: community development groups, support groups, educational groups, and focus groups. Each of these is formed to meet a specific community or individual need. Before examination of these groups and the community health nurse's role within each, it is important to explore first what a group is and how it is formed.

DEFINITION OF GROUP

The term **group** is defined in a variety of ways; however, the following definition is particularly appropriate to nursing: "A group is an open system composed of three or more people held together by a common interest or bond. The individuals who make up the group are its subsystems" (Tappen, 1983, p. 149).

It is believed that a minimum of three individuals constitute a group because only then can the complex **relationships** develop that characterize a group. A triad, or three-person group, permits four relationships. A group of four per-

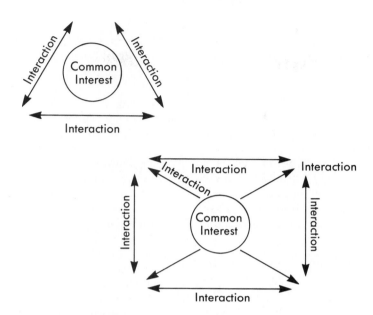

FIGURE 10-1 A group of three permits four possible relationships, and a group of four permits eleven possible relationships.

mits eleven possible relationships (Figure 10-1). In a three-person group a power relationship can develop between two of its members to win their position over the lone third member. In a dyad (a relationship between two individuals), a power relationship of this sort cannot exist. There is some evidence that suggests that larger groups produce less member satisfaction. This lower level of satisfaction may be related to the time available for members to participate. However, the larger the size of the group the greater the availability of the resources among members (Tubbs, 1988).

FUNCTIONS OF GROUPS

Some of the basic functions of a community may be provided to its members through group formation. These functions include safety and security, mutual support, networking for distribution of resources, socialization, and a sense of belonging. Safety and security refer to protection of community members from crime, natural disasters, and threats against their physical safety. Groups that meet these needs include volunteer rescue squads, the American Red Cross, and neighborhood crime-watch groups.

Other groups may provide mutual support such as physical or psychological support during a crisis situation. Examples of such groups are Alcoholics Anonymous, Friendly Visitors, or Parents Without Partners. Communities provide networks for the distribution of resources, whether in the form of exchange of information or materials, or services through groups such as the Salvation Army, the Cystic Fibrosis Association, and religious charity organizations.

Communities also provide opportunities for socialization by which values, beliefs, and attitudes can be shared. Community groups of this type include Kiwanis clubs, Chamber of Commerce groups, nutrition centers, and the community Y. Furthermore, groups may provide an individual with a sense of belonging and an opportunity to contribute services; for example, participation as a hospital or nursing home volunteer or as a member of a political action group.

Most of us have participated in one group or another, whether it was a school committee, a social club, or a religious organization. Perhaps you may have noticed that some groups you were involved with functioned better than others. Was this because of the leaders, the group members, the tasks involved, or a combination of all three factors? By the conclusion of this chapter you will be better prepared to understand the dynamics that contribute to a group's effectiveness.

CHARACTERISTICS OF GROUPS

Obviously, there is a difference between a group of individuals waiting at a bus stop and a group of nurses who meet each month as part of an honor society. The latter example is that of a formal group. Formal groups usually have three basic characteristics. Not all groups, however, serve the same function; thus not every group possesses each of the following characteristics:

> *Structure or organization.* Individuals who compose a group have different functions. For example, one person in the group may be the leader; one may be a task master (concerned with how to best tackle the problem); one may be the maintainer (maintains good and harmonious working relationships); yet another may be the joker.
> *Shared goals.* Members of a group work together to accomplish a shared goal that could not be achieved by individuals working alone. They may come together to solve a problem, to produce something, to reach a decision, or to enjoy one another's company.
> *Common sense of identity.* Members of a group have a sense of belonging and feel the distinctiveness of their group compared with other groups.

Many similarities exist between small groups and the larger society. The group has rules and traditions, and a hierarchy of leaders and followers. The group is affected by its environment, and the group must change and adapt to survive. Last, groups, like societies, also have periods of difficulty and transition and may decline (Llewelyn & Fielding, 1982).

GROUP DEVELOPMENT

The manner in which all groups grow refers to group development. According to Tuckman and Jensen (1977) there are five stages of group development: forming, storming, norming, performing, and adjourning. These stages of group devel-

opment may be compared to the steps of the nursing process (assessing, analyzing, planning, implementing, and evaluating).

Stage 1: Forming (Assessing)

Forming is the process in which the group members assemble and come together as a group. Discovery takes place as individuals examine their backgrounds, attitudes, and personal styles. During the forming stage, individuals are gathering information about each other. This is similar to the assessment component of the nursing process, in which pertinent information about a client is assessed. Typically during the forming stage, individuals exercise their best behavior to create a good impression. There is usually a great deal of stress during this time because members are not clear what the group will be like nor what will be expected of them. Communication within the group is usually formal and polite, and members tend to talk only about safe topics such as the weather or traffic. Even though uncomfortable feelings may exist, there is generally an underlying perception of optimism within the group. By the end of this stage, members have a sense of common identity and begin to define the boundary between the group and the environment.

Stage 2: Storming (Analyzing)

Storming can be an uncomfortable stage because there may be conflict between the needs of the individuals in the group and the needs of the group as a whole. Bargaining begins as members jockey for positions within the group. Individual members explore what they might be able to contribute to the group. This stage represents the analysis portion of the nursing process because it is at this point that the members review information obtained in the forming stage. The weak organizational structure developed in the first stage may have to be reworked. As the name implies, the group climate is unstable and emotional. Communication may become openly hostile and angry. Some group members may even leave the group altogether. Individual differences among group members may become more apparent and may lead to the development of subgroups or factions. Power struggles also may occur, in which two or more people may try to compete for the leadership position.

Stage 3: Norming (Planning)

Eventually, if the group members are able to satisfactorily resolve their individual differences, **norming** will take place. At this time, group "norms" or rules for participation are established. These norms must be established if the group is to form a cohesive unit. During this stage the group develops ways of achieving its goals and decides who will do what and how it is to be done. Members begin to feel more relaxed, more a part of the group. They have made a decision to remain with the group and have begun to redefine their positions within the group. The group climate is characterized by more relatedness among members and therefore more purposeful and constructive action. This stage is comparable to the planning aspect of the nursing process, in which ideas are generated in an attempt to solve the problem identified in the previous stage. The group begins to mature, with discussions focusing on suggestions and ideas and with movement away from conflicts. Decisions are now made in a more democratic manner.

Stage 4: Performing (Implementing)

Once the norming stage is completed, the group can begin to work on the task at hand. The group can function as a unit, be productive, and work well together. As in the implementation phase of the nursing process, in the **performing** stage various strategies are tested. This is the most enjoyable stage because the group has achieved consensus on its purposes and objectives. Each member feels like a part of the group and knows what behavior is expected of him or her. The climate is one of openness, in which members are cooperative and relaxed. Differences among group members still exist, but the mature group can deal with individuality and disagreement. Conflicts that arise can be resolved through negotiation, and feedback within the group is constructive.

Stage 5: Adjourning (Evaluating)

In this final stage the group comes to some kind of closure. A summary or an evaluation of the group takes place to determine if the original purposes were met. Similar to the evaluation phase of the nursing process, the objectives are reexamined with the possibility of having to develop new strategies. If the group does not achieve complete closure, members may leave feeling dissatisfied. The **adjourning** stage may be characterized by ambivalent feelings because members are pleased that the tasks are completed but at the same time feel sad that the group is ending. Some groups may feel threatened by this stage and thus either avoid it or rush through it.

ROLE DIFFERENTIATION

In his study of role differentiation, Bales (1959) suggests that there are two major specialist roles within all groups. He refers to these as task roles and socioemotional or maintenance roles. The individual identified as a task specialist is one who is interested in one or more of the aspects of getting the job done. The task specialist exhibits behavior that contributes to the completion of a group task. The socioemotional specialist attempts to keep the group working together in harmony by relieving tension with a joke. This specialist also will make peace after conflicts and will control the more assertive group members so that the less confident can be heard.

An addition to Bales' work involves a third specialist role referred to as individual functions (Benne & Sheats, 1948). This third role includes those roles that serve individual members' own needs rather than those of the group as a whole. These three specialist roles complement each other. Those groups that are the most effective have members with different specialities. The box on p. 222 provides a summary of several examples of different roles within groups.

THE GROUP LEADER

An effective group leader is one who can influence others to work harmoniously and productively to attain the goals of the group. A group leader is also aware of the group's total resource potential and how to use it.

Four qualities are necessary in an effective group leader (Sampson & Marthas, 1981; Tappen, 1983). These qualities include the ability to set

ROLES WITHIN GROUPS

Task roles

Initiator/energizer: proposes new ideas or tasks to the group

Information giver: provides facts from personal knowledge or experience that might assist the group in its deliberations

Opinion seeker: seeks clarification by asking for opinions, judgments, or feelings of other group members

Disagreer: points out problems with the information given; presents different points of view

Elaborator: expands on existing information or suggestions being made

Evaluator: critically evaluates ideas and proposals for their practicality and effectiveness

Social/maintenance roles

Encourager: offers praise to those who have made contributions and demonstrates acceptance of ideas and suggestions

Gatekeeper: attempts to obtain contributions from other members; may suggest ways to ensure that all members have an opportunity to speak

Norm keeper: expresses standards or guidelines for the group to use in its deliberations

Harmonizer: mediates conflicts and disagreements through humor, conciliation, and mediation

Consensus taker: states opinions and decisions made by the group to test group's agreement or disagreement

Expressor: describes feelings and reactions held by group members

Individual roles

Aggressor: criticizes others and makes hostile remarks

Blocker: can obstruct progress made by the group by being negative and unreasonable

Recognition seeker: uses the group as a personal audience and calls attention to himself or herself

Monopolizer: talks often and long, thereby preventing others from participating

Definitions from "Task roles and social roles in problem-solving groups" by R.F. Bales. In E.E. Maccoby, T.M. Newcomb, & E.L. Hartley (Eds.). *Readings in Social Psychology* (3rd ed.) New York: Holt, Reinhart & Winston; and "Functional roles of group members" by P. Sheats, 1948, *Journal of Social Issues, 4*, pp. 41-49. Copyright . . . by Holt, Rienhart & Winston. Reprinted by permission.

goals, the ability to think critically, the ability to help the group become aware of its own resources, and the ability to motivate and initiate action.

Ability to Set Goals

A leader becomes involved in three types of goals: individual-level or personal goals, group-level goals, and organization-level goals. For example, Sue attends a morning meeting to discuss the discharging of a client. Sue's personal goal is that the meeting concludes so that she does not miss her lunch appointment. Group-level goals may often be different from individual goals. The group may be more interested in discussing weekend plans than interventions for the client's discharge. Finally, organizational goals may also affect the leader's action. In this case the organization is anxious not only to have the client discharged but to be able to provide continuity of care. The group leader can be instrumental in helping group members find common ground in making compromises and in formulating clear and common goals.

Ability to Think Critically

A group leader is one who not only has knowledge about a problem but is able to analyze it rather than just complain about it. Possessing knowledge about nursing gives the leader credibility and self-confidence when working with others. The leader also needs to be aware of behavior and what motivates individual group members. In the previous example the group leader can help members "brainstorm" in identifying possible community resources that might assist the client at home.

Ability to Help the Group Become Aware of Its Own Resources

The leader recognizes the strengths that individual members bring to the group and how they can best be used. In the discharge planning example, the leader attempted to match each member's talents with necessary tasks. Joan, the group's occupational therapist, was assigned to explore which structure modifications might be needed in the client's home. Betty, the group's physical therapist, was assigned to teach the client transfer techniques.

Ability to Motivate and Initiate Action

The leader has to be able not only to listen to group members but also to encourage the flow of information. The leader may notice, for example, that a group member has not made any contributions to the discussion. Rather than assuming that the individual is bored or unconcerned, the leader could attempt to bring him or her into the conversation. A group with a good idea or suggestion may not be a productive group without a leader who can guide and help members see their ideas come to life. The leader facilitates openness to ideas that may be new and different so that the group does not become immobilized by conflict.

SHARED LEADERSHIP

The same elements that make an effective leader also apply to situations that involve **shared leadership.** Although some leaders prefer to work alone, others enjoy sharing leadership responsibility. For example, a community health nurse and a physician might co-lead a group by contributing their individual perspectives of the health problem under discussion.

There are both advantages and disadvantages of shared leadership. Some of the advantages include the following:

1. The novice group leader can learn from the more experienced leader through observation and role modeling.

2. The group can benefit in seeing co-leaders communicate, cooperate, and disagree in an effective manner.

3. After each group meeting, co-leaders can share their perceptions and provide feedback to each other on the group process.

Shared leadership is more complex than leadership by one individual, a fact which can result in some of the following disadvantages:

1. Group members may play one leader against the other, just as a child may go first to the mother and then to the father when denied a request.

2. One leader may be perceived by group members as having more authority or power, which can lead to tension between the leaders.

3. Shared leadership may be less efficient because leaders must share responsibility for decision making.

SOCIAL POWER AND GROUP CONFLICT

Social **power** and **conflict** are two additional concepts that the community health nurse needs to examine to enhance his or her leadership ability. Social power can be defined as the exercise of actual or potential power to influence another person's behavior, whether that individual wants it changed or not (Cartwright & Zander, 1968). Although social power is not evenly distributed to all group members, everyone has some power. The occupant of the group leader position is often given added social power. French and Raven (1968) have distinguished five types of social power: attraction power, reward power, coercive power, legitimate power, and expert power.

Attraction power refers to a "liking" relationship; that is, a person who is liked in a group has more power than a person who is disliked. *Reward power* is based on the ability of a group member to provide rewards to other members. The reward can be in the form of money or information. *Coercive power* is the ability of one person to inflict harm on another by threatening public embarrassment, loss of prestige, or loss of popularity. The belief that one person has the right to dictate the behavior of another person is referred to as *legitimate power.* Finally, *expert power* is based on an individual's education, skills, and experience. It may be helpful for the community health nurse to assess the social power of a group, especially if the goal is to bring about change. The nurse, for example, can use expert power to encourage group members to follow directions on health matters.

Group conflict is almost an inevitable process, but it is not necessarily harmful because it can stimulate creativity and growth. A group leader should attempt neither to avoid nor to stimulate conflict, but rather to try to manage it.

There are many potential sources of conflict, including value and cultural differences among group members; conflict of loyalties within and outside of the group; power struggles; dislike of members for one another; and involvement in the group task itself. A group leader can take some preventive steps before conflicts arise by encouraging an atmosphere in which individual differences are considered normal. Open communication among group members is another measure that can be helpful in preventing destructive conflict by constructively managing it. Conflicts also can be reduced when leaders attempt to meet the needs of group members. Once a conflict has developed, the leader can help group members analyze it to determine its source so that solutions can be generated (Tappan, 1983).

GROUP COHESION

Group **cohesion** refers to a member's sense of belonging and the degree to which one feels that he or she fits into the group and is included by others. When members feel included in a group, they are more likely to identify with and commit to the group's goals. A group that is cohesive can often tolerate differences in the opinions, attitudes, behaviors, and feelings of its members, thereby making the environment safer to participate without fear of being ostracized (Marram, 1978). Sometimes the more cohesive the group is, the more productive and successful it will be.

There are several techniques that may be used for improving relations and group cohesiveness, such as using initial meetings to share ideas and beliefs. For some groups it may be beneficial to have the member write down perceptions of himself/herself, of the other members, and of how they think others view them. Another alter-

native to develop or improve group cohesiveness is a group retreat, in which members go to a neutral location and develop a "we-ness" through discussion of individual beliefs, and listening to each other and compromising in areas where there are diverse opinions.

Group solidarity can be threatened by conflict over the nature of authority in the group and the delegation of leadership. This dilemma may be resolved by using the strategy of negotiation technique, in which leadership and delegation of tasks are continuously negotiated on the basis of interests and member expertise. Finally, it is important that each group member's presence and contributions are acknowledged. This enhances the cohesiveness of the group because it helps give each individual a sense of positive self-esteem (Singhaus, Brennan, & MacKay, 1990).

MOTIVATIONAL THEORY

One of the most widely used frameworks for exploring motivation at all organizational levels is the motivation maintenance theory (Herzberg, Mausner, & Synderman, 1959). This theory identifies five major "dissatisfiers": company policy and administration, supervision, salary, interpersonal relations, and working conditions. These factors are termed *hygiene factors* because of their similarity to the principles of medical hygiene; they have a preventive rather than a curative potential. For example, interpersonal relations among group members are not directly related to the group's task; however, these relationships can affect the environment or condition under which the group must function. According to the motivation maintenance theory, a second group of factors, identified as "satisfiers," includes satisfying job content, task achievement, responsibility for a task, and professional achievement. These satisfiers are termed *motivators* because they provide impetus for superior performance.

Three principles of the **motivational theory** are applicable to groups. Regardless of how much recognition and status are provided, hygiene factors need to be reasonably satisfied or the productivity of group members will be diminished. The second principle is based on the premise that the talents and abilities of most individuals are not fully used and that many persons want to undertake new responsibilities. Therefore individual enrichment is likely to lead to a highly motivated group member. The third principle relates to developing goals or objectives, or both, that are not only clear to group members but will spur them to higher levels of productivity. This principle becomes important in the delegation of tasks. When tasks are assigned to group members, the significance of the task, and the reasons why an individual or group has been selected to complete the project, should be explained (Veninga, 1982).

Motivational theory takes into consideration the needs of group members to enhance the group's productivity.

TYPES OF GROUPS

As already indicated, nurses are expected to understand group process and to be able to function competently both as group participants and as group leaders. Nurses who function in community settings may become involved in one of four types of groups: community development groups, support or self-help groups, educational groups, and focus groups.

Community Development Groups

Community development groups are special groups that come together to support advocacy. Advocacy is action that is designed to help individuals who feel unable to acquire and use power to make social systems more responsive to their needs. Community development groups may be formed for persons all along the age continuum. A Parent-Teacher Association (PTA) may be formed to ensure that teenagers are informed about acquired immunodeficiency syndrome (AIDS) and its transmission. A group of senior citizens may join together to form a Gray Panthers organization, the purpose of which may be to educate older adults about their rights regarding rent control.

An example of a successful community development group is presented in the box to the right.

Support, or Self-Help, Groups

Many **support groups** in the United States have been formed to meet a variety of needs for both

---

COMMUNITY DEVELOPMENT GROUP SUCCESSFUL IN NUTRITION CENTER CONFLICT

Several years ago in a small urban community, a neighborhood nutrition center was to be closed for budgetary reasons. The nutrition center had operated in the basement of a church for more than 7 years. The older participants were able to walk from their homes and apartments. They felt comfortable in attending because the center was an established part of the neighborhood. They were confused and angry over the closure, which would force them to travel greater distances and require the use of public transportation.

A few of the older adults formed a community development group to decide on the best course of action. The manager of the nutrition center and the nurse provided support and feedback to the group. Strategies were established, such as circulating a written petition, writing letters to city councilmen and letters to the editor, and inviting councilmen for whom the participants had voted to visit the nutrition center. With a local election soon approaching, the final strategy proved to be the best. The nutrition center is still flourishing and meeting the needs of the local neighborhood.

---

the layperson and the professional. Support, or self-help, groups may consist of persons of all ages. The groups are usually self-regulating, with an emphasis on peer cohesiveness rather than formal structure (Burnside, 1984). The members often provide specific help in handling members' problems or conditions that require attention.

Four categories of support, or self-help, groups can be categorized as follows (Levy, 1976):

1. *Behavioral control.* The focus is on behavior modification and includes such groups as Alcoholics Anonymous, Weight Watchers, and Gamblers Anonymous.

2. *Stress, coping, and support.* Members share a common condition or life experience in such groups as arthritis clubs, Reach for Recovery, and the Parents' Association for Retarded Children.

3. *Survival oriented.* These groups advocate

self-reliance and individual responsibility and include such groups at the National Organization for Women, Latch-key Programs, and the American Association of Retired Persons.

4. *Personal growth or self-actualization.* Groups that fit into this category provide socialization and promote self-expression for persons with common life values; for example, golden agers clubs, Big Brothers/Big Sisters, and the Young Women's Christian Association and Young Men's Christian Association are a few personal growth support groups.

Individuals isolated from social or emotional resources may benefit from the establishment of a newly organized support group that promotes their health and self-esteem. The support group approach has been used in addressing teenage pregnancy. This type of group can provide a supportive milieu that offers socialization, education, discussion, and problem solving. Pregnant teenagers often have many psychological problems that may be ignored in an impersonal clinic atmosphere. Pregnant teenaged girls are at greater risk for the development of complications such as pregnancy-induced hypertension (PIH) and premature delivery because they are still maturing themselves. Many pregnant teenagers lack knowledge concerning the significance of symptoms, which causes them to delay seeking medical intervention. The community health nurse is in a good position to establish a support group for pregnant teenagers. The group could be scheduled while patients are waiting in

the clinic to see the physician. The nurse, however, also would need to work closely with the clinic staff members to obtain their support by acquainting them with the goals of the group (Everett, 1980).

Educational Groups

Although community development and support groups can provide an exchange of information, this exchange is the main focus of educational groups. **Educational groups** provide opportunities for continuing education in the area of preventive health. Figure 10-2 shows a nurse leading a prenatal class. With the growing concern for relevant and meaningful instruction in health care, community nurses will find themselves being asked to lead such a group. Nurses in community settings may also be asked to provide educational material to other nurses and health care workers on such topics as discharge planning, community resources, and the use of high technology equipment in home care.

The leader of educational groups often takes on the role of teacher, but this does not mean that the leader has to dominate the session. The educational group leader can present some basic facts about the topic and then encourage group members to participate by stating their opinions and ideas or by asking questions.

There are several advantages to health teaching in groups. One advantage is that it is more cost effective than one-on-one teaching. A second advantage is that a group setting stimulates

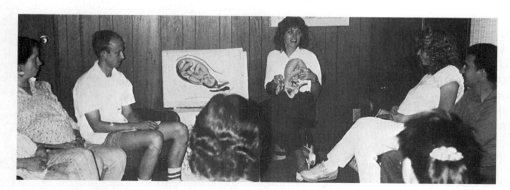

FIGURE 10-2 Example of an educational group. The nurse uses a model and pictures to illustrate labor and delivery to a group of expectant parents.

an organized presentation, which means more consistency in giving information. Finally, teaching a group can affect and alter attitudes and behavior toward health practices. As group members begin to share personal experiences and discuss realistic approaches to health problems, they may modify their attitudes.

For the community health nurse involved in an educational group—whether the group's focus is prenatal instruction, chronic lung obstruction, or stress reduction—the principles are the same. The leader first must assess the characteristics and the needs of the population before the program begins. Realistic and appropriate objectives need to be selected for the group. Finally, there is a need to evaluate the educational process either formally by questionnaires or tests, or informally by observations and interviews (Lewis, 1984).

The community health nurse working in an area with many older adults may choose to use the group approach to provide health information. A senior citizen apartment complex may have an appropriate space for such health conferences. The nurse can survey the older adults to determine topics of greatest interest and most convenient times. Posters advertising the conferences might provide helpful reminders to the participants. Titles of the conferences should be simple but also attention grabbing, such as "Meet your Feet," "Drug Use and Misuse," "Fitness For Fun," and "Are You Losing Your Senses?" Given the opportunity, older adults are usually eager to learn what they can do to enhance their health.

Focus Groups

A **focus group** may be used by community health nurses to obtain information about clients' feelings and opinions about a given problem, experience, service, or phenomenon. Focus groups can provide a safe environment in which clients can share their thoughts and perceptions without fear of being criticized. One advantage of focus groups is group synergy, which is similar to brainstorming. Clients not only respond to questions, but they can listen to what others say and add to or validate the information given (Krueger, 1988).

Although in the past focus groups have been used mostly in marketing research, they may be a valuable tool to the nurse who wants to develop a health education program. Small group discussions have assisted individuals to modify or maintain health-related behavior, such as with smoking cessation, maintaining exercise and weight-control programs, and managing stressful life events. The National Cancer Institute has used focus groups to pretest their educational materials on cancer prevention (Basch, 1987). More recently a nurse (Gray-Vickrey, 1993) conducted a focus group with caregivers of individuals with Alzheimer's Disease. The purpose of this group was to determine the caregiver experience to develop interventions that could reduce their burdens.

In general a focus group is composed of 4 to 12 participants who have similar backgrounds. For example, in Gray-Vickrey's (1993) group all members were caregivers. A focus group session may last from 1 to 3 hours; therefore, the session should be conducted in a comfortable environment. Usually the dialogue is captured by using a tape recorder. The nurse acting as the moderator of the focus group would be responsible for developing open-ended questions; facilitating the session by encouraging expression of different opinions; documenting by taking brief notes to validate contents of the tape; and analyzing and interpreting the results (Kingry, Tiedje & Friedman, 1990).

INITIATING A SMALL GROUP

The community health nurse may have noticed an increase in his or her caseload of patients with a particular disease process. The nurse decides that instituting an educational or a support group would not only enhance the members' knowledge of the disease but would provide mutual support to combat feelings of isolation. The group might be a Better Breathers Club for those with chronic obstructive pulmonary disease, a stroke club for those with cerebral vascular accidents, or a Reach for Recovery group for women who have had mastectomies. Regardless of the group, the nurse leader must complete three important tasks before the first meeting.

The first task involves administrative issues such as finding a convenient place to hold the

— RESEARCH ◆ HIGHLIGHT —

Focus Group Responses of New Mothers

Forty-one English-speaking new mothers (not all primiparas) between 15 and 22 weeks postpartum in six representative focus groups (place of residence and medical care, health insurance and socioeconomic status) met for approximately two hours in waiting rooms of closed physicians' offices or a conference room at a research institution to describe their birth experiences. This sample of convenience was procured through invitations by obstetricians, friends, or a notice at a breast-feeding center.

Four of the six groups responded to a brief questionnaire that sought demographic information and data associated with their pregnancies and deliveries. The mothers described their feelings and their babies at 3 points in time (immediately after birth, at 1 week, and 1 month postpartum). The remaining two groups were requested to think about these events. The mothers in these two groups were not asked to disclose their feelings in writing. While the four groups completing the questionnaire were viewed as representing a cross-section of new mothers in terms of education and socioeconomic status, their known routes of delivery (cesarean section) exceeded the national average. It was stipulated that this result, which was a limitation, held for the six groups as well.

Focus group meetings were tape-recorded, and transcripts for analysis resulted in the identification of the following five themes common to all, but not identical in reactions across the groups: (1) loss of autonomy and control, (2) unexpected physical pain, (3) unexpected emotional reactions, (4) financial pressures, and (5) support during labor and birth. Transcriptions for each theme were provided, and limitations preceded the discussion, which centered on the exploration of the participants' negative responses (potential bias) and which included substantiation from previous research.

The investigators suggest that the five themes be used in close-ended interviews and questionnaires to examine women's responses to the clinical and psychosocial elements of birth. Since the findings suggest some recommendations, they provide concrete examples for immediate implementation by caregivers, childbirth educators, and expectant parents in an effort to improve birthing experiences for the five dimensions. In addition, objective data should be obtained in relation to strategies for intervention that extend to external resources in the provision of care.

From Narratives of birth and the postpartum: Analysis of the focus group responses of new mothers by M.R. DiMatteo, R.L. Kahn, & S.H. Berry, 1993, *Birth, 20*(4), 204-211.

meeting. Finding a meeting place may require the nurse to negotiate with a hospital, school, or church administrator. There may possibly be resistance from the administrator or small community agencies that requires time and energy to resolve. The nurse may have to persuade administrators and agency personnel that he or she can function as a group leader. Resistance can be decreased if the nurse is prepared to present specific objectives for the group experience.

The second task in establishing a group requires making decisions about the group itself. The nurse needs to decide who will comprise the group. Will the group consist of patients with

acute or chronic illness? Will family members be included? What will the group size be? These are all important decisions that must be made before the initial meeting. It has been recommended that the group size be maintained at four to twelve members if the objectives are interaction and group cohesiveness. The nurse leader also needs to decide on how often the group will meet, at what time, and the length of each meeting. Answers to these questions depend on the composition of the group and its purposes. For some educational groups it may be beneficial to establish the total number of group sessions on the basis of the topics to be presented.

Preparing the prospective group members is the third task of the community health nurse. When possible it is best for the nurse to speak to each potential member individually. In this way the leader can prepare the member with information concerning what to expect from the group sessions. Later, written materials such as a summary of the content and topics to be covered can be sent (Clark, 1987). Starting any small group takes persistence, energy, and collaboration on the part of the nurse leader, but the members' responses often make the effort worthwhile.

Chapter Highlights

- A group is an open system composed of three or more persons held together by a common interest or bond. A minimum of three individuals is needed to allow the development of the complex relationships that characterize a group.

- Some functions of groups include safety and security, mutual support, networking for distribution of resources, socialization, and a sense of belonging.

- Characteristics common to most groups include a typical structure or organization, shared goals, and a common sense of identity.

- The five stages of group development are forming, storming, norming, performing, and adjourning. These steps parallel the five steps of the nursing process.

- The major specialist roles within groups are task roles, social/maintenance roles, and individual roles.

- Effective group leadership requires the ability to set goals, think critically, help the group become aware of its own resources, motivate others, and initiate action.

- Shared leadership in a group has both advantages and disadvantages. Although it may be more effective in some groups, it also may be more complex and less efficient.

- Social power is the ability to influence another person's behavior. The five types of social power are attraction power, reward power, coercive power, legitimate power, and expert power.

- Herzberg's motivational theory, as applied to groups, takes into consideration that the needs of group members must be satisfied to enhance the group's productivity.

- Community health nurses may become involved with community development groups, self-help or support groups, educational groups, or focus groups.

 ## CRITICAL THINKING EXERCISE

A nurse manager working in a rehabilitation unit for chemically dependent clients notes that the success rate of the program, based on the number of clients who return two or three times, is not high. The nurse decides to form a focus group of six to ten clients to determine what their perception of their treatment program should be.

1. Outline and give examples of the stages the group may go through before it can function productively. Use the description of group process in the chapter.

2. Write examples of the types of questions the nurse will ask to move the group forward and accomplish the goal.

REFERENCES

Bales, R.F. (1959). Task roles and social roles in problem solving groups. In E.E. Maccoby, T.M. Newcomb, & E.L. Hartley (Eds.). *Readings in social psychology* (3rd ed.). New York: Holt, Rinehart & Winston.

Basch, C.E. (1987). Focus group interview: An underutilized research technique for improving theory and practice in health education. *Health Education Quarterly, 14,* 411-448.

Benne, K., & Sheats, P. (1948). Functional roles of group members. *Journal of Social Issues, 4,* 41-49.

Burnside, I. (1984). *Working with the elderly* (2nd ed.). Monterey, CA: Wadsworth Health Sciences.

Cartwright, D., & Zander, A. (Eds.). (1968). *Group dynamics* (3rd ed.). New York: Harper & Row.

Clark, C. (1987). *The nurse as group leader* (2nd ed.). New York: Springer.

Everett, M. (1980). Group work in the prenatal clinic. *Health and Social Work, 5,* 71-74.

Gray-Vickrey, P. (1993). Gerontological research: Use and application of focus groups. *Journal of Gerontological Nursing, 19,* 21-27.

Herzberg, F., Mausner, B., & Synderman, B. (1959). *The motivation to work.* New York: Wiley & Sons.

Kingry, M.J., Tiedje, L.B., & Friedman, L.L. (1990). Focus groups: A research technique for nursing. *Nursing Research, 39,* 124-125.

Krueger, R.A. (1988). *Focus groups: A practical guide for applied research.* Newbury Park, CA.: Sage.

Levy, L. (1976). Self-help groups: Types and psychological process. *Journal of Applied Behavioral Sciences, 12,* 310-312.

Lewis, S. (1984). Teaching patient groups. *Nursing Management, 15*(5), 49-56.

Llewelyn, S., & Fielding, G. (1982). Group dynamics: Forming, storming, norming and performing. Pt. 1. *Nursing Mirror, 155*(July 21), 14-16.

Marram, G. (1978). *The group approach in nursing practice* (2nd ed.). St. Louis, MO: Mosby.

Sampson, E., & Marthas, M. (1981). *Group process for the health professions* (2nd ed.). New York: Wiley & Sons.

Singhaus, M., Brennan, I., & MacKay, C. (1990). Achievement of group cohesion through the development of a psychiatric seminar. *Clinical Nurse Specialist, 4*(3), 158-161.

Tappen, R. (1983). *Nursing leadership: Concepts and practice.* Philadelphia: F.A. Davis Co.

Tubbs, S. (1989). *A systems approach to small group interaction* (3rd ed.). New York: Random House.

Tuckman, B., & Jensen, M. (1977). Stages of small group development revisited. *Group and Organization Studies, 2,* 419.

Veninga, R. (1982). *The human side of health administration.* Englewood Cliffs, NJ: Prentice Hall.

11

QUALITY ASSESSMENT AND IMPROVEMENT IN THE COMMUNITY

June A. Schmele ◆ Margo MacRobert

The nursing process is dynamic in that evaluation of outcomes either confirms goals or serves as a basis for formulation of new goals.

Betty Neuman

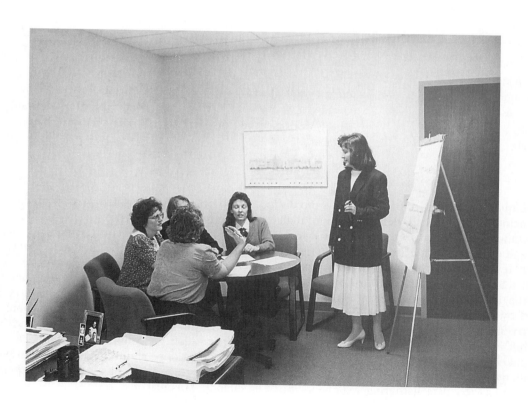

OBJECTIVES

At the conclusion of this chapter, the student will be able to:

1. Define the key terms listed.
2. Discuss the social context that influences the quality of care.
3. Discuss the concept of quality.
4. Identify selected models of quality assessment and improvement.
5. Define the steps of the American Nurses' Association Quality Assurance Process.
6. Discuss the transition of quality assurance to quality assessment and improvement.
7. Discuss selected models for quality assessment and improvement.
8. Discuss selected processes that are related to quality management in health care.
9. Describe the role of the community health nurse in quality health management.
10. Describe future health care trends and issues that will have an effect on quality management in the community.

KEY TERMS

Accountability
Accreditation
Certification
Continuous quality improvement
Licensure

Outcome
Process
Program evaluation
Quality
Quality assessment and improvement

Quality assurance
Standard
Structure
Total quality management
Utilization management

The quest for quality of patient care is rapidly influencing the health care delivery system in all organizations and settings. One of the most troubling and often disruptive aspects of this current quality revolution is the absence of common quality related terminology. The term **quality assurance** is falling into disuse and is being replaced by the phrase **quality assessment and improvement.** There are two major reasons for this shift in terminology. First, experts agree that it's unlikely if not impossible to assure quality. Second, traditional use of the term quality assurance emphasized data gathering mainly for accreditation and certification purposes, which often resulted in overlooking the identification of

the problem and the subsequent problem solving and improvement of care.

In spite of the shift in terminology, the term quality assurance will be used selectively in this chapter to represent and preserve the original concepts that have led to present day practice of quality assessment and improvement. It is important to recognize that certain geographic areas, such as the European communities, and certain settings such as community health, have been more cautious about changing terminology; therefore they may still use the term quality assurance. This may also represent the state of the science of quality management, specifically in community health nursing. For example, current literature about specific quality improvement projects in community settings is relatively scant. This may be a result either of the current practice or of a lack of publication about quality assurance programs in community settings.

ENVIRONMENTAL CONTEXT

One of the events that had a major effect on health care quality was the development of the Joint Commission on the Accreditation of Hospitals, which was formed in 1951 to carry out institutional accreditation and ultimately improve the quality of health care. This accrediting body was formed under the joint sponsorship of the American College of Surgeons, the American College of Physicians, the American Medical Association, and the Canadian Medical Association. In 1959 Canada established its own accreditation system apart from the Joint Commission (Jonas & Rosenburg, 1986).

In 1961 the National League for Nursing (NLN) developed accreditation standards and criteria for home health agencies and community health services. The American Public Health Association (APHA) collaborated in the early development of this accreditation process. The current NLN accreditation requirements reflect the trend away from assessing structure (resources) and process (activities) toward the assessment of outcomes (results) (NLN, 1987).

Since the 1960s, Donabedian, has been one of the most respected physicians and often quoted experts in the field of health care quality assessment and improvement. His classic and often cited early publication, Evaluating the Quality of Medical Care (1966), continues to be a foundational work in the study of quality. Although his discipline is medicine, the description and discussion of methods apply to other disciplines as well.

During the late 1960s, nursing leadership in quality assessment and improvement became increasingly evident. Phaneuf (1972) developed the nursing audit evaluation method, which focused on the functions of nursing as determined in the retrospective review of client records. During the same period the Slater nursing competency scale, which focused on nurse performance, was developed and published (Wandelt & Stewart,

1975). Wandelt and Ager (1970) published the quality patient care scale, which was a concurrent appraisal of patient care. Although these quality assessment and improvement approaches were developed some time ago, they remain useful today.

The 1960s marked the involvement of the federal government in health care access. In the 1965 Social Security Amendment, Medicare (see Chapter 4) and Medicaid were created to fund health care for the elderly and the indigent.

Since the mid-1960s the American Nurses' Association (ANA) has been committed to the development of standards of nursing practice (see Chapter 1), which is reflected in various nursing practice specialties. During the 1970s the ANA Model for Quality Assurance was developed with Norma Lang's participation (ANA, 1975). Also during this decade Hegyvary and associates developed a method of monitoring quality to investigate the relationship between the nursing process and patient outcomes. Their findings suggested that there was a need to study both process and outcome in relationship to other variables (Haussman, Hegyvary, & Newman, 1976).

The state of the art of quality assurance in the 1980s was largely governed by accreditation requirements or legislation directed toward cost containment. The rapid rise in the number of home health agencies and the demand for increasingly sophisticated levels of patient care have resulted in an accompanying concern for quality. The concerns about quality or lack of quality in home care were well-summarized in the landmark American Bar Association (1986) report to Congress entitled The "Black Box" of Home Care. Although this report was published several years ago, the concerns remain relevant today and have given rise to major efforts to maintain and improve quality in home care. Meisenheimer's 1989 publication, Quality Assurance for Home Care, presents the status of quality assessment and improvement in home care. Although there is a sparsity of literature devoted to the subject of quality in community health nursing, Flynn and Ray (1987) summarize the state of the art and suggest the importance of recognizing the interactive components of structure, process, outcome, and environment to measure quality. These authors refer to some of the best-known community health quality assessment and improvement programs, such as those of the Colorado and Minnesota departments of health; the Visiting Nurse Association (VNA) of New Haven, Connecticut; the VNA of Omaha, Nebraska; and the Ramsey County Public Health Nursing Service (Flynn & Ray, 1987). These programs were recognized as models for quality assessment and improvement in the community setting. For example, the long-term effort of the Omaha VNA was to develop a patient classification system that places a major emphasis on the systematic measurement of quality (Martin & Scheet, 1992).

In the 1990s, delivery of cost effective and quality health care remains a strong national focus. The Joint Commission on Accreditation of Healthcare Organizations introduced its *Agenda for Change,* which emphasized the need for a quality improvement approach based on the feedback of health care consumers (Joint Commission, 1992).

An additional important change of focus in quality assessment and improvement is the movement toward total quality management and continuous quality improvement. Health care organizations that were modeled after larger successful corporations adopted new philosophies of quality improvement such as those espoused by Deming (1982), Juran (1989), and Crosby (1979). Additional health care applications of the concepts of total quality management and continuous quality improvement are reflected in the works of Berwick, Godfrey, and Roessner (1991), Gaucher and Coffey (1993), the Joint Commission (1992), and Donabedian (1993). This important change of focus will be discussed in greater detail later in this chapter.

SOCIAL CONTEXT

The major forces that influenced the development of quality assurance are found within the social context. These influences have been felt even more strongly by health care providers within the last few years with the advent of drastic changes in the health care field. Bull's model (Figure 11-1) shows the social forces and the ma-

jor relationships between them. New technology, consumer demands, government legislation, methods of financing, cost, and competition require increasing professional accountability. Some of these influences include implicit or explicit quality management mechanisms, such as professional accountability measures and accreditation processes. These social forces will be briefly described.

Professional Accountability

The concept of **accountability** implies being answerable to someone for something. Professional nurses are answerable to the public (their clients) for the safe and professional practice of nursing. The ANA has developed professional nursing standards that are applicable to community health nursing practice (ANA, 1986a), home health care (ANA, 1986b), and other community specialties such as school health programs (ANA, 1983), hospice (ANA, 1987), and others. The generic standards for clinical nursing practice have recently been revised (ANA, 1991). These standards contain professional guidelines that direct practice and are applicable across all specialty areas to guide the practitioner and ensure professional accountability.

Licensure

Licensure is a legal process that is meant to assure the public of a minimum level of competent care. Licensure is controlled by state laws called nurse practice acts, which are interpreted and enforced by an arm of government, the State Boards of Nursing. The National Council Licensure Examination is the means by which the State Boards (the public) evaluate the applicants' qualifications for practice.

Certification

Common use of the term **certification** implies the recognition of an individual's qualifications in a nursing specialty practice by attesting that the individual possesses the "predetermined skills and knowledge in a specialized field of study" (Jones, 1981, p. 353). Criteria are specified by the certifying agency. Qualifications may include the following: "(a) graduation from an accredited or approved program, (b) acceptable performance

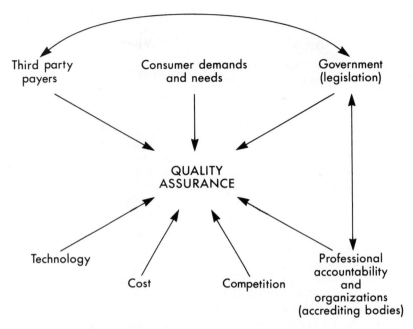

FIGURE 11-1 Societal forces influencing quality assurance. *(From Quality assurance: Professional accountability via continuous quality improvement (1992) by M. Bull. In C.G. Meisenheimer (Ed.).* Improving quality *(p. 4), Gaithersburg, MD: Aspen. Copyright 1992 by Aspen Publishers. Reprinted by permission.)*

on a qualifying examination or series of examinations, and/or (c) completion of a given amount of work experience" (ANA, 1975, p. 5). Although there are other organizations that certify nurses, the ANA is the major certifying agency. According to the ANA, in 1993 there were 82,733 ANA-certified nurses. Of these 2471 were certified in community health nursing. The three specialty areas with the highest number of certified nurses were psychiatry and mental health, medical-surgical, and gerontological nursing. The newest certification programs are in perinatal nursing and gerontological clinical specialist nursing practice (ANA, 1993). A comparison of the major differences in the processes of licensure and certification is shown in Table 11-1.

Accreditation

Accreditation is a voluntary process in which institutions or organizations are recognized as having met the predetermined standards of an accrediting body. Probably the best known example is the Joint Commission on Accreditation of

Healthcare Organizations (Joint Commission). Although accreditation is voluntary, federal funding may be contingent upon it; thus in reality the voluntary nature may be somewhat of a token process. This is frequently the case with hospitals accredited by the Joint Commission. The Joint Commission also extends to community

TABLE 11-1 Comparison of licensure and certification

	Licensure	Certification
Regulatory agency	Governmental	Nongovernmental
Action	Mandatory	Voluntary
Level of practice	Entry	Advanced
Area of practice	Basic	Specialized
Purpose	Protection of public	Career advancement
Testing process	National council licensure examination	Certifying examination

health in the form of home health care accreditation. Before 1988 the Joint Commission had accredited hospital-based home care as part of the hospital accreditation program (Joint Commission, 1991). In 1988 the Joint Commission began a new accreditation process for all home health agencies.

Other accrediting bodies also affect community health and include the NLN accreditation process for community health agencies, which is called The Community Health Accreditation Program (CHAP). CHAP's purpose is "to employ accreditation to evaluate the quality of home care in this country and to counter public fears about a quality crisis in this increasingly crucial health care arena" (NLN, 1989, p. 1). The CHAP standards place a strong emphasis on organizational management and client outcomes (NLN, 1989).

Accrediting agencies have a strong effect on the health care delivery system. Some accrediting bodies have been given the authority to ensure that a health care agency has met the Medicare requirements, thus certifying the agency for Medicare reimbursement. The agency is then recognized to have preferred or deemed status. Currently, the CHAP program and the Joint Commission have been judged to have status for home health accreditation programs.

The rise in health care consumerism, that is, the public's increasing knowledge about health care matters, is greatly influencing the roles of consumers and providers in the health care system. Whether the consumer is prepared and ready to make health care decisions remains an issue. Some believe that the majority of consumers are inadequately prepared and perhaps too ill-informed to make appropriate health care decisions. The contrasting and perhaps more popular view is that consumers have not only a right, but a responsibility, to be actively heard in decisions relating to their health care. These opposing views affect approaches to quality management. For example, a community health agency that supports the value that consumers should actively participate in health care matters will review the extent and quality of consumer participation. This review is frequently accomplished by determining the consumer's perceptions, expectations, and met or unmet needs.

Those agencies that do not value consumer participation will review other aspects of quality instead.

QUALITY

The emphasis on excellence and **quality** is widespread throughout today's corporate sector. Although the health care arena in general has increasingly emphasized quality matters, the corporate sector appears ahead in many ways. Only recently have health care personnel begun to consider the successful corporate developments in quality management. Some of the best-known corporate ideas have implications for the future because of their applicability to the health care field.

In the post-World War II era, Japan's recognition of its serious deficiencies in quality and productivity led to the use of a consultant from the United States. W. Edwards Deming, a widely recognized international consultant, is given credit for the current success of Japanese industry. Deming's idea was that improved quality would lead to increased productivity and ultimately to a more highly competitive position in the market (Deming, 1982). The work of Deming and his approaches to the improvement of quality have been very visible in the industrial sector and are increasingly seen in the health care sector.

Philip Crosby, also a well-known quality-improvement consultant, is known for his writings, which are well-summarized in the following quotation: "Quality is free. It's not a gift, but it is free. What costs money are the unquality things — all the actions that involve not doing jobs right the first time." (1979, p. 1). Crosby insists that the beginning of any quality improvement program must begin with top management. The quality principles of Philip Crosby are also becoming well-known in the field of health care quality management.

QUALITY ASSESSMENT AND IMPROVEMENT IN HEALTH CARE

Donabedian states that "for purposes of assessment the definition of quality must be made precise and operative in the form of specific criteria and standards which respectively specify the desirable attributes and their quantitative measurements" (1978, p. 113). Donabedian is credited with the development of the three approaches to assessment: (1) structure; (2) process; and (3) outcome. **Structure** refers to resources that are used to provide care. Examples of structure are staff (qualifications, number, and mix); space; equipment; and other physical facilities. **Process** means those activities that are performed in the delivery of care. Examples include the nursing process (assessing, planning, implementing, and evaluating) or other activities or tasks that may be performed, such as teaching, counseling, or physical care activities. **Outcome,** which refers to results, often is reflected in the measurement of health status in such areas as functional ability, mortality, mobility, and recidivism (Donabedian, 1978). During the past 30 years, in his numerous writings, Donabedian seldom used the words *quality assurance.* Only recently he stated that "the term 'quality assurance,' though firmly ensconced is a misnomer; quality at best can be protected and enhanced but not assured" (1988, p. 184). It is important to recognize the soundness of Donabedian's theory that there really can be no assurance of quality.

Lang, a nurse who is well-known for her early work in the improvement of quality, states that the broadest meaning of quality assurance includes all activities aimed at defining and measuring multiple aspects of quality nursing care and those activities that are planned and implemented as a result of the measurement of care (ANA and Sutherland Learning Associates, 1982, p. vii). Burgess and Ragland offer a succinct summary statement by indicating that quality assurance "was adopted as the commonly accepted title for programs that assessed, evaluated and improved care given to consumers in the health care system" (1983, p. 442).

Special application is made to community health by Donabedian, who states that when the focus of quality assessment and improvement is on population groups,

the quality of care depends first on access to care, then on the performance of practitioners in case finding, diagnosis, and treatment, and then on the performance of patients and family members through participating in care. Equal access to and enjoyment of the

highest level of quality in care may now become the community's ideal (1988, p. 174).

Donabedian's view is in keeping with ANA statements that direct the practice of community health nursing toward the promotion of the public's health.

The programs, services, and institutions involved in public health emphasize promotion and maintenance of the population's health, the prevention and limitation of disease. Public health activities change with changing technology and social values, but the goals remain the same: to reduce the amount of disease, premature death, discomfort, and disability (ANA, 1986a, p. 2).

THE QUALITY IMPROVEMENT MOVEMENT

During the early 1990s, most acute-care health care organizations have seriously concerned themselves with the pursuit of quality of health care. Driven by escalating costs and high levels of competition, this quality revolution is known at the organizational level as **total quality management,** and at the process improvement level as **continuous quality improvement.** There are also a multitude of other acronyms, such as quality assurance, quality leadership, and many others that represent this current drive for quality. Although documentation of these total quality management programs mainly describes those programs in the acute care setting, this movement will likely gain momentum in the community, especially when the effects of health care reform are felt.

In most health care settings, quality improvement constitutes a shift in paradigm. This is a movement away from inspection and isolated blame for a defect, toward the focus on evaluation of an entire systems process (Berwick, 1989). The process is studied, and groups identify ways to make the process better; that is, less costly, less time consuming, and more satisfying to the customer. The inherent philosophic change in total quality management organizations is a focus toward both the customer receiving health care and the need for organizational accountability for cost, effectiveness, and customer satisfaction.

W. Edwards Deming was sometimes considered the father of the quality improvement movement. The method he developed was widely used in the 1950s by Japanese industry and began a resurgence toward improvement in this country in larger corporations and the health care industry in the late 1980s and early 1990s. This movement has gained a strong foothold in most modern acute health care agencies. It is evident that Deming's 14 points (1986) directed at quality improvement are equally as applicable to community settings of today (see box).

Deming advocates employee involvement in the improvement process. Through the employees' shared ownership of the process, Deming believes that quality will increase and costs will decrease. Although Deming's work was and still is foundational in the development of the quality improvement programs, the work of others such as Crosby (1979), and Juran (1989) is also important.

DEMING'S 14 POINTS OF QUALITY IMPROVEMENT

1. Create constancy of purpose for improvement of product and service.
2. Adopt a new philosophy.
3. Cease dependence on inspection.
4. Stop the practice of awarding business based on the price tag alone.
5. Constantly improve every process for planning, production, and service.
6. Institute job training.
7. Promote leadership.
8. Eliminate fear.
9. Break down barriers between staff and work areas.
10. Eliminate slogans and expectations.
11. Eliminate numeric quotas and management goals.
12. Remove barriers that take joy out of work; eliminate the annual evaluation system.
13. Initiate a specific program of education and improvement for all employees.
14. Put everybody in the company to work to accomplish the transformation.

From *Out of Crisis* by W.E. Deming, 1986, Cambridge, MA: M.I.T. Center for Advanced Engineering Study.

MODELS OF QUALITY ASSESSMENT AND IMPROVEMENT

A variety of traditional quality assessment and improvement models provide the user with an operational framework for implementation. Although quality assessment and improvement are being integrated with a larger quality management program in most health agencies, it is important for the community health nurse to understand the key components of representative models. These three representative models are those of the Joint Commission, the traditional program evaluation approach, and the ANA. Each of these models, as well as several others, have applicability to community health. The ANA model will be discussed in greatest depth because of its generic applicability to all levels of service in community health nursing (individual, family, group, and community).

Joint Commission Model

The quality assessment and improvement model developed by the Joint Commission can be used as a generic model for community settings. Because the Joint Commission has a home health accreditation program, this model is especially applicable to home health. The Joint Commission model, which is considered a monitoring and evaluation model, provides the following step-by-step approach:

1. Assign responsibility.
2. Delineate scope of care and service.
3. Identify important aspects of care and service.
4. Identify indicators.
5. Establish a means to trigger evaluation.
6. Collect and organize data.
7. Initiate evaluation.
8. Take action to improve care and service.
9. Assess the effectiveness of actions and ensure that improvement is maintained.
10. Communicate results to relevant individuals and groups (Joint Commission, 1992, p. 14).

The following example illustrates how the Joint Commission quality assessment and improvement model was used in one specific home health setting. It is not a comprehensive application of the model for a total home health program; rather it includes only representative selected items for each step of the process.

1. **Assign responsibility.** The nursing supervisor for the home health agency was made accountable for the quality assessment and improvement program by the agency's administrator. She then formed a committee of interested staff nurses.

2. **Delineate scope of care and services.** The scope of care, which was identified in the agency mission statement, included the delivery of nursing care in the home to medical-surgical, maternity, elderly, and pediatric clients.

3. **Identify important aspects of care and services.** The quality assessment and improvement committee met to determine the diagnostic and therapeutic activities that have the greatest effect on the quality of care. Based on Joint Commission recommendations (1988a) to include high-risk, high-volume, and problem-prone situations, the following important aspects of care were identified:

- Ventilatory care — high risk
- Mobility of the elderly — high volume
- Catheter care — problem prone

4. **Identify indicators.** Mobility of the elderly population was identified as the aspect of care for study; thus the following indicators (criteria) were developed:

- Structure: Assistive devices will be provided.
- Process: A functional assessment will be performed by means of the mobility section of a tool (LaLonde, 1986).
- Outcome: Clients' mobility will be maintained or improved as shown by functional status.

5. **Establish a means to trigger evaluation.** It was predetermined that if more than 20% of the clients had a decline in their mobility level, an in-depth evaluation would be performed.

6. **Collect and organize data.** An audit of the clinical records of 30 patients older than the age of 65 years was performed by quality assessment and improvement committee members.

7. **Initiate evaluation.** Data from the records showed that 40% of the clients declined in mobility level. Because the trigger for evaluation was exceeded, nurses were involved in an in-depth prob-

lem-solving session to determine the cause of the diminished mobility. The cause was determined to be the lack of client involvement in the identification and ownership of the goal of maintenance of mobility.

8. **Take action to improve care and service.** The selected action recommended by the quality assessment and improvement committee was for the nurse to include the client or significant other in mutual goal setting related to mobility.

9. **Assess effectiveness of and ensure that improvement is maintained.** The nurse made deliberate efforts to include clients in mutual goal setting. Data again were gathered after 3 months and showed that only 11% of the clients now had a decline in mobility level. Because this percentage was now below the threshold for evaluation, no further action was taken. It was then decided that mobility levels would again be monitored in 3 months.

10. **Communicate results to relevant individuals and groups.** A summary report of the findings was sent to the agency administrator in charge of the organization-wide quality assessment and improvement program.

The impact of the Joint Commission approach to quality assurance is felt most strongly in the acute care setting. With the advent of Joint Commission accreditation of home health agencies, however, the use of the 10-step model will likely become more prevalent in community health agencies. It is noteworthy that the model may be considered a generic model and may be used in any setting to improve the quality of care.

Program Evaluation Model

A program is a systematically designed set of activities that are performed to bring about a certain outcome. Evaluation is a cognitive process of placing a value on something. It has been defined as "the attaching of meaning to data. This process is usually based on a series of measurements or a specific set of data that are interpreted on the basis of the professional judgment of the faculty or supervisor" (Litwack, Linc, & Bower, 1985, p. 5). Thus **program evaluation** may be considered a systematic collection of "information about how the program operates, about the effects it may be having and/or to answer other questions of interest" (Herman, Morris, & Fitz-Gibbon, 1987, p. 8). The three major purposes of program evaluation activities are planning programs, monitoring program implementation, and assessing program utility (Rossi & Freeman, 1985 and 1989; and Sandefer, Freeman, & Rossi, 1986).

There are two major types of program evaluations. One is formative evaluation, which is the process of making judgments about each phase of the program in an ongoing manner from beginning to end. The other is summative evaluation, which is the judgment about whether a program outcome was met. An example of formative evaluation of a community-based support group for unwed mothers is the judgment about whether the group's ground rules are helpful to the group's interactive processes. Because formative evaluations take place throughout the entire process, there is an opportunity to make needed changes at any stage of the program. An example of a summative evaluation is the determination, based on data, of whether the support group met its predetermined outcome objectives.

In some instances neither a formative nor a summative evaluation is indicated; rather a needs assessment related to the specific program area is needed (Herman, Morris, & Fitz-Gibbon, 1987). This type of assessment would uncover problem areas or concerns that future programs may address. An example of this is a concern for bereaved parents of deceased children. Thus an assessment would be made of the occurrence of bereavement within a defined geographic area, and the community resources available to that area. The needs assessment may indicate that the number of bereaved clients who are not already receiving bereavement counseling is minimal and thus a counseling group is not indicated at this time. It is vital, therefore, that the sponsor (one who requests the evaluation) clarify the purpose of the evaluation, whether it be assessment, formative, summative, or any combination of these three. In addition, it is imperative for the sponsor and the evaluator to reach consensus about the precise purpose of the evaluation.

The boxes on this page and on page 241 present questions that can be asked during assessment, formative, and summative program evaluations. These questions, which differentiate

GUIDELINES FOR NEEDS ASSESSMENT

Questions on the minds of the sponsors and audiences

What needs attention?

What should our program(s) try to accomplish?

Where are we failing?

Kinds of questions the evaluator might pose

What are the goals of the organization or community?

Is there agreement on the goals from all groups?

To what extent are these goals being met?

What do clients perceive they need? What problems are they experiencing?

What do staff perceive they need? What problems are they experiencing?

How effective is the organization in addressing problems perceived by clients?

What are the areas in which the organization is most seriously failing to achieve goals?

Where does it need to plan special programs or revise old programs?

From *Evaluator's handbook* (p. 16) by J.L. Herman, L.L. Morris, & C.T. Fitz-Gibbon, 1987, Newbury Park, CA: Sage. Copyright 1987 by The Regents of the University of California. Reprinted by permission of Sage Publications, Inc.

between needs assessment and formative and summative evaluations, can be used as guidelines to evaluate specific community concerns and programs. After the evaluation is completed, it is appropriate to formulate a summary report that will meet the needs of the sponsor.

In summary, the major considerations of program evaluation are as follows:

1. Determine focus (target population and program).

2. Establish purpose.

3. Define appropriate type of evaluation (assessment, summative, or formative).

4. Formulate data-gathering questions.

5. Gather data.

GUIDELINES FOR FORMATIVE EVALUATION

Questions on the minds of sponsors and audiences

How can the program be improved?

How can it become more efficient or effective?

Kinds of questions the evaluator might pose

What are the program's goals and objectives?

What are the program's most important characteristics — materials, staffing, activities, administrative arrangements?

How are the program activities supposed to lead to attainment of the objectives?

Are the program's important characteristics being implemented?

Are program components contributing to achievement of the objectives?

Which activities or combination best accomplish each objective?

What adjustments in the program might lead to better attainment of the objectives?

What adjustments in program management and support (staff development, incentives, etc.) are needed?

Is the program or some aspects of it better suited to certain types of participants?

What problems are there and how can they be solved?

What measures and designs could be recommended for use during summative evaluation of the program?

From *Evaluator's handbook* (p. 17) by J.L .Herman, L.L. Morris, & C.T. Fitz-Gibbon, 1987, Newbury Park CA: Sage. Copyright 1987 by The Regents of the University of California. Reprinted by permission of Sage Publications, Inc.

GUIDELINES FOR SUMMATIVE EVALUATION

Questions on the minds of sponsors and audiences

Is Program X worth continuing or expanding?

How effective is it?

What conclusions can be made about the effects of Program X on its various components?

What does Program X look like and accomplish?

Kinds of questions the evaluator might pose

What are the goals and objectives of Program X?

What are Program X's most important characteristics, activities, services, staffing, and administrative arrangements?

Why should these particular activities reach Program X's goals?

Did the planned program occur?

Does the program lead to goal achievement?

What programs are available as alternatives to Program X?

How effective is Program X? In comparison with alternative programs?

Is the program differentially effective with particular types of participants and/or in particular locales?

How costly is the program?

From *Evaluator's handbook* (pp. 16-17) by J.L. Herman, L.L. Morris, & C.T. Fitz-Gibbon, 1987, Newbury Park CA: Sage. Copyright 1987 by The Regents of the University of California. Reprinted by permission of Sage Publications, Inc.

6. Make a data-based judgment.
7. Formulate report.

The role of the staff nurse is usually that of a participant or data gatherer or both, under the direction of the evaluator. The evaluator should be someone who is prepared at a master's level or has had special training or experience in evaluation.

Program evaluation may be relatively simple or highly sophisticated, depending on the complexity of the program and the purpose of the evaluation. The program evaluation model is particularly relevant for community health programs. For those nurses who become heavily involved with program evaluation, a variety of resources are available. The program evaluation kit consists of nine publications that offer a step-by-step evaluation approach (Herman, Morris, & Fitz-Gibbon, 1987). The nine books have varying degrees of sophistication and can be used singly or as a package. In addition, the classic evaluation research work of Rossi and Freeman (1989) comprises a well-known approach to evaluating social programs.

The following is an evaluation plan based on the program evaluation model:

1. **Determine focus.** The nutritional program for low-income mothers and children (women, infants, and children [WIC]) will be the focus of the evaluation.

2. **Establish purpose.** The evaluation will be performed to determine the outcome of the WIC program.

3. **Define appropriate type of evaluation.** A summative evaluation to determine the outcome of the program will be completed.

4. **Formulate questions to gather data.** Guidelines for Summative Evaluation (p. 241) will be used.

5. **Gather data.** The program head will respond to the questions, using available program reports and client visits.

6. **Make a data-based judgment.** The information obtained will show whether the program is meeting the outcomes objectives.

7. **Formulate report.** A brief summary report will be prepared and directed to the administrative head.

American Nurses' Association Model

The ANA has developed and popularized the ANA quality assurance model. This model has widespread applicability in any health care setting and may be used as a guide to implement a quality assessment and improvement program in the community. The model was developed in 1974 and modified and adapted to its present form as shown in Figure 11-2. The model is a circular step-by-step approach that is ongoing and may be entered at any point. However, the identification of values is the logical entry point because values provide the basis for actions that follow. The ANA offers the following succinct overview of the model:

Once values have been identified, structure, process, and outcome criteria can be developed. These criteria are made operational by tools of measurement. When the measurements have been taken, the data can be interpreted. With these interpretations in mind, the nursing staff identifies possible courses of action and chooses the action most likely to resolve the problems. When the action has been taken, the model suggests that continued evaluation and review can determine the effectiveness of the action and the progress of health care delivery. Values and criteria are also reevaluated (ANA & Sutherland, 1982, p. 112).

The ANA has developed various publications to assist the nurse in using the model. The publication that is probably the most well known is still applicable. *A Plan for Implementation of the Standards of Nursing Practice* (1975) presupposes the extremely important, but often neglected, basic idea that standards can be implemented through a quality assessment and improvement program. A second, more recent set of three self-contained publications offers step-by-step workbooks to implement the ANA quality assurance model. These workbooks are guides that direct the various roles of persons involved with the quality assurance program: staff nurses, quality assurance committee members, coordinators, and administrators. One of the workbooks, which was written for committee members, is directed specifically to community health agencies (ANA & Sutherland, 1982).

The steps of the ANA model can be summarized as follows:

1. Identify values.
2. Identify structure, process, and outcome standards and criteria.
3. Secure measurements.
4. Make interpretations.
5. Identify courses of action.
6. Choose action.
7. Take action.
8. Reevaluate.

Resource material from the aforementioned ANA publications will be used to examine the steps of the model in more detail.

Step one: identify values. The importance of reflecting on individual, professional, and agency values cannot be overstated. Rapid changes in the environment surrounding the delivery of health care strongly influence and impinge on these values, which in turn influence both the

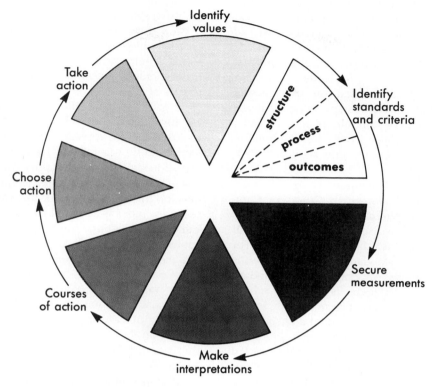

FIGURE 11-2 The ANA model for quality assurance in nursing. *Note.* From *Workbook for nursing quality assurance committee members: Community health agencies,* p.4, by ANA and Sutherland Learning Associates, 1982, Kansas City, MO: ANA. Copyright 1982 by the American Nurses' Association. Reprinted by permission.

way health care is delivered and the focus of quality assessment and improvement activities. For example, in a given home health agency if the nursing process is valued as the basis of professional nursing practice, the evaluation of this process will emerge as a vital part of the quality assessment and improvement program. In contrast, if in another home health agency the major value is placed on carrying out physician orders, this action will receive major attention. These values can be determined in various ways: by reading, discussing, and redefining the nursing philosophy or by identifying the key aspects of nursing practice within the agency. It is important to articulate the values that relate to the specific quality assessment and improvement focus or program.

Step two: identify structure, process, and outcome standards and criteria

Focus. Initially the focus of the quality assurance activity must be defined. The focus may be the staff, the clients, the organization, or all three, or any combination of the three. Another way to look at focusing is to decide which program is to be evaluated. For example, in an agency that values the importance of health promotion in schools, the focus might be on the clients and the staff in a health program designed for a school.

Standards and criteria. After the focus of the quality assessment and improvement activity is decided, standards must be selected or formulated. **Standards** are defined as an "agreed upon level of practice" (ANA, 1986a, p. 1). (ANA community health nursing standards are discussed in Chapter 1.) These standards generally are broad statements that reflect values and the level of care. There are many sources of standards, such as professional organizations, accrediting bodies, and agency policies and procedures. The ANA practice standards are based on the nursing process and include various specialties that are applicable to areas of community nursing practice. Examples of these areas are community health, hospice, home care, and schools (1983, 1986a, 1986b, 1987).

Another source of community health standards is the *Model Standards: A Guide for Community Preventive Health Services,* which was developed in 1985 as a collaborative project of several community health organizations (APHA et al., 1985). These standards deal with various community programs. An example of a standard with a school health focus is that the school health program will be planned and implemented to ensure that each student and staff person is provided with a healthful environment in which to work and study, together with needed preventive health services and health instruction (APHA et al., 1985, p. 145). If standards that are already written are used, it is desirable to discuss them thoroughly and ratify them with staff members so that ownership of the standards will be established.

After identification of standards, the criteria or items by which to measure the accomplishment of the standard will be formulated. To continue the school health example, the following criteria illustrate the three types of assessment measures:

- *Structure:* A problem-oriented health record will be maintained for each student.
- *Process:* The nurse will document problem-related data, using the POHR format.
- *Outcome:* The student health record will serve as a comprehensive data source for educational health team conferences.

The number of standards and criteria developed and used depend on professional judgment based on identification of priority standards and criteria. Generally, the development of a small, manageable number of priority standards and criteria that will accurately identify the key aspects

of care is considered more effective than an all-inclusive agenda.

Step three: secure measurements. "The degree to which actual practice conforms to established criteria provides the information used for making judgments about the strengths and weaknesses of nursing practice" (ANA & Sutherland, 1982, p. 113). Thus the predetermined criteria are formulated into some type of a measuring tool that will be applicable to whatever data collection method is chosen; for example, audit, observation, and client self-report. The methods are discussed in greater detail later in this chapter. To develop the measuring tool, an appropriate set of response types is assigned to each item. There is value in selecting simple, easily marked responses such as "yes/no," "criterion met/criterion not met," or a scale from 1 to 5 that indicates "least desirable care to most desirable care." A numeric value may be assigned to the total responses, which sums up the final evaluation of attainment of criteria. In addition, it is helpful to specify on the measuring tool what the source of the data will be. A simple example is shown in Figure 11-3.

After the measuring tool is developed or selected, the data are then gathered from a representative sample of the unit of study by means of the chosen method.

Step four: make interpretations. The degree to which the predetermined criteria are met is the basis for interpretation of the strengths and weaknesses of the program. The rate of compliance is compared with the expected level of criteria accomplishment. The expected level may be determined in various ways, such as a realistic improvement over previous rates. In some instances national norms are available, such as the norms presented in the previously discussed model standards. For example, the compliance rate expressed according to these norms might be that 90% of the two-year-old population will have completed primary immunization for the officially designated vaccine-preventable diseases (APHA et al., 1985, p. 41).

Step five: courses of action. If the compliance level is above the norm or the expected level, there is great value in conveying positive feedback and reinforcement to those delivering

Instructions: Please indicate whether or not each criterion was met.

Criteria

1.   Structure: A Problem–Oriented
       Health Record (POHR) will
       be maintained for each
       student. (See student
       health file.)   _____ Met   _____ Not
                                                                                         met

2.   Process: The nurse will
       document problem–related
       data using the POHR
       format. (See student
       health file.)   _____ Met   _____ Not
                                                                                         met

3.   Outcome: The student health
       record will serve as a
       comprehensive data
       source for educational
       health team conferences.
       (Observe health team
       conference.)   _____ Met   _____ Not
                                                                                         met

FIGURE 11-3   Example of section of measuring tool for school health program quality assurance audit.

the care. On the other hand, if the compliance level is below the expected level, it is essential to improve the situation. A necessary first step is to identify the cause of the deficiency. Then it is important to identify various solutions to the problem.

Step six: choose action. Usually various alternative courses of action are available to remedy a deficiency. Thus it is vital to weigh the pros and cons of each alternative while considering the environmental context and the availability of resources. In the event that more than one cause of the deficiency has been identified, actions may be needed to deal with each contributing cause. For example, the compliance level of immunizations was below the norm of 90% in the example in step four. Causes were identified as (1) parents' lack of awareness about the need for immunizations; and (2) the lack of accessibility of the immunization clinic in a certain geographic area. Of the possible solutions, an intensive media

campaign to raise the awareness level of the clients was chosen, and well-publicized immunization clinics were set up in a nearby shopping center on two consecutive weekends.

Step seven: take action. It is important to firmly establish accountability for the action to be taken. In other words, it is essential to answer the questions of who will do what by when? This step then concludes with the actual implementation of the proposed course(s) of action.

Step eight: reevaluate. The final step of the quality assessment and improvement process involves an evaluation of the results of the action. This reassessment is accomplished in the same way as the original assessment and begins the cycle again. Careful interpretation is essential to determine whether the course of action improved the deficiency. If the deficiency was remedied, positive reinforcement is offered to those who participated and the decision is made about when to reevaluate this aspect of care. If the deficiency was not remedied, the problem-solving process is repeated.

Application. The following example applies the ANA quality assurance process to a school health program. The example is not intended to be complete; only selected items for each step are included for illustrative purposes. Assume that a school nurse task force with an administrative representative has been designated to develop the quality assurance program.

Step one: identify values. On the basis of the ANA standards for school nursing practice, the task force identified the key value: that the main purpose of the school health program was "to enhance the educational process by the modification or removal of health related barriers to learning and by promotion of an optimal level of wellness" (ANA, 1983, p. 1).

Step two: identify standards and criteria. Various sets of standards, policies, and procedures were reviewed in preparation for the development of standards and criteria. A standard with accompanying criteria was established by the task force for structure, process, and outcome:

- *Standard:* A component of the school health program will be directed toward the prevention of disease.
- *Structure criterion:* An updated immunization record will be maintained for each student.
- *Process criterion:* The nurse will assess the immunization status of students.
- *Outcome criterion:* 100% of the students will have received mandatory immunizations before attending school.

Step three: secure measurements. The method chosen to measure the standards was a record audit. The rating response selected for each criterion was "met/not met." A simple tool was developed by using the format shown in Figure 11-3.

Steps four, five, and six: make interpretations, identify courses of action, and choose action. The data gathered from the school files revealed the following: (1) immunization records were maintained for 100% of the students; (2) the nurse assessed the immunization status of each first grade student during the enrollment

process; and (3) 90% of the students had received their required immunizations. Data was interpreted as showing that there were no problems in the area of criteria 1 and 2, and positive reinforcement was given to school nurses for the fulfillment of these criteria. However, it was noted that there was a deficiency in the lack of accomplishment of the outcome criteria related to mandatory immunizations (criterion 3). A problem-solving session of the task group explored several possible reasons: parents had not been informed of the necessity of immunizations, immunization records had not been retained by parents, parents were not aware of readily available immunization clinics, and parents had misinformation about the cost of the immunization. It was determined that the cause of the problem was lack of parent accountability for immunization of their children. The short-term solution decided upon was to obtain the vaccines from the health department, secure permission from the parents, and immunize the children on the first day of school. The long-term plan was to prepare a parent information packet dealing with the necessity of the mandatory immunizations. Evidence of immunization was required before any child could be enrolled in the first grade.

Step seven: take action. The school nurse, who carried out both the short-term and long-term plan as described in step 6, updated the immunization records accordingly. Plans were made to reaudit the immunization criteria on an annual basis thereafter.

Note that the preceding example consisted only of selected aspects of the program. If the entire program was to be evaluated, a similar process would be used for prioritized key aspects of the school health program.

After identifying the key aspects, the task force might then prioritize them according to importance. For example, during the first year, the task force may decide to emphasize the elements of the nursing process (assessment, planning, implementation, and evaluation) and selected outcomes such as immunizations, school attendance, dental health, first aid, and needs of the handicapped. It is considered more effective to evaluate a small number of the high-priority standards and criteria rather than to attempt an all-encompassing evaluation. The ability to prioritize according to the program values is vital to effective completion of the quality assessment and improvement process.

DATA SOURCES AND METHODS

There are various ways to accomplish quality assessment with a variety of data sources and methods of gathering data. The same criteria can be used or modified for the various data-gathering methods. Some of the most common methods applicable to community health are discussed briefly here.

Audit

Audit is defined as

a review of clinical records used to determine the presence or absence of predetermined criteria. A retrospective audit deals with the clinical record after the discharge from the service, while a concurrent audit is accomplished while the client or patient is still receiving services (Schmele, 1989a, p. 73).

It is important to recognize that audit is only one of several methods of gathering data; it is, however, one of the most frequently used methods when the individual is the unit of service, such as in home health care. The audit method receives a great deal of emphasis from evaluators, especially third-party payers, because the quality of care is considered to be reflected in the documentation. Reimbursement for nursing services such as home health is contingent on the documentation that demonstrates the client's specific need for skilled nursing services. Some federally mandated quality assessment and improvement processes for home health call for periodic audit of the clinical record. According to Blaha and Smith,

Examination of the documentation of care in clinical records and minutes of patient care conferences should provide the surveyor with information to measure the agency's adherence to its stated standards in acceptance, continuance of care, and discharge of patients (1986, p. 19).

Direct Observation

Direct observation is the watching or viewing of the nurse-client interaction, usually by a nonparticipating observer. This method may be used for various levels of service, such as for individuals, families, or groups. Most frequently the observation method involves visual inspection of the process of care. An advantage of the method is that the actual giving of care is observed. A disadvantage is the probability that the presence of an additional person may affect the nurse-client relationship by causing a change in the nurse's behaviors and/or the client's responses. A second disadvantage of the method is the additional resource expenditure of the time and cost of the presence of an additional professional person during the care.

Peer Review

Peer review is defined as a quality assessment and improvement method in which "a professional of equal standing reviews the quality of care" (Schmele, 1989a, p. 73). An example of peer review is the use of the quality assessment and improvement process by a group of nurses who are caring for clients with AIDS; they would predetermine standards and criteria and then use the criteria to evaluate each other's practice. An advantage of peer review is that clinical nurses who have the greatest expertise develop the standards and criteria rather than nurse managers or administrators who may lack clinical expertise. There also is value in using a participative approach to help establish ownership of the quality assessment and improvement process and the subsequent investment in the program.

Supervisory Evaluation

In supervisory evaluation the performance of the nurse is reviewed by the employee's superior. Performance appraisal, sometimes called employee evaluation, is commonly a management function. In terms of the broad definition of quality management, however, supervisory evaluations are directed toward the improvement of practice. Thus it is important that the criteria used in performance evaluations reflect nursing practice standards and criteria.

Self-Evaluation

Sometimes, in addition to supervisory evaluation, individuals may be asked to evaluate their own performances. For example, Knox has developed a system of self-appraisal and goal setting for community health nurses (1985). Her system, which is based on the nursing process, emphasizes nurses' accountability for their own professional performances. This is accomplished by comparing one's own behavior with predetermined criteria of the expected practice behaviors. When combined with goal setting, self-appraisal provides direction for professional development and helps measure progress toward performance goals.

Client Satisfaction

With the rise in consumerism and competition, there is growing interest in assessing the client's level of satisfaction with the care received. This is usually achieved through a survey in which clients are asked to respond to a number of criteria about their care. Although recent literature indicates a lack of consensus about the precise role of consumer satisfaction as a measure of quality, it substantiates client satisfaction as an essential part of the evaluation of quality of care (Donabedian, 1987; Flynn & Ray, 1987; Schroeder, 1988; Schroeder, 1993).

One of the drawbacks of client satisfaction surveys is the likelihood of biased responses. That is, the clients may tell the providers what they think providers want to hear, particularly if the client is from a culture that perceives the health care provider as an authority figure or someone the client should please. With the increasing knowledge and sophistication of consumers, it is likely that clients will express their health care expectations more openly in the future. In addition, in the future clients themselves may have an active, albeit temporary, role on the health care team in determining what the quality of care should be.

Tracers

The tracer method (Kessner, Kalk, & Singer, 1973) requires the selection of a similar set of specified health problems in a given population. For example, in a given community the selected tracer was the diagnosis of AIDS. There are predictable health problems that may appear in this population (see Chapter 20). "By evaluation of the diagnostic, therapeutic, and follow-up

processes of the set of tracers and the outcome of treatment, it is possible to assess the quality of routine care provided in a health care system" (p. 189).

Trajectory

The trajectory method of assessment begins with a cohort of persons who share a distinguishing characteristic, such as a diagnosis, a laboratory finding, or a set of signs and symptoms. It then follows the path of this company of people through the health care system, noting what happens at important junctures along the way, and what outcomes are achieved by the end of the journey (Donabedian, 1985, p. 311). An example of this method in the community is the follow-up of prenatal care throughout the pregnancies of a group of women who are below the poverty level. The final step would be to look at the outcome of the care provided.

Staging

Staging is defined as "the measurement of an adverse outcome and the investigation of its antecedents" (Donabedian, 1985, p. 311). For example, if a client's disease process, such as tuberculosis, had progressed to an extreme stage, it may indicate that care was inaccessible. This of course would require further retrospective probing into the situation and follow-up problem solving.

Criteria Mapping

Criteria mapping, also known as decision trees or flow diagrams, is a branching framework that is used to chart points of discussion about a strategy of care (Donabedian, 1985; Wilbert, 1985). The most well-known use of criteria mapping is seen in the process of case management. A case management plan and critical path are used to "map, track, evaluate, and adjust the patient's course and achievement of outcome" (Zander, 1988, p. 23).

Sentinel

The sentinel approach involves the monitoring of factors that may result in disease, disability, or complications (Donabedian, 1985). An example of this approach is the monitoring of incidences and prevalence of influenza before and after establishment of a comprehensive care program in the community.

Utilization Management

Utilization management, also known as utilization review, is directed toward the monitoring of health care services for appropriate use. For example, utilization management programs are developed to control costs through cost-effective use of services. Federally funded home health agencies that participate in Medicare/Medicaid programs are required to perform a clinical record audit to comply with utilization management guidelines. Although the goal of utilization management is to provide cost-efficient services, there is a need for integration and coordination of these activities that are similar to the objectives of quality assessment and improvement. For example, a home health utilization management audit shows that clients with in-dwelling urinary catheters are requiring prolonged home health coverage because of a high rate of urinary tract infections. This information is valuable to the nurse manager because it indicates that the quality of care of these particular clients needs to be assessed and followed closely. A problem-solving approach may lead to interventions that are directed toward earlier removal of the catheter. Removal of the catheter decreases the exposure to the agent that causes the infection. Fewer infections would reduce the number of costly home health visits.

QUALITY MANAGEMENT ROLES

With the advent of total quality management and continuous quality improvement, there are increasing opportunities for nurses to participate in the improvement of quality. Every professional nurse who practices in the community is accountable for both personal nursing practice and the maintenance of standards of practice. The ANA standards that govern community health nursing practice apply to all community health nurses (see Chapter 1). It is important to note that this set of standards contains a specific standard on quality assurance and professional development (ANA, 1986). More recently, the ANA has revised the generic standards of clinical nursing

practice. This important document is applicable across specialties and contains standards of care based on the nursing process, and standards of professional performance. The latter includes a standard on quality of care, which is presented in the box below. This standard presents guidelines

---

THE AMERICAN NURSES ASSOCIATION STANDARDS OF CLINICAL NURSING PRACTICE

Standards of professional performance

Standard I. Quality of Care

The nurse systematically evaluates the quality and effectiveness of nursing practice.

Measurement Criteria

1. The nurse participates in quality of care activities as appropriate to the individual's position, education, and practice environment. Such activities may include:

   • Identification of aspects of care important for quality monitoring.
   • Identification of indicators used to monitor quality and effectiveness of nursing care.
   • Collection of data to monitor quality and effectiveness of nursing care.
   • Analysis of quality data to identify opportunities for improving care.
   • Formulation of recommendations to improve nursing practice or client outcomes.
   • Implementation of activities to enhance the quality of nursing practice.
   • Participation on interdisciplinary teams that evaluate clinical practice or health services.
   • Development of policies and procedures to improve quality of care.

2. The nurse uses the results of quality of care activities to initiate changes in practice.
3. The nurse uses the results of quality of activities to initiate changes throughout the health care delivery system as appropriate.

From *Standards of Clinical Nursing Practice* (p. 13) by the American Nurses' Association, 1991, Kansas City, MO: Author. Copyright 1991 by the A.N.A. Reprinted by permission.

for all professional nurses to use to evaluate their practice.

In addition, there are various ways in which nurses can actively participate in quality assurance program activities such as problem solving, participation in work groups to identify work processes, data collection, assisting with development of standards and criteria, interpreting results of studies, and implementing corrective action. Some activities are performed on an individual basis and others as peer-group activities. Additional roles that community nurses may assume depend on their competence, education, experience, and interest.

In some instances nurses may have opportunities to become quality assessment and improvement committee members, participate on CI councils, or even serve on total quality management task forces. Committee membership and responsibility is usually designated by an administrative head. The makeup of the committee may vary from a peer group to a multidisciplinary or interdisciplinary group. Committee functions also may vary from total accountability for a program to a specific assignment such as evaluating a particular program. In agencies in which a quality assessment and improvement coordinator position is in place, that coordinator usually chairs or facilitates the work of the committee. In agencies without a coordinator position, a committee member usually is designated as chairperson. Ideally, the chairperson of the quality assessment and improvement committee would be a community nurse specialist with a master's degree. It is essential that nurses who perform key quality management functions and activities have a strong interest in and enthusiasm for the improvement of quality.

RESEARCH

The current research emphasis is on outcome of care. An example of this type of research is the work of LaLonde (1986), who developed, tested, and refined outcome measures of quality in home health in the following areas: general symptom distress, discharge status, taking pre-scribed medications, care giver strain, and functional status. Rinke and Wilson (1988), under the auspices of the NLN, published an anthology that contains selected approaches to the use of outcome measures in home health, and Waltz and Strickland (1988) are the authors of two volumes of research findings related to nursing outcomes. Several of these studies apply either explicitly or implicitly to community health nursing. More recently, the National Center for Nursing Research convened a conference dealing with current research on patient outcomes. The proceedings of this conference represent the state of the science of patient outcomes research with major applicability to community health nursing (U.S. Department of Health and Human Services, 1992).

An important demonstration project that was recently funded by the WK Kellogg Foundation has the objective of improving health care delivery in the home setting. Research-related approaches have been used to: 1) define consumer-based outcome measures; 2) develop a system to use the outcome measures; and 3) incorporate 1 and 2 above into the CHAPS Home Health Accreditation program. There are strong possibilities for using selected elements of this project for additional research and for other quality improvement processes (Peters, 1993).

It can be anticipated that there will be an even greater emphasis on research related to quality. Two vitally important research questions yet remain unanswered: (1) What is the relationship among structure, process, and outcome? (2) What is the relationship between cost and quality? Research in quality measurement in community health nursing holds many challenging opportunities for the future. (The student who wishes to explore this further is referred to Schmele, 1993.)

The community health nurse is in a position to take a leadership role in planning the health care system of the future. This system, which may bear only minimal resemblance to the present system, will have many opportunities for both client advocacy and quality management of care.

Chapter Highlights

- Quality assurance includes all clinical and management functions that are directed toward the improvement of health care delivery.

- The current total quality management movement is a primary influence on quality of health care.

- Quality assessment and improvement will become even more important in the future as rapid changes continue to take place within the health care system.

- The availability of classic documents, such as the Agency for Health Care Policy and Research guidelines for clinical care and ANA Standards of Clinical Nursing Practice provide sound guidelines to direct the delivery of quality nursing care in a reformed health care system.

- The Joint Commission for Accreditation of Healthcare Organizations, established in 1951, continues to have a major effect on the development of quality management programs.

- The Joint Commission model of quality assessment and improvement is a monitoring and evaluation model that uses a step-by-step approach to improve quality.

- Joint Commission and CHAP enjoy deemed status as accreditors of home health agencies; thus, agencies accredited by either of these accreditors are automatically in compliance with Medicare regulations.

- Methods of evaluation that may be used within the quality assessment and improvement cycle include audit, observation, peer review, patient satisfaction surveys, supervisory evaluations, and self-evaluations. Other more complex and less commonly used methods are criteria mapping, staging, sentinel, tracers, and trajectory.

- The ANA model of quality assurance is a cyclical quality improvement model that includes the steps of identifying values, identifying standards and criteria, securing measurements, making interpretations, identifying courses of action, choosing a specific action, and taking action.

- Licensure is a legal process designed to assure the public that an individual or institution has met minimum requirements. Certification is a voluntary process designed to indicate that an individual has reached a specified level of expertise in a given area of practice.

- The program evaluation model may be used to plan programs, monitor program implementation, and assess the program's use.

- Risk management and utilization review are two quality management processes that are related to the quality assessment and improvement process.

- All professional nurses are held accountable for their own nursing practice.

- The research process is frequently used in studies that relate to the quality of care. A current research emphasis is on outcome of care.

CRITICAL THINKING EXERCISE

A community health nurse has been making daily visits to a client with advanced multiple sclerosis to change dressings on pressure areas and maintain a supra pubic tube. The client's private insurance company has been pressuring the client to cut back on the nursing visits. There is a potential caregiver in the home, but his extreme anxiety has made the nurse reluctant to ask him to assist.

1. What might be a reasonable goal for this nurse?
2. Using the technique criteria mapping, develop a strategy, or plan of care, that might accomplish the nurse's goal.

REFERENCES

American Bar Association. (1986). *The "black box" of home care* (A report presented by the Chairman of the Search Committee of Aging, House of Representatives, Ninety-Ninth Congress, Second Session). Washington, DC: U.S. Government Printing Office (Publication No. 99-573).

American Nurses' Association. (1975). *A plan for implementation of the standards of nursing practice.* Kansas City, MO: Author (Publication No. NP-98).

American Nurses' Association. (1983). *Standards of school nursing practice* (Publication No. NP-66). Kansas City, MO: Author.

American Nurses' Association. (1986a). *Standards of community health nursing practice* (Publication No. CH-2). Kansas City, MO: Author.

American Nurses' Association. (1986b). *Standards of home health nursing practice* (Publication No. CH-14). Kansas City, MO: Author.

American Nurses' Association. (1987). *Standards and scope of hospice nursing practice* (Publication No. CH-16). Kansas City, MO: Author.

American Nurses' Association. (1991). *Standards of clinical nursing practice* (Publication No. NP-79, 20M). Washington, DC: Author.

American Nurses' Association. (1993). *American Nurses Credentialing Center Certification Catalog.* Washington, DC: Author.

American Nurses' Association and Sutherland Learning Associates. (1982). *Workbook for nursing quality assurance committee members: Community health agencies.* Kansas City, MO: Author.

American Public Health Association, Association of State and Territorial Health Officials, National Association of County Health Officials. U.S. Conference of Local Health Officers, and Department of Health and Human Services, Public Health Service Centers for Disease Control. (1985). *Model standards: A guide for community preventive health sources* (2nd ed.). Washington, DC: Author.

Blaha, A.J., & Smith, A.S. (1986). Medicare standards for home health agencies: A basic approach. *Caring, 5*(8), 18-20.

Berwick, D.M., Godfrey, A.B., & Roessner, J. (1991). *Curing health care.* San Francisco: Jossey-Bass Publishers.

Berwick, D.M. (1989). Continuous improvement as an ideal in health care. *The New England Journal of Medicine, 320*(1), 53-56.

Burgess, W., & Ragland, E.C. (1983). *Community health nursing.* Norwalk, CT: Appleton-Century-Crofts.

Crosby, P.R. (1979). *Quality is free.* New York: New American Library.

Deming, W.E. (1982). *Quality, productivity, and competitive position.* Cambridge, MA: M.I.T. Center for Advanced Engineering Study.

Deming, W.E. (1986). *Out of Crisis.* Cambridge, MA: M.I.T. Center for Advanced Engineering Study.

Donabedian, A. (1966). Evaluating the quality of medical care. *Millbank Memorial Fund Quarterly, 44,* 166-204.

Donabedian, A. (1978). The quality of medical care: Methods for assessing and monitoring the quality of care for research and for quality assurance programs. In *Health United States* (DHEW Publication No. [PHS] 78-1232, pp. 111-126). Hyattsville, MD: U.S. Department of Health, Education, & Welfare.

Donabedian, A. (1985). *Explorations in quality, assessment and monitoring* (Vol. 3). Ann Arbor, MI: Health Administration Press.

Donabedian, A. (1987). Five essential questions from the management of quality in health care. *Health Management Quarterly, 9*(1), 6-9.

Donabedian, A. (1988). Quality assessment and assurance: Unity of purpose, diversity of means. *Inquiry, 25,* 173-192.

Donabedian, A. (1993). Continuity and change in the quest for quality. *Clinical Performance and Quality Health Care, 1*(1), 9-16.

Flynn, B.C., & Ray, D.W. (1987). Current perspectives in quality assurance and community health nursing. *Journal of Community Health Nursing, 4*(4), 187-197.

Gaucher, E.J., & Coffey, R.J. (1993). *Total quality in health care.* San Francisco: Jossey-Bass Publishers.

Haussman, R.K., Hegyvary, S.T., & Newman, J.F. (1976). *Monitoring quality of nursing care, Pt. II* (DHEW Publication No. HRA 76-7). Bethesda, MD: U.S. Department of Health, Education, & Welfare.

Herman, J.L., Morris, L.L., & Fitz-Gibbon, C.T. (1987). *Evaluator's handbook.* Newbury Park, CA: Sage.

Joint Commission on Accreditation of Healthcare Organizations. (1988a). *Assuring quality care in nursing services.* Chicago: Author.

Joint Commission on Accreditation for Healthcare Organizations. (1991). *Accreditation manual for home care.* Oak Brook Terrace, IL.: Author.

Joint Commission on Accreditation for Healthcare Organizations. (1992). *Using quality improvement tools in a health care setting.* Oak Brook Terrace, IL.: Author.

Jonas, S., & Rosenberg, S.N. (1986). Measurement and control of the quality of health care. In S. Jonas (Ed.), *Health care delivery in the United States* (3rd ed., pp. 416-464). New York: Springer.

Jones, F.M. (1981). ANA's certification for specialization. In J. McCloskey, & H. Grace (Eds.), *Current issues in nursing* (pp. 353-359). Oxford: Jones, Blackwell Scientific Publications, Inc.

Juran, J.M. (1989). *Juran on leadership for quality: An executive handbook.* New York: The Free Press.

Kessner, D.M., Kalk, C.E., & Singer, J. (1973). Assessing health quality — The case for tracers. *New England Journal of Medicine, 288,* 189-194.

Knox, L.J. (1985). *The Knox guide to self-appraisal and goal setting for community health nurses.* Ottawa: Canadian Public Health Association.

LaLonde, B. (1986). *Quality assurance manual of the Home Care Association of Washington* (1st ed.). Edmonds WA: Home Care Association of Washington.

Litwack, L., Linc, L., & Bower, D. (1985). *Evaluation in nursing: Principles and practice.* (Publication No. 15-1976). New York: National League for Nursing.

Martin, K., & Scheet, N.J. (1992). *The Omaha System.* St. Louis: Mosby.

Meisenheimer, C.G. (Ed.). (1989). *Quality assurance for home health care.* Rockvill, MD: Aspen.

National League for Nursing. (1987). *Accreditation criteria, standards, and substantiating evidence* (Publication No. 21-1306). New York: Author.

National League for Nursing. (1989). *Standards of excellence for home care organizations* (Publication No. 21-2327, p. 1). New York: Author.

Peters, D. (1992). A new look for quality in home care. *Journal of Nursing Administration, 22*(11), 21-26.

Phaneuf, M.C. (1972). *The nursing audit: Profile for excellence* (p. 15). New York: Appleton-Century-Crofts.

Rinke, L.T., & Wilson, A.A. (Eds). (1988). *Outcome measures in home health.* (Publication No. 21-2195). New York: National League for Nursing.

Rossi, P.H., & Freeman, H.E. (1985). *Evaluation: A systematic approach* (3rd ed.). Beverly Hills, CA: Sage.

Rossi, P.H., & Freeman, H.E. (1989). *Evaluation* (4th ed.). Newbury Park, CA: Sage.

Sandefer, G.D., Freeman, H.E., & Rossi, P.H. (1986). *Workbook for evaluation.* Beverly Hills, CA: Sage.

Schmele, J.A. (1985). A method to evaluate nursing practice in a community setting. *Quality Review Bulletin, 11*(4), 116-122.

Schmele, J.A. (1989a). Data collection mechanisms. In C. Meisenheimer (Ed.). *Quality assurance for home health care* (pp. 72-80). Rockville, MD: Aspen.

Schmele, J.A. (1993). Research and total quality. In A.F. Al-Asaf, & J.A. Schmele (Eds.). *Textbook in total quality.* Delray Beach, FL: St. Lucie Press Corporation.

Schmele, J.A., & Donabedian, A. (In press). The application of a model to measure quality of nursing care in home health. In J.A. Schmele (Ed.). *Quality management in nursing and health care.* New York: Delmar Publishers, Inc.

Schroeder, P. (Ed.). (1988). The consumer's view of quality. *Journal of Nursing Quality Assurance, 2*(3).

Schroeder, P. (1993). *Improving quality and performance.* St. Louis: Mosby.

Shepherd, T. (1988). Cadillac care: Advances in technology raise cost control questions. *Healthcare Financial Management,* November, *42* (11):23-28.

U.S. Department of Health and Human Services (1992). *Patient outcomes research: Examining the effectiveness of nursing practice* (NIH Publication No. 93-3411). Washington, DC: U.S. Government Printing Office.

Waltz, C.F., & Strickland, O.L. (Eds). (1988). *Measurement of nursing outcomes* (Vol. 1). New York: Springer.

Wandelt, M.A., & Ager, J. (1970). *Quality patient care scale.* Detroit: Wayne State University.

Wandelt, M.A., & Stewart, D.S. (1975). *Slater nursing competencies rating scale.* New York: Appleton-Century-Crofts.

Wilbert, C.C. (1985). Selecting topics/methodologies. In C. Meisenheimer (Ed.). *Quality assurance: A complete guide to effective programs* (pp. 103-131). Rockville, MD: Aspen.

Zander, K. (1988). Nursing care management: Strategic management of cost and quality outcomes. *Journal of Nursing Administration, 18*(5), 23-30.

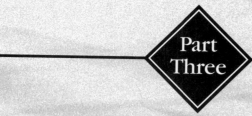

Caring for the Individual in the Community

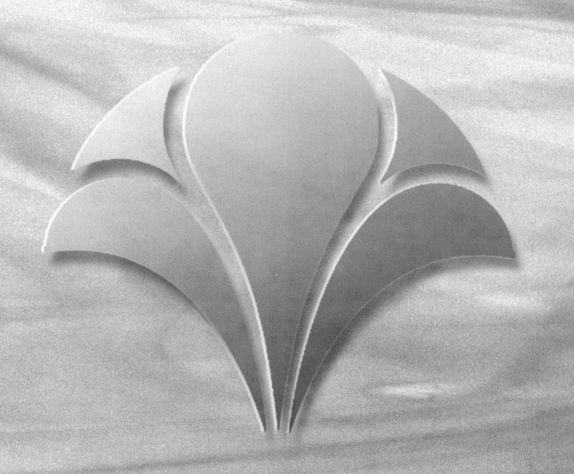

Across their life span, individuals have varying health care needs related to both age and gender. Chapter 12 describes the care of the newborn and postpartum mother in the framework of primary, secondary, and tertiary prevention. The special problems related to the care of the toddler and preschooler are described using the nursing process in Chapter 13. Chapter 14 describes the nursing care required to manage the biological and emotional concerns of adolescents. The specific health care needs of women and men are described in Chapters 15 and 16. Chapter 17 deals with health-related life events commonly experienced by the elderly.

The nurse's role in caring for individuals in the community is enhanced by knowledge of the life processes experienced by individuals from birth to death. Part III supplies information that will contribute to that knowledge and assist the nurse in planning health interventions at primary, secondary, and tertiary levels across the life span.

CARING FOR THE
MATERNAL-INFANT CLIENT

Karen Piotrowski

Infant mortality is not a health problem. Infant mortality is a social problem with health consequences.

Marsden Wagner, pediatrician, WHO

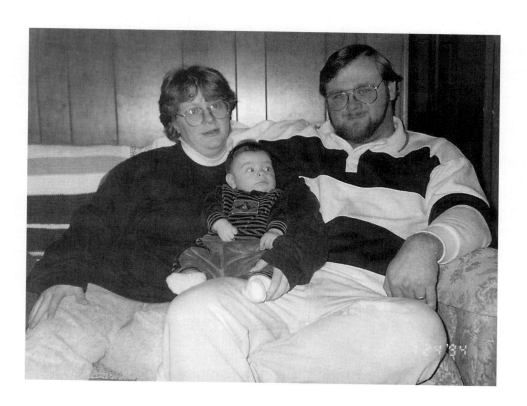

OBJECTIVES

At the conclusion of this chapter, the student will be able to:

1. Define the key terms listed.
2. Describe the roles of the community health nurse as a provider of health care services to the maternal-infant client.
3. Discuss maternal and infant mortality trends in the United States.
4. Discuss changes in fertility and birth rates in the United States.
5. Identify the major barriers facing women as they seek health care during pregnancy.
6. Discuss the concept of risk as it applies to the maternal-infant client.
7. Describe the impact of primary, secondary, and tertiary prevention services on the health and well-being of the mother, infant, and family.
8. Describe the impact of social, political, and economic forces on the delivery of health care to the maternal-infant client.
9. State the components of preconception, prenatal, and postpartum health care.
10. Discuss the importance of research as a basis for improving the delivery of health care to the maternal-infant client.
11. Use the nursing process when planning community-based health care for the maternal-infant client.

KEY TERMS

Birth rate	Low birth weight	Preconception care and
Early postpartum discharge	Maternal mortality rate	counseling
Fertility rate	Neonatal mortality rate	Prenatal care
Infant mortality rate	Postneonatal mortality rate	Very low birth weight

Nurses have a long tradition as caregivers, advocates, and leaders in the area of maternal-infant health. Historically, much of this care took place in the community, with the home as a major site. As early as 1900, concern was expressed regarding an infant mortality rate of approximately 150 deaths per 1000 live births (Starfield, 1985). Even then, prenatal care was recognized as a possible measure to reduce infant mortality and to assure more positive pregnancy outcomes. Home visits by a public health nurse became an essential component of some prenatal health services, providing education, emotional support, and direct care (Stevens, 1920).

Lillian Wald, founder of the Henry Street Settlement and advocate for children, brought home health care to the poor. In an effort to reduce infant mortality, new mothers were visited by Henry Street nurses and instructed about appropriate infant care measures. Margaret Sanger's experiences as a public health nurse caring for poor pregnant women and newly delivered mothers opened her eyes to their lack of knowledge concerning safe and effective birth control methods. This discovery compelled her to take on the role of political activist for a woman's right to know about and have access to contraceptive measures. Overcoming many legal obstacles, Margaret Sanger founded Planned Parenthood, an organization that still provides birth control education and services. In 1925, Mary Breckinridge recognized that women living in the remote rural areas of Kentucky were in need of perinatal health care services (see Figure 1-4, p.13). To meet this need she founded the Kentucky Frontier Nursing Service, which still provides not only professional nurse midwifery care throughout the childbearing period but also well-child care services in the form of parental education, immunizations, and health assessments (Kalisch & Kalisch, 1986). Significantly, the high-risk population receiving care from this service continues to demonstrate lower infant mortality and low birth weight rates than the rest of Kentucky and even the United States (ANA, 1987).

Over the years, numerous commissions and studies have recommended the development of a comprehensive system of maternal-infant health services that targets all women and infants, especially those at greatest risk. The ultimate goal of the various recommendations was to significantly reduce maternal-infant morbidity and mortality—a goal only partially met especially with regard to the poor, isolated, and minority populations in the United States.

New objectives for the year 2000 have been formulated for all people in the United States, including the maternal-infant population (see box on this page). Objectives are also defined for specific high-risk target groups within the maternal-infant population using a variety of factors, including minority status, age, and income. The efforts of health care professionals need to be directed toward achieving these objectives in a cooperative manner with individuals, families, community agencies, businesses, the media, and of course, government at the local, state, and federal level (U.S. Department of Health and Human Services, 1992).

This chapter focuses on the care of the mater-

HEALTHY PEOPLE 2000: SELECTED OBJECTIVES FOR THE MATERNAL-INFANT CLIENT

- Reduce the infant mortality rate to no more than 7 per 1000 live births and the neonatal mortality rate to no more than 4.5 per 1000 live births.
- Reduce low birth weight to no more than 5% of live births and very low birth weight to no more than 1% of live births.
- Reduce the maternal mortality rate to no more than 3.3 per 100,000 live births.
- Reduce severe complications of pregnancy to no more than 15 per 100 deliveries.
- Increase first trimester prenatal care to at least 90% of all pregnant women.
- Increase to at least 90% the proportion of pregnant women and infants who receive risk-appropriate care.
- Increase abstinence from tobacco use by pregnant women to at least 90%.
- Increase abstinence from alcohol, cocaine, and marijuana by pregnant women by at least 20%.
- Increase to at least 75% the proportion of mothers who breastfeed their babies in the early postpartum period and to at least 50% who continue until their babies are 5 to 6 months old.
- Reduce pregnancies among girls aged 17 and younger to no more than 50 per 1000 adolescents.
- Reduce unintended pregnancies to no more than 30% of pregnancies.

From *Healthy people 2000: Summary report* by the United States Department of Health and Human Services, 1992. Copyright 1992, Boston: Jones and Bartlett. Adapted by permission.

---

nal-infant client within the community. The community is becoming a major setting for health care services, as less costly alternatives to in-hospital care are sought. It is critical that the alternative services created meet the needs of the maternal-infant client in a safe, caring, and cost-effective manner. The survival of a society depends on the health and well-being of its children. A major factor in ensuring this is to provide for the health and well-being of the mothers, fathers, and families before conception, during pregnancy, and in the period of recovery and adjustment following birth.

ROLES OF THE COMMUNITY HEALTH NURSE IN MATERNAL-INFANT CARE

The community health nurse is in a powerful position to influence the creation, provision, and evaluation of health care services for the maternal-infant client. Nurses must be *advocates* to ensure that all women receive risk specific care regardless of socioeconomic, racial, or cultural status. Risk specific care is an individualized approach to health care that is based on a holistic assessment of each woman's risk for a complicated pregnancy, birth, or postpartum recovery. This care should be provided before, during, and after pregnancy. Acting individually and through professional nursing organizations, nurses need to convince policy makers in government, business, and the community that funding for preventive health services will help to ensure the health and well-being of the maternal-infant client. Additionally, preventive health services are cost effective when compared with the cost of technologically sophisticated in-hospital care and long-term follow-up of low birth weight infants. Prenatal care, a major preventive health service, saves approximately $3 for every $1 spent (National Commission to Prevent Infant Mortality, 1988).

Nurse *researchers* can initiate and conduct appropriate studies that will provide data to guide the creation of new and innovative services that target populations at greatest risk for adverse outcomes and that stimulate participation in these services. Commission reports have emphasized the critical need for interdisciplinary research and have made numerous recommendations regarding the aspects of maternal-infant health care delivery requiring scientific inquiry (COPH, 1993; Institute of Medicine, 1988) (see box below).

As *communicators,* nurses can use interactions with health care consumers as an opportu-

---

SUGGESTED RESEARCH TOPICS: MATERNAL-INFANT HEALTH

Reduction of infant morbidity and mortality:
- factors that influence fetal/newborn growth and development
- factors that influence maternal health and well-being
- interventions to motivate healthy lifestyles before, during, and after pregnancy
- risk factors for preterm labor
- measures to facilitate early identification and suppression of preterm labor

Preconception care and counseling:
- effectiveness
- content

Prenatal care:
- care models: scheduling of care, content, intervention techniques
- incentives to stimulate use and reduce barriers
- casefinding and outreach methods
- nature of social support required during pregnancy

- effect on decreasing unwanted pregnancies and child abuse/neglect
- effect on increasing use of primary prevention care and enhancing parenting skills

Home visitation programs:
- care models: content, nurse vs. non-nurse visitors, criteria for enrollment, cost-saving measures, frequency of visits
- comparison of the impact of home care vs. hospital care on adjustment of the mother, her family, and the newborn; safety considerations
- benefits vs. cost
- alternatives to home visits such as telephone follow-up

Advanced nursing practice
- effectiveness of nurse practitioners, midwives, and clinical nurse specialists as providers of maternal-infant health care
- nurses as entrepreneurs

nity to market maternal-infant health services, including the location of these services, application processes, and of course their importance for health and well-being. These interactions can occur through the media, at health fairs, in churches and schools, in primary health care agencies, and in the nurse's own practice. Nurses can also use outreach workers and neighborhood residents as collaborators in the effort to reach women in need of health care services related to childbearing (May, McLaughlin, & Penner, 1991).

Nurse *entrepreneurs* are becoming more common as nurses establish community-based private practices to meet the growing care needs of the maternal-infant client (Stern, 1991). Home-based services that provide care to postpartum mothers and to infants with special needs, and lactation consultation services that support breastfeeding mothers are two examples of the direction private practices can take.

Nurses must be *educators* not only for the pregnant client but also for the public and for the policy makers from government, business, and community. Nurses need to emphasize the importance of preventive health care as one means of ensuring the well-being of pregnant women and the optimal growth and development of their infants. Throughout the childbearing period the nurse teaches the pregnant woman and her family about pregnancy and its impact, self care and infant care measures, healthy lifestyle behaviors to promote health and prevent illness, and parenting skills.

Community health nurses are of course *caregivers,* using their professional skills to develop, implement, and evaluate a plan of care. Creativity in problem solving is often required as technological sophistication is transferred from the hospital to the home setting. As *case managers,* community health nurses are uniquely qualified to coordinate the often complex needs of the pregnant woman, infant, and family that are at risk. Community-based nurse managers employed in the New Mexico Families FIRST project use the nursing process and standards of care to ensure that high-risk families receive comprehensive, individualized, quality care. These nurses developed a prenatal risk assessment tool and care standards for each high-risk category identified. Once a family's risk categories are identified, the standards of care are used to develop, implement, and evaluate the family's care plan (Mawn & Bradley, 1993).

BIOSTATISTICAL DATA RELATED TO THE MATERNAL-INFANT CLIENT

There is an extensive amount of statistical data related to the maternal-infant client compiled and reported by the National Center For Health Statistics in weekly and monthly morbidity and mortality reports (Table 12-1). An examination of available data reveals the status of maternal-infant health and well-being in terms of changes in the morbidity and mortality rates, factors that influence the health status of the maternal-infant client, and trends in birth and fertility rates. Additionally, health practices of pregnant women are examined, including their use of primary prevention health care services such as prenatal care. Trends in the rates of morbidity, mortality, and birth are influenced by a population's access to basic needs for shelter, food, employment, education, and health care (Arnold & Grad, 1992). In fact, it is a widely held belief that a country's infant mortality rate reflects the health status of its people. Statistical analysis can provide direction to health care providers by revealing risk factors, identifying populations to target for specific health care services, and suggesting solutions to problems of limited access and use. In an era of rising costs and diminishing resources, the use of available data when planning care is critical if we are to provide cost-effective health care to all maternal-infant clients, especially those at highest risk for adverse outcomes.

Infant Morbidity and Mortality

Between 1970 and 1991, the **infant mortality rate,** or the number of deaths in the first year of life per 1000 live births, declined from 20 to 8.9 (Figure 12-1). Provisional data predict an infant mortality rate of 8.5 in 1992. Overall, the four leading causes of death in 1991 were congenital anomalies, sudden infant death syndrome, disorders related to short gestation and unspecified low birth weight, and respiratory distress syndrome. It should be noted that the leading cause

TABLE 12-1 Perinatal biostatistical data for the United States

Biostatistical measurement	Rate
Infant mortality rate:	
Number of deaths in the first year of life per 1000 live births. (1991)*	8.9 all infants 17.6 Black infants 7.3 White infants
Neonatal mortality rate:	
Number of infant deaths in the first 28 days of life per 1000 live births. (1991)	5.6 all infants 11.2 Black infants 4.5 White infants
Postneonatal mortality rate:	
Number of infant deaths after the first 28 days of life per 1000 live births. (1991)	3.3 all infants 6.4 Black infants 2.8 White infants
Low birth weight:	
Infants born weighing less than 2500g, shown as percent of births. (1990)	7.0% all births 13.3% Black births 5.6% White births
Fertility rate:	
Number of live births per 1000 women between the ages of 15 and 44. (1990)	70.9 all women 89.0 Black women 62.8 White women
Maternal mortality rate:	
Number of maternal deaths related to complications of pregnancy, birth, and the puerperium per 100,000 live births. (1991)	7.9 all women 18.4 Black women 5.6 White women

* Above rates reflect the most recent year for which statistics are available as reported by the National Center for Health Statistics (NCHS, 1993a,b,c,d).

of death for White infants was congenital anomalies, whereas for Black infants the leading cause was disorders related to short gestation and unspecified low birth weight. Despite progress in reducing the infant mortality rate, the United States has not kept pace with many other industrialized nations. In 1989, it ranked 24th in infant mortality among countries or geographic areas with a population of at least 1 million people.

This ranking represents a decline from 20th place in 1980 (NCHS, 1993a,d).

Approximately 67% of infant deaths occur during the first 28 days of life, which is called the *neonatal period* (NCHS, 1991b). The **neonatal mortality rate,** or the number of infant deaths during the first 28 days of life per 1000 live births, is closely associated with intrauterine events and low birth weight. **Low birth weight** (birth weight < 2500 g) infants are 20 times more likely to die during this period than neonates of an appropriate weight, and **very low birth weight** (birth weight < 1500 g) infants are 200 times more likely to die (McCormick, 1985). During the 1980s, the **postneonatal mortality rate,** or the number of infant deaths after the first 28 days of life per 1000 live births, remained stable at 3.6. Postneonatal deaths are closely associated with inadequate social and environmental conditions resulting from poverty, namely unsafe and unsanitary housing and limited resources to provide for the infant's needs in terms of health care, nutrition, and developmental stimulation. Many of these households are maintained by single parents who have limited educational backgrounds and inadequate social support systems. The four major causes of postneonatal death are sudden infant death syndrome (SIDS), congenital anomalies, accidents, and infectious diseases. Accidents have increased in number during the first year of life, and the rate of immunizations is estimated at only 70% to 80% nationwide for children under 2 years of age (Rosenbaum, Layton, & Lew, 1991; NCHS, 1991a).

Closer analysis of infant mortality data reveals some disturbing trends. First, the infant mortality rate for Black infants is 17.6, more than twice that for White infants, which is 7.3. A similar relationship is apparent when examining neonatal and postneonatal mortality statistics. In addition, infant mortality rates are significantly higher in the inner city and remote rural areas, especially in southern states. Second, the rate of decline in the infant mortality rate stabilized in the 1980s. Experts attribute the slowing of progress to the fact that the regionalization of perinatal care and the technological and treatment advances of the 1960s and 1970s reached peak effectiveness (NCHS, 1993a,d). Health care providers need to

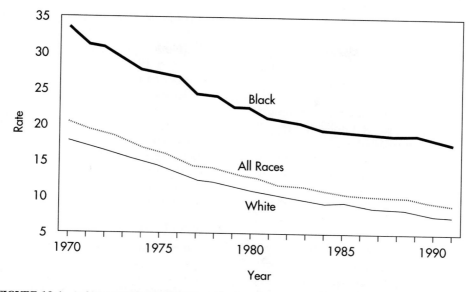

FIGURE 12-1   Infant mortality rates,* by race† of mother: United States, 1970-1991. *(From Infant Mortality, United States, 1991. By National Center for Health Statistics Morbidity and Mortality Weekly Report, 42(48). Copyright: Massachusetts Medical Society. Reprinted with permission.)*

* Deaths at < 1 year of age, per 1000 live births in specified group.
† Includes Hispanic and non-Hispanic infants; rates are presented only for Black and White infants because the Linked Birth/Infant Death Data Set (used to more accurately estimate infant mortality rates for other racial groups) was not available for 1990 and 1991.

look beyond technology and neonatal intensive care units (NICU) for interventions that can help to stimulate further declines in the infant mortality rate to the year 2000 goal of no more than 7 deaths per 1000 live births.

Prevention of low birth weight, the factor most closely associated with neonatal deaths, may be the key to further reducing the infant mortality rate. It has been found that the risk of neonatal mortality increases as the weight at birth decreases (York & Brooten, 1992). Low birth weight and very low birth weight are also major risk factors associated with morbidity in terms of congenital anomalies, developmental problems, and cerebral palsy. Since low birth weight can result from preterm birth (birth before completion of 37 weeks gestation) or from intrauterine growth retardation, or both, efforts to reduce low birth weight must focus on factors that influence fetal growth in utero as well as the early detection of preterm labor and prompt

treatment to suppress it. Low birth weight is a multifaceted problem that requires an interdisciplinary effort to reach a solution. The greatest number of low birth weight infants are born to non-white women, adolescents, women over 40 years of age, and women who experience reproductive or medical problems such as placental and reproductive abnormalities, anemia, infections, and hypertension. Poverty, unemployment, limited education (< 12 years), and inadequate prenatal care are social problems associated with low birth weight (Arnold & Grad, 1992). Low birth weight is also more likely to occur among women who are physically abused before or during their pregnancies (Parker & McFarlane, 1991). One study found that the incidence of low birth weight for battered women was nearly twice that of non-battered women (Bullock & McFarlane, 1989). Research studies now indicate that certain unhealthy behaviors are linked to low birth weight. Such behaviors include smoking, drug and alcohol abuse, inappropriate nutritional intake, and a stressful lifestyle (Institute of Medicine, 1985; Meis, Ernest, & Moore, 1987).

The cost of low birth weight can be viewed in both human and financial terms. Parenting an infant with special needs can take a toll on the caregivers and other family members, creating a stressful environment that is unhealthy for all concerned. Often these caregivers are the least capable of coping with a difficult situation. The financial ramifications of low birth weight are equally staggering. A low birth weight neonate can incur hospital costs ranging from $14,000 to more than $100,000. Continuing care costs can be as high as $400,000 over a lifetime. A major factor associated with low birth weight is inadequate prenatal care. If all women received adequate prenatal care, the incidence of low birth weight and infant mortality would decrease. Estimates of the average cost of prenatal care for one woman ranges from $400 to $600 (Arnold & Grad, 1992; Institute of Medicine, 1988; Office of Technology Assessment, 1988).

Birth and Fertility Rates

When **birth rates** (the number of live births per 1000 population) are examined from 1970 to 1989, a slight increase from 15.5 to 16.3 has been noted. In 1990, the **fertility rate** (the ratio of the number of live births per year to the number of women of child-bearing age) was 70.9 live births per 1000 women between the ages of 15 and 44. While the birth rate for women in their twenties showed only a slight increase, for young teens (age 15 to 17) there was an increase of 6% from 1975 to 1988. The birth rate, in 1989, for young teens was 36.5 per 1000 women, an increase of 8% from 1988. In 1990, the birth rate for this population increased by another 3% to 37.5. At the opposite end of the reproductive age range, the birth rate for women between the ages of 35 and 39 rose 50% in the 1980s to 29.7 in 1989 and 31.7 in 1990. For women aged 40 to 44 a 20% increase in the birth rate was noted from 1975 to 1985; in 1989 the rate was 5.2 and in 1990 it was 5.5. An interesting trend in childbearing can be noted when analyzing the birth rates for married and unmarried women. While childbearing declined slightly for married women, in 1989 it increased dramatically among unmarried women to 41.8 per 1000 women aged 15 to 44. In 1980 the percentage of births to single women was 18.4% compared with 28% in 1990. A large percentage of this increase is among Caucasian women, a significant number of whom are college educated professionals (NCHS, 1991a, 1993b). The rise in the birth rate among unmarried women and women in their young teens needs to be carefully examined in terms of the effect this trend might have not only on the health and well-being of the mother but also on the growth and development of her infant.

Maternal Morbidity and Mortality

The **maternal mortality rate** in 1991 was 7.9 maternal deaths per 100,000 live births caused by complications of pregnancy, childbirth, and the puerperium. The disproportionate number of Black women who die is reflected in a maternal mortality rate that is 3.2 times higher than for White women (NCHS, 1993c). Pregnancy induced hypertension, hemorrhage, embolism, and ectopic pregnancy account for the majority of deaths (Rochat, Koonin, Atrash, & Jewett, 1988). While 40% of pregnant women experience no medical or obstetrical complications during the antepartum, intrapartum, and postpartum periods, 60% do. About 50% of the women who have a complicated pregnancy experience health problems serious enough to require special medical care. Both poverty and young and older age (adolescents and women aged 35 years and older) increase a woman's risk for pregnancy-related complications (Gold, Kenny, & Singh, 1987).

Infant and Maternal Mortality in Canada

Canadian infant and maternal mortality rates present an interesting contrast to those in the United States (Table 12-1). Infant mortality rates have steadily declined in Canada. In 1991, the rate was 6.4 per 1000 live births as compared with 9.6 in 1981 and 7.9 in 1986. Neonatal and postneonatal mortality rates have declined in a similar fashion. The neonatal mortality rate in 1991 was 4.1 and the postneonatal mortality rate was 2.3.

Maternal mortality rates are also lower in comparison to the United States. In 1990, the rate was 0.2 per 100,000 live births, and in 1991 it was 0.3. The Canadian health care system, which emphasizes health care of mothers and children, may account for Canada's more favorable infant and maternal mortality rates when compared with the United States (Statistics Canada, 1994).

MATERNAL-INFANT HEALTH CARE SERVICES IN THE COMMUNITY
Primary Prevention

Primary prevention refers to health care aimed at health promotion and disease prevention. According to Lawton Chiles, chairperson of the National Commission to Prevent Infant Mortality, "Our fight against infant mortality has stalled because we have not reached the mothers and children at risk. We need to invest in the kind of resources that provide preventive health care rather than waiting to provide costly 'rescue' treatment later" (1988, p. 3). It is estimated that as many as 50% of infant deaths could be prevented and many of the long-term disabilities requiring costly lifetime care could be avoided with an organized, comprehensive system of preventive maternal-infant health care services that includes the participation of the pregnant woman in early and ongoing **prenatal care** (health care that occurs during pregnancy). The health care system in the United States must be more effective in providing universal access to early maternity and pediatric care for all mothers and infants, in eliminating barriers that limit access to and use of this care, and in targeting those clients most at risk and in need of care (National Commission to Prevent Infant Mortality, 1988).

Prenatal care

Beneficial outcomes of prenatal care. Studies have demonstrated an association between poor pregnancy outcome and inadequate prenatal care. Conversely, early comprehensive and ongoing prenatal care can be a critical factor in reducing the incidence of low birth weight infants and preterm birth. The benefits of prenatal care have been noted for both low-risk and high-risk pregnancies (McCormick et al., 1989; Hulsey Patrick, Alexander, & Ebeling, 1991). The positive effects attributed to prenatal care may in part be related to two factors (Tyson et al., 1990). These factors are as follows:

1. Women who participate in prenatal care throughout their pregnancies tend to exhibit fewer risk factors such as poverty and low educational levels.

2. Women who participate in organized health care are more likely to comply with and help to plan their health care regimens.

Beyond the positive effects related to low birth weight and infant mortality, it is important to determine how prenatal care might influence the development of parenting skills, increase knowledge and use of preventive health care services, decrease the number of unwanted pregnancies, and reduce the incidence of child abuse and neglect (McCormick et al., 1989).

Despite its beneficial effects, the proportion of women beginning prenatal care in their first trimester remained stable at approximately 76% between 1979 and 1988 and even declined slightly to 75.8% in 1990. Women at highest risk for poor pregnancy outcomes are the women who have the potential to derive the most benefit from prenatal care, yet they are the least likely to receive it. In 1990, 83.3% of White women, 81% of Hispanic women, 60.7% of Black women, and 57.9% of Native American women participated in prenatal care that began in the first trimester. Maternal age, unemployment, minority or migrant status, geographic location, high parity, single marital status, and low educational level are demographic factors associated with a late start to prenatal care (after the fifteenth week of pregnancy) or no prenatal care at all. Approximately, 6.1% of all pregnant women in 1990 had late or no prenatal care. Specifically, 3.4% of White women, 9.3% of Hispanic women, 11.2% of Black women, and 12.9% of Native American women had late or no prenatal care. Unfortunately, it is these very factors that place pregnant women at greatest risk for fetal loss, preterm birth and low birth weight, maternal morbidity and mortality, and infant death (Horton, 1992; St. Clair, Smeriglio, Alexander, & Celentano, 1989; Buekens et al., 1993; NCHS, 1993b).

Barriers. Analysis of the data from numerous surveys of pregnant women reveals a variety of factors that can create barriers to obtaining prenatal care (see box on page 266). Knowledge of

BARRIERS TO PARTICIPATION IN PRENATAL CARE

Demographic barriers:

Age (< 20 or > 40)
Education (< 12 years)
High parity (> 3)
Geographic location
Single marital status
Minority/migrant status
Employment status

System barriers:

Inadequate capacity
Limited number of providers
Attitude/behaviors of providers
Cultural insensitivity
Communication/language differences
Casefinding methods
Clinic environment
Appointment scheduling

Financial barriers:

Poverty
Inadequate health insurance
Medicaid
Complicated enrollment process
Eligibility determination delays

Client barriers:

Personal/cultural views
Knowledge deficit
Stressful life experiences
Transportation and child care
Attitude toward the pregnancy
Influence of family
Previous experience with care
Fear

Donald & Coburn, 1988; Young, McMahon, Bowman, & Thompson, 1989).

Financial barriers have increased along with the unemployment rate. The number of Americans, particularly women and children, living in poverty has grown, leaving them without adequate insurance coverage for health care. Adolescents often are dependent on their parents for health care, having no insurance and limited financial resources of their own. Reluctant to reveal their pregnancies, adolescents are likely to delay the start of prenatal care or to not seek it at all. Even for women covered by employer health insurance plans, benefits may not reimburse for maternal-infant health care. Health care providers need to appreciate that using public assistance and public health care may be humiliating and stigmatizing, especially for the "new poor." In addition, application for public assistance is time consuming and confusing with long, complicated forms to complete. It is important to note, however, that public prenatal clinics may actually offer higher quality care with access to a larger referral network than the private care offered to the poor. Yet women forced to use public clinics may delay entry simply because of a bias against public care and the status assigned to those who use private care (Handler & Rosenberg, 1992).

Commissions designated to improve prenatal care recommended a streamlining of the Medicaid enrollment process, the eligibility determination, and the reimbursement system. The Omnibus Budget Reconciliation Act (OBRA-86) allows individual states to alter Medicaid in an attempt to foster greater participation in prenatal care. Presumptive Medicaid eligibility provides pregnant women with immediate short-term eligibility while full Medicaid eligibility is being determined. Continuous Medicaid eligibility guarantees that eligible women will remain covered throughout their pregnancies even if family income and resources fluctuate. Application is facilitated when Medicaid workers are available at the sites where primary care and prenatal care are provided. Finally, employers and insurance carriers need to recognize the cost effectiveness of preventive health care services for the maternal-infant client and provide for coverage of

the most common barriers is of importance when preventive health services during pregnancy are planned, implemented, and evaluated. Rarely is one single factor responsible for pregnant women receiving inadequate care. Rather, it is a combination of many factors that limit access to and participation in prenatal care. Solutions, therefore, must incorporate many different approaches (National Commission to Prevent Infant Mortality, 1988; Institute of Medicine, 1988; Mc-

these services (Hill, 1988; Institute of Medicine, 1988).

Prenatal care services, especially those in the public sector, must share a major responsibility for the creation of *system barriers* that prevent women from obtaining the health care that they need. A system stretched to the limit means that women are often frustrated by delays in scheduling the first visit and long appointment waiting times sitting in overcrowded waiting rooms only to experience a short, impersonal "check up" by the health care provider. These same providers, often short staffed and overworked, have been described by their clients as rude, inhospitable, and insensitive to client feelings, needs, and cultural beliefs. Communication barriers exist when the language of the provider is not the language of their client. Clinics are often open during hours that conflict with the work or school schedule of its pregnant clients.

The removal of system barriers begins with expansion of services and recruitment and retention of qualified health care professionals. Obviously, the frustration that women experience with waiting lists and appointment delays can be overcome if more health care providers become a part of the system, including nurses working in advanced practice who take on major caregiving responsibilities. If casefinding is to be successful, and women are to be enrolled, then there must be a health care system in place that meets their needs and encourages their continuing participation. Inservice education programs can help health care providers, and ancillary workers can develop effective communication techniques and sensitivity to their clients' cultural values and beliefs. Waiting times can be used to present valuable information through videos, reading materials, and group classes. "One stop" care can provide on-site participation, as needed, in smoking cessation groups, substance abuse counseling, and social support programs (ANA, 1987).

Prenatal programs that are based within the community of its clients are more likely to be used because they will be more accessible and culturally sensitive. Members of the community can be of assistance in providing social support

and casefinding services, in role modeling appropriate behaviors for pregnant women and new parents, and in conducting group sessions to facilitate the sharing of feelings, needs, and experiences among pregnant women and new parents. Businesses can become active partners in the prenatal care effort by advertising services, providing space for satellite clinics, donating materials for mobile clinics, and offering incentives in the form of merchandise and service vouchers to pregnant women who continue to participate in prenatal care (Affonso, Mayberry, Graham, Shibuya, & Kunimot, 1993; Helton, 1990).

Client barriers must also be a concern of health care providers. Many factors influence a woman's care-seeking pathway to achieve a safe passage through pregnancy for herself and her baby (see research highlight box, p. 268). Not all women appreciate the value of prenatal care. Culturally they may define pregnancy as a healthy state requiring medical intervention only if a problem occurs. The attitudes and beliefs of a woman's support group can also influence a woman's entry and participation in prenatal care. If this support group values prenatal care, then it will serve as a positive stimulus. However, research conducted by St. Clair et al. (1989) found that women who came from very close social networks composed primarily of family members living in close proximity to one another were more likely to underuse prenatal care services. Although further research is needed, it is obvious that health care providers need to be aware of the pregnant woman's social network and incorporate them into recruitment strategies and educational interventions. Women who encounter difficulties with transportation, child care problems, and meeting the basic needs of food and shelter for their families may not see preventive health care services as a priority. Multiparous women, especially those with previously uneventful pregnancies, may use experience-based self diagnostic measures to determine their state of well-being during pregnancy and enter prenatal care late as the time to arrange for the birth of their baby draws near. Some women may lack knowledge about the signs of pregnancy or where to go for care. A woman's feelings about her pregnancy play a role in seeking prenatal care; an unplanned or unwanted pregnancy may result in denial, depression, and ambivalent feelings regarding how to proceed, whether to continue with the pregnancy or to have an abortion. Fear can be a barrier, with the source of the fear varying from woman to woman. Women may fear discovery of their pregnancy by family and friends, fear health care providers and medical procedures, and fear sanctions regarding "bad" habits such as smoking, drinking, and drug abuse. According to McFarlane (1993), women who are physically abused are twice as likely to delay enrollment in prenatal care until the third trimester. These women stated that the abuser blocked access to prenatal care by denying them transportation and often interfered with healthy practices during pregnancy by destroying vitamins and other required medications. Another powerful deterrent in seeking prenatal care could be previously negative experiences with the health care system.

Women and their communities need to be made aware of the importance of healthy behavior during pregnancy and the participation in prenatal care. The media — television, radio, and print — can be used to disseminate the information as can community outreach volunteers. Door-to-door, person-to-person contact may be needed for those who are homeless or who live in remote rural areas. Telephone hotlines can be used to give information and to make the first prenatal appointment. Community groups and churches can be encouraged to provide transportation and child care services. Social service referrals can help women deal with major life stressors so preventive health care can assume importance. The prenatal care system needs to operate in conjunction with other health care agencies, social services, and even employers that have contact with women of childbearing age as a means of encouraging preconception counseling, early entry into prenatal care, and compliance with appointments. Social support such as "buddy" systems and incentive programs can be used to encourage pregnant women to continue

 RESEARCH 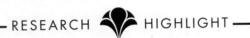 HIGHLIGHT

Seeking Health Care During Pregnancy

Twenty-seven women were interviewed to explore the care-seeking pathway each took to achieve a safe passage through pregnancy. Analysis of interview data revealed that seven processes were used. Searching for prenatal care could be as simple as a telephone call or as difficult as struggling through a maze of red tape that could end the search. Consulting was achieved by the gathering of information and opinions from spouses/partners, relatives, friends, and colleagues. Transferring from one care provider to another occurred when expectations were not met or circumstances changed. Criteria for care were identified and used to guide the search. Criteria included financial considerations, location, quality, and reputation of the care provider, and the nature of preexisting relationships with a provider. Waiting periods often occurred during care seeking. Waiting was most common with multiparous women and women who were forced to consider public care. Waiting ended as a result of a perceived change in health status or the prodding of a significant other. Women who self diagnosed their pregnancies and believed that prenatal care was not necessary used contingency planning. They determined that care would be sought at the onset of labor or at the self detection of a threat to safe passage for themselves or their babies. Self care—efforts to take care of self by making healthy changes in lifestyle—was engaged in to some degree by all women in the sample regardless of their participation in prenatal care. Major themes emerging from the study were that women do assume personal responsibility for seeking safe passage and that they are more likely to seek care if they have choices and can afford private care.

From Seeking safe passage: Utilizing health care during pregnancy by E. Patterson, M. Freese, & R. Goldenberg, 1990, *Image*, 22(1), 27-31.

When making a home health care visit to an elderly woman, a community health nurse met the client's 20-year-old granddaughter, Susan. While speaking to Susan about the care requirements of her grandmother, Susan stated that she was concerned about how she would manage to continue to care for her grandmother "after the baby comes." Further discussion with Susan revealed that Susan was about 4 months pregnant. When the nurse asked Susan if she had received any health care related to her pregnancy, Susan replied that she felt fine and did not have time to look into the matter because she worked part-time, went to school, and helped to take care of her grandmother. Susan also stated, "I don't know where to go to see a doctor but I'll find out when the time to have the baby comes closer. Anyway, I need to get some money together to pay for the hospital, since the father of my baby refuses to have anything to do with me and I don't have any health insurance." Realizing the importance of prenatal care for a healthy outcome for Susan and her baby, the nurse used the nursing process to develop a plan to help Susan obtain the health care and support she needs.

NURSING DIAGNOSIS: Altered health maintenance during pregnancy related to a lack of knowledge regarding the importance of prenatal care and the presence of factors that interfere with ability to obtain prenatal care.

Client goals	Nursing interventions	Evaluation
Susan will: • identify the benefits of prenatal care for herself and her baby. • enroll in the prenatal care program in her neighborhood within 1 week. • meet prenatal care appointments as scheduled. • participate in the pregnancy, childbirth preparation, and parenting classes offered by the clinic. • apply for the community support services that she needs.	**Discuss** the benefits of prenatal care: • Pregnancy is a dynamic state and risk status can change; therefore, ongoing assessment of her health status and that of her baby is critical. • Prenatal care is effective in preventing low birth weight and reducing maternal-infant morbidity and mortality. • Referrals can be made to other community support services such as WIC, well baby clinics, Medicaid. • Classes are available to teach her about pregnancy, childbirth, and postpartum and newborn care. **Arrange** to meet Susan at the prenatal clinic located within a short distance of her home. Introduce her to the nurses at the clinic, orient her to the services offered by the clinic, and initiate the enrollment process **Refer** Susan to a social worker at the clinic so eligibility and need for community support services can be determined and application initiated.	• Susan enrolled in prenatal care and met her scheduled appointments or called to reschedule if she could not. • Susan stated the benefits of prenatal care and encouraged a pregnant classmate to make an appointment at her clinic. • Susan signed up for childbirth preparation classes with her sister who will be her coach during labor. • Susan applied for and is now covered by Medicaid. • Susan arranged for home care for her grandmother since her grandmother was eligible for this service. • Susan plans to join the parenting support group after she has her baby.

in prenatal care. Women who are currently enrolled or who have participated in prenatal care can be enlisted to encourage friends, relatives, and neighbors to seek appropriate care. Comprehensive family planning services need to be made available as a means of decreasing the number of unplanned and unwanted pregnancies.

Special consideration must be given to the needs of pregnant adolescents in an effort to help them continue with their education, participate in prenatal care, and become responsible parents, if that is their decision. Peer counseling and support groups can be especially effective with regard to adolescent sexuality, pregnancy, and parenting (National Commission to Prevent Infant Mortality, 1988; PHS, 1989; COPH, 1993).

The community health nurse is in an ideal position in terms of casefinding and promoting participation in early and ongoing prenatal care. The nursing process can be used as an organizing framework to identify and overcome barriers to prenatal care, facilitate enrollment in prenatal care, encourage ongoing participation, and make referrals to appropriate community support services.

The components and content of prenatal care. The content of each prenatal contact needs to be relevant, individualized, and its value appreciated by the pregnant woman if health care providers expect them to continue with care. The planning, implementation, and evaluation of care must involve the active participation of the pregnant woman and her support group. Although the method of delivery may vary, all prenatal care programs should incorporate three basic components, namely early and continuous risk assessment, health promotion activities, and medical and psychosocial intervention and follow-up (PHS, 1989).

Assessment of risk status is an important component of prenatal care and must use a holistic approach. Risk factors can arise from any aspect of a woman's life, in fact, many of these factors occur together. Although most risk factors are present before or appear early in pregnancy, some can appear at any time. Thus, health assessments must not only occur early but must continue throughout pregnancy targeting times when specific risk factors are most likely to appear. Major categories of risk factors or characteristics that assist in the identification of women who are more likely to experience adverse pregnancy outcomes include:

1. Medical and genetic disorders present prior to pregnancy such as hypertension, diabetes, cardiovascular disease, and sickle cell disease

2. History of reproductive problems such as preterm birth, short interpregnancy intervals, and uterine malformations

3. Nutritional deficits such as low maternal weight, obesity, anemia, inadequate dietary practices, and inappropriate weight gain during pregnancy

4. Health problems arising during pregnancy such as pregnancy-induced hypertension, multiple gestation, placental anomalies, and infection

5. Psychosocial deficits such as single marital status, lack of participation by the father of the baby, limited education, inadequate support system, psychiatric disorders, abusive relationships, and high stress level

6. Economic deficits such as poverty, unemployment, and inadequate health insurance

7. Adverse health behaviors such as smoking and alcohol and drug abuse

8. Environmental problems such as inadequate housing, safety hazards, and exposure to teratogens in the home or workplace

As part of the risk status assessment, the pregnant woman's level of health must be determined. Use of a prenatal self-assessment questionnaire, such as the one developed by Moore and colleagues (1986), would be helpful in obtaining the client's view regarding their health status as well as their feelings and concerns regarding their pregnancy. Thus, a more individualized approach to care is facilitated, with the client as an active participant. Data gathered from the questionnaire can be used to identify learning needs, lifestyle habits and health practices, composition and quality of support system, coping mechanisms, and expectations regarding pregnancy and parenting.

Health promotion activities constitute the second required component of prenatal care. Parents who are healthy themselves and are part of a supportive network of family and friends that value health care are more likely to give birth to and raise healthy infants who exhibit optimal growth and development. Health care providers must be skilled in the communication, counseling, and teaching techniques to successfully motivate the prenatal client and her support group to participate in activities that promote healthy living before, during, and after pregnancy and to acquire the knowledge to develop effective child care and parenting practices. Implementation of specific health promotion strategies needs to take into consideration the client's readiness to make a change or to learn. For example, counseling regarding nutritional practices and the impact of physical changes that accompany pregnancy is best accomplished during the preconception period or early in the first trimester. On the other hand, the best time to educate the client about childbirth techniques, self-care needs during the early postpartum period, and newborn care would be the third trimester.

Medical and psychosocial intervention and follow-up need to reflect a multidisciplinary approach because client needs are likely to occur in a number of areas including physical, psychological, social, environmental, economic, and educational. Health care providers must be aware of the variety of health care and social services that are available in the community to assist their clients so that appropriate referrals can be made. Home care agencies, drug and alcohol rehabilitation centers, family planning clinics, child care services, and employment counseling programs are the types of services the prenatal client may need. Case managers can be effectively enlisted to oversee and coordinate the plan of care designed for each pregnant woman. In this manner, continuity of care can be assured, and individualized needs can be met. With the case management approach, one person is in charge and available both to the interdisciplinary team and to the prenatal client (ANA, 1987).

The content of prenatal care should also reflect the seven components of prenatal care identified by the ANA Consensus Conferences (1987). The components are risk assessment, individualized care, nutrition counseling, education to reduce or eliminate unhealthy habits, stress reduction, social support services, and health edu-cation. Ideally care begins within 1 year before pregnancy with **preconception care and counseling.** This approach provides the opportunity to perform a baseline assessment and to identify and modify health problems, personal behaviors, and environmental hazards that could adversely affect pregnancy before conception occurs. Parents experiencing a high level of wellness as they begin pregnancy and then parenting are more likely to experience positive outcomes. Early entry into prenatal care can be encouraged, or, if necessary, pregnancy postponed. Preconception care and counseling should be a component of the health care given to men and women during the reproductive years with primary care agencies, family planning clinics, schools, well-child clinics, substance abuse, and STD (sexually transmitted disease) clinics as possible settings. Care of the pregnant client then continues through the three trimesters and postpartum period (from conception through the recovery period following birth) and for the infant client through the first year of life. The student is advised to consult a comprehensive maternity nursing textbook for specific assessment measures, laboratory and diagnostic testing, and interventions during pregnancy and the postpartum period.

A variety of approaches can be used to meet the care requirements of the prenatal client. Successful programs often combine a number of the following approaches:

1. Traditional appointments with a health care provider at a prenatal care site
2. Home visits by community nurses, paraprofessional home visitors, and community volunteers
3. Telephone contacts for missed appointment follow-up, assessment of current status and concerns, and provision of information
4. Group classes and support groups

Scheduling care. The frequency and timing of prenatal care contacts are currently being debated. The American College of Obstetricians and Gynecologists (ACOG, 1988) recommends a visitation schedule that begins in the first trimester of pregnancy, with monthly visits until 28 weeks, then every 2 weeks until week 36, and finally weekly visits until birth occurs for an average of 13 visits if the pregnancy reaches full term at 40 weeks' gestation. On the other hand, the Public Health Service Expert Panel on the Content of Prenatal Care (1989) recommends a contact schedule similar to the French model of seven visits (Buekens et al., 1993). The healthy nulliparous woman (first pregnancy) would be scheduled for nine visits and the healthy multiparous woman (more than one previous delivery) would experience an average of seven visits. The panel highly recommends the initiation of preconception care and counseling within 1 year of conception and an early start to prenatal care at no later than 6 to 8 weeks' gestation. The purpose of this recommendation is to provide information concerning a client's level of health and risk status that can then be used as the basis for determining the content and scheduling of prenatal care contacts. Thus a cost effective approach is used that targets high-risk clients for the most intensive care. Central to any prenatal care scheduling is providing the client with the opportunity to contact their health care provider should concerns arise or changes in their condition occur.

Home care services

Home visiting by community health nurses during and after pregnancy is a highly effective method of providing primary prevention care not only for the maternal-infant client but also for the family (Figure 12-2). This method of care delivery offers advantages both for the nurse and for the client (Hyde-Robertson, 1992). These advantages can include:

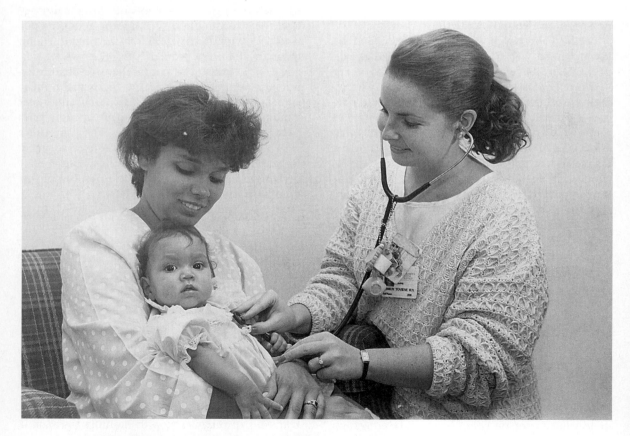

FIGURE 12-2 A professional nurse makes a home visit to assess the health status of a mother and her young infant. (*Photograph courtesy of Children's Hospital Home Care, Buffalo, New York.*)

1. The client and family receive care in an environment where they are often more comfortable, in control, and together.

2. Because the home is a more private environment, questions can be asked and concerns can be expressed freely. Confidential matters related to such topics as sexuality and family planning can be discussed more openly and in a less rushed manner.

3. Readiness for learning is enhanced as the family faces the realities of pregnancy and postpartum changes, newborn care, and family adjustments including sibling rivalry.

4. Anxiety is often reduced by the presence of a knowledgeable, caring professional nurse in the home. Additionally, positive outcomes can be facilitated including the creation of a healthier home for all.

5. Nurses have the opportunity to assess the client's environment for safety, cleanliness, and adequacy for family needs.

6. Nurses can observe the interactions of the client and her support group, especially the father of the baby, in an environment where they may feel more free to be themselves.

7. Nurses can adapt instructions to the resources available in the client's own environment. Health teaching can occur at a more leisurely pace with the active participation of both the client and her family.

8. Referrals can be made based on a more exact assessment of the client's needs.

Home visiting can be costly, so the benefits of preventive health care services must be documented, and limited resources must target those families at greatest risk for problem development. Assessment of continuing progress during health care appointments and in telephone follow-up can be used to determine the need for and frequency of home visits. In addition, a determination can be made as to the most effective visitor: professional nurse, paraprofessional, or lay volunteer. Regularly scheduled home visits to women at increased risk have been found to be effective in meeting the objectives of prenatal care by providing interventions that promote health and positive pregnancy outcomes, including a reduction in low birth weight and infant mortality (PHS, 1989; York & Brooten, 1992).

An analysis of home visitation programs indicates that prenatal visitation must be followed up with postnatal visitation if lasting positive effects are to be achieved. When at-risk families received both prenatal and postnatal visits, substantial improvements were noted in maternal health, infant growth and development, parenting techniques, and the incidence of child abuse and neglect for at least 2 years following delivery. It is interesting to note that visitation programs that include nurse visitors were more likely to have positive outcomes because families viewed the nurse as a professional with knowledge and experience to share (see box on page 274). Although the most successful programs provided a series of visits, the long-term benefits seemed to outweigh the expense. In many European countries, home visitation is offered to all families. Because this may not be feasible in the United States, targeting families in greatest need—families exhibiting high-risk factors and families experiencing their first pregnancies—may be a cost effective alternative (Olds & Kitzman, 1990).

Some home visitation programs found creative solutions to the problem of limited resources. One solution effectively matched the skill levels of professional nurses, paraprofessionals, and peer counselors with the degree of client risk and the nature of their needs (Peoples-Sheps, Ejird, & Miller, 1989). A program on a U.S. Army base used volunteer nurses to provide home visitation for low-risk postpartum families. Community health nurses who monitored the program and served as mentors for the volunteers were then used more effectively as care providers for families at high risk (Misener & Knox, 1990). In an effort to enroll pregnant teens into prenatal care and enhance their life and parenting skills, the Resource Mothers Program was established. In this program, nonprofessional women work as home visitors in their community. Under the supervision of professional nurses, these women counsel, support, assist, and advocate for pregnant teens living in their community (Heins, Nance, & Ferguson, 1987).

Early postpartum discharge

A major concern facing maternal-infant health care providers is the growing trend toward **early postpartum discharge.** What began in the mid

HOME VISITATION DURING THE PRENATAL PERIOD

Assessment:

- Health status of the maternal-fetal unit
- Maternal adaptation to pregnancy and its changes
- Family responses to pregnancy
- Cultural influences on health care patterns and behaviors
- Knowledge regarding pregnancy, its impact, healthy behaviors, and self-care requirements
- Need for community support services

Interventions:

- **Teach:** importance of early, ongoing prenatal care, signs of effective and ineffective adaptation to pregnancy, signs of labor, self-care and healthy lifestyle behaviors during pregnancy, infant care measures and preparation, parenting techniques
- **Discuss:** feelings regarding pregnancy, formulation of a birth plan, arrangements for postpartum care of the mother and her newborn
- **Counsel:** lifestyle changes to promote health in terms of nutrition, stress, and use of tobacco, alcohol, and drugs
- **Encourage:** continuing participation in prenatal care and the plan of care developed
- **Use:** community support agencies by making referrals as needed to such services as Medicaid, child care centers, family violence counseling and shelters, expectant parents classes, housing support, smoking cessation and substance abuse rehabilitation programs
- **Involve:** family in the process of assessment and care

1970s as a successful voluntary program involving women who were healthy and had adequate economic, housing, health care, and family support has now become a mandate of a growing number of insurance carriers, with a prediction of universal implementation over the next few years. Today, many insurance policies will cover only a 24-hour hospital stay after an uncomplicated vaginal birth (in the 1950s the stay was for 10 days) and 3 days after an uncomplicated cesarean birth. The rationale for this trend is not only its cost-saving implications but also the belief that recovery and family attachment and adaption to the newborn are facilitated within the comfort of a home environment. However, there have been a number of concerns expressed by health care providers regarding early discharge. These concerns include missed maternal complications (infection, hemorrhage, fatigue, and depression) and infant complications (jaundice, cardiac and respiratory disorders, infection, hypothermia), inadequate family preparation for maternal and infant care in the home, and limited time to establish skill and confidence with breastfeeding. In addition, the safety of early discharge for a disadvantaged population with fewer resources needs to be investigated more fully. The studies conducted to date have indicated positive outcomes with no increase in the occurrence of maternal or infant morbidity or mortality. However, the effect of early discharge on family processes and the adaptation of its members has received limited study (Vrazo, 1993; Norr & Nacion, 1987; Williams & Cooper, 1993).

Early discharge programs need to incorporate strategies that address the concerns expressed by health care providers. Attention must be given to the very dramatic changes that occur during the postpartum period (the 6- to 8-week period following birth). These changes require as much support and intervention as the prenatal and intrapartum periods, therefore services should extend through this period (Lukacs, 1991; Donaldson, 1991). Nursing diagnoses typical of the early postpartum period should be considered when planning discharge, preparing the family, and designing a program of telephone and home care follow-up (see box on page 275).

The components of early postpartum discharge programs should include:

1. Criteria to ensure that only healthy maternal-infant clients are discharged. Most criteria that are currently used relate both to a low-risk status maintained throughout pregnancy and to the birth process. In addition, the birth recovery progress up to discharge must be uncomplicated for both the mother and the infant as indicated by stable vital signs and postpartum assessments (fundus, lochia, episiotomy), lab values within normal ranges (Hct, Hgb, Coombs, bilirubin, glucose), adequate elimina-

COMMON NURSING DIAGNOSES OF THE EARLY POSTPARTUM PERIOD

Mother:

- High risk for fluid deficit related to blood loss associated with vaginal birth and uterine atony.
- High risk for infection related to effects of vaginal birth on the genitourinary tract.
- Fatigue related to demands of recovery and newborn care.
- Pain related to episiotomy and uterine cramping (afterpains).
- Alteration in nutrition: less than body requirements related to concern regarding effects of pregnancy weight gain on appearance.
- Constipation related to slowed peristalsis and painful episiotomy.
- Moderate anxiety related to responsibilities of family and newborn care.

Newborn:

- High risk for ineffective breathing pattern and airway clearance related to limited reserve capacity of newborn respiratory system and limited protective function in terms of coughing and ability to clear airway.
- High risk for infection related to immature immunologic function and presence of healing umbilical cord/circumcision.
- Ineffective breastfeeding related to maternal inexperience with breastfeeding techniques and newborn feeding behaviors.
- High risk for injury related to elevated bilirubin levels.
- High risk for alteration in body temperature related to immature thermoregulatory mechanism associated with newborn status.

Family:

- High risk for altered parenting related to inexperience and lack of adequate family support.
- Altered family processes related to addition of newborn.
- Parental role conflict related to need of mother to return to work following a 6-week maternity leave.

tion patterns, tolerance of oral intake, and positive progress in parental attachment to the newborn. It is also important to determine if the mother has basic knowledge and ability regarding her own self-care and the care of her infant and an available support system and adequate housing (Halloran & Zickler, 1988).

2. Participation in comprehensive prenatal care throughout pregnancy.

3. Participation in prenatal classes that prepare parents for postpartum events and care measures. The content taught prenatally needs to be the foundation for a teaching plan that continues during the 24-hour hospital stay and in the home after discharge. Planning content for health teaching is important for continuity and the avoidance of duplication.

4. Establishment of a post discharge follow-up program that includes telephone contacts and at least one home visit by a qualified nurse who specializes in maternal-infant care. Ideally, this nurse visitor has contact with the client prenatally and during the hospitalization. The first phone call should occur within 24 hours (see box on page 276) and the first visit within a few days of discharge (see box on page 276). It is during the first week following birth, before recovery is complete, that the new mother and her family face the full force of postpartum demands. Today it is not unusual for the new family to be separated from their extended family by distance, financial constraints, and various other commitments. Thus an important source of support, nurturing, and care is unavailable. The nurse visitor is in an ideal position to meet this need and assist the family during this transition period (Evans, 1991). The frequency of postpartum follow-up visits has not been established and requires further study. As with prenatal care, the scheduling of postpartum visits should be risk specific. Home care can continue even when problems arise since phototherapy for hyperbilirubinemia and IV antibiotics for infections can be administered in the home setting. It is also helpful if a 24-hour information hotline is included in the follow-up service to provide immediate response to questions and concerns.

5. Arrangements for follow-up care should be made during the third trimester and during the period of hospitalization. Provisions for care of the maternal-infant client should include ongoing

---

POSTPARTUM TELEPHONE FOLLOW-UP: SUGGESTED FORMAT FOR ASSESSMENT OF MATERNAL-NEWBORN AND FAMILY STATUS

- Describe how you are feeling today.
- What have you been doing to take care of yourself?
- How does the baby seem to you?
- Describe how the baby has been eating and sleeping.
- What has been the greatest source of happiness for you since coming home?
- What has been the greatest source of stress for you since coming home?
- What are your concerns?
- How are the other members of your family doing since you and the baby came home?
- How can I help to make things easier for you?

From Postpartum follow-up: A nursing practice guide by the Nurse's Association of the American College of Obstetrics and Gynecology, 1986, *OGN Nursing Practice Resource.* Washington, DC: NAACOG: The Organization for Obstetrical, Gynecological, and Neonatal Nurses. Adapted by permission.

HOME VISITATION FOLLOWING EARLY POSTPARTUM DISCHARGE

Assessment:
- Maternal recovery following pregnancy and birth
- Newborn adaptation to extrauterine life
- Family adaptation to birth and the newborn
- Cultural influences on health care patterns and behaviors for the mother and her newborn
- Environmental adequacy, safety, and cleanliness
- Knowledge regarding postpartum recovery, maternal-infant care
- Need for community support services

Interventions:
- **Teach:** signs of effective and ineffective recovery for mother and infant, action to take if signs of ineffective recovery are noted, maternal and infant care measures, breastfeeding, process of infant growth and development, measures to promote positive family attachment/adaptation to newborn, family planning measures
- **Discuss:** feelings/concerns regarding the birth experience, postpartum recovery, and infant care; provide support and reassurance
- **Encourage:** participation in primary prevention health care services for all family members including evaluation of health status on a regular basis, use of healthy lifestyle practices, immunizations
- **Use:** community support services by making referrals as needed to such services as WIC, lactation consultants, well-child clinics, child-care centers, family planning clinics, parenting support groups
- **Involve:** family in the process of assessment and care

---

health guidance, course of action if warning signs appear, preventive activities such as immunizations, and methods to adequately space pregnancies.

6. Establishment of a network of support services that can meet the individual needs of families. Such services could include group parenting classes and support groups, breastfeeding groups such as LaLeche League, and lactation consultation services.

The value of home visitation as a method of providing primary prevention care has been demonstrated by a number of programs and research studies. Evaluation of the effectiveness of this approach for maternal-infant health care needs to continue since data that reveals positive effects can be used to influence health care policy and funding.

SECONDARY PREVENTION

The focus of secondary prevention health care services is the early detection of health problems and the initiation of prompt treatment. As less-

costly alternatives to inhospital care are sought, many more high-risk pregnancies are being managed on an outpatient basis and in the pregnant woman's home.

The success of home care after the early discharge of uncomplicated vaginally delivered mothers and infants has added further impetus to the movement away from long hospitalizations for women experiencing a complicated pregnancy. Today, hospitalization is most often used for a pregnant woman whose condition is unstable and requires continuous, intensive monitoring. Once stabilized and responsive to treatment, the client is discharged to her home where care continues.

Hospitalization can be a stressful experience, especially if prolonged and at a distant location from the client's home (a major consideration for women living in rural communities). Loss of identity, privacy, control, and familiar surroundings, separation from support group, and worry about self, fetus, and family are all stressors that are difficult to cope with. These women often feel well and are bored, restless, and restricted by hospital routines. The impact of stress and anxiety on the outcome of a high-risk pregnancy and ultimately on attachment to the newborn has not been fully examined.

Hospitalization also disrupts family processes. Women may feel guilty about their inability to meet the needs of partner and children. Family routines are altered, substitute care takers are sought, and financial resources are strained. Additionally, families may feel left out of the care plan and feel isolated from the hospitalized client by rules and regulations that limit visitation (Murphy & Robbins, 1993; Middlemiss et al., 1989).

Home care, on the other hand, can limit the amount of family disruption while enhancing a sense of control and participation in the care of the maternal-fetal unit. Safety, as a primary concern, is addressed by assisting the family to devise a system that encompasses the care and bedrest requirements of the pregnant woman. To this end, setting priorities, simplifying tasks, and identifying sources of support among relatives and friends are helpful interventions. Nurses can identify community resources such as home and child care agencies and laundry and shopping services. Diversional activities and phone call networks can help a woman on bedrest pass the time (Monahan & DeJoseph, 1991). In addition, the woman and her family need to learn how to monitor her condition, how to implement the treatment plan, and how to take action should warning signs develop. A diary or journal that describes day-to-day progress and concerns can be used by the community health nurse to set the focus and priorities for each visit (Dahlberg, Parker, & Knox, 1989).

The cost effectiveness of home care is of great concern to the health care system and third-party payers. It is estimated, for example, that 10 weeks of home care for preterm labor including tocolysis (labor suppression treatment), bedrest, visits by a high-risk perinatal nurse specialist, and weekly nonstress tests would cost approximately $2100 as compared with approximately $24,500 for 10 weeks of hospital care (Dahlberg et al., 1989).

Many home care agencies have been established for the high-risk pregnant woman. These agencies encompass assessment of maternal-fetus status, implementation of treatment measures, and provision of support for the pregnant woman and her family. Home fetal assessment is now possible since monitoring units can be safely transported to the home setting (Figure 12-3). Monitoring of fetal heart patterns, nonstress testing, and even ultrasonographic examination can be conveniently done in the home (Goodwin, 1992).

Today diabetic women are instructed about home blood glucose monitoring. Data concerning glucose levels, diet, activities, and insulin intake can be compiled by the woman and brought to weekly outpatient visits for evaluation. Thrombophlebitis can be treated at home with subcutaneous heparin therapy. Pregnant women experiencing hyperemesis can be stabilized in the hospital and discharged to home care while still receiving total parenteral nutrition. Bedrest requirements for a woman with pregnancy-induced hypertension can be maintained at home while she and her family monitor her blood pressure, count fetal movements three times a day, and observe for the warning signs of a worsening condition. Nursing visits and family access to 24-hour-a-day nursing contact via telephone make these health care approaches safe and effective.

The success of home management of women at risk for or actually experiencing preterm labor in the prevention of preterm birth is well documented (Hill, 1990). Because low birth weight related to preterm birth is associated with infant morbidity and mortality, interest in cost-effective

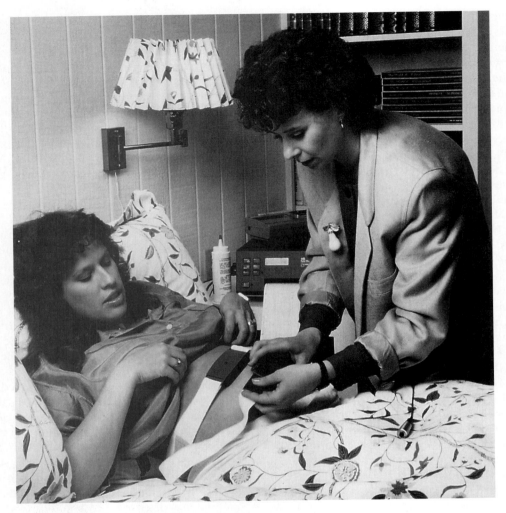

FIGURE 12-3 A professional nurse performs a nonstress test in the home of a pregnant woman. *(Photograph courtesy of Tokos Medical Corporation.)*

measures to prevent preterm birth has grown. Factors that place a woman at risk for preterm labor include a previous history of preterm labor or birth, multiple gestation, uterine anomalies, and stressful living conditions and lifestyles. These women are placed on a regime of activity reduction, external uterine activity monitoring, and daily telephone contact with a nurse who evaluates transmitted uterine activity tracings and discusses maternal concerns (Figure 12-4). This approach facilitates the early identification of preterm labor before major cervical changes

have occurred. It has been found that tocolysis is most effective when begun at this early stage. Research findings indicate that the combination of uterine monitoring and nursing support are the most critical components of this approach to preterm labor management and results in a reduction of preterm births (Hill et al., 1990; Koehl & Wheeler, 1989). If preterm labor is detected while at home, the woman is hospitalized for tocolysis. Once labor is suppressed she is discharged to home on subcutaneous pump or oral maintenance dosages of tocolytic medication,

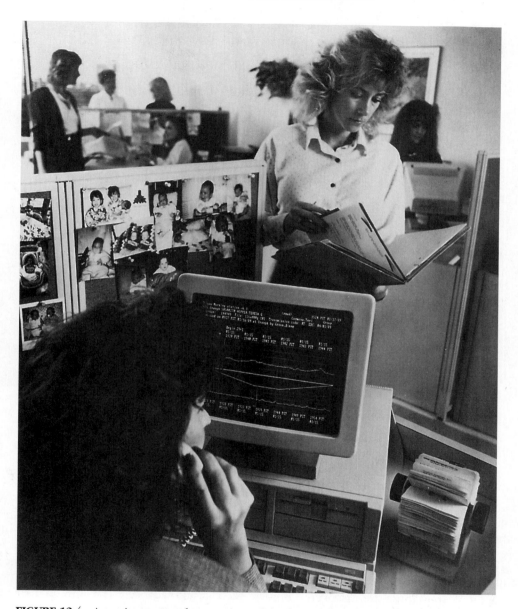

FIGURE 12-4 A nursing center where uterine activity data transmitted from the home of a client experiencing preterm labor is displayed on a computer screen and evaluated by professional nurses. *(Photograph courtesy of Tokos Medical Corporation.)*

while nursing support, uterine monitoring, and reduced activity continue (Figures 12-4 and 12-5). Nursing support of the woman and family experiencing preterm labor has been found to be a critical factor in the success of labor suppression because compliance with the treatment regime is more likely to occur (Watson et al., 1990).

TERTIARY PREVENTION

Tertiary prevention involves health care services that assist individuals and families to limit the

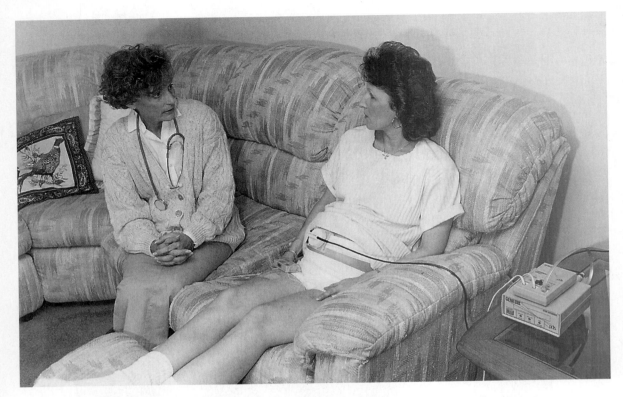

FIGURE 12-5   A professional nurse makes a home visit to a pregnant woman experiencing preterm labor. A subcutaneous pump attached to the client's thigh infuses terbutaline (a tocolytic medication to suppress labor), and an external monitor attached to the client's abdomen over the uterine fundus assesses uterine activity. *(Photograph courtesy of Children's Hospital Home Care, Buffalo, New York.)*

spread of disease or disability, improve health, and/or maintain stability.

For the maternal-infant client, the need for tertiary prevention health services must not only be identified but these services must also be available. When unhealthy behaviors such as smoking and alcohol and drug abuse are discovered during preconception or prenatal assessment, prompt referral to appropriate rehabilitation centers, cessation programs, and support groups must be made. Unfortunately, such services are not always available in sufficient numbers to meet the demand. Waiting lists for admission can delay cessation and expose the woman and her fetus to harmful substances for a much longer period. The consequences of alcohol, drug, and tobacco use during pregnancy in terms of human

and financial cost are well documented. The incidence of congenital anomalies, low birth weight, preterm birth, infections including AIDS and Hepatitis B, and infant growth and developmental problems is higher when a pregnant woman uses these substances. Nurses must be politically active and advocate for the establishment of more services, especially those designed specifically for pregnant women. It must also be recognized that fathers need to participate in cessation programs because their use of these substances has the potential for adversely affecting their offspring.

The relatively high incidence of low birth weight and preterm birth in the United States coupled with the advanced technology that can save even very low birth weight infants has forced the health care system and health care providers to examine the potentially long-term care requirements of these infants and how these requirements can best be met. The cost of continuing hospitalization, especially the time spent in neonatal intensive care units, is very high. As a result, programs that provide for earlier discharge of these infants to supported home care are being developed. Many studies indicate that earlier discharge programs are cost effective and in the long run safe and beneficial to both family and infant (Damato, 1991). However, care providers have found that the transition period surrounding discharge can be very stressful for parents who express feelings of fear and inadequacy. Addressing these issues by working with and providing support for families can be helpful in fostering attachment and optimal growth and development of the infant. In addition, child abuse and accidents can be prevented. Unfortunately, most health care dollars for sick infants are allotted to in-hospital care with little left for home care and family support services (Butts et al., 1988).

A number of interventions have been identified and used successfully by early discharge programs. These interventions recognize the stress experienced by these families and the value of support measures to raise parental confidence (Arnold & Grad, 1991). The most frequently cited interventions include:

1. Discharge Planning: Many infants are discharged still requiring some of the technological support that helped them to survive. Caring for these infants requires preparation of both the parents and their home. If the discharge is to be accomplished with the least amount of stress and confusion, then it must begin early, ideally at the time of admission. A teaching plan must be established that provides time for parents to practice caring for their infant in the supervised hospital setting. The timing of teaching sessions needs to take into consideration the emotional status of the parents and must incorporate time for the development of attachment to the infant. The community health nurse who will be the home visitor should be a part of the discharge planning and teaching sessions so that continuity of care occurs. A predischarge home visit provides the opportunity to evaluate the adequacy of the home and initiate changes that may be required to accommodate the special needs of the infant (Baker, Kuhlman, & Magliaro, 1989).

2. Telephone Follow-up: Maintaining contact with the newly discharged infant's family can be a cost-effective method of insuring continuity of care, providing support and information, enhancing self confidence, and reducing anxiety. Nurses can call parents to inquire about the status of the infant and how they are managing. Parents also have the option of calling the nurse when concerns or questions arise. Butts et al. (1988) discovered that the greatest numbers of client-initiated calls occurred during the first 5 months. The three major reasons for calling were to discuss newborn health problems and issues relating to normal infant care, and to give information concerning the status of their infant.

3. Home Visitation: On-site assessment of the status and progress of the infant, ability of the parents to care for the infant, adaptation of family members to the presence of an infant with special needs, and the functioning of the equipment being used are critical if safety is to be maintained. Following discharge, the task of caring for the infant may become overwhelming. Specialists in such areas as perinatal nursing, respiratory care, and physical therapy are often needed to reinforce hospital instructions, adapt infant care to the home environment, and of course offer encouragement and support to the parents and family members.

4. Community Support Network: Families need to be in touch with support services available in their community. Respite services and support groups of parents caring for infants with special needs are important to help the family develop and use effective coping strategies to deal with stress. Early intervention programs are an important aspect of avoiding or minimizing the developmental delays that these infants often experience. Emergency phone numbers for police, rescue squads, primary health care provider, equipment vendors, and even utility companies should be readily available (Damato, 1991).

Chapter Highlights

- Nurses have a long tradition as caregivers, advocates, and leaders in the area of maternal-infant care.

- The United States Department of Health and Human Services has specified goals for the year 2000 that relate to the health of and health care services for the maternal-infant client.

- Today's community health nurse must take on a variety of roles including that of advocate, researcher, communicator, entrepreneur, educator, caregiver, and case manager to ensure that all maternal-infant clients receive comprehensive, high-quality, risk-specific health care.

- Maternal-infant morbidity and mortality rates in the United States are too high, especially among populations that are disadvantaged.

- Low birth weight and very low birth weight newborns are more likely to die than infants who are born at an appropriate weight.

- A larger proportion of unmarried women are giving birth.

- Primary prevention health care services including preconception care and prenatal care can significantly reduce the infant mortality rate and the incidence of low birth weight.

- Despite its benefits, many women delay entry into prenatal care or receive no prenatal care at all.

- Demographic, financial, system, and client barriers influence a woman's entry into prenatal care.

- The content and scheduling of prenatal care should be individualized, relevant, and risk-specific.

- Earlier discharge of women following birth, women experiencing complications of pregnancy, and infants with special needs are factors that have stimulated the growth of home care services for the maternal-infant client.

- A decrease in the use of hospitals as the site for secondary and tertiary health care services for the maternal-infant client has been facilitated by the development of programs that incorporate discharge planning, home visitation and telephone follow-up, and community-based support services.

 CRITICAL THINKING EXERCISE

You have been asked to testify before a congressional committee that is investigating health care reform. Describe three strategies you would propose as effective measures to reduce the incidence of maternal-infant morbidity and mortality rates in the United States.

REFERENCES

Affonso, D., Mayberry, L., Graham, K., Shibuya, J., & Kunimot, J. (1993). Prenatal and postpartum care in Hawaii: A community based approach. *Journal of Obstetric, Gynecologic, and Neonatal Nursing, 22*(4), 320-325.

American College of Obstetricians and Gynecologists (ACOG). (1988). *Guidelines for prenatal care.* Washington, DC: ACOG.

American Nurses Association. (1987). *Access to prenatal care: Key to preventing low birth weight.* Report of Consensus Conference. Kansas City, Mo.: ANA.

Arnold, L., & Grad, R. (1992). Low birth weight and infant mortality: A health policy perspective. *NAACOG's Clinical Issues in Perinatal and Women's Health Nursing, 3*(1), 1-12.

Baker, K., Kuhlmann, T., & Magliaro, B. (1989). Homeward bound: Discharge teaching for parents of newborns with special needs. *Nursing Clinics of North America, 24*(3), 655-664.

Buekens, P., Kolelchuck, M., Blondel, B., Kristenson, F., Chen, J., & Masuy-Stroobant, G. (1993). A comparison of prenatal care use in the United States and Europe. *American Journal of Public Health, 83*(1), 31-36.

Bullock, L., & McFarlane, J. (1989). The birth-weight/battering connection. *American Journal of Nursing, 89*(9), 1153-1155.

Butts, P., Brooten, D., Brown, L., Bakewell-Sachs, S., Gibbons, A., Finkler, S., Kumar, S., & Delivoria-Papadapoulis, M. (1988). Concerns of parents of low birthweight infants following hospital discharge: A report of parent-initiated telephone calls. *Neonatal Network, 7*(2), 37-42.

Committee on Perinatal Health (COPH). (1993). *Toward improving the outcome of pregnancy—the 90s and beyond.* White Plains, NY: March of Dimes Birth Defects Foundation.

Dahlberg, N., Parker, L., & Knox, G. (1989). The high-risk antepartal client. *Caring, 8*(10), 24-30.

Damato, E. (1991). Discharge planning from the neonatal intensive care unit. *Journal of Perinatal and Neonatal Nursing, 5*(1), 43-53.

Donaldson, N. (1991). A review of nursing intervention research on maternal adaptation in the first 8 weeks postpartum. *Journal of Perinatal and Neonatal Nursing, 4*(4), 1-11.

Evans, C. (1991). Description of a home follow-up program for childbearing families. *Journal of Obstetric, Gynecologic, and Neonatal Nursing, 20*(2), 113-118.

Gold, R., Kenny, A., & Singh, S. (1987). *Blessed events and the bottom line: Financing maternity care in the United States.* New York: Alan Guttmacher Institute.

Goodwin, L. (1992). Home fetal assessment. *Journal of Perinatal and Neonatal Nursing, 5*(4), 33-45.

Halloran, P., & Zickler, C. (1988). Early postpartum discharge for mothers and infants. *Pediatric Nursing Forum, 3*(1), 3-8.

Handler, A., & Rosenberg, D. (1992). Improving pregnancy outcomes: Public versus private care for urban, low income women. *Birth, 19*(3), 123-130.

Heins, H., Nance, N., & Ferguson, J. (1987). Social support in improving perinatal outcome: The Resource Mothers Program. *Obstetrics and Gynecology, 70,* 263-266.

Helton, A. (1990). A buddy system to improve prenatal care. *American Journal of Maternal Child Nursing, 15,* 234-237.

Hill, I. (Ed.). (1988). *Reaching women who need prenatal care.* National Governor's Association: Health Policy Department, Human Resources Policy Division, Center for Policy Research.

Hill, W., Flemming, A., Martin, R., Hamer, C., Knuppel, R., Lake, M., Watson, D., Welch, R., Bentley, D., Gookin, K., & Morrison, J. (1990). Home uterine activity monitoring is associated with a reduction in preterm birth. *Obstetrics and Gynecology, 76*(1) [suppl], 13s-18s.

Horton, J. (Ed.). (1992). *The women's health data book: A profile of women's health in the United States.* Washington, DC: The Jacob's Institute of Women's Health.

Hulsey, T., Patrick, C., Alexander, G., & Ebeling, M. (1991). Prenatal care and prematurity: Is there an association in uncomplicated pregnancies? *Birth, 18*(3), 146-150.

Hyde-Robertson, B. (1992). The necessity for maternal-infant perinatal home care. *Caring Magazine, 11*(12), 26-31.

Institute of Medicine. (1988). *Prenatal care: Reaching mothers, reaching infants.* Washington, DC: National Academy Press.

Kalisch, P., & Kalisch, J. (1986). *The advance of American nursing.* Boston: Little, Brown, & Co.

Koehl, L., & Wheeler, D. (1989). Monitoring uterine activity at home. *American Journal of Nursing, 89,* 200-203.

Lukacs, A. (1991). Issues surrounding early postpartum discharge: effects on the caregiver. *Journal of Perinatal and Neonatal Nursing, 5*(1), 33-42.

Mawn, P., & Bradley, J. (1993). Standards of care for high-risk prenatal clients: The community nurse case management approach. *Public Health Nursing, 10*(2), 78-88.

May, K., McLaughlin, F., & Penner, M. (1991). Preventing low birth weight: Marketing and volunteer outreach. *Public Health Nursing, 8*(2), 97-104.

McCormick, M. (1985). The contribution of low birth weight to infant mortality and childhood morbidity. *New England Journal of Medicine, 312,* 82-90.

McCormick, M., Brooks-Gunn, J., Shorter, T., Holmes, J., Wallace, C., & Heagarty, M. (1989). Outreach as casefinding: Its effect on enrollment in prenatal care. *Medical Care, 27*(2): 103-111.

McDonald, T., & Coburn, A. (1988). Predictors of prenatal care utilization. *Social Science and Medicine, 27*(2), 167-172.

McFarlane, J. (1993). Abuse during pregnancy: The horror and hope. *AWHONN's Clinical Issues in Perinatal and Women's Health Nursing, 4*(3), 350-362.

Meis, P., Ernest, J., & Moore, M. (1987). Causes of low birth weights in public and private patients. *American Journal of Obstetrics and Gynecology, 156,* 1165-1168.

Middlemiss, C., Dawson, A., Gough, N., Jones, E., & Coles, E. (1989). A randomized study of domiciliary antenatal care scheme: Maternal psychological effects. *Midwifery, 5,* 69-74.

Misener, T., & Knox, P. (1990). Symbiotic and synergistic community-based volunteer home visiting program for postpartum families. *Public Health Nursing, 7*(3), 169-174.

Monahan, P., & DeJoseph, J. (1991). The woman with preterm labor at home: A descriptive analysis. *Journal of Perinatal and Neonatal Nursing, 4*(4), 12-20.

Moore, L., Burns, A., Thomas, L., & Skaria, M. (1986). Self-assessment: A personalized approach to nursing during pregnancy. *Journal of Obstetric, Gynecologic, and Neonatal Nursing, 15*(4), 311-318.

Murphy, J., & Robbins, D. (1993). Psychosocial implications of high-risk pregnancy. In R. Knuppel & J. Drukker (Eds.). *High risk pregnancy: A team approach.* (pp. 244-261). Philadelphia: W.B. Saunders.

NAACOG. (1986). Postpartum follow-up: A nursing practice guide. *OGN Nursing Practice Resource.* Washington, DC: NAACOG, The Organization for Obstetrical, Gynecological, and Neonatal Nursing.

National Center for Health Statistics (NCHS). (1991a). Advance report of final natality statistics, 1989. *Monthly Vital Statistics Report. 40*(8), [suppl]. Hyattsville, Maryland: Public Health Service.

National Center for Health Statistics (NCHS). (1991b). *Health, United States, 1990.* Hyattsville, Maryland: Public Health Service.

National Center for Health Statistics (NCHS). (1993a). Infant Mortality, United States, 1990. *Morbidity and Mortality Weekly Report, 42*(9), Massachusetts Medical Society.

National Center for Health Statistics (NCHS). (1993b). Childbearing patterns among selected racial/ethnic minority groups, United States, 1990. *Morbidity and Mortality Weekly Report, 42*(20), Massachusetts Medical Society.

National Center for Health Statistics (NCHS). (1993c). Mortality Patterns, United States, 1991. *Morbidity and Mortality Weekly Report, 42*(46), Massachusetts Medical Society.

National Center for Health Statistics (NCHS). (1993d). Infant Mortality, United States, 1991. *Morbidity and Mortality Weekly Report, 42*(48), Massachusetts Medical Society.

National Commission to Prevent Infant Mortality. (1988). *Death before life: The tragedy of infant mortality.* Washington, DC: Author.

Norr, K., & Nacion, K. (1987). Outcomes of postpartum early discharge 1960-1986: A comparative review. *Birth, 14*(3), 135-140.

Office of Technology Assessment. (1988). *Healthy children: Investing in the future.* Washington, DC: U.S. Government Printing Office.

Olds, D., & Kitzman, H. (1990). Can home visitation improve the health of women and children at environmental risk? *Pediatrics, 86*(1), 108-116.

Parker, B., & McFarlane, J. (1991). Identifying and helping battered pregnant women. *American Journal of Maternal Child Nursing, 16*(3), 161-164.

Patterson, E., Freese, M., & Goldenberg, R. (1990). Seeking safe passage: Utilizing health care during pregnancy. *Image, 22*(1), 27-31.

Peoples-Sheps, M., Efird, C., & Miller, C. (1989). Home visiting and prenatal care: A survey of practical wisdom. *Public Health Nursing, 6*(2), 74-79.

Public Health Service Expert Panel on the Content of Prenatal Care. (1989). *Caring for our future: The content of prenatal care.* Washington, DC: Department of Health and Human Services, Public Health Service.

Rochat, R., Koonin, L., Atrash, H., & Jewett, J. (1988). Maternal mortality in the United States: Report from the maternal mortality collaborative. *Obstetrics and Gynecology, 72,* 91-97.

Rosenbaum, S., Layton, C., & Lew, J. (1991). *The health of America's children.* Washington, DC: Children's Defense Fund.

St. Clair, P., Smeriglio, B., Alexander, C., & Celentano, D. (1989). Social network structure and prenatal care utilization. *Medical Care, 27*(8), 823-831.

Starfield, B. (1985). Giant steps and baby steps toward child health. *American Journal of Public Health, 75,* 599-604.

Statistics Canada, Canadian Center for Health Information. (1994). *Deaths, 1991.* Ottawa, Ontario, Canada: Minister of Industry, Science, and Technology.

Stern, T. (1991). An early discharge program: An entrepreneurial nursing practice becomes a hospital-affiliated agency. *Journal of Perinatal and Neonatal Nursing, 5*(1), 1-8.

Stevens, S. (1920). The public health nurse in the extension of maternity nursing. *Public Health Nursing, 12,* 497-501.

Tyson, J., Guzick, D., Rosenfeld, C., Lasky, R., Grant, N., Jiminez, J., & Heartwell, S. (1990). Prenatal care evaluation and cohort analysis. *Pediatrics, 8*(2), 195-204.

US Department of Health and Human Services. (1992). *Healthy people 2000: Summary report.* Boston: Jones and Bartlett Publishers.

Vrazo, F. (1993, August 21). Hospitals want new moms out quickly. *The Buffalo News,* p. A1 & A3.

Watson, D., Welch, R., Mariona, F., Lake, M., Knuppel, R., Martin, R., Johnson, C., Bently, D., Hill, W., Flemming, A., & Morrison, J. (1990). Management of preterm labor patients at home: Does daily uterine activity monitoring and nursing support make a difference? *Obstetrics and Gynecology, 76*(1) [suppl], 32s-35s.

Williams, L., & Cooper, M. (1993). Nurse managed postpartum home care. *Journal of Obstetric, Gynecologic, and Neonatal Nursing, 22*(1), 25-31.

York, R., & Brooten, D. (1992). Prevention of low birth weight. *NAACOG's Clinical Issues in Perinatal and Women's Health Nursing, 3*(1), 13-24.

Young, C., McMahon, J., Bowman, V., & Thompson, D. (1989). Maternal reasons for delayed prenatal care. *Nursing Research, 38*(4), 242-243.

13

CARING FOR CHILDREN

Janet T. Ihlenfeld

Train a child in the way he should go; and when he is old, he will not depart from it.

Proverbs 22:6

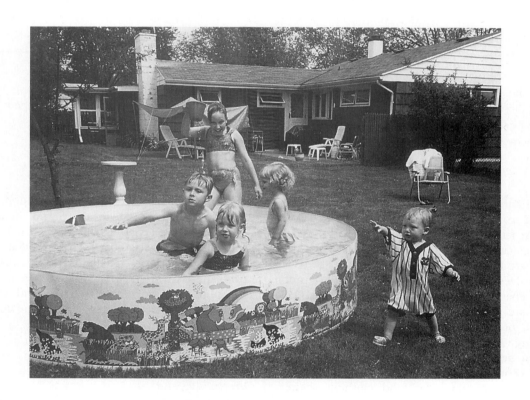

OBJECTIVES

At the conclusion of this chapter the student will be able to:

1. Define the key terms listed.
2. Recall concepts of growth and development in children ages 1 to 11 years.
3. Describe nursing care of children related to growth and development, immunizations, nutrition, accident prevention, dental care, and concerns about AIDS.
4. Describe nursing care of children related to violence, child abuse, lead poisoning, and iron deficiency anemia.
5. Describe nursing care of children in poverty and the lack of health care access.

KEY TERMS

Autonomy versus doubt and shame

Child abuse and neglect

Concrete operations

Dental caries

Denver developmental screening test

Industry versus inferiority

Initiative versus guilt

Iron deficiency anemia

Plumbism

Pre-operational phase

Sensorimotor development

Therapeutic play

Trust versus mistrust

Children are exposed to everything in the world around us. Within their own point of view, they react to what they experience, and these reactions can influence the rest of their lives. Children are being bombarded by various events in their lives including war, poverty, health problems, changes in the family, and other issues. Children are at risk for being seriously affected by health problems and are very vulnerable to becoming victims of violence and child abuse. Society in general places children at risk because they cannot take care of themselves, so they must rely on others for food, clothing, shelter, health care, and love. The physical environment in some communities places children at risk because of factors such as poverty. But poverty alone is not the only way children are vulnerable in society today. All children are at risk.

As has been outlined in earlier chapters, primary prevention is the prevention of problems, secondary prevention is the detection and treatment of problems, and tertiary prevention is the attempt to help individuals regain high-level functioning. This chapter will discuss the nursing care of children related to growth and development. Immunizations, accident prevention, dental problems, AIDS, nutrition, iron deficiency anemia, plumbism, violence, child abuse and neglect, and poverty from the perspective of the community health nurse.

GROWTH AND DEVELOPMENT
Assessment

Progressive and continued growth and development in children is essential for optimal functioning. The highest rate of growth in the human being occurs during the first year of life. Although general rates of growth include coupling the birth weight by 6 months of age and tripling it by 1 year of age, growth rates for each individual child are variable. As the infant grows, the degree of gross motor skill increases as do fine motor skills. By 13 months, the toddler should be able to take approximately 10 unaided steps. Between 8 months and 2 years, the teeth begin to appear and the toddler graduates to solid foods. The development of teeth also helps the newly communicating toddler to copy and make specific sounds necessary in acquiring language skills. From 2 to 3 years of age, the rate of growth slows; however, the intellectual and neurologic capacity continues to grow and develop (Whaley & Wong, 1991).

The infant develops cognitively as well during the rapid growth period of the first few years. According to Piaget (1974/1978), the child from birth to age 2 years is in a period of **sensori-motor development** in which the infant explores the environment through the five senses, especially taste, touch, and sight. The infant develops patterns of action called schemes in which ways of doing things are explored and tried out. The concept of object permanence begins during this period and is fully in place by age 2 years.

Erikson (1963) calls the infancy period in the child's life the time of **trust versus mistrust,** when the infant develops and interacts with parents and learns that the parents care for its needs. Consequently, should the baby not have a stable caretaker, the infant learns mistrust of the world. The next stage of development, according to Erikson, is that of **autonomy versus doubt and shame.** Here the toddler wishes to gain control of the world but doubts whether it can be attained. It is also the period of toilet training in which the toddler wishes to please the parent but still sometimes feels ashamed following "toileting accidents."

The child from 3 to 5 years of age becomes leaner and not as chubby as the active toddler. He or she becomes more coordinated and the head and face develop more adult proportions from that of the round-headed, large-eyed infant and toddler.

The 3-to-4-year-old child is often called the preschooler because of the nearness to kindergarten and elementary school ages. The preschooler is theorized by Piaget (1974/1978) to be in the **pre-operational phase** of development. This is a period when representational thought develops and the child learns to solve simple problems. Language becomes more defined, and communication difficulties ease.

According to Erikson (1963), the preschool age group is dealing with **initiative versus guilt** in their efforts to grow up. This is the age when the child begins to spend more time with peers and explores the ability to be independent. This conflict between independence and dependence on the parents is the central part of initiative versus guilt. The desire to decide things for oneself is important, and the ability to say "No" to another's requests brings a source of control to the child. Hence, there is also guilt because the child's search to have some control also brings conflict when the control is exerted by others. This control is often held by the parents or other adults, and the child reacts because of a belief that he or she has done something wrong.

These years are still egocentric ones for the child and are filled with fantasy and other types of make-believe. Children at this age have very vivid imaginations and can play for hours seemingly without food or sleep. The preschool child is very busy playing all the time and learns at a very fast pace (Meer, 1985).

As the child grows during the elementary school years, ages 5 to 11 years, steady growth continues and fine motor skills are refined. Cognitive growth continues in the school-age years, according to Piaget (1974/1978), with the development of **concrete operations.** This is where the child looks at all occurrences in life at face value, literally defining the world as it occurs. Erikson (1963) also recognizes this period as that of **industry versus inferiority** where the child likes to be busy accomplishing things related to projects and mimicry of the adult world. There is little or no interpretation of meanings or results. Should those tasks not be completed, the child generates a poor self-esteem related to the lack of development of lifelong skills.

Diagnosis

The community health nurse should always consider the proper growth and development of each child encountered. This constitutes primary prevention. However, should the assessment show deficiencies requiring secondary prevention, the following NANDA nursing diagnoses (Carroll-Johnson, 1991) are the ones usually identified: anxiety, body image disturbance, impaired verbal communication, diversional activity deficit, fear, altered growth and development, impaired physical mobility, and altered sensory perception.

Planning

Once nursing diagnoses have been made, the community health nurse should investigate the appropriate screening programs to determine the need for further intervention. As a part of secondary prevention, screening tests do not diagnose how far a child is behind his or her peers; rather, screening functions to indicate areas where further evaluation of the child is needed by other health professionals.

The **Denver Developmental Screening Test (DDST)** is the most widely used screening test for young children. Its categories of personal-social, fine motor adaptive, language, and gross motor serve to indicate generalized standing for the child on the basis of average development for children of that child's age (O'Pray, 1980).

Screening tools should be sensitive to cultural and residential backgrounds. For instance, a child in an urban area might not know about cows because their frame of reference is the city. The nurse should always be aware of the possibility that biased questions may result in lower scores for some children, hence the caution that developmental screening tests should be used only as a general guideline and not as a diagnostic tool (O'Pray, 1980).

The community health nurse also screens children for vision and hearing defects, immunizations, and assessment for child abuse and neglect (Fleming, 1986). Screening programs exist in the community to help families with low incomes obtain additional access to health services. The nurse should be aware of the Head Start facilities in the community, which screen for vision, hearing, and anemias (Aronson, 1986).

Implementation

The community health nurse should institute referrals to health care agencies for any child whose growth and development are not appro-

priate. These interventions would also include parent education related to the reason for the health care referral and the health care consequences of the referral for both the child and the family.

The nurse may use play to help teach the preschooler and school-aged child concepts of health promotion. The play setting makes learning easy and applicable to the child's world. For instance, a lesson on tooth brushing could begin first by having the preschoolers fashion a crude tooth in clay and then, while the nurse demonstrates, use a stick to "brush" the clay tooth. The child could also help the nurse make up a poem or a song to help remember to brush and have him or her recite or sing it before brushing. Drawing posters to help the child remember would also be fun. This way of using play as the mode for learning is perfect for most health promotion teaching for children.

Therapeutic play or medical play is used to help children learn about and prepare for health care procedures and activities. It is very useful to help hospitalized children deal with their experiences, but it is also useful in preparing children who are well for experiences that they may have with the health care system (Meer, 1985), such as preoperative teaching.

Children can use therapeutic play under the supervision of the nurse to dress up as nurses or physicians. They can use puppets to play out hospital or clinic scenes. Children can also give injections, under adult supervision, to dolls and stuffed toys to work out why these activities are done to them. Preschoolers can handle plastic syringes, without the needle, under the supervision and aid of the nurse to work through the immunization process and other instances where they are given "shots" or medicine. It is used to help prepare children for hospitalization and is particularly beneficial to children who will be having tonsillectomies and other surgical procedures. They can pretend to give an anesthetic to stuffed animals and dolls to prepare for surgery. The ability of the child to concentrate on make-believe and fantasy helps make therapeutic play a very important and easily learned way to deal with the health care system.

The community health nurse is also in an excellent position to help teach parents about health promotion activities related to infants, toddlers, preschoolers, and school-aged children. The nurse can help parents understand the elements of nutrition that are so important to this age group and the need for disease prevention, including education regarding the immunizations required and recommended for all children.

Parents also need to be taught the usual developmental milestones of their young children so that they can anticipate them. Many times parents expect too much too soon from children, and this tends to leave a family at risk for child abuse because of the lack of understanding of the child's capabilities and frustration over their "perceived" lack of development.

Evaluation

The community health nurse may make home visits or follow-up contacts with the family of the referred child to assess the compliance with the health care regimen and to further assess the situation. Further referrals may be necessary in cases where the initial contact with the health care system was not sufficient.

IMMUNIZATIONS
Assessment

As an essential part of primary prevention, children must be immunized against communicable diseases. The diseases for which there are vaccinations include measles, mumps, rubella, poliomyelitis, diphtheria, pertussis (whooping cough), tetanus, *Haemophilus influenzae* type b, hepatitis B, influenza virus (changes yearly), pneumococcal virus, and meningococcal virus. School entrance requirements include the following immunization series: MMR (measles, mumps, and rubella), OPV (oral polio vaccine), and DPT (diphtheria, tetanus, and pertussis). Newer vaccines for hepatitis B and *Haemophilus influenzae* type b (PRP-OMP [PedvaxHIB] and HbOC [HibTITER]) are not required for school admission at this time; however, they may be required in the near future as society realizes the importance of protection from these diseases. Children can now be vaccinated against *Haemophilus influenzae* type b, which has been documented to be one of the major causes of morbidity and mor-

tality in infants and young children (Reece, 1991). Immunization against hepatitis B would prevent future development of this serious and potentially fatal blood-borne disease.

Assessment of children regarding immunizations determines whether each child has had the appropriate series of vaccinations (Table 13-1). The Centers for Disease Control and Prevention (CDC) reported in 1985 that only 64.9% of children ages 1 to 4 years had had the DPT series, and only 73.7% of 5-to-14-year-olds had the series (United States Department of Commerce, 1992).

Compliance with measles vaccinations in 1985 was even lower than for the DPT series: only 60.8% of 1-to-4-year-olds had the measles vaccine, and 71.5% of 5-to-14-year-olds had one (United States Department of Commerce, 1992). These low rates of protection mirror the increase in measles cases from 18,193 cases in 1989 to

TABLE 13-1 Immunization Practices Advisory Committee (ACIP) recommendations for childhood vaccination

Age at vaccination	Vaccination
0-2 days	Hepatitis B (dose #1)
1-2 months	Hepatitis B (dose #2)
2 months	Hib + DPT (dose #1), OPV (dose #1)
4 months	Hib + DPT (dose #2), OPV (dose #2)
6 months	Hib + DPT (dose #3), OPV (dose #3)
6-18 months	Hepatitis B (dose #3)
12-15 months	Hib + DPT (dose #4)
15 months	MMR (dose #1)
4-6 years	MMR (dose #2)

DPT, Diphtheria, pertussis, tetanus vaccine; *Hib, Haemophilus influenzae* type b vaccine; *MMR,* Measles, mumps, rubella vaccine; *OPV,* Oral polio vaccine.

Due to rapidly changing recommendations regarding vaccinations, the reader is cautioned to check the latest literature before proceeding with a vaccination schedule and to consult the latest pharmacologic information for side effects and contraindications.

Compiled from ACIP Recommendations published in the *Morbidity and Mortality Weekly Reports.*

27,786 cases in 1990 (Summary of Notifiable Diseases, 1992). There were 11 major outbreaks of measles in the United States in 1991; however, the total numbered 9,643 cases partially due to increased emphasis on immunization in 1991 after the large increases in the number of cases between 1989 and 1990 (Atkinson, Hadler, Redd, & Orenstein, 1992).

Diagnosis

Nursing diagnoses for children found lacking in immunizations include potential for infection, impaired health maintenance, knowledge deficit (of the parents), and noncompliance (of the parents).

Planning

When carrying out the planning phase, parental education and investigation of health care sites where immunizations are given are important parts of the nursing process. The community health nurse needs to be aware that children may not have been immunized because the family does not have access to health care or there is no health insurance to pay for the expensive vaccines. Some parents also may be fearful because of stories related to uncommon severe side effects of the vaccinations.

Implementation

The community health nurse often is the primary care provider who gives the vaccinations to children in clinics and other health care agencies. The nurse should remember to give the vaccination only after thoughtful and careful explanation of the procedure to both the child and the parents. Written informed consent to receive the immunization must be obtained from the parent prior to administration. The appropriate education should also be given at the developmental level of the child so that they understand the reason for the "shot." Children should not be told that "it won't hurt" because there will be some discomfort. The children should be told that the injection will be like an insect bite and be over very quickly. Truth will provide trust in the nurse from both the child and the parents and will serve to promote return for subsequent booster injections and other types of health care.

Evaluation

Maintenance of proper immunization records for all children will aid in the tracking of children who do not complete all of the vaccination schedules. Many of the vaccinations require multiple doses, including the DPT, OPV, MMR, Hepatitis B, and both types of *Haemophilus influenzae* type b vaccines (Reece, 1991). The community health nurse needs to be aware of the community's way of keeping immunization records and follow-up contacts.

ACCIDENTS AND ACCIDENT PREVENTION
Assessment

Motor vehicle accidents involving automobiles, buses, trucks, all-terrain vehicles, snowmobiles, boats, and jet-skis as well as accidents from drowning, fires, burns, falls, bicycle accidents, or ingestion of foreign objects are the most serious health problems of children. The U.S. National Center for Health Statistics found that there were 7900 deaths from all types of accidents in 1989 to children under age 15 years (U.S. Department of Commerce, 1992). At highest risk for accidents are those children in low income, poorly educated families who live in substandard housing. In addition, the younger the mother, the higher the risk of an accident to the child.

Diagnosis

Community health nurses see children in urban, suburban, and rural areas and can easily assess situations where accidents are likely to occur. The nursing diagnoses that are important for accident prevention include potential for trauma, potential for poisoning, potential for suffocation, and knowledge deficit.

Planning

The nurse needs to develop accident prevention and risk identification strategies for communities with children. Educational seminars based on primary prevention, the development of literature for families to follow, and community outreach projects are ways to do this.

Implementation

As part of secondary prevention, nurses often treat injuries from accidents in clinics. The community health nurse can emphasize that neighborhood clinics exist and encourage those who are injured to seek health care at those sites. Nurse-run treatment clinics that give immediate health care to those with minor injuries have been developed in a community in Great Britain (Garnett & Elton, 1991). In addition, community health nurses surveyed in Great Britain indicated that they could increase the awareness of families about accident prevention by teaching the families during their home visits (Carter, Bannon, & Jones, 1992).

Within educational programs, the nurse must emphasize safety in all areas. The high activity level of infants, toddlers, preschoolers, and elementary school-aged children increases the likelihood that accidents will occur. Falls, burns, poisonings, and other accidents may occur in many settings such as homes, grandparents' homes, schools, and day care centers. Steps should be taken by all caretakers to prevent their occurrence.

The nurse must assess the home for apparent dangers and then teach safety measures as part of health promotion. The nurse needs to look for functioning smoke alarms and determine the family's fire evacuation plan. Should no plan exist or if there are no functioning smoke detectors, the nurse should intervene immediately by providing smoke alarms and/or batteries and developing an evacuation plan with the family.

Poison control interventions must include educating parents to lock and/or seal medicine and kitchen cabinets where children can reach medicines, cleansers, and other potential sources of poisoning. Poisoning information and the presence of poison control centers and educational seminars in community centers are ways to promote prevention in the community (Brannan, 1992).

Stairwell openings need to be fenced off where toddlers and infants may fall, and windows need screens and/or mechanisms that prevent them from being opened wide enough for young children to crawl through. There should be non-skid rugs in high-traffic areas, and running should be prohibited. Preventing children's access to areas where food is prepared is also very important to prevent burns. "Child-proofing" electrical outlets, use of safety electrical outlets in all areas of the home, quick wipe-up of spills, and the use of child-proof cupboards and locked cabinets where detergents, pesticides, and other chemicals are stored is also essential to prevent accidents. Community health nurses can help parents cope with these changes in their homes.

Kitchen safety needs to be addressed as well. The nurse should teach caretakers to turn all pot and pan handles away from the edge of the stove or range to prevent accidental spilling. This is especially important for all types of cooking vessels that contain hot or boiling fluids. Coffee makers, tea pots, and kettles of boiling water, jelly, or sauce pose serious threats to children. Young ones can easily pull the containers down on themselves, spilling the scalding liquid on them and causing serious burns. Flame burns can also occur to children who get too close to unattended barbecues or to natural gas-fueled ranges that have been left on. Clothing can catch fire easily resulting in serious, and maybe fatal, burns. Children can also be burned by hot metal parts of slides and swings (*The Buffalo News,* 1993).

Children can also drown in the home. Young children have been known to drown in as little as 1 inch of water and have been found dead in open toilets and unattended bathtubs and sinks. Many parents believe that swimming pools pose the highest drowning risk for their children. Although that is the case, other areas of potential tragedy include neighborhood streams, ponds, sewers, wading pools, fountains, washtubs, pails, sump pump holes, and irrigation ditches (see box on page 292). The community health nurse's intervention should focus on parent education relating to supervising children around water, providing barriers around water to prevent accidental falls into it, and knowledge about emergency procedures such as cardiopulmonary resuscitation should near-drowning occur (Coffman, 1991).

Home hazards have been reduced in families who have been assessed by community health nurses. The Hennepin County Burn Center in Minneapolis, Minnesota, in cooperation with the public health department made home visits to educate parents related to burn prevention, poison control, and other areas with the potential

DROWNING HAZARDS

Drainage ditches
Swimming pools
Sinks
Bathtubs
Toilets
Streams, rivers, and lakes
Ponds
Sewers
Wading pools
Fountains
Washtubs
Pails
Sump pump holes
Irrigation ditches
Washing machines
Septic ponds/cesspools

for injury. The researchers found a decrease in home hazards in households visited (Sullivan, Cole, Lie, & Twomey, 1990).

A study by Jones (1992) found that when nurse practitioners did health teaching, information related to car seats for children was given less than 30% of the time, information on smoke detectors less than 15% of the time, and information on firearms less than 7% of the time. The researcher recommended that nurses routinely provide such information to caretakers to prevent accidents before they happen.

Children are especially prone to injury while playing. Because they are so absorbed in their play activities or are developmentally unaware of dangers, accidents occur even when there is adult supervision. Studies have shown that most injuries are a result of one of two contributing factors: either the child came into direct contact with an object such as falling from a piece of play equipment, or a child behaves aggressively when toys are used inappropriately (Chang, Lugg, & Nebedum, 1989). Researchers have also found that in a survey of one university day care center, injuries occurred more often to children ages 3 to 4 years and that these injuries were related to horseplay, running, or fighting (Lee & Bass, 1990).

Injuries from playground accidents are the most frequently cited injury to children in day care centers. Severe injuries may be sustained by falls from climbers or jungle gyms, slides, swings, and other climbing apparatus and from running and falling or tripping over objects in the playground (Aronson, 1985, 1986). Nurses should make sure that play apparatus is safe and that no sharp edges on wooden or metal structures are unshielded. Rules should be set up and enforced regarding use of these apparatus. Insurers of day care centers often recommend that jungle gyms be removed to reduce liability claims since they are involved in a great many accidents. Shock absorbing surfaces such as sand or foam may be installed under playground equipment to cushion falls from the apparatus (Chang, Lugg, & Nebedum, 1989).

It is also important for the nurse to stress to children the need to be safe when they are passengers in any vehicle whether car, van, truck, boat, bus, or airplane. This teaching can begin with preschoolers and continue with the parents (Aronson, 1986). Children need to be taught to remain in their seats and to obey the directions of adults when riding in a vehicle. In addition, children need to be taught now to safely cross a street.

Most governments require that passengers in cars be restrained by the seat belts and shoulder harnesses in the vehicles. In addition, car seats are required in the United States for infants and small children up to 40 pounds or 4 years of age because their body size does not allow for proper restraint by the belts that are installed by the automobile manufacturers. These infant or child seats should meet the guidelines established by the government and usually are listed on the product as conforming to Federal Motor Vehicle Safety Standards.

The nurse should emphasize that children should buckle up every time they are in a car, and parents should help by being role models for their children. Parents who do not usually wear seat belts should be encouraged to do so not only for their own safety but also to model ideal behavior for their children. Seat belt and car seat use also reduces the sometimes "active" behavior of children while riding in cars. The nurse can use this fact to further explain the benefits of belt use to resistant parents. Block (1991) found that the incorrect use of child car seats was frequent in a study of 149 mothers. The research recommended that health care providers explain the use of car seats and the rationale for their use to parents. It was also recommended that car seat manufacturers provide better instructions for parents so that they are used properly in the vehicles.

One aspect of teaching vehicular safety may be difficult for the nurse. The children may ride a bus — either a large schoolbus or a van — to a day care center or school. Many school buses are not equipped with restraint systems, whereas some vans are equipped with car seats. This safety requirement for buses has not caught up with those for cars, and many legislatures are currently discussing laws regarding restraints in buses. However, at this time it would be best for the nurse to emphasize that children in such vehicles always hang on to the handles on the seats in the buses, always remain seated, and always face forward in the bus. This will help emphasize

order and promote use of belts when they are available in buses. The nurse in the community is the logical one to lobby for legislation in that area.

Children can also be seriously injured in bicycle accidents in which they either fall off the bicycle or are hit by other vehicles. All children riding bicycles should wear helmets (see Figure 13-1). This would minimize head injuries should the child fall off the bike and hit his or her head on the ground, pavement, or other hard surface. Bicycle helmet laws are gaining acceptance in many states including California, Georgia, New Jersey, and New York (*The Buffalo News,* 1993), and those communities where laws are not in place often see activities promoting voluntary helmet use.

Bicycle riding safety should also be part of the health education stressed by the community health nurse. Children should be taught to abide by the rules of the road relating to riding bicycles. Motorists in communities also need to be re-

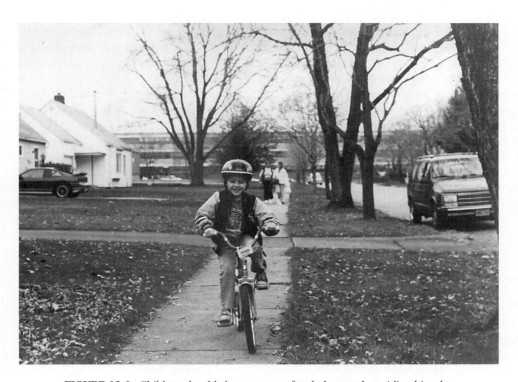

FIGURE 13-1 Children should always wear safety helmets when riding bicycles.

minded to watch for children on bicycles, especially in good weather and during vacations from school.

Evaluation

Community health nurses can evaluate their interventions related to safety by surveying the accident statistics for children in their community. A low number of accidents and/or a decrease in the accidents in their areas would signal a positive effect of all of the nurse's health promotion and teaching. However, the prevention of accidents is an ongoing process for the community health nurse.

DENTAL PROBLEMS
Assessment

Poor dental hygiene is a health threat to children of all ages. Once teeth appear, the threat of developing dental caries exists. Many parents send their child to bed with a bottle of milk or a sugary liquid predisposing an infant or toddler to the "nursing bottle syndrome." Here, the maxillary anterior teeth are destroyed and the rest of the teeth form **dental caries** because of the presence of milk in the mouth while the child sleeps. These teeth may need to be extracted because of severe tooth decay.

As an aspect of primary prevention, parents should be taught to begin gently brushing the child's teeth daily as soon as the teeth appear. They should also be taught not to send the child to bed with a bottle to prevent further cavities and tooth decay (Clemen-Stone, Eigsti, Gerber & McGuire, 1991). The establishment of good dental hygiene in the early years will help ensure healthy adult teeth.

Diagnosis

The nursing diagnosis related to the primary prevention of dental problems in children is bathing/hygiene self-care deficit.

Planning

The community health nurse should plan to give tooth-brushing lessons to parents and children related to dental hygiene. These sessions should be tailored to the developmental levels of the child, and they should be given to the parent as well. The nurse should also plan referrals to dentists and dental clinics and set up educational activities in which routine dental screening by a dentist is stressed.

Implementation

The nurse can easily carry out teaching plans related to tooth brushing and other dental activities in day care centers, schools, churches, scout meetings, or other settings in which children are gathered into groups. These lessons should include detailed pictures of the mouth. Children should be allowed to use their own tooth brush and toothpaste during the discussions so that they can have a feel for the procedure themselves.

Children should also be taught what to do if a tooth gets dislodged from their mouth. The tooth should be gently placed back into the tooth socket in the mouth, and the child should seek adult help immediately. The caretaker should immediately take the child to a health agency where emergency dental services are available.

The nurse also needs to be reminded that the early elementary school years are when the child loses the baby teeth. Discussions about the "Tooth Fairy" are always common in the 4-to-7-year-old age group. Children need to be reassured that losing baby teeth is a normal process and that their adult teeth will grow into place.

Evaluation

The absence of dental caries and/or other dental problems and a schedule of regular visits to the dentist would signal an appropriate response to the nurse's health teaching. Revision of the process can be accomplished as the child grows and develops.

ACQUIRED IMMUNODEFICIENCY SYNDROME (AIDS)
Assessment

Children are also affected by the AIDS epidemic. By 1990, there were estimated to be over one half million children infected with AIDS worldwide as reported by the World Health Organization. Over 1 million additional cases of HIV in children are estimated to occur between the years 1991 and 2000 (Department of Economic and Social Development Statistical Office, United Nations, 1992).

In 1991 in the United States there were 147 deaths from AIDS in children under 5 years of age (death rate of 1/100,000), and there were 44 deaths in children ages 5 to 12 years (less than 0.5% of all deaths in this age group) (United States Department of Commerce, 1992). For children under 5 years there were 535 cases of AIDS reported in 1991 and 624 cases reported in 1992, an increase of 16.6%. For children ages 5 to 12 years there were 157 reported cases of AIDS in 1991 and 146 in 1992, a 7% decrease (Update-AIDS, 1993). Many of these children were exposed to HIV through prenatal exposure or breastfeeding exposure from HIV-positive mothers, or they were children with hemophilia who were exposed to HIV through blood products, especially Factor VIII transfusions, prior to the current practice of extensive blood product testing.

Elementary school children are aware of AIDS in the community through the media and required lessons in the schools. They are often concerned that they are at risk for developing AIDS.

Diagnosis

Children who are concerned about AIDS need to be reassured about the disease related to their age group. The nursing diagnoses of note for this health problem are knowledge deficit and potential for infection. The children need to be taught about AIDS early in life so they can prevent their personal exposure to HIV.

Planning

The community health nurse should plan activities in which children have the opportunity to question health care providers about AIDS. Their normal curiosity will easily begin discussions. In addition, community health nurses should be aware that the children may be especially worried about AIDS because of the illness and/or death caused by the HIV virus of a parent or other significant person in their lives. Children

whose parent or parents are ill with or have died of AIDS require special attention from the community health nurse.

Implementation

Children need primary prevention programs in which they are taught about AIDS. Age-specific health promotion activities are the best. Activities in which children can ask questions of health providers are helpful.

Educating children about "safer sex" is an area of controversy in many communities. The nurse should be aware of all governmental and school board regulations in the community so that appropriate information is given. The nurse should seek guidance from the local school board, school system, churches, and other community groups such as scouts, youth centers, and sports groups and enlist their help in the health promotion process.

Counselling for children who will lose or may have already lost a parent to AIDS is essential. The child will need to work through his or her feelings of abandonment and grief. The child may feel that the parent became ill and/or died because of the child's own bad behavior. The child needs to be repeatedly reassured that the parent did not become ill because of anything that the child did. Children should be reassured that unlike catching a cold, they will not catch AIDS from the parent and die also. The child's view of death should also be explored. Age-specific views of death should be taken into account in all aspects of this nursing intervention.

Truthful information is essential for all children in this instance. Children who have lost a caretaker to AIDS already distrust adults because they feel abandoned by them. Trust with the nurse must be developed to further the children's own grief process.

Evaluation

The nurse would be able to evaluate whether the information on AIDS is understood by the children by letting them review their own views on AIDS. Then the nurse can revise any teaching plans and develop additional activities for each age group.

NUTRITION
Assessment

Children ages 1 to 11 years must receive adequate nutrition to grow and develop properly. Assessment of a child's nutritional status begins with measurements of height and weight. In addition, a diary of the child's daily food intake helps to see the amount of calories, nutrients, and fluids that the child consumes.

The 1-to-2-year-old infant may still be on a formula diet. Although the American Academy of Pediatrics recommends that mothers breastfeed their babies for the first year, many do not. Many infants are placed on solid diets long before their first year. Assessment of the child in this age group would include whether the food assortment is appropriate for this age group.

Toddlers like to feed themselves. Foods are generally the same as those eaten by the rest of the family but in smaller portions and in smaller sizes. Finger foods are appropriate here because the child's level of growth and development necessitates independent feeding practices. Toddlers love to eat all types of small foods. Of particular importance, however, is the potential for the toddler to choke on these small foods. Toddlers should never be given foods that are the size of the diameter of their trachea and that, if inhaled, could result in choking and death. Toddlers should not be given peanuts, grapes, raisins, cherries, hard candies, popcorn, jelly beans, miniature marshmallows, weiners or hot dogs (they should be cut in half length-wise if given to toddlers), or other small foods (see box on this page).

Preschoolers sometimes refuse to eat. This age group likes to play so much that they do not have time to eat. Parents are often concerned about this behavior and contact the nurse for advice. Usually, these children will eat when they are hungry, and parents should be reassured that this stage of development usually does not last long enough for nutritional deficiencies to occur.

School-age children generally eat what the parents do. Children in school may eat the lunch purchased from or provided by the school, or they may take their own lunch. Many children take their lunch to school but trade it to other children or even throw most of it out. Parents rarely can tell whether the child is eating what they were sent to school with.

Peer pressure even in the elementary school years influences food choices. Fast food products are very high in fats and low in overall nutritional value. Children should be assessed for the amount of "junk" food that they eat each day and each week. One survey noted that 10% of the school-aged sample skipped breakfast and most ate snacks containing junk food (Graham & Uphold, 1992).

Some nutritionists recommend that children over age 2 years have their blood cholesterol levels tested so that the amount of dietary fat in their diet can be altered to cut down on their risk of heart disease in later life (O'Brien, 1991).

Diagnosis

The nurse can determine which nursing diagnoses are appropriate for the child. They may include altered nutrition: less-than-body requirements, altered nutrition: more-than-body requirements, potential for more-than-body requirements, knowledge deficit, and feeding self-care deficit.

HEALTHY SNACKS CHILDREN LIKE TO EAT

Toddlers

Fruit
Gelatin dessert
Pudding

Preschoolers

Fruit
Fruit juice
Celery and carrots
Cheese
Chocolate milk

School-aged Children

Pizza
Pasta
Fruit
Vegetables and salads

Planning

Community health nurses can develop nutritional plans and sample meals for the parents of young children as part of a program of primary prevention. These plans can be used as guidelines in food selection.

Implementation

Parents and school-aged children can be instructed about the appropriate food groups. The dietary guidelines for each group should be covered, and an understanding about children who are either underweight or overweight should be made.

Nurses in the United States should be ready to refer appropriate families to the WIC Program (The Special Supplemental Food Program for Women, Infants, and Children) so that children under 5 years who are in low-income families can receive food vouchers and nutritional counselling and other health care services (Sargent, Attar, Meyers, Moore, & Kocher-Ahern, 1992). Community health nurses in other countries should investigate governmental programs related to nutrition for lower income families.

Evaluation

Evaluation of proper nutrition in children can be made by maintaining proper records of height and weight. Frequent measurements can help parents and health providers immediately see results of proper nutrition or point out weight changes that can be alleviated by the start of an appropriate diet.

IRON DEFICIENCY ANEMIA
Assessment

Iron deficiency anemia is the most common nutritional problem of children today. It is mostly found in children up to 3 years of age. Infants and toddlers of this age group are generally poor eaters and may not get enough iron in their daily food intake. In addition, some of these children may have had reduced levels of iron in their blood since birth because their mothers may also have been deficient in iron and passed along these lower iron blood levels to the infants during fetal development (Whaley & Wong, 1991).

Lack of an appropriate blood level of iron is seen in children who are susceptible to infection, who have poor weight gain, and who lag behind with their peers on height/weight charts. Poor oxygenation is another adverse effect of low iron blood levels and tends to negatively affect the school performance of these children.

Diagnosis

Nursing diagnoses that may be made regarding iron deficiency anemia include altered growth and development, altered health maintenance, self-care deficit: feeding, altered nutrition: less-than-body requirements, and altered circulation: impaired tissue perfusion.

Planning

Nutritional educational materials should be developed for implementation by the community health nurse. Parents will need to be taught how to choose the correct foods for their children and how to prepare them appropriately so that nutrients and iron are not lost in the cooking process. Easy-to-follow guides for parents regarding the administration of oral iron supplements will also need to be developed and access to the medication for families who do not have health care insurance will have to be provided.

Implementation

As part of a primary prevention program, the nurse should emphasize proper nutrition and a diet including red meats, fruits, vegetables, grains, and dairy products. Many parents do not like to give their children red meat because of the idea that these meats are not good because of their link to future heart disease and high cholesterol levels. The nurse needs to emphasize to the parents that all children need various nutrients to grow and develop appropriately and that the lack of iron in the body from not giving the child cooked red meat is more deliterious than the future potential for heart disease from excessive red meat ingestion. The nurse must also teach the caretakers how to give the prescribed oral iron supplements.

Evaluation

The community health nurse should follow up on all nutritional protocols to ensure compliance. Secondary prevention in the form of frequent measurements of height and weight of the child as well as complete blood counts (CBC) should be taken to help monitor the iron level in the blood as evidenced by the red blood cell counts (RBC), and hematocrit (HCT) and hemoglobin (Hgb) levels.

LEAD POISONING/PLUMBISM
Assessment

More than 3 to 4 million children in the United States are exposed to lead (Bodenhorn, 1991). Because of the severity of the problem of **plumbism,** in 1991 the CDC reduced from 25 mcg/dL to 10 mcg/dL the level of lead in the blood requiring treatment (Feldman & White, 1992).

Children are exposed to lead all over the world (Lee & Moore, 1990). Children exposed to lead in the environment are not only from the lower income groups in urban areas, but from all socioeconomic groups in all areas including industrialized cities, suburbs, and even rural areas (Barker & Lewis, 1990). Children in wealthy families may be exposed to lead in the dust from renovation of old houses or in the water supply as it courses through lead-lined pipes. Others may pick up lead dust on their clothes as they play in areas where the soil has lead dust blown in from industrial areas. Lead is also in the environment in homes with stained glass or where jewelry-making activities call for using lead (Brown, Bellinger, & Matthews, 1990). All children are at risk. Because infants and toddlers explore the world largely by tasting everything, these are the age groups at highest risk from lead exposure.

Children are exposed to lead in a number of ways. Children may eat paint chips from woodwork in their homes (pica) or they may inhale automobile emissions in urban areas where leaded gasoline is still available for purchase. In addition, children may ingest lead from dietary sources such as water contaminated with lead from the solder in plumbing joints or the solder in the seams of food cans. In 1993, the United States Environmental Protection Agency announced that 819 municipal water systems in the United States had above-normal lead levels (Zremski, 1993). This illustrates the subtle risk of lead ingestion for all persons. Children living near industrial lead smelters are also at risk for lead exposure from contaminants in the air and the soil (Letourneau & Gagne, 1992) (see Research Highlight box). In addition, many children are exposed prenatally to lead because their mothers had ingested lead themselves. Exposure in pregnant women is particularly problematic because the chelating agents to remove excessive lead from the blood can cause birth defects (Brown, Bellinger, & Matthews, 1990) (see box on page 299).

Children who are at highest risk for plumbism

 RESEARCH 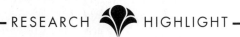 HIGHLIGHT

Blood Lead Levels of Children in Rouyn-Noranda, Quebec

Blood lead levels in children ages 2 to 5 years living near a lead smelter in Rouyn-Noranda, Quebec, Canada were assessed. The researchers completed a survey of the preschool-aged children living in the area in 1979 (N = 29) and again in 1989 (N = 124). The results showed that there were fewer children with high lead levels in 1989 but that there was still lead in the soil surrounding the smelter in the community. During this 10-year pe-

riod, the amount of lead emissions from the smelter decreased, and unleaded gasoline was also phased in, resulting in a subsequent decrease in leaded exhaust emissions. The researchers posed the question whether reduced exposure to airborne lead played a role in the decreased blood lead levels in the children, which, if true, would necessitate action to remove lead in the soil around the smelter plant to further reduce lead exposure.

From "Blood lead level in children living close to a smelter area: 10 years later" by G.G. Letourneau & D.J.P. Gagne, (1992), *Canadian Journal of Public Health, 83*(3), 221-225.

include those who are also at the highest risk for nutritional deficiencies and iron deficiency anemia: low-income urban families. Children who have nutritional deficiencies are at high risk because their bodies will hold all minerals for growth, even heavy metals such as toxic lead. Elevated lead levels are insidious to detect; however, any child who is developmentally delayed should be evaluated for the presence of lead in the blood (Whaley & Wong, 1991).

Children with high lead levels have been found to have behavior problems, perhaps related to its effect on the brain. Evidence of this was found after a study of 201 African-American children ages 2 to 5 years (Sciarillo, Alexander, & Farrell, 1992). Educational problems such as learning difficulties caused by brain damage from lead have also been found (Bellinger, Stiles, & Needleman, 1992; Feldman & White, 1992; Leviton, Bellinger, Allred, Rabinowitz, Needleman, & Schoenbaum, 1993).

Research has found that damage from chronic exposure to lead is irreversible (Chao & Kikano, 1993). The best way to treat lead poisoning is to prevent it (DeRienzo-DeVivio, 1992). The environment must be screened for lead, and the lead must be eliminated (Mushak, 1992; Wartenberg, 1992).

Diagnosis

Nursing diagnoses related to the child with lead poisoning after the screening process include al-

tered growth and development, impaired home maintenance management, knowledge deficit, altered nutrition: less-than-body requirements, and potential for poisoning.

Planning

The community health nurse should plan to refer the child who has been identified as having a lead exposure to the appropriate health care agency where treatment can begin. The nurse must also plan an educational session with the parents or caretakers to help them understand how their child obtained this heavy metal and how it was transferred to their blood. Parents' educational plans need to include information allowing parents to learn that there is no single source of lead to blame for their child's exposure. In addition, the child must be fully informed about what is going on.

Implementation

If untreated, lead poisoning may result in regressed mental development, severe anemia, and mental retardation. Chelation therapy with $CaNa_2EDTA$ (calcium disodium edetate) is the treatment of choice to eliminate the lead from the child's system. However, this treatment will not reverse any preexisting physical or brain damage caused by the high lead levels in the blood (Whaley & Wong, 1991).

The community health nurse must help the family cope with the process of monitoring the child's blood lead levels and if required, the process of the chelation therapy. The child may be hospitalized for the intravenous $CaNa_2EDTA$ therapy or may receive D-penicillamine (Cuprimine, Depen) orally for the chelation process. Each of these medications binds with the heavy metal to aid in its excretion from the body (Whaley & Wong, 1991).

Evaluation

Continued monitoring of the child's blood lead levels over several years is an important responsibility for the community health nurse. Repeated home visits, clinic follow-ups, or telephone contacts must be made to ensure compliance with the monitoring schedule. Because repeated chelation treatments may need to be given to the affected child, it is important that parental education and support continue.

VIOLENCE
Assessment

Violence is pervasive in today's society. Violent crime such as murder and armed robbery is increasing. In 1989 it was reported that over 22 million American households had had experience with crime (United States Department of Commerce, 1992). Children are also the victims of crime; there were 1200 homicide deaths of children under 15 years of age in the United States in 1989 (United States Department of Commerce, 1992). Child abuse and neglect, discussed later in this chapter, are also pervasive.

Violence is not only experienced by children, but it is also viewed by them in television programs, news reports, cartoons, and action and horror films. Many children relate to the super-hero whose purpose is the destruction of an evil enemy. There is controversy at this time about whether the exposure to violence in the media has an affect on the viewers (Pergament, 1993). Some parent groups believe that television violence promotes violent behavior in the child (Ridley-Johnson, Surdy, & O'Laughlin, 1991). However, other research has found that viewing violent television programs did not affect the children's behavior; in fact, behavior problems in the children actually followed the viewing of nonviolent television programs (Sawin, 1990).

Steps are being taken regarding violence in television programming as the result of United States Senate Hearings with television network executives in May, 1993 (Duston, 1993a, 1993b). The television networks reportedly devised a plan to place warning messages in television listings and on the television screen before the beginning of violent programs (TV Networks, 1993); however, children's cartoons will not have these warnings (Scanlan, 1993). This caused lawmakers to call for a blocking device on televisions so that parents could restrict the reception of violent programming in their homes (Duston, 1993c). By February, 1994, the cable and broad-cast networks announced the development of a system to monitor TV violence (Gunther, 1994; Schmid, 1994). This controversy will undoubtedly continue into the future.

In recent years children have been increasingly exposed to war and other armed conflict. Children in Eastern Europe and parts of Africa and Asia are experiencing war first-hand. They have been the victims of civil strife and "ethnic cleansing" in Bosnia and other areas of the former Yugoslavia. Children in Northern Ireland are routinely exposed to terrorist attacks. A study of children in Ulster, Ireland, found that the children there were affected by viewing news reports of the violence around them. Children living in high-violence areas were most affected by the reports of violence (Cairns, 1990).

Children from areas of strife in the world are often refugees in the United States, Canada, and other countries. They have experienced the violence in their homelands and now need to adjust to a different culture and environment.

Children in areas of the world that are not directly affected by war and strife see the effects of the conflict on television and in magazines and newspapers. Children in "safe" areas may feel that they are vulnerable to the violence also because developmentally they are unable to see the separation between themselves and the actual violence.

Children also see reports of murders and attacks in their cities, towns, and neighborhoods. Some children may also live in areas where these events occur and may witness the police investigations and view the bullet casings, blood stains, and other remnants of violence. They may be children of abused mothers who witness domestic violence and often flee with their mothers to shelters to get away from the violence (Hollenkamp & Attala, 1986). Some children attend schools where weapons are found or even carry the weapons themselves for protection. Shootings and knifings in schools are not uncommon. Children are afraid.

Diagnosis

The nursing diagnoses that relate to children affected by all types of violence include anxiety, ineffective coping, fear, potential for injury, and potential for trauma.

Planning

The community health nurse can anticipate reactions from children to violence in all aspects of health care. The nurse should develop a plan of primary prevention as well as reality orientation to aid children when they are exposed to violence, whether actual violence or viewed violence.

Implementation

Nurses can use therapeutic play to help children work through their feelings of fear and anxiety related to violence.

Research has shown that while television violence may influence the behavior of children negatively, instruction on what television programs to watch does reduce the risk (Comstock & Strasburger, 1990). The nurse can easily work with the children and families to help choose the programming that they feel is best.

Nurses can also help families choose appropriate movies, since the film ratings have been found not to relate to the effects of the violence on young children (Wilson, Linz, & Randall, 1990).

The nurse should also teach children about personal safety and how to deal with strangers and attempts from drug dealers to get them to experiment with drugs. The children should be taught how to call police and fire/rescue departments and should also be able to give their own

◼ CASE STUDY

January 16, 1991. The sights and sounds of battle in Baghdad, Iraq, are broadcast live on the evening news as television news anchors speak to correspondents over the telephone.

January 17, 1991. The sights of anxious news correspondents desperately struggling to put on gas masks as air raid sirens wail in Israel and Saudi Arabia during live interviews with television anchors.

All through these experiences and more over the following days and nights, Nancy, age 6 years, was watching war — Desert Storm — on television. Nancy is frightened about what she sees on the television.

Assessment: Nancy is literally being bombarded by viewing bombing and destruction in another country being carried out by her country as part of an Allied Coalition Force. Nancy sees the destruction on the television and it is hard for her to imagine that these images are taking place far away from her. Her sense of security is shattered. Nancy does not understand that these bombs cannot hurt her. Because of her developmental stage, she sees these events as happening close to her.

Diagnosis: Anxiety related to viewed war and developmental level.

Planning: The nurse will develop a therapeutic play session so that Nancy can work out her anxiety. Therapeutic play will help Nancy understand her feelings and to learn about the war.

Implementation: The community health nurse provides sheets of blank paper, crayons, construction paper, pencils, and an uninterrupted length of time of about 20 minutes. The nurse explains that this is a time to draw some pictures. Nancy is asked to draw 4 pictures, one for each of the following themes:

1. Draw how you feel right now.
2. Draw you and your family as you are right now.
3. Draw what you think war is.
4. Draw what you think is going on in other children's families in countries where the war is going on.

Once Nancy has time to draw the pictures, the nurse and Nancy discuss what the pictures mean and the reality behind any misconceptions.

Evaluation: After this exercise, Nancy understood that the war was a long way away and that the war would not spread to her home.

name, address, and telephone number to appropriate officials. Safety should be stressed as positive and not as a defensive, frightening aspect of life.

Evaluation

The community health nurse can see the consequences of nursing interventions by assessing whether children have decreased reactions to perceived violence. Helping children cope with neighborhood violence can be evaluated by looking at the level of violence and fear that the children are experiencing.

CHILD ABUSE AND NEGLECT
Assessment

Infants, toddlers, preschoolers, and school-aged children may all become victims of **child abuse and neglect.** Both of these acts are also called child maltreatment. Abuse constitutes the physical or psychological damage inflicted upon a child by the parent or caretaker (Humphreys & Ramsey, 1993a). There were over 2 million cases of child abuse reported in the United States in 1987. This reflects a rate of 8.3 cases per 1000 population (United States Department of Commerce, 1992).

Sexual abuse involves incest, promotion of the child's prostitution by the parent, or other sexual acts forced on a child under 18 years of age (Charnizon, 1990). There were 15,700 cases of sexual abuse reported in the United States in 1986, and evidence then showed that the rate of reporting these cases was increasing dramatically (United States Department of Commerce, 1992).

Neglect is the absence of reasonable care required by a child, such as shelter, food, supervision, or health care (Charnizon, 1990). Leaving a young child (under 12 years of age) alone also constitutes child neglect.

Factors that indicate a high risk for child abuse or neglect include history of the child being born prematurely or with a low birth weight, and a history of chronic illness in the child (Charnizon, 1990).

Factors placing the family at high risk for becoming abusers include alcoholic or substance abusing parents, the absence of the natural parent in the home, violence or excessive stress in the family, unemployment, financial difficulties, single parents without a situational support system, history of abuse of the parents as children, and immature parents who have unrealistic expectations for the child (Charnizon, 1990).

While completing the assessment, the nurse must be aware of how the culture of the family influences parenting styles and the disciplining of children. Spanking children may be acceptable in some communities while in others it is seen as abusive. Some cultural groups practice procedures (i.e., coining) that leave bruises (Devlin & Reynolds, 1994). Having an understanding of familial practices with children is essential so that suspected instances of child abuse, maltreatment, or neglect can be accurately identified and distinguished from circumstances that do not indicate violence toward children.

Diagnosis

Nursing diagnoses for the abused and/or neglected child include anxiety, fear, hopelessness, ineffective coping, post-traumatic response, potential for injury, potential for trauma, powerlessness, and unilateral neglect.

Nursing diagnoses for the family involved are altered parenting role performance, altered family processes, anxiety, fear, hopelessness, ineffective family coping, potential for violence, powerlessness, and social isolation.

Planning

Children who have been identified as possibly being abused or neglected must be helped. The nurse can plan as a part of secondary prevention to help restore the physical and psychosocial well-being of the child. The child may feel betrayed by the parents but does not want to implicate the parent in the abusive behavior. The nurse should be ready to help children who are blaming themselves for their "punishments" by helping them see that they did nothing themselves to warrant such treatment.

Implementation

Helping the child who has been neglected, maltreated, or abused is of paramount importance. Long-term effects of child abuse include depression, withdrawal, and a tendency to abuse one's own children later in life.

Because registered nurses functioning in their professional role are mandated reporters for suspected cases of child abuse and/or neglect, it is the responsibility of the nurse to always be on the lookout for children who may have been abused or for families where the potential of abuse is suspected. The nurse should intervene by obtaining documented facts and alerting the appropriate authorities by calling the government's child abuse hotline listed in the telephone book or by informing the local social services or child welfare agency. Nurses who suspect child abuse outside of their professional role are encouraged to report the abuse as any private citizen would.

Play therapy is often used to help children through the stressful process of treatment for child abuse. This is where the children are encouraged to work through their abusive experiences through play. Specially educated counsellors help the children through the process. Anatomically correct dolls and other play things are provided for the children so that they can act out what happened to them (Humphreys & Ramsey, 1993b).

Evaluation

Proper follow-up of all reported cases of possible child abuse and neglect must be made. Routine surveillance of the family by regular contacts from the community health nurse and other health care personnel can help families break the cycle of child abuse. Continued support of the abused or neglected child can help the child restore his or her shattered self-esteem and grow up trusting others.

POVERTY
Assessment

Poverty is a long-term problem necessitating tertiary prevention. In 1990, there were 12.7 million children living under the poverty line in the United States. Of these children, over 5 million were less than 6 years old (United States Department of Commerce, 1992). Many children live in single parent families, in shelters for the homeless, and in other areas in which their lives are

managed despite poverty. Unemployment and global recession adds more children to this toll as their parents are left without means to support them.

Many children live in industrial areas where the lack of proper food, shelter, and other necessities results in an increased potential for poor health (Goodwin, 1991). Homeless children are particularly at risk for developmental, nutritional, and educational problems (Shulsinger, 1990). In addition, children living in poverty have the potential to become drug addicts, become members of gangs, and experience teenage pregnancy (Kaplan-Sanoff, Parker, & Zuckerman, 1991) at as young as 10 or 11 years of age.

In 1988, 16.9 million children in the United States were without any kind of health insurance (United States Department of Commerce, 1992). Many European countries and Canada provide health care for all their citizens; however, even in these countries access to health care remains a problem for the poor.

Many children are refugees from violent areas of the world, are immigrants seeking a new start, or are members of migrant families trying to find work in an uncertain economy. These children are all underserved by the health care system (Drapo, Patrick, & Kemp, 1987).

Diagnosis

Nursing diagnoses appropriate for children living in poverty include impaired home maintenance management, hopelessness, powerlessness, and social isolation.

Planning

The goal of the nurse is to help the child and family climb out of poverty. This is very difficult and requires massive education, job training, health insurance, and governmental support.

Implementation

The community health nurse needs to work with the children and families within the means available. The nurse should be ready to refer all to the appropriate government support systems for which the family qualifies. "Safety nets" do exist within all governmental systems, and the nurse should help the family through the maze of bureaucracy.

Evaluation

Evaluation of poverty for the community health nurse involves conscientious maintenance of data on children in poverty. Families and children cannot be "lost in the system" or "lost through the cracks." Efforts must continue to help these children grow and develop despite monumental roadblocks set before them.

Chapter Highlights

- Childhood is a time of rapid physical and cognitive development.

- Therapeutic play can be used as a health promotion tool.

- All children must receive immunizations against communicable diseases.

- Accidents are a leading cause of childhood morbidity.

- Nurses must teach parents and caretakers accident prevention.

- Children are affected by AIDS: physically through prenatal exposure and breastfeeding from HIV positive mothers and emotionally through the AIDS-related death of a parent/caretaker.

- Proper nutrition in children can enhance growth and development and prevent iron deficiency anemia.

- Environmental exposure to lead can cause learning deficiencies and brain damage.

- Children are affected by violence both in their neighborhoods and through the media.

- The incidence of child abuse and neglect is increasing.

- Many children lack access to health care and health care insurance.

 CRITICAL THINKING EXERCISE

A community health nurse gives a brief presentation about nutrition at a parent-teacher meeting. The presentation leads to a request for a day-long workshop to be presented to the parents of toddlers and preschoolers. There is also to be a session for school-aged children that will be presented to the children themselves.

Plan a workshop that will include:

1. Information to be presented to parents about developmental ability related to eating behaviors and nutritional needs of all age groups.
2. Information about good nutrition that will be presented to the school-aged children in such a way that they will enjoy the presentation and learn from it.

REFERENCES

Aronson, S.S. (1985). Health care providers and daycare. In M.C. Sharp, & F.W. Henderson (Eds.). *Daycare: Report of the sixteenth Ross roundtable on critical approaches to common pediatric problems* (pp. 71-82). Columbus, OH: Ross Laboratories.

Aronson, S.S. (1986). Maintaining health in child care settings. In N. Gunzenhauser, & B.M. Caldwell (Eds.). *Group care for young children: Considerations for child care and health professionals, public policy makers, and parents, Pediatric Round Table Series: 12,* (pp. 137-146). New Brunswick, NJ: Johnson & Johnson Baby Products Co.

Atkinson, W.L., Hadler, S.C., Redd, S.B., & Orenstein, W.A. (1992). Measles surveillance—United States 1991. *Morbidity and Mortality Weekly Report, 41*(SS-6), 1-12.

Barker, P.O., & Lewis, D.A. (1990). The management of lead exposure in pediatric populations. *Nurse Practitioner, 15*(12), 8-10, 12-13, 16.

Bellinger, D.C., Stiles, K.M., & Needleman, H.L. (1992). Low-level lead exposure, intelligence and academic achievement: A long-term follow-up study. *Pediatrics, 90*(6), 855-861.

Block, D.E. (1991). Correctness of child safety seat usage and rental program participation. *Dissertation Abstracts International, 52*(03-B), 1347.

Bodenhorn, K.A. (1991). Lead poisoning: The foremost preventable disease of childhood. *Journal of Pediatric Health Care, 5*(3), 156-157.

Brannan, J.E.. (1992). Accidental poisoning of children: Barriers to resource use in a Black, low-income community. *Public Health Nursing, 9*(2), 81-86.

Brown, M.J., Bellinger, D., & Matthews, J. (1990). In utero lead exposure. *American Journal of Maternal Child Nursing, 15*(2), 94-96.

Cairns, E. (1990). Impact of television news exposure on children's perceptions of violence in Northern Ireland. *Journal of Social Psychology, 130*(4), 447-452.

Carroll-Johnson, R.M. (Ed.). (1991). *Classification of nursing diagnoses. Proceedings of the Ninth Conference, North American Nursing Diagnosis Association.* Philadelphia: J.B. Lippincott.

Carter, Y.H., Bannon, M.J., & Jones, P.W. (1992). Health visitors and child accident prevention. *Health Visitor, 65*(4), 115-117.

Chang, A., Lugg, M.M., & Nebedum, A. (1989). Injuries among preschool children enrolled in day-care centers. *Pediatrics, 83,* 272-277.

Chao, J., & Kikano, G.E. (1993). Lead poisoning in children. *American Family Physician, 47*(1), 113-120.

Charnizon, M. (Ed.). (1990). *NYSPCC Professionals' handbook: Identifying and reporting child abuse and neglect.* New York: The New York Society for the Prevention of Cruelty to Children.

Clemen-Stone, S., Eigsti, D.G., & McGuire, S.L.. (1991). *Comprehensive family and community health nursing* (3rd ed.). St. Louis: Mosby.

Coffman, S.P. (1991). Parent education for drowning prevention. *Journal of Pediatric Health Care, 5*(3), 141-146.

Comstock, G., & Strasburger, V.C. (1990). Deceptive appearances: Television violence and aggressive behavior. *Journal of Adolescent Health Care, 11*(1), 31-44.

Cuomo signs helmet law for young bicyclists. (1993, July 23). *The Buffalo News,* p. A-8.

Department of Economic and Social Development Statistical Office, (1992). *Statistical yearbook 1988/1989 (Annuaire statistique 1988/1989),* 37th issue. New York: United Nations.

DeRienzo-DeVivio S. (1992). Childhood lead poisoning: Shifting to primary prevention. *Pediatric Nursing, 18*(6), 565-567.

Devlin, B.K., & Reynolds, E. (1994). Child abuse. How to recognize it, how to intervene. *American Journal of Nursing, 94*(3), 26-31.

Drapo, P.J., Patrick, C.R., & Kemp, C. (1987). Addressing the needs of underserved populations in community health nursing education. *Public Health Nursing, 4*(4), 236-241.

Duston D. (1993a, May 22). TV executives vow to mend violent ways. Officials spurred by a warning. *The Buffalo News,* p. A-3.

Duston, D. (1993b, June 26). Ted Turner blames TV for violence. *The Buffalo News,* p. A-3.

Duston, D. (1993c, July 2). Lawmakers seek TV device to block access by children, *The Buffalo News,* p. A-13.

Erikson, E.H. (1963). *Childhood and society,* (2nd ed., rev.). New York: Norton.

Feldman, R.G., & White, R.F. (1992). Lead neurotoxicity and disorders of learning. *Journal of Child Neurology, 7*(4), 354-359.

Fleming, J.M. (1986). Nursing education to meet child care needs. In N. Gunzenhauser, & B.M. Caldwell (Eds.). *Group care for young children: Considerations for child care and health professionals, public policy makers, and parents. Pediatric Round Table Series: 12,* (pp. 114-123). New Brunswick, NJ: Johnson & Johnson Baby Products Co.

Garnett, S.M., & Elton, P.J. (1991). A treatment service for minor injuries: Maintaining equity of access. *Journal of Public Health Medicine, 13*(4), 260-266.

Goodwin, S. (1991). Breaking the links between social deprivation and poor child health. *Health Visitor, 64*(11), 376-380.

Graham, M.V., & Uphold, C.R. (1992). Health perceptions and behaviors of school-age boys and girls. *Journal of Community Health Nursing, 9*(2), 77-86.

Gunther, M. (1994, February 4). Simon, networks strike deal on TV violence. *The Buffalo News,* p. A-4.

Hepatitis B virus: A comprehensive strategy for eliminating transmission in the United States through universal childhood vaccination. Recommendations of the Immunization Practices Advisory Committee (ACIP). *Morbidity and Mortality Weekly Reports, 40*(RR-13), 1-25.

Hollenkamp, M., & Attala, J. (1986). Meeting health needs in a crisis shelter: A challenge to nurses in the community. *Journal of Community Health Nursing, 3*(4), 201-209.

Humphreys, J., & Ramsey, A.M. (1993a). Child abuse. In J. Campbell & J. Humphreys (Eds.). *Nursing care of survivors of family violence* (2nd ed.), (pp. 36-67). St. Louis: Mosby.

Humphreys, J., & Ramsey, A.M. (1993b). Nursing care of abused children. In J. Campbell & J. Humphreys (Eds.). *Nursing care of survivors of family violence* (2nd ed.), (pp. 211-247). St. Louis: Mosby.

Jones, N.E.. (1992). Injury prevention: A survey of clinical practice. *Journal of Pediatric Health Care, 6*(4), 182-186.

Kaplan-Sanoff, M., Parker, S., & Zuckerman, B. (1991). Poverty and early childhood development: What do we know, and what should we do? *Infants and Young Children, 4*(1), 68-76.

Lee, E.J., & Bass, C. (1990). Survey of accidents in a university day-care center. *Journal of Pediatric Health Care, 4*(1), 18-23.

Lee, W.R., & Moore, M.R. (1990). Low level exposure to lead: The evidence for harm accumulates. *British Medical Journal, 301*(6751), 504-505.

Letourneau, G.G., & Gagne, D.J.P. (1992). Blood lead level in children living close to a smelter area: 10 years later. *Canadian Journal of Public Health, 83*(3), 221-225.

Leviton, A., Bellinger, D., Allred, E.N., Rabinowitz, M., Needleman, H., & Schoenbaum, S. (1993). Pre- and postnatal low-level lead exposure and children's dysfunction in school. *Environmental Research, 60*(1), 30-43.

Measles prevention: Recommendations of the Immunization Practices Advisory Committee (ACIP). (1989). *Morbidity and Mortality Weekly Reports, 38*(S-9), 1-18.

Meer, P.A. (1985). Using play therapy in outpatient settings. *American Journal of Maternal Child Nursing, 10*(6), 378-380.

Mushak, P. (1992). Defining lead as the premiere environmental health issue for children in America: Criteria and their quantitative application. *Environmental Research, 59*(2), 281-309.

O'Brien, S. (1991). Panel recommends blood cholesterol health screening and education guidelines for children and adolescents. *Journal of the American Association of Occupational Health Nurses, 39*(6), 296.

O'Pray, M. (1980). Developmental screening tools: Using them effectively. *American Journal of Maternal Child Nursing, 5*(2), 126-130.

Pergament, A. (1993, June 30). Are TV networks to be blamed for too much sex, violence?, *The Buffalo News,* p. B-10.

Piaget, J. (1978). *Success and understanding* (A.J. Pomerans, Trans.). Cambridge, MA: Harvard University Press. (Original work published 1974.)

Recommendations of the Immunization Practices Advisory Committee (ACIP). (1992). Pertussis vaccination: Acellular pertussis vaccine for reinforcing and booster use—Supplementary ACIP statement. Recommendations and reports. *Morbidity and Mortality Weekly Reports, 41*(R-1), 1-10.

Recommendations of the Immunization Practices Advisory Committee (ACIP). (1993). Recommendations for use of Haemophilus b conjugate vaccines and a combined diphtheria, tetanus, pertussis and Hb vaccine. *Morbidity and Mortality Weekly Reports, 42*(RR-1), 1-15.

Reece, S.M. (1991). New protection against *Haemophilus influenzae* type b infections in infants and young children. *Nurse Practitioner, 16*(11), 27, 31-36.

Retrospective assessment of vaccination coverage among school-aged children—Selected U.S. cities, 1991. (1992). *Morbidity and Mortality Weekly Reports, 41*(6), 103-107.

Ridley-Johnson, R., Surdy, T., & O'Laughlin, E. (1991). Parent survey on television violence viewing: Fear, aggression, and sex differences. *Journal of Applied Developmental Psychology, 12*(1), 63-71.

Sargent, J.D., Attar-Abate, L., Meyers, A., Moore, L., & Kocher-Ahern, E. (1992). Referrals of participants in an urban WIC program to health and welfare services. *Public Health Reports, 107*(2), 173-178.

Sawin, D.B. (1990). Aggressive behavior among children in small playgroup settings with violent television. *Advances in Learning and Behavioral Disabilities. A Research Annual, 6,* 157-177.

Scanlan, C. (1993, July 1). Labels won't apply to daytime children's programs, *The Buffalo News,* p. A-3.

Schmid, R.E. (1994, February 2). Television dodges action by Congress with self-policing. *The Buffalo News,* p. A-4.

Sciarillo, W.G., Alexander, G., & Farrell, K.P. (1992). Lead exposure and child behavior. *American Journal of Public Health, 82*(10), 1356-1360.

Shulsinger, E. (1990). Needs of sheltered homeless children. *Journal of Pediatric Health Care, 4*(3), 136-140.

Sullivan, M., Cole, B., Lie, L., & Twomey, J. (1990). Reducing child hazards in the home: A joint venture in injury control. *Journal of Burn Care and Rehabilitation, 11*(2), 175-179.

Summary of notifiable diseases, United States, 1991. (1992). *Morbidity and Mortality Weekly Report, 40*(53), 1-12.

Too hot for tots? (1993, July 20). *The Buffalo News,* p. C-3.

TV networks to run program warnings. Message to precede violent shows. (1993, June 30). *The Buffalo News,* p. A-1, A-8.

United States Department of Commerce. (1992). *Statistical abstract of the United States. The national data book,* (112th ed.). Washington, DC: United States Department of Commerce: Economics and Statistics Administration, Bureau of the Census.

Update: Acquired immunodeficiency syndrome—United States 1992. (1993). *Morbidity and Mortality Weekly Report, 42*(28), 547-557.

Wartenberg, D. (1992). Screening for lead exposure using a geographic information system. *Environmental Research, 59*(2), 310-317.

Whaley, L.F., & Wong, D.L. (1991). *Nursing care of infants and children* (4th ed.). St. Louis: Mosby.

Wilson, B.J., Linz, D., & Randall, B. (1990). Applying social science research to film ratings: A shift from offensiveness to harmful effects. *Journal of Broadcasting and Electronic Media, 34*(4), 443-468.

Zremski, J. (1993, May 12). Tests reveal elevated lead levels. *The Buffalo News,* p. A-7.

14

CARING FOR ADOLESCENTS AND YOUNG ADULTS

Joan M. Cookfair

My heart leaps up when I behold
   a rainbow in the sky:
So was it when my life began;
   So it is now I am a man.
So be it when I grow old,
   or let me die!
The child is father of the man. . . .

William Wordsworth

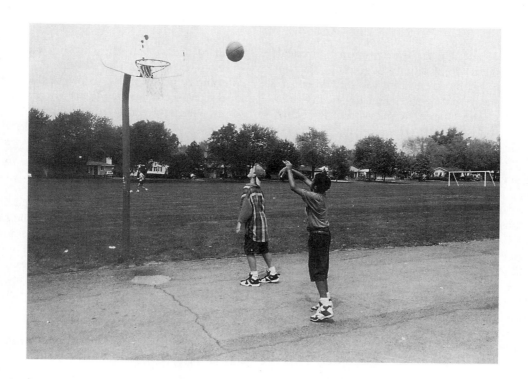

OBJECTIVES

At the conclusion of this chapter the student will be able to:

1. Describe the health and development of adolescents and young adults.
2. Describe health concerns of adolescents and young adults.
3. Discuss primary, secondary, and tertiary interventions to promote wellness in the age group.
4. Describe the major causes of mortality and morbidity in adolescents and young adults.
5. Discuss the lack of health insurance as a contributing cause for a lack of wellness.
6. Describe and discuss some social concerns relating to adolescents and young adults.

KEY TERMS

Acne vulgaris
Adolescence
Adolescent kyphosis
Alienation
Altered growth pattern
Anorexia nervosa

Bulimia
Developmental task
Jumper's knee
Little leaguer's elbow
Menarche
Osgood Schlatter's disease

Puberty
Risk-taking behavior
Spirituality
Substance abuse
Suicide

The adolescent years are a time of physical growth and emotional lability. Beginning at about age 12 years in most cultures, the individual experiences hormonal changes that drastically alter appearance and body chemistry. At the same time there may be too little knowledge absorbed and a lack of experience on which to base decisions affecting well-being and long-term health. **Adolescence** begins with puberty (about 11 to 14 years of age for girls and 13 to 18 years of age for boys). Late adolescence, or young adulthood, continues in Western civilizations until about 24 years of age. This is a very stressful time in the life process because of rapid changes in body image and feelings.

There are, in addition, stressors being encountered by this group that are unique in history. Adolescents and young adults must learn to live in a world of political upheaval, AIDS, pollution, and constant change in the external environment.

An awareness of the internal and external stressors experienced by them will enable the community health nurse to plan interventions at a primary, secondary, and tertiary level to help adolescents and young adults achieve a state of wellness and a realization of their full potential.

MAJOR CAUSES OF MORTALITY AND MORBIDITY IN ADOLESCENCE

During the past 30 years, the causes of death have changed for the 12- to 24-year-old age group. The percentage of youth who die has not. Alone among the age groups, they have not experienced an overall decrease in the rate of mortality. A rise in the death rate from violence, injury, and what may be described as risk-taking behavior is the reason. Figure 14-1 illustrates the leading causes of death for youth aged 15 to 24 years.

The number of motor vehicle accidents in this age group is increasing. Three quarters of injury

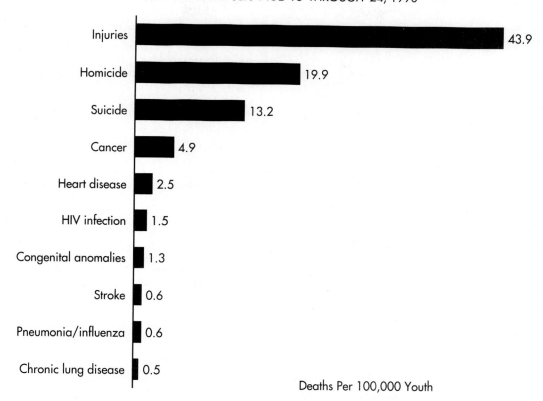

MAJOR CAUSES OF DEATH FOR ADOLESCENTS
AND YOUNG ADULTS AGE 15 THROUGH 24; 1990

Injuries — 43.9
Homicide — 19.9
Suicide — 13.2
Cancer — 4.9
Heart disease — 2.5
HIV infection — 1.5
Congenital anomalies — 1.3
Stroke — 0.6
Pneumonia/influenza — 0.6
Chronic lung disease — 0.5

Deaths Per 100,000 Youth

FIGURE 14-1 Major causes of death for adolescents and young adults. *From* Prevention '93/'94, *by U.S. Department of Health and Human Services, Public Health Service, Office of Disease Prevention and Health Promotion, Washington, DC: U.S. Government Printing Office (in press).*

deaths among young people 15 to 24 years of age are a result of motor vehicle accidents. It is generally recognized that alcohol is often a causative factor in motor vehicle accidents. However, the trends in alcohol use vary among age levels. As a result of school programs, increasing parental awareness, and media coverage, the use of alcohol is decreasing among adolescents. However, among persons in the 18- to 24-year age group, drinking is more prevalent than ever (U.S. Department of Health and Human Services, 1991). This group might be helped by educational programs in secondary schools and colleges.

For a young person suspected of experimenting with drugs or alcohol, a counseling session with the family may be in order. For young adults who have become habitual drinkers, Alcoholics Anonymous might be helpful. Chronic substance abusers of any age should be referred for medical intervention and rehabilitation.

NUTRITIONAL STATUS IN ADOLESCENCE

During late adolescence and young adulthood, fast foods and stress can place individuals at high risk for altered nutritional status. Education as to the importance of a balanced diet may have a long-term positive effect on health and well-being. A balanced diet for an adolescent should consist of at least four servings of milk and milk products per day, three servings of meat or other protein sources, and four servings of fruits and

DAILY BALANCED DIET FOR ADOLESCENTS

Four servings of milk and milk products
Three servings of meat or other protein source
Four servings of fruits and vegetables
Four servings of bread and cereals

TABLE 14-1 Stature, weight, and age as indications of nutritional status

Comparison	Potential interpretation
Steady linear growth and weight gain within expected rate	Good long-term nutritional status
Very low weight for height	Recent weight loss or slowed weight gain
Weight and height low for age	Long-term malnutrition; reflects parents' stature or growth hormone deficiency
Excessive weight for height	Obese child (resulting from behavioral, genetic, or systemic disease)

From *Pediatric nutrition in clinical practice* by W.E. Maclean & G.G. Grahm, 1982. Menlo Park, CA: Addison-Wesley. Copyright 1982 by Addison-Wesley. Reprinted by permission.

vegetables, one of which is a source of vitamin C and one a source of vitamin A. In addition, four servings of bread or cereals should be a part of the diet (Surgeon General's Report on Nutrition and Health, 1987). See the box above.

If altered nutritional status is suspected, further assessment can be conducted by asking the individual to keep a 24-hour diary of all foods consumed. Most effective is a follow-up interview. Some young people may not record their daily food consumption accurately for a number of reasons. During an interview, the validity of the diary can be assessed, and suggestions may be made as to foods to substitute that would be more appropriate for the young person to consume. Care should be taken to remain within the cultural and/or financial restrictions of each person. It may be necessary to request a parent conference for younger adolescents. Even with older adolescents, a family-oriented approach to making changes in eating habits and exercise behavior may have the best chance of success (Cousins et al., 1992).

Comparison of an adolescent's height for age, weight for age, and weight for height can offer important clues about his or her nutritional status. Table 14-1 describes some potential interpretations of a lack of steady linear growth and development. An **altered growth pattern** may indicate a need for further assessment as to nutritional status and general well-being.

Primary Prevention

Counseling about what constitutes proper nutrition is especially challenging with this age group. This is a time when the need for independence and autonomy is strongly felt. Convincing adolescents that good nutrition will improve their appearance and raise their energy level may be one way to enlist their cooperation. For many adoles-

cents the calories provided from snacks is a significant part to the total daily diet. A recognition that snacking behavior can be healthy if the right snacks are provided may help them to maintain a balanced diet.

Secondary Prevention

If the altered nutritional status needs further intervention because of excessive weight for height or low weight for height, further screening is indicated. A family history may indicate genetic predisposition for obesity. A conference with family members may also be of value to determine if the problem is behavioral. Further screening to determine the presence of systemic disease may be indicated. Low weight for height may indicate a need for a family conference as well. The family may be genetically predisposed to small body frame and slightness of build. If the family is on a very restricted budget, it may be possible to arrange for food stamps or other supplementary food programs. If the family expresses concern about the individual, a further physical examination followed by referral for laboratory testing may be indicated. Pallor, pale conjunctiva, and lethargy are reasons to screen for

────── RESEARCH ❀ HIGHLIGHT ──────

Consequences of Overweight in Adolescents

Overweight in adolescents may have deleterious effects on their subsequent self-esteem, social and economic characteristics, and physical health. We studied the relation between overweight and subsequent educational attainment, marital status, household income, and self-esteem in a nationally representative sample of 10,039 randomly selected young people who were 16 to 24 years old in 1981. Follow-up data were obtained in 1988 for 65% to 79% of the original cohort, depending on the variable studied. The characteristics of the subjects who had been overweight in 1981 were compared with those for young people with asthma, musculoskeletal abnormalities, and other chronic health conditions. Overweight was defined as a body-mass index above the 95th percentile for age and sex.

In 1981, 370 of the subjects were overweight. Seven years later, women who had been overweight had completed fewer years of school (0.3 year less; 95% confidence interval, 0.1 to 0.6;

$p = 0.009$), were less likely to be married (20% less likely; 95% CI, 13% to 27%; $p \neq 0.001$), had lower household incomes ($6710 less per year; 95% CI, $3942 to $9478; $p \neq 0.001$), and had higher rates of household poverty (10% higher; 95% CI, 4% to 16%; $p \neq 0.001$) than the women who had not been overweight, independent of their base-line socioeconomic status and aptitude-test scores. Men who had been overweight were less likely to be married (11% less likely; 95% CI, 3% to 18%; $p \neq 0.005$). In contrast, people with the other chronic conditions we studied did not differ in these ways from the nonoverweight subjects. We found no evidence of an effect of overweight on self-esteem.

Overweight during adolescence has important social and economic consequences, which are greater than those of many other chronic physical conditions. Discrimination against overweight persons may account for these results.

From "Social and Economic Consequences of Overweight in Adolescence and Young Adulthood" by S. Gortmaker, A. Must, J. Perrin, A. Sobol, & W. Dietz (1993). *New England Journal of Medicine, 329*(14), 1008.

──────────────────────────────────

anemia or protein calorie malnutrition. A test for hematocrit and hemoglobin levels, as well as a test for serum total protein levels, are important. Depending on the family history, the laboratory tests, and the nurse's assessment as to the possibility of an eating disorder, it may be advisable to refer the young person for medical evaluation.

Adolescents and young adults who are below the mean for height or are excessively tall may be concerned about being different from their parents. Once again, a family conference can determine if the status of their physical development is familial. They may also be experiencing a simple constitutional delay. There may be a familial history of late maturation. In such a case, no treatment is indicated beyond explanation and family support. If the individual is extremely distressed because of factors such as personality sensitivity or lack of achievement in other areas,

referral for psychological counseling may be indicated. Overweight in adolescents may place them at risk for poor social and economic achievement, according to a study done by researchers from Harvard University and the New England Medical Center (Gortmaker, Must, Perrin, Sobol, & Dietz, 1993).

Tertiary Prevention

If an altered growth pattern is the result of growth hormone deficiency, long-term malnutrition, psychiatric disturbance, or systemic disease, in-depth follow-up, teaching, counseling, and encouragement of compliance with medical regimens will assist the young person to maintain the highest level of wellness.

PUBERTY

Puberty begins at about 11 to 14 years of age for girls and 13 to 18 years of age for boys. **Menar-**

che signals the start of puberty for girls. Maturation of sexual characteristics may take 2 to 8 years (Murray & Zentner, 1989).

Emotional Development

Emotional development is a process that depends on maturation, experience, social interaction, and internal regulation. It is influenced by innate intelligence, environment, and culture.

According to Piaget (1963), adolescents between the ages of 12 to 15 years enter the formal operational stage, when they begin to think in terms of concepts and abstractions. Exceptions to this progression are those who are developmentally delayed or whose innate intelligence does not allow them to think conceptually.

The **developmental task,** according to Erikson (1963), is identity versus diffusion for the young adolescent. How well the task is completed depends on whether the developmental tasks preceding it have been successfully completed and a support system is in place. Young adolescents need to discover where they fit within the family and with their peers. Most importantly, they need to firmly develop a sense of presence. They need to experience a definite feeling of personhood, a cognitive and affective knowledge of their own identity. Failure to accomplish this task may result in identity diffusion, a feeling of not belonging anywhere. This can lead to alienation, insecurity, and antisocial behavior (Murray & Zentner, 1989).

The late adolescent (18 to 24 years of age) experiences a need for personal intimacy, according to Erikson (1963). With physical growth completed, they are functioning at the peak of their physical potential. Developing a true and mutual psychosocial relationship with another person, be it friendship, erotic encounters, or joint inspiration, at this stage is important to develop a healthy personality. Without such a relationship, the individual may suffer from severe feelings of isolation (Erikson, 1963).

Havighurst's (1972) developmental tasks for adulthood include selecting a mate, beginning a family, and assuming civic responsibilities. Young adults have the tasks of making an occupational choice and negotiating a successful transition from childhood to a clear sense of adult role

identity. They also must become minimally sensitive to criticism, conquer major fears, and establish sincere friendships. Sheehy (1976) links her hallmarks of well-being to Erikson's developmental stages. And Gallagher and Kreidler (1987) maintain that leaving the family home and establishing physical, financial, and psychological independence are a part of normal young adult development.

Table 14-2 compares several developmental theories of young adulthood. Most of the theorists emphasize the importance of forming a separate family unit from the family of origin as a means of establishing a firm identity. Because of the economy in the 1990s this task has become very difficult for some young people. Some choose to remain at home for extended periods to acquire education beyond high school in the hope that it will lead to job security (Figure 14-2). Some put off marriage and child bearing until they can attain financial security. Others marry and move home to establish an extended family network in one household. Nurses working with extended family networks need to be aware of the stressors inherent in the situation both to the young persons involved and to their middle-aged parents.

Spiritual Development

The adolescent who is a member of a family involved in an organized religious group will absorb historical and contemporary religious concepts believed by that group. **Spirituality** is not necessarily the same as religion. For some, participation in an organized religion may seem an empty action (Hill & Smith, 1990). The young person, searching for identity, may find stabilizing forces in rituals and religious practices outside of organized religion. During this period the vulnerable adolescent may be influenced by cults and very formalized sects, such as the Hari Krishna. Young adults, searching for a clear sense of identity, may reject parental values for a time as they attempt to define a personal philosophy. Spirituality is rarely fixed and may change throughout a lifetime. It may be defined as "a component of health related to the essence of life" (Hill & Smith, 1990, p. 184). Nurses must be able to set aside their own sense of spirituality to be able to

TABLE 14-2 Comparison of developmental tasks of young adulthood

Erickson's stages (1963)	Havighurst's developmental tasks for adulthood (1972)	Levinson's stages (1977)	Gould's stages (1972)	Sheehy's stages (1976)
Identity vs. confusion Commencing adult tasks Focusing on an occupation Reviewing of ideals and idols Preserving sense of continuity during psychologic turmoil Imposing a moratorium period if feasible **Intimacy vs. isolation** Undertaking specific affiliations Developing sexual relationships and achieving orgasm	**Early adulthood** Mate selection Learning to live with a partner in marriage Beginning a family Raising children Managing a home Starting an occupation Assuming civic responsibility Selecting a social group	**Separating from family (16-24)** Leaving family home and establishing physical, financial, and psychologic distance **Moving into adult world (20-27/29)** Exploring adult roles in interpersonal occupational areas; making provisional commitments and beginning to develop a life structure **Age 30 transition** Reevaluating and changing commitments **Settling down (28-32)** Making deeper commitments Achieving occupational fulfillment	**Ages (18-22)** Peer group support in separating from family Moving away from family with anxiety Receptive to new ideas **Ages 22-28** Feelings of autonomy and self-reliance Resolution of separating from family Opportunity for expansiveness, (i.e., living, growing, and building) **Ages 29-34** Feelings of doubt, questioning of activities Weariness about established status Reawakening of strivings Stressful marriage	**Pulling up roots (18-22)** Becoming part of a peer group Adopting a sex role Selecting an occupation Developing a world view/ideology Leaving home physically Beginning emotional distancing Deidealizing parental figures **Trying twenties (22-28)** Clearer definition of major goals Selecting a mentor Testing occupational and interpersonal relationships **Ages 30** Coping with restless feelings Reviewing relationships Becoming more introspective Searching for identity Increased awareness of mortality related to signs of biological aging **Rooting and extending (early thirties-mid-thirties)** Renewed moderation Committing and investing oneself

From *Nursing and health: Maximizing human potential throughout the life cycle* by L. Gallagher & M. Kreidler, 1987, Norwalk, CT: Appleton and Lange, p. 348. Modified from *Continuations: Adult development and aging* by L. Troll, 1982, Monterey, CA: Brooks-Cole and *Psychosocial caring throughout the life span* by I.M. Burnside, 1979, New York: McGraw-Hill. Adapted with permission.

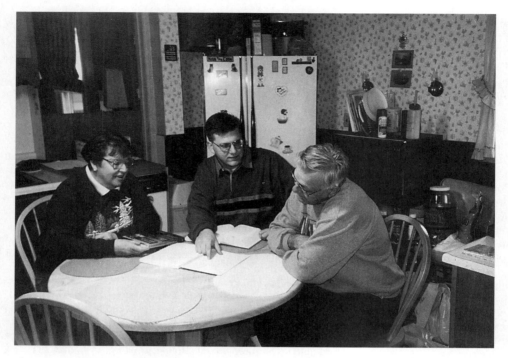

FIGURE 14-2 Young adult remaining at home to complete school.

assist a struggling young client trying to find meaningful answers for themselves.

HEALTH CONCERNS OF ADOLESCENTS AND YOUNG ADULTS
Acne

Acne is an inflammatory papulopustular skin eruption occurring usually in or near the sebaceous glands on the face, neck, shoulders, and upper back. Its cause is unknown but involves bacteria breakdown of sebum into fatty acids that are irritating to surrounding subcutaneous tissue (Glanze, Anderson, & Anderson, 1990). Sebaceous glands are mostly controlled by direct hormonal stimulation with androgens, derived from gonads in both sexes. If not treated or kept under control, the lesions may progress to a condition called **acne vulgaris,** characterized by noninflammatory papules called comedones. These may be in the form of blackheads or whiteheads. If closed, there is a possibility that the comedones may form cysts. These cysts can

cause permanent scarring (Thorn, Adams, Braunwald, Isselbacher, & Petersdorf, 1977). The initial stimulus to the formation of comedones is not known, but because it occurs predominantly in adolescents and young adults, it is viewed as a common health problem of individuals experiencing the hormonal changes connected with puberty.

Primary prevention. There is no method of prevention that completely eliminates the incidence of acne vulgaris. Some young people experience severe episodes; others do not. Educating 12- and 13-year-olds to cleanse the skin two or three times a day with warm water and a mild soap, encouraging them to shampoo daily, and advising them to drink lots of liquids will help them prevent the formation of closed comedones or cysts. No diet restrictions are indicated, but if the person notices that certain foods aggravate the acne, those foods should be avoided.

Secondary prevention. Should the acne progress to the formation of comedones, both the parents of the young adolescent and the older adolescent should be encouraged to obtain drying or peeling lotions that can be used overnight. In addition, prudent exposure to sun and wind will help keep the skin clean and dry. Comedone removal by the use of an extractor will assist in clearing the pores of possible infection (Vaughan, McKay, & Behrman, 1979).

Tertiary prevention. In the event that the acne becomes severe, the individual should be referred to a dermatologist. Incision and drainage can prevent scarring, and systemic antibiotics can be helpful. Because appearance is of great importance to young people trying to establish identity and intimate relationships, the young adult who has scars from acne vulgaris may be referred to a plastic surgeon. Scars can be removed by a fairly simple procedure.

Adolescent Kyphosis

Adolescent kyphosis, a mild curvature of the spine, is usually self-limiting and often undiagnosed. It may be precipitated by poor posture during a rapid growth spurt. If it progresses, it can lead to mild back pain and/or abnormal curvature of the thoracic spine (Glanze et al., 1990).

Primary prevention. Teach proper posture to young adolescents, most particularly girls in whom kyphosis seems more common. Teach spine stretching exercises and recommend sleeping without a pillow to prevent abnormal curvature from developing.

Secondary prevention. Any routine examination of an adolescent, particularly girls, should include screening for the development of adolescent kyphosis. Observe the individual for differences in the level of shoulders, scapula, and hips while standing erect. Observe from the side and back to assess abnormal curvature. Refer for medical evaluation if curvature is extreme or progressive.

Tertiary prevention. In some instances, a brace is recommended as a temporary measure during growth spurts. Teaching the reasons for compliance and encouraging daily stretching exercises will be helpful. Recommendation of maintaining good posture when sitting and standing should continue. If a medical evaluation determines that the young person has severe kyphosis or congenital scoliosis, teaching and counseling in collaboration with medical treatment may be indicated.

Adolescent Girls and Menstruation

Problems can arise for young adolescent girls during menstruation because of lack of information and hormonal imbalance. Among these problems are amenorrhea (delay in onset of menses), dysmenorrhea (cramping or back pain during menses), and anxiety about the whole process to name a few. Chapter 15 goes into detail about some of the nursing interventions that may be helpful.

Young Adults and Recurrent Infections

Young adults must be cautioned about maintaining prudent lifestyles. The need to excel in school or work two jobs to support a young family often causes excessive fatigue that can lead to a weakening of the immune system. Recurrent infections lead to lifetime problems. Young adults, perhaps no longer subject to parental prompting, may also need to be reminded to properly brush their teeth and get frequent dental checkups to prevent periodontal disease. Young women who suffer from debilitating premenstrual tension will need teaching and counseling to assist them to cope (see Chapter 15).

EMOTIONAL CONCERNS OF ADOLESCENTS AND YOUNG ADULTS

Failure to establish an identity during early adolescence can lead to periods of confusion and possible **alienation.** Failure to develop a close relationship during late adolescence may cause a sense of isolation (Erikson, 1963). Prolongation of either of these situations will place the individual at risk for depression and subsequent emotional disorders. Poor health, poverty, or disability may also lead to a chronic sense of hopelessness. It is crucial to identify prolonged depression in this age group. It is a time when emotions are acute and every failure is a disaster. The incidence of suicide among 12- to 19-year-olds is rising, and it is the third leading cause of death in 15- to 24-year-olds according to the Centers for Disease Control and Prevention.

Suicide

Primary prevention. Be particularly observant of young people who have vague chronic complaints of illness, particularly in a school setting. Be aware of adolescents who have repeated episodes of trauma (burns or accidents). Alert teachers to the danger of depression in young people who write notes and poetry on themes related to death. Consider strong intervention if the person begins giving away prized possessions. Be particularly alert if there is a family history of **suicide.**

Secondary prevention. Nurses who work in community settings, for example, emergency rooms, schools, and primary care settings, are the first to see young people who have made suicidal gestures. The parents and the individual must be made to understand that any suicide attempt is a serious and life-threatening event. No verbal threat of suicide or acting out behavior should be ignored, especially in this age group. Referral to crisis intervention centers and professional help for counseling can be very helpful, and, in some instances, prevent disaster.

Tertiary prevention. If a suicide attempt results in physical disability or death, ongoing counseling will be needed for the family and the peers of the individual involved. Support groups are available in some communities, and nurses should facilitate family access to them. Sometimes crisis intervention groups go into the schools to assist with grief counseling.

Eating Disorders

Anorexia nervosa occurs initially in adolescent females, but rarely occurs in males. It may begin with a major life change, such as moving away from home or a first sexual encounter (Gallagher & Kreidler, 1987). The onset can also be triggered by the start of menstruation. The cause of the disturbance remains unclear, although certain personality traits are frequently observed, such as a tendency toward perfectionism and obsessive-compulsive behavior. Evidence of an organic cause has been accumulated that may lead to the possibility of an abnormality of the hypothalmic-pituitary and end function in persons with the disorder (Whaley & Wong, 1987).

There is often a feeling of personal ineffective-

ness, an inaccurate confused interpretation of hunger stimuli, and a disturbance of body image and body concept (Bruch, 1976). The illness can be life threatening and requires aggressive intervention.

Primary prevention. Assess for dietary insufficiency young girls who exhibit extreme anxiety with a weight gain of 1 or 2 pounds. Follow their progress carefully to determine pathology. Confer with family members to further assess behaviors associated with anorexia nervosa, such as perfectionism, mood disturbances, or anxiety about a recent life change. Monitor for continued weight loss. Refer for medical assessment if weight loss is progressive to the point of poor nutritional status.

Secondary prevention. If the person is diagnosed as being anorexic, counsel him or her about the various services available. Often the most effective intervention is a behavior modification program in conjunction with ongoing individual and family therapy. Refer to support groups available in the area. Continue to monitor for continued weight loss. Should the condition progress to be life threatening and the young girl or boy develops secondary amenorrhea, bradycardia, or altered electrolyte status, refer for medical intervention and possible hospitalization.

Tertiary prevention. Medical intervention may include psychotherapy aimed at the resolution of the adolescent identity crisis, particularly as it relates to altered body image (Whaley & Wong, 1987). The young person and the family must be informed that excessive stress can bring on a recurrence of the disorder and that intermittent counseling and medical treatment may be lifelong in some persons.

Bulemia is characterized by binge eating. The young person rapidly consumes large amounts of food and then induces vomiting. He or she may also take laxatives and diuretics. Bulemia may accompany some of the behaviors of anorexia or exist as a separate behavior (Gallagher & Kreidler, 1987). Treatment is very similar.

ADOLESCENT SEXUAL DEVELOPMENT

Counseling about the normal progression of sexual development will assist the young adolescent and the young adult to progress through puberty with a minimum of anxiety. Information about sexually transmitted diseases (Chapter 20), the dangers of unwanted pregnancy, and the risk of acquiring the HIV virus may also discourage sexual risk-taking behavior. If a young person is known to be sexually active, information concerning safe sexual practices might prevent infection or pregnancy. Adolescents need information about all aspects of sexual development: the anatomy and physiology of normal development, concerns about masturbation, the menstrual cycle, and reproduction, to name a few. The nurse needs to be knowledgeable and informed about these topics to be able to assist young people through this difficult developmental stage.

ADOLESCENTS AND SPORTS

The potential benefit of a sports program to the development of youth is generally recognized. However, there is a flip side that is too often overlooked. The potential benefit is balanced by a potential danger to the vulnerable adolescent.

A well-managed youth sports program should help to build self-esteem, reinforce values and concepts such as teamwork and fair play, and aid the physical development of young participants. However, a poorly managed program — one that has not been well planned and carefully monitored by parents, teachers, and youth participants — can result in emotional abuse from poorly trained coaches and unnecessary physical injury to the youthful participants. There is evidence to suggest that some coaches model their behavior after media portrayals of coaches on adult professional teams. Coaches have a significant impact on vulnerable young people, and those same young people may be the ones who perform the most poorly. Self-esteem is the issue. Coaches with skill in the sport and effectiveness training are the most appropriate (Mellion, 1988).

In addition to considering the age-appropriateness of a particular youth sports program, the physical condition of each participant should be carefully evaluated. A complete physical examination should be required of each new member to make certain there are no physical problems that would mitigate against the young person's participation.

Some of the injuries to be concerned about in prepubertal and pubertal athletes are related to rapid growth spurts in long bones and connecting cartilages. Injuries involving the bony growth plate, particularly the knee, may cause epiphysites or apophysites. The most common result of recurring injury is **Osgood-Schlatter's disease,** which occurs at the insertion of the patella tendon and often produces painful hypertrophy of the tibial tubercle. The injury may respond to rest and immobilization, but in some cases surgical intervention will be necessary. Any injury to the knee should be carefully evaluated (Mellion, 1988). Another sports injury that presents a particular hazard to young athletes is **little leaguer's elbow.** Repetitive stress from overhead throwing will cause lateral compression and medial traction on the elbow. This can lead to abnormal growth of the bones of the elbow and/or permanent flexion contractions (American Academy of Orthopedic Surgeons, 1991). **Jumper's knee,** another disorder that may result from repetitive trauma (to the knee), may occur in connection with basketball, track, or gym-

THE BILL OF RIGHTS FOR YOUNG ATHLETES

Right to participate in sports

Right to participate at a level commensurate with each child's maturity and ability

Right to have qualified adult leadership

Right to play as a child and not as an adult

Right of children to share in the leadership and decision-making of their sport participation

Right to participate in safe and healthy environments

Right to proper preparation for participation in sports

Right to an equal opportunity to strive for success

Right to be treated with dignity

Right to have fun in sports

FIGURE 14-3 The bill of rights for young athletes. *From* Sports Injuries and Athletic Problems (1988) *by M. Mellion (Ed.), St. Louis: Mosby. Copyright 1988 by Mosby - Year Book, Inc. Reprinted by permission.*

nastics. Inflammation is usually resolved by rest and immobility. All overuse injuries are helped by stretching and reconditioning after the pain subsides. Resumption of the activity should not begin before the injured area is completely rehabilitated.

Nurses in schools and primary health settings can advocate for safe sports activity. If an injury occurs, a careful assessment, intervention, and appropriate referral should take place.

There is much pressure on today's young people to compete and develop their full potential. Youth sports programs can be safe and can benefit the development of the young participants if they are well planned by coaches, parents, and participating individuals. Figure 14-3 describes a Bill of Rights for Young Athletes. In particular it is well to remember that they have a right to play as a child and not an adult.

SUBSTANCE ABUSE IN ADOLESCENCE

Substance abuse has become a frightening phenomenon, particularly in urban areas of the United States. Increasingly, teens are involved in drug-related violent crimes not just because they take drugs but because they sell them.

DRUG-RELATED BEHAVIOR

Primary and general signs of drug abuse in the young person include:

- Decrease in quality of school work without a valid reason. Reasons given may be boredom, not caring about school, not liking the teachers.
- Personality changes, behaving in unexpected ways; becoming more irritable, less attentive, less affectionate, secretive, unpredictable, uncooperative, apathetic, depressed, withdrawn, hostile, sullen, easily provoked, oversensitive.
- Less responsible behavior, not doing chores or school homework, school tardiness or absenteeism, forgetful of family occasions such as birthdays.
- Change in activity, antisocial pattern, no longer participating in family activities, school or church functions, sports, prior hobbies, or organizational activities.
- Change in friends, new friends who are unkempt in appearance or sarcastic in their attitude; the youth is secretive or protective about these friends, not giving any information.
- Change in appearance or dress, in vocabulary, music tastes to match that of new friends, imitating acid rock and roll musicians.
- More difficult to communicate with, refuses to discuss friends, activities, drug issues; insists it is all right to experiment with drugs; defends rights of youth, insists adults hassle youth; prefers to talk about bad habits of adults. Irrational behavior, frequent explosive episodes, driving recklessly, unexpectedly stupid behavior.

- Unaccounted for loss from the home of money, credit cards, checks, jewelry, household silver, coins.
- Addition of drugs, clothes, money, albums, tapes, or stereo equipment that are suddenly found in the home.
- Presence of whisky bottles, marijuana seeds or plants, hemostats, and rolling papers. There may also be unusual belt buckles, pins, bumper stickers, or T-shirts, and the *High Times* magazine in the car, truck, or home.
- Preoccupation with the occult, various pseudoreligious cults, satanism, or witchcraft; and evidence of tattoo writing of 666, drawing of pentagrams on self or elsewhere, or misrepresentation of religious objects.
- Signs of physical change or deterioration; including pale face; dilated pupils; red eyes; chewing heavily scented gum; using heavy perfumes; using eye wash or drops to remove the red; heightened sensitivity to touch, smell, or taste; weight loss, even with increased appetite (marijuana smoking causes the "munchies"—extra snacking).
- Signs of mental change or deterioration, including disordered thinking or illogical patterns, decreased ability to remember or in rapid thought processes and responses, severe lack of motivation.

From *Nursing assessment and health promotion strategies through the life span* (4th ed.) (p. 368) by R. Murray & J. Zenter, 1989, Norwalk, CT: Appleton & Lange. Copyright 1989 by Appleton & Lange. Reprinted by permission.

In 1988, the firearm death rate for Black males aged 15 to 19 years reached an all-time high of 18 per 100,000, a 42% increase since 1984. Violence has become the leading cause of death for black males, aged 10 to 24 years. The data show a strong link between crime and alcohol or illegal drugs (Simons, Finlay, & Young, 1991). Lack of economic opportunity and the romanticizing of the drug culture by the media may be a part of the reason. Parents need to be educated to identify drug-related behavior in teens and young adults. The box on page 318 outlines some behaviors that may be seen in young persons experimenting with drugs. Permanent disability and/or involvement in drug-related crimes may result. Death can occur from some substances such as crack or cocaine. When they are made aware of this, young people and parents may modify their own behavior or intervene for their children.

Alcohol and tobacco are still being seen as health threats for many teens and young adults despite the efforts of the media and the schools to discourage their use. In a survey of 7891 ninth-grade students, researchers found the use of so-called legal drugs to be prevalent in all the schools. Forty-five percent of the students said they had used alcohol and 275 said they had used tobacco in the 30 days prior to being questioned. By comparison, 8% said they had used marijuana, 2% used cocaine, and 1% used steroids in the previous 30 days. The survey was carried out in 26 schools, both public and private. The researchers found that alcohol and tobacco use mirrored national statistics. Figure 14-4 demonstrates the findings.

Other findings from the study include the information that:

- Only small differences exist in the use by girls and boys. For instance, smokeless tobacco is almost exclusively used by boys.
- Tobacco use begins early. Sixty percent of those who had tried cigarettes reported having first smoked by age 12 years.
- Many more cigarette smokers reported using drugs and alcohol than did nonsmokers.
- Students said it was easy to obtain alcohol and cigarettes despite laws that restrict the sales.
- Most teen-agers obtained alcohol from their homes. When they did buy it at a store, they most often chose beer and wine coolers.
- Forty-four percent of the smokers said they had shoplifted cigarettes from counter-top displays.
- More than one-third of the students said they owned clothing labeled with cigarette ads. A quarter of them said they had received free packs of cigarettes in the mail. (Cummings, 1992)

It would appear that promoting tobacco-free and drug-free environments must start early in the lives of many individuals. For adolescents who wish to behave like adults, it makes sense to promote acceptance of a drug-free environment around them. Obviously strict enforcement of laws on the sale of cigarettes and alcohol to minors would help to prevent their consumption. Nurses can promote support groups in the

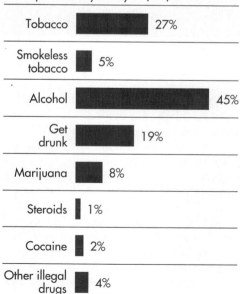

NINTH-GRADE DRUG USE

Survey of 7891 ninth-grade students from Erie County's public and parochial schools

In the past 30 days did you (use)...

Tobacco — 27%
Smokeless tobacco — 5%
Alcohol — 45%
Get drunk — 19%
Marijuana — 8%
Steroids — 1%
Cocaine — 2%
Other illegal drugs — 4%

FIGURE 14-4 Ninth grade drug use. *From* Survey of county teens *by M. Cummings, 1992, Buffalo, NY: Roswell Park Cancer Institute. Reprinted by permission.*

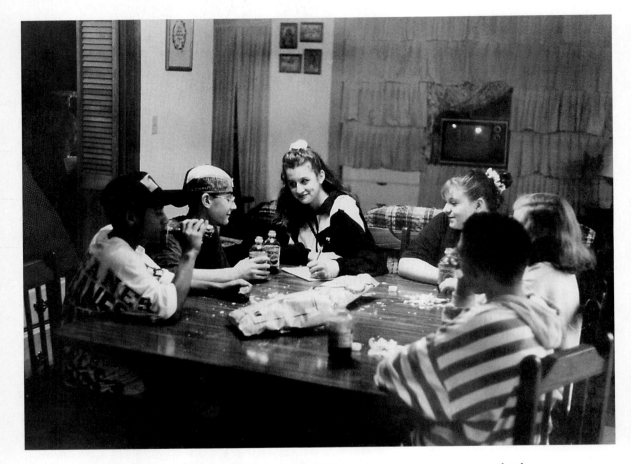

FIGURE 14-5   Group of junior high school students who sign contracts to support each other.

schools that make it worthwhile to stay drug-free. Figure 14-5 shows a group of junior high-school students who sign contracts to support each other. The school sponsors social events, counseling sessions, and educational sessions to assist them.

RISK TAKING BEHAVIOR IN ADOLESCENCE

Risk taking behavior may have tragic consequences for some. Increased violence among teenagers and young adults is of concern, especially in urban areas. Much of it seems to be connected with involvement in drug dealing and accessibility to weapons. Efforts to pass laws to stop drug dealing and control gun sales have received much publicity. The number of homicides and murders in the under-25-year-old group is much higher than ever before.

AIDS, a fatal disease not included in mortality and morbidity rates 10 years ago, is now an ominous threat. In spite of the publicity concerning its method of transmission, 1301 cases were reported in the United States in individuals 13 to 19 years of age as of June, 1993. For those between 20 and 24 years of age, 11,840 cases were reported (Centers for Disease Control and Prevention AIDS Surveillance Hotline). It is probable that most young adults in the 20- to 24-year-old group acquired the virus during adolescence, given the average 5- to 10-year period from initial HIV infection to AIDS diagnosis. Chapter 20 explains in detail primary, secondary, and tertiary interventions for nurses to use against AIDS.

SOCIAL CONCERNS RELATING TO ADOLESCENTS AND YOUNG ADULTS

"The number of adolescents without a defined role in society is growing, and these are our alienated youth" (Farrow, 1993, p. 509). The economic recession in the United States has effected access to health care. Thirty-one percent of all Americans are without health care (*Healthy People 2000*, 1990). Primary and secondary prevention are seldom sought when there is no ability to pay. Immunizations, counseling, and screening for potential health problems frequently does not happen.

According to a survey done in 1985, 445 nurses engaged in community health practice identified skill deficiencies related to adolescent health issues. In particular they were not comfortable with needs of psychosocial origin (Bearinger, Wildey, Gephart, & Blum, 1992).

Throughout the 1990s, the number of teenagers in the United States is estimated to increase to 24.1 million. Many of the health problems they experience increasingly are of psychosocial origin. The present Surgeon General's public remarks identify the problem of youth alienation, particularly in urban centers, as a public health issue (Farrow, 1993). Monitoring and assisting parents to understand the healthy emotional, moral, and spiritual development of adolescents and young adults is essential to their well-being, particularly in light of evidence that morbidity and mortality for them seems to relate increasingly to risk-taking behaviors.

Nurses need to be aware of health concerns specific to the age group, such as acne, adolescent kyphosis, recurrent infections, and possible depression. Suicide is the third leading cause of death in young people ages 15 to 24 years. Any suicidal gesture should not be ignored. Eating disorders, on the rise particularly in young adolescent girls, should be dealt with at a primary level if possible. Assessing for dietary insufficiency in young girls who express extreme anxiety over a weight gain of 1 to 2 pounds may be an effective way to begin. Counseling the adolescent and the young adult as to normal sexual development and the dangers inherent in risk-taking sexual behavior may prevent unwanted pregnancy and infection with human immune deficiency virus.

Early identification and anticipatory guidance to high-risk families, particularly in urban centers, and establishing accessible health clinics for adolescents where primary and secondary care and crisis intervention are available would seem to be an effective method for helping to upgrade wellness in adolescents and young adults, particularly those at high risk. Lobbying for such services and becoming aware of the changing health care needs occurring in the age group are a priority for nurses. This is especially true for those working in the community.

Chapter Highlights

- Adolescence begins at about 11 to 14 years of age in girls and 13 to 18 years of age in boys with the onset of puberty.

- Adolescence extends in developed countries to about age 24, young adulthood.

- Physical growth should be carefully monitored during this period because of rapid growth spurts to determine altered growth patterns.

- Health concerns such as acne and adolescent kyphosis should be dealt with at primary, secondary, and tertiary levels.

- Osgood Schlatter's disease, little leaguer's elbow, and jumper's knee can result from injuries incurred in sports activity.

- Coaches should be adept at building self-esteem in this vulnerable group and should not emphasize competition.

- Drug abuse, including alcohol and smoking, are considered high-risk behavior in this group.

- The causes of death in the 12- to 24-year-old age group have changed to violence and injury resulting from high-risk behavior. Alone among all age groups, they have not experienced a decrease in mortality.

- Nurses, working with youth, have identified a need for increased skills in the psychosocial area.

 CRITICAL THINKING EXERCISE

As a school nurse in a middle school you have noted an alarming increase in the number of sports injuries in the school since a new coach has been hired. The new coach is a former well-known successful basketball player who has no experience in education, although he has the credentials to be a coach. Speaking to him about your concerns has not been effective.

1. Prepare an appeal to the principal that expresses your concern. Include information about the injuries that could cause permanent damage.
2. Relate your positive thoughts about the kind of sports program that would be beneficial to the students. Include physical and developmental needs of both the boys and the girls.

REFERENCES

American Academy of Pediatrics. (1988). *Report of the committee on infectious diseases* (21st ed.). Elk Grove Village, IL: Author.

Bearinger, L., Wildey, L., Gephart, J., & Blum, R. (1992). Nursing competence in adolescent health: Anticipating the future needs of youth. *Journal of Professional Nursing, 8*(2), 80-86.

Bruch, H. (1976). Anorexia nervosa. In J. Gallager, F. Heald, & D. Garell (Eds.). *Medical care of the adolescent* (pp. 343). New York: Appleton-Century-Crofts.

Centers for Disease Control and Prevention. (1993). *HIV/AIDS surveillance report, 2nd quarter edition, vol. 5, no. 2.* Atlanta, GA: Department of Health and Human Services.

Cousins, J., Rubovits, D., Dunn, K., Reeves, R., Ramirez, A., & Foreyt, J. (1992). Family versus individually oriented intervention for weight loss in Mexican American women. *Public Health Reports, 107*(5), 549.

Cummings, M. (1992). *Survey of county teens.* Buffalo, NY: Roswell Park Cancer Institute.

Erikson, E. (1963). *Childhood and society.* New York: Norton.

Farrow, J. (1993). Youth alienation as an emerging pediatric health issue. *American Journal of Diseases in Children, 147*(5), 509.

Gallagher, L.P., & Kreidler, M. (1987). *Nursing and health: Maximizing human potential throughout the life cycle.* East Norwalk, CT: Appleton & Lange.

Glanze, W., Anderson, K., & Anderson, L. (Eds.). (1990). *Mosby's medical, nursing, and allied health dictionary.* St. Louis: Mosby.

Gortmaker, S., Must, A., Perrin, J., Sobol, A., & Dietz, W. (1993). Social and economic consequences of overweight in adolescence and young adulthood. *New England Journal of Medicine, 329*(14), 1008.

Havighurst, R.J. (1972). *Developmental tasks and education* (3rd ed.). New York: McKay.

Healthy People 2000. (1990). U.S. Department of Health and Human Services.

Hill, L., & Smith, N. (1990). *Self-care nursing: Promotion of health* (2nd ed.). Norwalk, CT: Appleton & Lange.

Hunter–Griffin, L.Y. (1991). *Athletic training and sports medicine of orthopedic surgeons.* Park Ridge, IL: American Academy of Orthopedic Surgeons.

King, E. (1984). *Affective education in nursing: A guide to teaching and assessment.* Rockville, MD: Aspen.

Maclean, W.E., & Grahm, G.G. (1982). *Pediatric nutrition in clinical practice.* Menlo Park, CA: Addison-Wesley.

Mellion, M. (Ed.). (1988). *Sports injuries and athletic problems.* St. Louis: Mosby.

Murray, R., & Zentner, J. (1989). *Nursing assessment and health promotion strategies through the life span* (4th ed.). Norwalk, CT: Appleton-Lange.

National Center for Health Statistics. (1987). *Health — United States.* (DHHS Publication No. PHS 84-1232). Washington, DC: U.S. Government Printing Office.

Piaget, J. (1963). *The origins of intelligence in children.* New York: Norton.

Sheehy, G. (1976). *Passages: Predictable crisis of adult life.* New York: Dutton.

Shils, M.E., & Young, V.R. (Ed.). (1988). *Modern nutrition in health and disease* (7th ed.). Philadelphia: Lea & Febiger.

Simons, J., Finlay, B., & Yang, A. (1991). *The adolescent young adult fact book. Children's defense fund* [pamphlet].

Surgeon general's report on nutrition and health. (1987). (Publication No. 88-50210). Washington, DC: U.S. Government Printing Office.

Thorn, G., Adams, R., Braunwald, E., Isselbacher, K., & Petersdorf, R. (1977). *Principles of internal medicine.* New York: McGraw-Hill.

U.S. Department of Health and Human Services, Public Health Service. (1991). *Healthy people 2000: National health promotion and disease prevention objectives, full report with commentary* (DHHS Pub. No. (PHS) 91-5212). Washington, DC: U.S. Government Printing Office.

U.S. Department of Health and Human Services, Public Health Service, Office of Disease Prevention and Health Promotion. *Prevention '93/'94.* Washington, DC: U.S. Government Printing Office, (in press).

Vaughan, V.C., McKay, R.J., & Behrman, R.E. (Eds.). (1979). *Nelson textbook of pediatrics* (11th ed.). Philadelphia: W.B. Saunders

CARING FOR WOMEN

Martha J. Yingling

The woman I am
   Hides deep in me
Beneath the woman
   I seem to be

Glen Allan

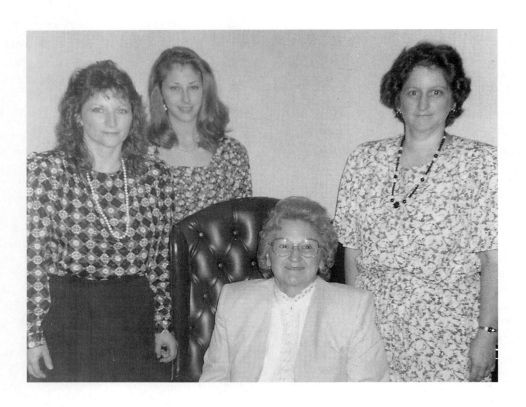

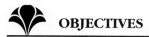 **OBJECTIVES**

At the conclusion of this chapter the student will be able to:

1. Identify the historical, social, political, and economics factors influencing women's health.
2. Apply the nursing process to women's health concerns in the community.
3. Identify the ways in which the nurse working in the community can meet the health needs of women in a variety of community settings.
4. State the role of the nurse in promoting self-concept and sexuality with the adolescent, midlife women, and pregnant women.
5. Discuss the reproductive hazards to women in the home and workplace.
6. Identify women who are most at risk for abuse and violence.

KEY TERMS

Body image
Menopause
National Women's Health Network

Office of Research on Women's
    Health
Sexuality

Women's health care movement
Women's Health Equity Act

Reproductive and gynecologic health care may be what most women seek when they enter the health care system. The special needs of women go beyond reproductive anatomy and function to include stresses associated with adolescence (image, peer acceptance), aging (menarche, loss), work, self-care (motivation and learning), abuse, sexuality, and more. This chapter will address the health needs of women from adolescence to old age. Evolution of women's health care, women's self-concept, sexuality, primary, secondary, and tertiary nursing care of women in the community. Reproductive hazards, and violence, abuse, and injury will also be discussed.

HISTORICAL, SOCIAL, AND POLITICAL FACTORS INFLUENCING WOMEN'S HEALTH CARE

An understanding of the historical, social, and political factors that affect women's health care is an essential component of community health nursing.

Historically, women have been perceived to be subservient, weaker, and less capable of self-direction than men (Kjervik & Martinson, 1986). Womens' health care has traditionally focused on reproductive anatomy and function and gynecologic needs. In 1870, Napheys wrote a book specifically for women who were married or about to be married. In the book he identified three phases in a woman's life: maidenhood, matrimony, and maternity. He also believed that a woman's physical makeup determined her destiny (Abrums, 1986; Napheys, 1870). In *Women: Their Diseases and Treatment,* a text for medical students and physicians, King (1896) stated that women's problems rose from the "sexual excesses" a woman was obligated to submit to during a marriage state. King also believed that most female complaints were associated with a sexual or reproductive disorder, a belief that was central to women's health care (Abrums 1986; King 1896). This belief still exists in many health care relationships today.

The Women's Movement of the 1960s and 1970s gave rise to the growth of the **women's health care movement** when groups of women's health activists "called attention to the failure of traditional medicine to deliver quality care to women" (Sloane, 1993). The women's health care movement grew rapidly, attracting large numbers of women who formed local groups of health collectives for the purpose of sharing their health experiences, increasing their knowledge about female anatomy and physiology; improving doctor-patient relationships, and identifying what constitutes quality health care. In the 1970s a group of health care activists founded The **National Women's Health Network,** a public interest group that currently represents more than 500,000 women. It is the most important national voice for women' health issues. (See box at top, right for a list of women's health issues.) The box at bottom, right lists the functions of the National Women's Health Network. During this time the traditional roles of women were being challenged. More women entered the workplace, which exposed them to new and varied stresses (Marieskind, 1980). Because of an increase in awareness and the changing roles of women, collaboration and an interdisciplinary approach are necessary to meet the health care needs of women. She also believes that the concepts of health promotion, disease and accident prevention, education for self-care, health risk identification, and coordination for illness care (when needed) are essential to the development of health care for women (Abrums, 1986). The 1990s have brought together the private and public sectors to address escalating health costs and the development of a strategy for improving the health of citizens during this decade. Some of the recommendations addressed were published in a document called *Healthy People 2000: National Health Promotion and Disease Prevention Objectives.* A summary of objectives related to women's health can be found in the box on page 327.

At the request of the Congressional Caucus for Women's Issues, in 1989 the General Accounting Office reviewed the National Institute of Health (NIH) policy about including women and minori-

---

WOMEN'S HEALTH ISSUES

- Quality of health care lacking for women.
- Women are subjects for new medical devices, surgical procedures, and drugs.
- Frequent, unnecessary, and excessive surgery is done.
- Increased managed pregnancies (ceasarean sections).
- Mental health is perceived as psychosomatic or psychotic.
- Women were seen as neurotic when treatment was requested.
- Solution to women's emotional problems was medication (Valium).

From *Biology of women* (3rd ed.) 1993, by E. Sloan, Albany, NY: Delmar. Copyright 1993 by Delmar Publishers Inc. Adapted with permission.

---

ties in clinical trials. The results of this study found that women and minorities were routinely excluded from these studies (Schroeder, 1993b). As a result, the Congressional Caucus for Women's Issues introduced the **Women's Health Equity Act,** a legislative package designed to bring women's access to health care, women's health care, and treatment and research in women's health into the twentieth century and to the forefront of American politics and science (Schroeder, 1993 p. 292; Bass & Howes, 1992). Because of their efforts, The **Office of Research On Women's Health** (ORWH) opened

---

FUNCTIONS OF THE NATIONAL WOMEN'S HEALTH NETWORK

- Monitors health policies affecting women.
- Distributes health information through a speaker's bureau, appearances on radio and TV programs.
- Publishes newsletter and resourse guides on various aspects of women's health.

From *Biology of women* (3rd ed.) 1993, by E. Sloan, Albany, NY: Delmar. Copyright 1993 by Delmar Publishers Inc. Adapted with permission.

SUMMARY OF *HEALTHY PEOPLE 2000* OBJECTIVES RELATED TO WOMEN'S HEALTH

- Reduce pregnancies among girls aged 17 and younger.
- Reduce overweight to a prevalence of 20% among people 20 years old and older, no more than 15% among adolescents aged 12 to 19 years, and 27% for women in general.
- Increase to 80% the proportion of women aged 40 years and older who have had a clinical breast examination and a mammogram.
- Increase by 50% the number of health promotions programs for students, faculty, and staff in postsecondary schools.
- Reduce hip fractures among people 65 years old and older.
- Increase by 30% the number of persons who regularly engage in light-to-moderate activity daily.
- Reduce rape and attempted rape of women aged 12 years and older.
- Reduce death rate for adolescents and young adults by 15%.
- Increase to 85% the proportion of people aged 10 to 18 years who have discussed human sexuality with their parents and/or have received information through another parent-endorsed source.

From: *Healthy people 2000: National health promotion and disease prevention objectives,* by the U.S. Department of Health and Human Services, DHHS Publication No. (PHS) 91-50212, 1991, U.S. Government Printing Office, Washington, DC.

1. Development of a women's health research agenda
2. Development of procedures to monitor NIH inclusion of women and minorities in clinical research studies
3. Recruitment and retention of women in clinical research studies
4. Recruitment and promotion of women in scientific careers
5. The establishment of the NIH Women's Health Initiative

A task force sponsored by the ORWH recommended a comprehensive plan for future directions for research on women's health. Financial support for the new research initiative and expansion of current studies to address priority areas in women's health came from the ORWH and increased funding from the federal government (Schroeder, 1993b). A summary of legislative action between 1990 and 1993 can be found in Table 15-1.

WOMEN'S ENTRY INTO THE HEALTH CARE SYSTEM

Women's entry into the health care system is influenced by a number of factors including perception of a need, the type of service needed (preventive, treatment), and the ability to pay for the service. Availability of services (time and transportation) and acceptability (language and cultural compatability) should also be considered as factors that impinge on women's access to the health care system (Chapin & Pereles, 1992).

Perception of a Need

Factors regarding women's health that are found consistently in the literature (Kjervik & Martinson, 1986; Chapin & Pereles, 1992) include the following:

- women use health services more often and for longer periods than men
- women report being sick more often than men
- women use more prescribed medications than men

Research has not shown how and why this is true, but a number of explanations have been of-

in September, 1990 (Massion, 1992). The ORWH goals included the following:

- Improve research related to diseases and conditions that affect women.
- Ensure that the NIH research adequately addresses women's health issues.
- Ensure that women are adequately represented in clinical research.

The initial efforts of the ORWH focused on five major areas (Massion, 1992):

fered. For example, women oversee the needs of their families and enter the health care system to meet those needs. They seek out preventive measures (immunizations), treatment for health problems, and help with sustentative care and rehabilitation (Kjervik & Martinson, 1986). Nathanson (1975) reported that the sick role is culturally more acceptable and compatible with the roles and responsibilities of women. He also stated that women's social roles are more stressful than men's roles, resulting in more illnesses for women (Kjervik & Martinson, 1986).

Women make more visits to a health care

TABLE 15-1   Summary of legislative action between 1990 and 1993

Year	Legislative action
1990	Mammography coverage under Medicare preserved
	Pap smears and mammographies made available to low-income women
1991	Office of Research on Women's Health (ORWH) opened
	Women's Health Equity Act expanded to include:
	• Office of Research on Women's Health at the Alcohol, Drug Abuse and Mental Health Administration
	• increased funding for research
	• improved federal standards for mammography screening facilities
	• reauthorizing the National Institute of Health (NIH) to include women and minorities in clinical trials and expand research on some vital women's health issues
1992	Funding for ORWH research on cancer, heart disease, and osteoporosis in older women from all races and socioeconomic groups increased
	Comprehensive gynecologic and obstetrical research program at the NIH funded
1993	The ORWH at the NIH permanently established
	Gag order lifted (information regarding family planning available again)

provider (physicians) than men, and the number of visits per year increases with age (Chapin & Pereles, 1992, p. 93). In addition, the types of physicians visited also varies with each age. For example, a survey of 2535 physicians found that women between the ages of 15 and 44 years visited general practitioners and gynecologist-obstetricians the most often, whereas women between the ages of 45 and 74 years visited general practitioners and internists more often. A summary of these visits can be found in Table 15-2 (Chapin & Pereles, 1992).

Women report being sick more often than men. Chapin and Pereles (1992, p. 95) reported that the differences in self-reported poor health may not reflect differences in illness rates but rather an inability to recognize illness. Not only do women live longer than men but they will live one third of their lives after menopause. They have more chronic diseases than men and are at increased risk for breast cancer, osteoporosis, anemia, eating disorders, autoimmune diseases (arthritis, Lupus), and chronic diseases such as diabetes, hypertension, and heart disease (p. 96).

Paying for Health Care

One of the major obstacles to health care for women is the inability to pay for the services. Women have fewer financial resources for health care and health maintenance and are more likely to be covered by public assistance health care programs (Chapin & Pereles, 1992). The number of women with private health insurance is slightly less than men, and women are less likely to have employment-related health insurance coverage (p. 97). Many women, particularly Hispanics, Blacks, and women who are widowed, separated, or divorced usually have public health insurance coverage (Medicaid) as their only source of coverage (p. 97). Type of work (part-time, self-employed workers, and those working in a small business) and escalating health care costs contribute to the increasing number of persons who are uninsured. Women hold more part-time jobs and more lower paying jobs with no coverage or with a lower level of insurance coverage than men (p. 97).

TABLE 15-2 Percentages of women making office visits

Type of practice	Age (yrs)				
	15 to 24	25 to 44	45 to 64	65 to 74	75 and older
General practice	34.0%	29.3%	33.4%	29.4%	30.7%
Internal medicine	6.0	8.2	14.9	18.8	22.0
Obstetrics/gynecology	28.1	29.2	7.0	2.4	0.8
Orthopedic	3.4	4.0	5.2	4.3	4.4

Adapted from "Women's access to the health care system", in *The women's health data book: A profile of women's health in the U.S.* (pp 93-107) by J.L. Chapin & S.A. Pereles, 1992, Washington, DC: The Jacobs Institute. Copyright 1992 by the Jacobs Institute of Women's Health.

Availability

Obstacles to accessing the health care system for women include lack of availability, time constraints, and lack of transportation. Almost 50% of the women in the U.S. labor force are mothers with children under 6 years old (Swanson & Albrecht, 1993). Time is especially problematic for urban women in accessing the health care system to meet their special health care needs and the health care needs of their families. A wide range of health care agencies and services are available to women in an urban setting, but most do not offer appointments at times that are accessible to working women. To seek health care, most women are required to take time off from work, a practice that most employers do not sanction. The problems of the women living and working in a suburban or rural area in accessing the health care system include time constraints and lack of transportation and availability. The availability of a wide range of health care providers and services may be lacking in suburban and rural areas, making it necessary for working women to seek help in urban centers. For both groups of women, loss of work time often results in loss of income. Women are confronted with the task of setting priorities in determining when and if they will enter the health care system.

Cultural Factors

Cultural values and beliefs are important factors to be considered when interacting with diverse cultural groups. The focal point for an effective therapeutic relationship begins with the nurses' understanding that the health beliefs and practices of a cultural group influence the way the group defines health. In addition, familiarity with common folk practices that are used by cultural groups to promote and maintain health, especially with regard to women's health, is an important factor in planning nursing intervention (Chapin & Pereles, 1992; Kozier, Erb, & Oliveri, 1991). See Chapter 3 for a more comprehensive discussion of culture and its impact on health.

THE NURSING PROCESS AND WOMEN'S HEALTH CARE

Wilkinson (1992, p. 3) states that the nursing process "provides the framework in which nurses use their knowledge and skills to express human caring." It is a special way of approaching client care for the purpose of promoting wellness, preventing illness, and restoring health. Both the nurse and the client benefit from the nursing process. For the client, nursing process provides continuity of care, individualized care, increased participation by the client, and assurance against omission or duplication of care. The nursing process helps the nurse increase self-confidence in the nursing role and meet the standards for nursing practice set by the American Nurses Association (ANA) and other standards set by specialty organizations such as Association of Women's Health, Obstetric, and Neonatal Nurses (AWHONN) (p. 12). The benefits of the nursing process become increasingly important to the nurse who is caring for women in a community health setting. It fosters effective communication between caregivers, clients, and families, thus supporting the benefits for the client and the nurse. The first step of the nursing process is assessment — collection of all data related to the client's health status. In addition to the information on an adult health history, the nurse uses an assessment especially targeted for women. The essential components of a health history targeted for women include the following:

1. Biographical data: age, marital status, number of children, nature of support system, occupation, and means of transportation
2. Perception of health status or the reason for seeking health care
3. History of present health status
4. Past health data including the following:

   - Childhood illnesses
   - Past surgeries/injuries
   - Menstrual history
   - Sexual history
   - Contraceptive history
   - Infertility history
   - Gynecologic history
   - Obstetric history

5. Family history
6. Review of systems
7. Health maintenance efforts (see box below, left)

8. Occupational/environmental history both at home and at work
9. Abuse assessment
10. Psychosocial history: body image, developmental stage, cultural aspects

A comprehensive assessment of women's health status can be very long and repetitive in some areas. The nurse should choose topics that are specific to the immediate health care needs of the client and should avoid repeating questions. The total assessment can be completed over time, with the most important questions being asked first. A listing of possible nursing diagnoses can be found in the box below, right.

MEETING WOMEN'S HEALTH CARE NEEDS IN THE COMMUNITY

Today's emphasis on cost containment measures has brought about the shift of health care from the hospital to the community (outpatient clinic, surgicenters, schools, workplace, and home) (Martinson & Widmer, 1989). The type of nursing care required by women in the community may include preventive health care, acute care, or chronic care. It can precede or follow acute care in an institutional setting, follow convalescent

---

QUESTIONS TO ASSESS WOMEN'S HEALTH PRACTICES

1. How often do you see a gynecologist or nurse practitioner for an examination and Pap smear?
2. Do you do a monthly self breast examination (SBE)?
3. What have you eaten during the past 24 hours?*
4. What vitamins or iron supplements do you take daily?*
5. How often do you exercise?

* Assess actions taken to prevent anemia and osteoporosis.

NANDA-APPROVED NURSING DIAGNOSES OF WOMEN'S HEALTH PROBLEMS

Body image disturbance
Self-esteem disturbance
Sleep pattern disturbance
Loss: spouse, reproductive function, or body part
Nutrition, altered: high risk for more-than-body requirements
Nutrition, altered: less-than-body requirements
Incontinence, stress (urinary)
Knowledge deficit
Altered growth and development
Hopelessness
Fear
Family coping, ineffective
Injury, high risk
Powerlessness
Rape-trauma syndrome
Role performance altered

DEFINING NURSES' ROLES IN WOMEN'S HEALTH CARE

Advocate: one who protects and supports a client's right to quality health care.

Caregiver: one who participates in nursing activity for the promotion, maintenance, and restoring of women's health status.

Change agent: one who purposefully and systematically implements change.

Counselor: one who gives guidance or assistance with problem solving.

Listening: a skill that involves both hearing and interpretation of what is said. It requires attention and concentration.

Role model: a person who inspires others to imitate his or her behavior.

Teacher: a provider of health-related information based on the client's needs.

TABLE 15-3 Summary of the women receiving preventive care

Type of preventive care	Percentage (%)
Blood pressure check	89
Clinical breast examination	67
Pap smear	65
Pelvic examination	64
Complete physical examination	61
Mammogram	56

Adapted from the commonwealth fund women's health survey: Selected results and comments by Warren H. Pearse, 1994, *Women's Health Issues* 4(1), 38-47.

care in a long-term setting, or be used in combination with out-patient care or in conjunction with respite care (Martinson & Widmer, 1989). The nurse working in the community is in a unique position to promote the health of women in a wide range of community settings. Using a variety of roles, the nurse can help women to meet their health care needs. The roles of the nurse are listed and defined in the box above.

PREVENTIVE HEALTH CARE AND WOMEN'S HEALTH

Pearse (1994) states that authorities agree that preventive care is the most important step in improving the overall health of the population: it is cost effective and a way to reduce rising health costs (p. 42). However, in a survey of 2500 women, fewer than two thirds of the women were found to have received the most basic preventive care (p. 43). A summary of women who received preventive services can be found in Table 15-3.

Health education is the principal nursing measure that is used in primary preventive nursing care for all clients. Women are receptive to health education because it leads to control of their bodies and promotes self-care. The nurse can focus the teaching-learning sessions on health-promoting behaviors that include health practices and health judgments. The teaching-learning sessions should be based on the needs of women, involve the family or significant others, and use a variety of teaching methods. The nurse assesses the women's ability to read and readiness to learn. Age, health status, language, and cultural influences are also important factors in a successful teaching-learning session. Mutually identified goals will be the basis for evaluating how much the women have learned (Craven & Hirnle, 1991).

Preventive health concepts can and should begin early in a woman's life. AWHONN's education committee has recently developed a flyer entitled "Teen's Guide to Women's Health" and recommends that it be used often. See the box on page 332 for the issues addressed in this flyer.

Since the Women's Health Movement in the 1960s and 1970s, women have been seeking information that will foster self-care and control over their own health. A change in philosophy, influenced by rising costs of health care, from treatment to prevention, has helped the growth in primary preventive measures and the amount of literature that is available to women. Health education and primary preventive measures can be found in the following community areas:

1. Schools: Both private and public schools have "the capability and responsibility to assist young people" in promoting health (Marcon-

TEEN'S GUIDE TO WOMEN'S HEALTH

It's your right and it just may save your life to have

- yearly check-ups with Pap smears after age 18 or when you become sexually active
- instructions for monthly breast examinations

Your health-care provider also can be available to answer your questions about sex, and provide

- help with decisions about whether or not to have sex
- testing for possible pregnancy and sexually transmitted diseases (STDs)
- advice on preventing pregnancy and decreasing your risk of getting a contagious disease while having sex
- help with unplanned pregnancy

You also can receive treatment for common problems including

- bladder infections
- vaginal yeast infections
- sexually transmitted diseases (STDs)
- problems with your menstrual periods and PMS
- help with problems like eating disorders; not eating right; feeling blue; sexual, physical, and mental abuse; family and boyfriend problems; and help with how to stop smoking, drinking alcohol, and taking drugs

And you can expect honest and accurate answers to any questions you have!

Prepared by the Association of Women's Health, Obstetric, and Neonatal Nurses *Consumer Education Committee*

---

tel & Chauvin, 1991, p. 171). Nurse educators in these settings can speak to adolescent health risks (injuries, both unintentional and intentional) and health risk behaviors (drug and alcohol use, unprotected sex, contraception). In addition, the nurse can address health concerns that affect the adolescent's self-concept (delayed onset of puberty, illnesses, developmental changes, nutritional status,

nesses, developmental changes, nutritional status, and physical changes) (Marcontel & Chauvin, 1991).

2. Hospitals in the community that provide outreach programs specific to the health care needs of women. These programs include both primary and secondary preventive activities. Participants in these programs are offered women's health education on topics of special interest to women (menopause, hormone replacement therapy, nutrition and exercise, and so on). Women have access to reference material (books, periodicals, videos, and brochures) and can get referrals when needed. Nurses working in these areas function as counselors, advocates, teachers, and role models.

3. Doctors' offices, HMOs, Planned Parenthood, women's clinics, and the workplace provide nurses with the opportunity to teach the client preventive care measures and to disseminate health related literature.

4. Preparation for admission to a hospital (preoperative teaching) can be taught in the home by the community health nurse. For example: Presbyterian Hospital, Charlotte, North Carolina, offers a prehysterectomy class for women scheduled for surgery. The class entitled "Understanding Your Hysterectomy" was started in 1992. As a result of this class, women became more self-directed with an increase in self-care, thereby decreasing the time spent on providing instructions (Vermillion, 1992).

5. Television, radio, and bookstores afford women the opportunity to learn positive health behaviors through special programing and a variety of literature.

6. Community voluntary services, including hotlines to provide counseling to battered women, rape victims, and those considering suicide (Swanson & Albrecht, 1993).

7. Since the 1970s women's health services and many self-help groups have emerged and new approaches to women's health care have been accepted.

8. The National Women's Health Network, which focuses on patient's rights, environmental safety, reproductive rights, and so on.

SUMMARY OF HEALTH RESOURCES FOR WOMEN

Adolescent Health Parents Too Soon
Illinois Department of Health
535 West Jefferson
Springfield, IL 62761
  provides information on teen pregnancy, healthy
  lifestyles, physical fitness, and HIV/AIDS prevention and care
Alan Guttmacher Institute
2010 Massachusetts Avenue
Washington, DC 20036
  public education in reproductive health and family planning
Food and Nutrition Center
Department of Agriculture
10301 Baltimore Boulevard
Room 304
Beltsville, MD 20705-2351
  provides information (videos, publications) about
  nutrition
National Coalition of Hispanic Health and Human
Services Organizations
1501 16th Street, NW
Washington, DC 20036-1401
  conducts national demonstration programs and
  contributes to the education and training of
  health professionals
Planned Parenthood Federation of America, Inc.
810 7th Avenue
New York, NY 10019
  sexuality education and family planning
National Women's Health Resource Center
2440 M Street NW
Suite 325
Washington, DC 20037
  education and information

Jacobs Institute of Women's Health
409 12th Street, SW
Washington, DC 20024
  education and health information and research
The American Fertility Society
1209 Montgomery Highway
Birmingham, AL 35216-2809
  information, education, and research
Resolve (National Office)
1310 Broadway
Somerville, MA 02144-1731
  infertility education, advocacy, and support
American Foundation for AIDS Research (AMFAR)
1515 Broadway, Suite 3601
New York, NY 10036-8901
  community and professional education
WARN (Women's AIDS Network)
P.O. Box 020525
Brooklyn, NY 11202
The following information on violence against
women:
National Council on Child Abuse and Family
Violence
1155 Connecticut Avenue, NW
Washington, DC 20036
National Displaced Homemakers Network
1625 K Street, NW #300
Washington, DC 20006
Sexual Assault and Domestic Violence Programs
6229 N. Charles Street
Baltimore, MD 21212
Batterers Anonymous
8485 Tamarind Avenue, #D
Fontana, CA 92335

The organization also undertook a special project to encourage health promotion among Black women. Self-help groups were established for the purpose of "raising the consciousness of women about the severity of and pervasiveness of Black women's health problems and to provide a comfortable, supportive atmosphere for women to explore health issues affecting them and their families" (Swanson & Albrecht, 1993, p. 248). A summary of health resources for women can be found in the box above.

Secondary Prevention For Women's Health Care

Screening, diagnosis, and treatment for existing health problems are the focus in secondary prevention. Screening activities include Pap smear and mammography for cancer, vision and hearing tests, and blood pressure tests. In the roles of teacher and counselor, the community health nurse can teach women how to do a breast self-examination by demonstrating the steps used and answering any questions that arise. The nurse will also recommend and encourage periodic screening for cancer as outlined by the American Cancer Society. New and innovative screening programs are being used among the socioeconomically disadvantaged, the elderly, rural populations, and racial and ethnic minorities—groups that are challenges for public health (McCoy, Khoury, Hermas, & Bankston, 1992). The University of Miami Mobile Mammography Program for the medically underserved women is such a program. This screening program has been in operation for the past 5 years and has been found to be cost effective and successful in reaching women who never before had a mammogram. Between September 1987 and December 1991, 12,456 women received mammograms. Seventy-two percent of the clients reported that this was their first mammogram (McCoy, et al., pp. 200-201).

The community health nurse's responsibilities regarding existing health problems include direct care as well as reviewing treatment modalities with the client and family such as the impor-

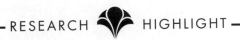

— RESEARCH ◆ HIGHLIGHT —

Mammographic Screening and Breast Cancer Risk

A Group Health Cooperative (GHC) in the western part of one state initiated a risk-based breast cancer screening program that included an invitation for screening subsequent to receipt of a survey that elicited data related to breast cancer risk factors, medical and screening history, and selected lifestyle behaviors. Based on self-reported risk factors, respondents were assigned to one of four risk categories: high, moderate, borderline, or no risk, which was conveyed in the letter of invitation along with a recommendation to perform monthly breast self-examination, to obtain an annual breast physical examination, and to appear for a mammogram at a specified interval (1, 3, 5 years) according to risk level.

The women (2422 of 2722) of this prospective study had reported no mammogram during the 1 year before being surveyed, were continuously enrolled at GHC, were between 50 and 79 years of age, were identified as high or moderate risk, and were given a minimum of 6 and maximum of 15 months to attend the center for their free screening examination. Reminders for attendance were not sent. The remaining 300 women and an additional 4498 women were not contacted (non-study subjects) and designated as no increased risk because their only risk factor was age.

In analyzing the 71% visitation rate for the association between participation in an organized screening program and six risk factors (age, family history of breast cancer, having a previous benign breast biopsy, nulliparity to age 30 years, early age at menarche, and late age at menopause) the hypothesis that those factors that might be readily identified by a woman as increasing her risk of breast cancer (*i.e.,* increased age, family history, and having needed a breast biopsy) would show positive associations with participation in screening was upheld. The sequence of factors in descending order was family history, previous biopsy, and age. In contrast, no association was found between participation and menopause at age 55 years or over, nulliparity to age 30 years, and menarche at age 10 years. This anticipated outcome, expressed as a hypothesis, was attributed to womens' decreased awareness that these factors increase their risk for breast cancer. The strongest association was between the risk category and participation in mammography. Increasing age was associated with participation only among women with moderate risk, a finding that was not consistent with previous reports that showed associations in the opposite direction. For high risk, participation was essentially the same or even slightly less among older women (60 to 79 years of age as opposed to 50 to 59 years). Because more women are living longer, and the incidence of cancer increases greatly with advancing age, primary care providers should use a variety of strategies to increase the rate of participation in screening programs by the elderly.

From "Breast cancer risk and participation in mammographic screening" by S. Taplin, C. Anderman, & L. Grothans, 1989, *American Journal of Public Health, 79*(11), 1494-1498.

tance of taking medications as prescribed and dietary restrictions. The nurse is also responsible for referring the women to agencies that will help to meet their health needs or to nurse practitioners and physicians who can offer the care needed (infertility control, abuse, or treatment for symptoms of menopause). An example of direct care given by the community health nurse is a multidisciplinary approach used in home care of the client who has had a mastectomy. On the day of discharge from the hospital, the community health nurse will visit the client to assess the client's status and to promote comfort. In the roles of caregiver, support person, teacher, and resource person, the nurse will facilitate the adjustment to the home environment and help to promote healing and recovery. The client will be referred to other health team members (social services, physician, or physiotherapist) as the need arises (Lesmond, 1990).

Tertiary Prevention For Women' Health Care

The community health nurse involved in tertiary prevention is concerned with rehabilitation and preventing the recurrence of health problems. Support and education are offered by the nurse to meet the health care needs of the client during this period. Referral to other health team members is done when necessary.

SELF-CONCEPT AND THE ROLE OF THE NURSE IN PROMOTING A POSITIVE SELF IMAGE

Body image, self-esteem, personal identity and role performance all play a role in how women perceive themselves (Craven & Hirnle, 1991). **Body image,** how one sees and feels about his or her body, is ongoing, subjective, and influenced by a variety of biologic, cultural, and social factors (Low, 1993; Craven & Hirnle, 1991, p. 1244). Adolescence, pregnancy, and menopause have been identified as critical periods in women's perception and feelings about their body (Low, 1993, p. 216; Marcontel & Chauvin, 1991). Although research and the literature concerning body image focus on diseases, surgery, eating disorders, and pregnancy, the diagnosis of body image disturbance can be applied to women with apparent good health who are dissatisfied with their body image (Low, 1993, p. 213).

Biologic Factors Affecting Body Image

Body build (height, weight), skin integrity, developmental changes, and actual or perceived unattractiveness are biologic factors that influences one's body image (Craven & Hirnle, 1991, p. 1244; Marcontel & Chauvin, 1991, p. 171). Adolescents are particularly vulnerable to the rapid changes that occur during this growth period (12 to 22 years). Low (1993, p. 216) states that physical appearance is especially important to adolescent girls in attracting friends and partners. Both young men and women are concerned about their self-image, but it is the young women who respond more often. The adolescent needs to accept the rapid body changes to establish a positive image. The combination of body changes and social pressures (dating, peer influence, role models, entry into junior high school) may have a negative impact on a girl's self-image resulting in such behaviors as chronic dieting, a behavior seen in 50% to 75% of all adolescent girls and adult women (Marcontel & Chauvin, 1991, Low, 1993).

The second critical period in a women's perception of her body image is pregnancy. Changes in body size, sensation, posture, movement, and feelings about the changes can be distressing for women, resulting in poor self-image (Flagler & Nichol, 1990, p. 269). A pregnant woman completes a rethinking and redefining of self to develop a maternal identity. The woman visualizes the ideal images, qualities, attitudes, and achievements of the ideal mother. For the actual self, the woman questions her behavior by asking such questions as How am I doing? The community health nurse interacting with the pregnant woman needs to assess the woman's understanding of the pregnancy and provide the information needed to support her. The nurse should also take time to point out something positive that the woman has done. For example: "You have done well with your weight gain, keep up the good work" (Curry, 1990). The body image provides structure and function to self concept.

Body changes occurring during pregnancy can be perceived as a threat, especially by the woman who knows little about the pregnancy. When working with pregnant women, the nurse has the opportunity to relieve anxiety and increase the women's knowledge about the changes in pregnancy (Flagler & Nicoll, 1990, pp. 269-270). For the pregnant adolescent who is coping with the developmental tasks of adolescence and peer pressure, the body changes of pregnancy can result in increased stress and a decreased self-concept. The nurse must remember that adolescence must be lived and not postponed or eliminated. Nursing intervention must focus on "supporting the completion of the adolescent process while providing prenatal care" (Reedy, 1991, p. 210).

Midlife is the third period in a woman's life that is critical to her well-being. Midlife is the period between ages 35 and 65 years, and this age group is the fastest growing segment of the population today (Garner, 1991). Midlife represents the more mature years between young adulthood but before the senior years and retirement (Frank, 1991, p. 421). It is during this time in women's lives that childbearing and menstruation end and myths about midlife, especially menopause, are rampant and generally unfavorable to women in our culture (Apbel, 1993, p. 1). Women during midlife are pictured as unattractive, depressed, and neurotic (p. 1); however, reality and myth do not mesh. Sarrell and Sarrell (1984, p. 255) state that one out of four women will not experience any major symptoms during menopause while the others will report one or more problems. The changes of midlife are both positive and negative. Women will experience more independence and increased interactions with others (family and friends), and for those who delayed childbearing to midlife, some may also have children (Apbel, 1993). Social class, cultural beliefs, economic background, educational level, and the media influence the way a woman will respond to the changes of midlife and menopause (Murray & Zentner, 1993). Aging accompanied by the symptoms of menopause (skin changes, hot flashes, headaches, fatigue, and nervousness) and the loss of reproductive function may result in a feeling of unattractiveness and/or

---

HEALTH CONCERNS OF WOMEN DURING MENOPAUSE

Heart disease
Cerebrovascular accidents (CVA)
Cancer:
    Lung cancer
    Breast cancer
    Reproductive system cancer
Alcohol and drug abuse
Accidents
Depression
Osteoporosis
Chronic diseases (arthritis, lupus)

---

uselessness. Those women who experience little or no problems often view this time as a period of freedom from menstruation and pregnancy, new vitality, and creativity while others feel it is a burden (Poorman, 1988; Low, 1993; Root, 1992). In addition to loss of reproductive function, women in this period of life are at increased risk for physical and emotional problems that also affect self-concept. See the box above for a list of health issues during midlife. Nursing strategies for women during midlife should focus on helping a woman to feel good about herself. Screening and education should be included to help women identify risk factors and to promote early diagnosis and treatment of any problem (Garner, 1991). Midlife and sexuality will be addressed later in this chapter.

Cultural and Social Factors Affecting Body Image

Women have faced criticism about their bodies from childhood to old age. Messages directly or indirectly sent to women pressure them to seek the "ideal" body weight (Lauer, 1990). Physical attractiveness is emphasized more in women than in men in the United States. Minority women face additional problems in identifying body image (Low, 1993, p. 214). For example, positive physical characteristics are identified by Caucasian standards, but this standard can decrease the woman's self-esteem and body image and "devalue" the woman's culture (Low, 1993, p. 214). An added stress for minority women is the pressure to conform to roles and beauty requirements of their culture (Low, 1993, p. 214). Another aggregate to consider when examining the changes in body image are lesbian women. In addition to those factors already mentioned, the lesbian woman is confronted with sexism and homophobia. Born female and in a society where homosexuality is not tolerated, the lesbian woman learns shame and guilt resulting in a negative self-image and feelings of being defective (Schoonmaker, 1993).

Historically, the changing ideal feminine figure has been identified by society, and women have been pressured to conform to an unrealistic standard (Low, 1993, p. 214). In today's society, the most influential message about an ideal body comes from the media (television and magazine advertisements) (Boering, 1991). Health risks that result from altered self-image may include chronic dieting, complications of cosmetic surgery, or other behaviors (sunbathing) used to reach and maintain the ideal body image (Low, 1993; Marcontel & Chauvin, 1991).

Role of the Nurse in Promoting Self-Concept

Murray and Zentner (1993, p. 375) stated that the role of the nurse is multifaceted. Effective use of the nurse's roles of teacher, counselor, role model, caregiver, and change agent creates a warm, accepting, supportive, and nonjudgmental relationship that fosters decision making in the adolescent and acceptance of body image in women of all ages. It is important for the nurse to listen to the patient as she expresses her concerns about her changing body image and to accept these concerns as an essential component to planning intervention. Some of the activities that would promote acceptance of body image and improve self-concept include letting teenagers identify the problem and encouraging women to choose entertainment that emphasizes the total woman (creativity, intelligence, and character) and does not focus on the media's portrayal of the "perfect woman" (Low, 1993). Exercise, focusing on internal sensations (massages, warm baths, physical closeness), and support groups are other activities the nurse can explore with women to promote a positive self-concept. In addition, the nurse can work through partic-

---

SUMMARY OF HEALTH MAINTENANCE ACTIVITIES TO PROMOTE WELLNESS IN MIDLIFE

- balanced diet with increased fiber
- decrease dietary fat
- increase exercise
- decrease alcohol and caffeine intake
- avoid/decrease use of medications
- relaxation techniques for stress reduction
- routine screening activities

Adapted from "Transition into midlife" by M. Frank, 1991, *Clinical Issues in Perinatal and Women's Health Nursing, 1*(3) 269-270.

---

ipation in professional organizations to establish agencies in the community that focus on the care of women. As an informed citizen, the community health nurse can become involved in activities that work to bring about change in the factors that affect women's self-concept (Low, 1993; Murray & Zentner, 1993). A summary of activities that promote health and self-concept can be found in the box above.

SEXUALITY

Sexuality has been defined by many experts in narrow terms. This definition has fostered two major misconceptions: 1) sexuality equals sex and reproduction, and 2) sexual learning is formal and has an agreed-on standardized content. This narrow definition of sexuality does not foster an understanding of the role that sexuality plays in the lifespan (Broering, 1991). It is the World Health Organization (WHO) that defines sexuality in much broader terms and allows for a holistic approach to nursing care. It states that sexual health is the "positive integration of somatic, emotional, intellectual, and social aspects of sexual being in ways that are positively enriching and that enhance personality, communication, and love" (Broering, 1991, p. 180; WHO, 1975).

Sexuality, a lifelong process, involves biologic functions, psychological factors, and sociocultural influences (Poorman, 1988; Bernhard, 1993; Broering, 1991). Biologic functions include the ability to give and receive pleasure (Broering,

1991, p. 180), and psychological factors include the woman's perception of self (body image) and her sexual identity. Sociocultural influences that affect a woman's sexuality include such things as the culture in which she lives, how she relates to the world around her, and how she chooses a sexual relationship (Broering, 1991; Bernhard, 1993).

Adolescence and Sexuality

The major task of adolescence is identity formation (Erickson's stage of identity formation versus identity confusion). During this period, the adolescent works toward a commitment to sexual orientation, takes on an ideological stance, and chooses a vocational direction (Poorman, 1988). Parents are devalued and the adolescent turns to peer groups and seeks out a heterosex-

ual partner (Poorman, 1988, p. 36). Teenage pregnancy, STD, and the lack of information regarding contraception are major problems confronting the adolescent. In the United States, most adolescents have become sexually active by the age of 19 years. By 1988 there was a 50% increase in teenage sexual activity. Sexual intercourse among teenagers is common and often unplanned, and the use of contraception is not usually considered. The number of sexually active adolescents who become pregnant each year is increasing; only 16% of these pregnancies were planned, and only 55% resulted in a birth. Among the reasons adolescents do not use contraception are lack of information about contraceptive methods, lack of availability of contraception, refusal to use contraception, and cost (Lommel & Taylor, 1992). The sexually active adolescent may prefer the

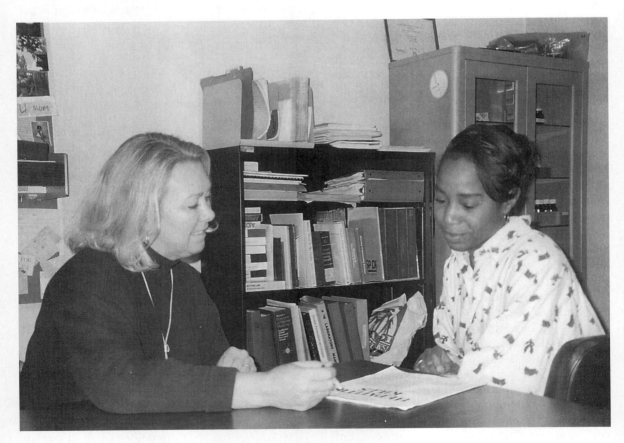

FIGURE 15-1   A student receiving counseling at a school health clinic.

risk of pregnancy rather than dealing with the immediate risk of not using birth control. Parental awareness, disapproval, and punishment for sexual activity are other reasons adolescents choose not to use contraception. In addition, selecting and using the correct contraceptive method requires partner involvement and cooperation. Nurses working in clinics, schools, doctors offices, or pediatric nurse practitioner offices, have the opportunity to identify the sexually active adolescents, provide counseling and education about high-risk behavior, help the adolescents make contraceptive decisions, and prescribe appropriate contraceptive methods (Lommel & Taylor, 1992; Keenan, 1991) (Fig. 15-1).

Nurses working in schools have the opportunity to participate in school-based sex education programs. Sex education in the schools is gaining new support. New surveys demonstrate a need for comprehensive sex education at earlier ages for today's youth and show a growing parental support for such a program (85% of United States adults favor such a program, up from 75% in 1975) (Broering, 1991, p. 182). The results of the 1988 National Adolescent Student Health Survey found that teenagers were not prepared to make informed decisions about their health. The Alan Guttmacher Institute (AGI) (1988, pp. 184-185) reported that only 17 states had mandatory sex education, each offering a variable program. A successful sex education program needs to combine organizational commitment, educational strategies, and the involvement of interested groups to plan and implement the program. Parent and community agency involvement would help in developing resources (financers, volunteers). Parental involvement will bring to the program family ideas, values, and attitudes and will enhance parent-child communication. Four levels of program development were identified by the AGI. They include state agencies, local school districts, professional educators (teachers & school nurses), and parent and community groups. Broering (1991, pp. 186-188) notes that while research is lacking to help us understand the way children are sexually socialized, influencing factors such as culture, family, peer group, and the media continue to contribute to child-

hood sexual learning. School-based sex education is a systematic approach to sex education intended to support the child's knowledge and is presented at a level that is consistent with the adolescent's cognitive development.

Midlife Women and Sexuality

The average age of **menopause** is 51 years, and fertility has ended if menstrual periods have stopped for 2 years or if the follicle stimulating hormone (FSH) is in premenopausal range (Root, 1992, p. 228). Women will experience and report a number of symptoms including hot flashes, numbness, palpitations, vertigo, headaches, fatigue, nervousness, insomnia, and depression, most of which will respond to hormone replacement therapy (HRT) (Poorman, 1988). As mentioned earlier, some women view this as freedom from menstruation and pregnancy, while others view menopause as the loss of sexuality and femininity (Bernhard, 1993). Most women will remain sexually active long after their ability or desire to have children diminishes. To prevent an unwanted pregnancy, the use of contraception for a period of 2 years if menses has stopped after age 50 years is recommended by some clinicians (Root, 1992). Research has shown that the incidence of elective abortion is higher between the ages of 40 and 50 years than at any other time of life except for the age of 15 years (Root, 1992, p. 228). More than 50% of pregnancies occurring after the age of 40 years ends in abortion (Root, 1992, pp. 228, 234). This is an opportune time for re-education and counseling. The community health nurse can help women make individual contraceptive choices, discuss STDs, and encourage them to examine how and why they made past decisions and to reflect on the consequences of those decisions.

Effective sexual counseling requires that the nurse has an understanding of and comfort with his or her own sexuality. Lack of a good knowledge base and the nurse's own developmental sexual history are two reasons why some nurses feel uncomfortable with sexual counseling. If nurses understand their own beliefs, values, and goals about sexuality and if their sexual experiences were positive, it will be easier to provide sexual counseling. Some nurses lack both knowl-

---

GUIDELINES FOR TAKING A SEXUAL ASSESSMENT

- be open to anything the woman may say
- be open to each woman's sexual orientation
- do not assume every woman is heterosexual
- learn what the woman has discussed with family or significant others
- identify the preferred types of sexual activity
- assess feelings and beliefs about gynecologic problems and health maintenance activities
- assess feelings regarding the effects of her problem on her sexuality and femininity
- assess feelings about childbearing

---

edge about gynecologic problems and surgery that affect sexuality and the techniques of sexuality counseling. Because many schools do not teach sexuality, the nurse should read current literature covering women's sexuality and other health-related issues to obtain the needed information (Bernhard, 1993). In sexual assessment each nurse must establish a unique personal style. With practice, the nurse can learn to be comfortable and consistent with data collection. The nurse's tone of voice, use of touch, and body language should communicate that the nurse is listening (Bernhard, 1993, pp. 253-254). Support of the nurse is perceived by the woman when she is encouraged to express her concerns and fears and they are acknowledged and included in the planning. Nurses working in women's clinics, offices, and women's health centers should include a sexual assessment for all women. A summary of guidelines for the nurse completing a sexual assessment can be found in the box above.

Reproductive Hazards

Reproductive hazards to women must be considered in the context of work and home environments. While 68% of women in the childbearing years work outside the home, a large number of women are fulltime homemakers and work at home, a place that has been traditionally considered "safe" (Ricci, 1990). Exposure to chemicals (metal, pesticides, anesthetic gases), physical hazards (ionizing radiation, hyperthermia), and bio-

logic hazards (infection, physical work) may result in infertility, spontaneous abortion, congenital anomalies, or transplacental carcinogenesis (Ricci, 1990, p. 227). Community health nurses are in a pivotal position to provide holistic care to women and their families in the home, community, and workplace by including an environmental and occupational history as part of their assessment. See the box below for a summary of an occupational/environmental health history. Analysis of this data will aid the nurse in identifying environmental health hazards affecting reproductive health. Through health education the nurse can help women identify the risks to reproductive health, identify their rights in the workplace, or refer women to the Federal Hazard Communication Standards Coordinator (Right-To-Know Coordinator) for further information. In the role of counselor, the nurse may assist the women by referring them for financial help or assisting women with grief work if an adverse reproductive outcome occurs.

The AWHONN (formerly NAACOG) publication *Reproductive Health Hazards: Women in the Workplace* (1985) states that nurses should work to educate legislators not to enact laws discriminating against women in the workplace. The legislator should be educated about the kinds and effects of workplace hazards that may in turn result in health-care policies that would promote the health of all concerned. See Chapter 27 for more information about Occupational

---

SUMMARY OF OCCUPATIONAL HEALTH HISTORY

- current occupation: describe job, work environment, number of years at the job
- past employment: describe full, part-time positions
- describe symptoms or illness related to work
- non-occupational behaviors that can affect health status such as smoking, drinking alcohol, certain hobbies, geographic area

Adapted from *Reproductive health hazards: Women in the workplace* by Association of Women's Health, Obstetric, and Neonatal Nurses, 1985, Washington, D.C.: Author.

Health Nursing and Chapter 29 for a discussion of environmental concerns.

VIOLENCE AND ABUSE OF WOMEN

Violence against women affects approximately 2 to 4 million women each year. Violence is the major cause of injuries to all women between the ages of 15 and 44 years. One out of every four households experience some form of domestic violence with 95% of the victims being women. Violence has become a major health issue (National Women's Health Report, 1993; Wolfe, 1991). The extent of abuse of women is not known. It is underreported in part because of threats, fear, feelings of guilt, and the stigma associated with the experience. Mounting evidence is showing that abuse of women may be the most common form of family violence during the perinatal period (King, et al., 1993, p. 163; National Women's Health Report, 1993). Current research studies of domestic violence and pregnancy show that rates of abuse of women during pregnancy ranges from 7% to 15% in the general population of pregnant women to 60% to 90% in the population of pregnant women who have a previous history of abuse (King et al., p. 164). Violence is nondiscriminatory; every woman is at risk, and most women experience more than one episode of violence. According to the American Medical Association (AMA), certain groups of women are at higher risk for abuse. They include women who are single, separated, or divorced, women between the ages of 17 and 28 years, women who abuse alcohol or drugs, women who are pregnant, or women whose partners are excessively jealous or possessive (NWHR, 1993, King et al., 1993). Stith (1991, p. 19) states that the most dangerous time for women is when they leave abusive situations or relationships. King et al. (1993, p. 163) state that violence can be categorized along a continuum ranging from emotional and psychologic abuse and harassment to homicide. A summary of the kinds of abuse experienced by women can be found in the box above. Violence of the older woman is a growing problem that is also underreported and not adequately recognized by clinicians (DeLorey & Wolf, 1993, p. 173). Living arrangements, age, health, lifestyles, and mobility

---

SUMMARY OF TYPES OF ABUSE WOMEN EXPERIENCE

Physical abuse: recurrent, increases in severity pushing, shoving, slapping, kicking
- assault with a weapon
- restraining
- refusing help

Emotional or psychological abuse: may precede or accompany physical abuse
- threats of physical harm
- isolation
- jealousy or possessiveness
- deprivation, intimidation, humiliation
- constant criticism

Sexual abuse: may include any form of forced sex or sexual degradation

Adapted from National Women's Health Report, September/October 1993, National Women's Health Resource Center 15(5): 1-3.

---

are factors that make older women vulnerable to violence (p. 175). See Chapter 31 for further discussion of abuse and violence.

Nursing Care-Violence and Abuse of Women

Nurses working in the community (clinics, doctor's offices, women centers, or schools) have the opportunity to identify women who are experiencing abuse and violence. Using their skills in assessment, therapeutic communication, counseling, advocacy, and referral, the nurse can work to promote the welfare of women by minimizing the effects of ongoing violence and teaching measures that would prevent violence. In the role of caregiver, the nurse is aware of the difficult choices women must make as they evaluate their relationships. An empowerment model of intervention as identified by King et al. (1993, p. 165) is the most effective approach for abused women. Using this approach, women's choices and the means to achieve their goals are respected. Nursing intervention includes primary, secondary, and tertiary measures. The goal of primary intervention in an abusive situation is to decrease the incidence of violence and abuse of women. The major focus is identifying abused women and increasing an awareness of the problem of violence and abuse at the group and community level. Secondary intervention includes assessing the abused woman and implementing an appropriate plan of care. Helping the abused woman in making long-term plans, providing continuous support for her decisions, and making effective referrals are all a part of tertiary intervention. In addition, the nurse needs to develop an awareness of how a woman's cultural perspective affects her response to abuse and nursing intervention (King et al., 1993; Delorey & Wolf, 1993).

Chapter Highlights

- Legislative action is being undertaken to promote women's access to health care and treatment.

- The Office of Research On Women's Health opened in September 1990 to ensure that women were represented in clinical research studies and that such studies adequately address women's health issues.

- Women's access to health care is hindered by availability of service, time, and cost.

- Women who are single, divorced, widowed, or are minorities have fewer resources for health care related to type of work and salaries.

- The community health nurse uses the roles of caregiver, teacher, counselor, advocate, and role model in meeting the health care needs of women.

- The nurse working in the community can be found in women's clinics, schools, doctor's offices, and hospital outreach programs.

- Nursing activities used by the community health nurse in meeting the health care needs of women include primary prevention, secondary prevention, and tertiary prevention.

- The roles of counselor, teacher, and advocate are effective tools the community health nurse can use to promote a positive body image and increased self-concept.

- Prevention of problems related to poor body image and decreased self-concept should be a focus of nursing intervention.

- There are three critical periods in a woman's life: adolescence, pregnancy, and midlife. The community health nurse is in a unique position to help women cope with the problems associated with each of these periods.

- The number of women experiencing violence and abuse is on the rise, especially the elderly.

- An empowerment model of intervention is the most effective approach for abused women.

 CRITICAL THINKING EXERCISE

Mrs. S. has recently undergone a mastectomy. On returning home she has developed an infection in her incision. A community health nurse has been requested to visit her daily to help her to change the dressings and assist her to promote healing. Mrs. S. has recently experienced menopause and between that and the mastectomy she is sure her husband will no longer be interested in her. Mr. S. seems attentive and concerned; he is very anxious about his wife's health.

1. Write several questions you might ask the woman concerning possible symptoms she might be experiencing related to menopause and not to her mastectomy.

2. How might you assist her in regaining her self-esteem?

REFERENCES

Abrums, M. (1986). Health care for women. *Journal of Obstetrics, Gynecology and Neonatal Nursing,* May/June, 250-251.

Apfel, R. (1993). Midlife: Triumph of hope over experience. *Developments: Center for Women's Development 2*(1), 1-5.

Association of Women's Health, Obstetric, and Neonatal Nurses (1985). *Reproductive health hazards: Women in the workplace,* Washington, D.C.: Author.

Bass, M., & Howes, J. (1992). Women's health: The making of a powerful new public issue. *Women's Health Issues,* Spring, *2*(3), 3-5.

Bernhard, L. (1993). Sexual counseling of women having gynecological surgical procedures. *Clinical Issues in Perinatal and Women's Health Nursing, 4*(2), 250-257.

Broering, J. (1991). Childhood sexual learning and sex education in schools. *Clinical Issues in Perinatal and Women's Health Nursing, 2*(2), 165-178.

Brundage, J., & Pachaloski, C. (1991). Guiding young women's health. *Clinical Issues in Perinatal and Women's Health Nursing, 2*(2), 191.

Campbell, J., Oliver, C., & Bullock, L. (1993). Battering during pregnancy. *Clinical Issues in Perinatal and Women's Health Nursing, 4*(3), 343-345.

Chapin, J.L., & Pereles, S.A. (1992). Women's access to the health care system. *The women's health data book: A profile of women's health in the U.S.,* Washington, D.C.: The Jacobs Institute of Women's Health, 93-107.

Chill, J., & Nightingale, E.O. (1991). Physicians and the basic human rights of women. *Women's Health Issues.* Washington, D.C.: The Jacobs Institute of Women's Health. *2*(4), 6.

Craven, R., & Hirnle, C. (1991). *Fundamentals of nursing: Human health and function.* Philadelphia: J.B. Lippincott.

Curry, M.A. (1990). Stress, social support and self-esteem during pregnancy. *Clinical Issues in Perinatal and Women's Health Nursing, 1*(3), 309.

Davis, H., et al. (1992). Culturally competent healthcare: AAN expert panel report. *Nursing Outlook,* Nov./Dec. *40*(6).

DeLorey, C., & Wolf, K. (1993). Sexual violence and older women. *Clinical Issues in Perinatal and Women's Health Nursing, 4*(2), 173-179.

Flagler, S., & Nicoll, L. (1990). A framework for the psychological aspects of pregnancy. *Clinical Issues in Perinatal and Women's Health Nursing, 1*(3), 269-270.

Frank, M.E.V. (1991). Transition into midlife. *Clinical Issues in Perinatal and Women's Health Nursing, 2*(4), 421.

Freeman, S.B. (1991). Management of perimenopausal symptoms. *Clinical Issues in Perinatal and Women's Health Nursing, 2*(4), 429.

Garner, C. (1991). Midlife women's health. *Clinical Issues in Perinatal and Women's Health Nursing, 2*(4), 473-481.

Hewitt, J.B., Misner, S.T., & Levin, P.F. (1993). Health hazards of nursing: Identifying workplace hazards and reducing risks. *Clinical Issues in Perinatal and Women's Health Nursing, 4*(2), 320.

Hibbard, J., & Pope, C. (1987). Women's roles, interest in health and health behavior. *Women and Health, 12*(2), 67-84.

Holt, K.A., & Langlykke, K. (Eds.). (1993). *Comprehensive adolescent pregnancy services: A resource guide.* Arlington, VA: National Center for Education in Maternal and Child Health.

Keenan, T. (1991). Adolescent health care and school-based clinics. *Clinical Issues in Perinatal and Women' Health, 2*(2), 956.

King, J. (1896). *Women: Their diseases and treatment* (7th ed). Cincinnati: John N. Scudder's Sons.

King, M.C., Campbell, D., Sheridan, D., Ulrich, Y., & McKenna, L.S. (1993). Violence and abuse of women: A perinatal health care issue. *Clinical Issues in Perinatal and Women's Health Nursing, 4*(2), 191.

Kjervik, D., & Martinson, I. (1986). *Women in health and illness: Life experiences and crisis.* Philadelphia: W.B. Saunders.

Kozier, B., Erb, G., & Oliveri, R. (1991). *Fundamentals of nursing: Concepts, process, and practice.* (4th ed). Reading, MA: Addison-Wesley.

Lauer, K. (1993) Transition in adolescence and its potential relationship to bulemic eating and weight control patterns in women. *Holistic Nursing Practice 4,* 8-16.

Lesmond, J. (1990). Homecare of mastectomy patients. *Home Health Care, 4*(4), 6.

Lommel, L., & Taylor, D. (1992). Adolescent use of contraceptives. *Clinical Issues in Perinatal and Women's Nursing. 3*(2), 199.

Low, M.B. (1993). Women's body image: The nurse's role in promotion of self-acceptance. *Clinical Issues in Perinatal and Women's Health Nursing, 4*(2), 213-219.

Lynch, M. (1993). When the patient is also a lesbian. *Clinical Issues in Perinatal and Women's Health Nursing, 4*(2), 196.

Marcontel, M., & Chauvin, V. (1991). Adolescence: Implications for preventive health care in schools. *Clinical Issues in Perinatal and Women's Health Nursing. 2*(2), 165-178.

Marieskind, H.I. (1980). *Women in the health system: Patients, providers, and programs.* St. Louis: Mosby.

Martinson, I.M., & Widmer, A. (1989). *Home health care nursing.* Philadelphia: W.B. Saunders.

Massion, C. (1992). Report on the National Institute of Health's Office of Research on Women's Health. *Health Form, 2*(1), 2.

McCoy, C.B., Khoury, E., Hermas, L., & Bankston, L. (1992). Mobile mammography: A model program for medically underserved women. *Women's Health Issues, 2*(4), 196-211.

McFarlane, J. (1993). Abuse during pregnancy: The horror and the hope. *Clinical Issues in Perinatal and Women's Health Nursing, 4*(3), 350.

McKenzie, S. (1992). Merger in lesbian relationships. *Women and therapy.* pp. 151-159, Binghamton, NY: Hayworth.

Murray, R.B., & Zentner, J.P. (1993). *Nursing assessment and health promotion: Strategies through the lifespan.* (5th ed). Norwalk, CT: Appleton & Lange.

Myeroff, W. (1993-1994). Caring for the young and restless. *Graduating Nurse,* 24-27.

Naphey, G. (1870). *The physical life of women: Advice to maiden, wife and mother* (4th ed). Philadelphia: George Macleon.

Nathanson, C. (1975). Illness and the feminine role: A theoretical review. *Social Sciences and Medicine 9,* 57-62.

National Women's Health Report. (1993). Violence against women. *National Women's Health Resources Center 15*(5), 1-3.

Pearse, W.H. (1994). The commonwealth fund women's health survey: Selected results and comments. *Women's Health Issues, 4*(1), 38-47.

Poorman, S. (1988). *Human sexuality and the nursing process.* Norwalk, CT: Appleton & Lange.

Redland, A. (1993). Strategies for maintenance of health-promoting behaviors. *Nursing Clinics of North America, 28*(2), 421.

Reedy, N.J. (1991). The very young pregnant adolescent. *Clinical Issues in Perinatal and Women's Health Nursing, 2* (2), 210.

Ricci, E. (1990). Reproductive hazards in the workplace. *Clinical Issues in Perinatal and Women's Health Nursing, 1*(2), 226-239.

Root, W. (1992). Contraception for midlife women. *Clinical Issues in Perinatal and Women's Health Nursing, 3*(2), 227.

Sarrell, L., & Sarrell, P. (1984). *Sexual turning points: The seven stages of adult sexuality.* New York: Macmillan.

Schoonmaker, C. (1993). *Aging lesbians: Bearing the burden of triple shame.* Binghamton, NY: Hayworth.

Schroeder, P. (1993a). In touch. *The Jacobs Institute of Women's Health Newsletter, 1*(1), 1-4.

Schroeder, P. (1993b). We've come a long way, maybe: Women's health and the 103rd congress. *Nursing and Health Care. 14*(6), 292-293.

Schroeder, P. (1992). Women's health: A focus for the 1990s. *Women's Health Issues. 2*(1).

Shalala, D. (1993). Nursing and society: The unfinished agenda for the 21st century. *Nursing and Health. 14*(6).

Sloane, E. (1993). *Biology of women.* (3rd. ed.). Albany, NY: Delmar.

Solberg, S. (1989). Women and their mental health: A social reflection of society's expectations and pressures. *Recent Advances in Nursing, 25,* 92-109.

Stith, S. (1991). Women at risk: The victim profile. *Violence Against Women,* 18-20.

Swanson, J., & Albrecht, M. (1993). *Community health nursing: Promoting the health of aggregates.* Philadelphia: W.B. Saunders.

Thompson, C.A. (1992). *Lesbian grief and loss issues in the coming out process.* Binghamton, NY: The Hayworth Press.

U.S. Department of Health & Human Services: *Healthy people 2000: National health promotion and disease prevention objectives: full report, with commentary,* DHHS Publication No. (PHS) 91-50212, 1991, US Government Printing Office, Washington, DC.

Vermillon, S.L. (1992). Presbyterian Hospital. Charlotte, N.C. Poster presentation. AWHONN National Meeting, Minn.

Wilkinson, J. (1992). *The nursing process in action.* Reading, MA: Addison-Wesley.

Wilton, J., & Noonan, M.D. (1991). A menopause center: Bridging the midlife gap. *Clinical Issues in Perinatal and Women's Health Nursing, 2*(4), 57.

Wolf, L. (1991). The epidemiology of battering. *Violence Against Women,* 14-17.

World Health Organization. (1975). *Education and treatment in human sexuality: The training of health professionals.* Report of WHO meeting. Technical report series, #372. Geneva.

CARING FOR MEN

Don Sabo

If you can fill the unforgiving minute
  With sixty seconds' worth of distance run—
Yours is the earth and everything that's in it,
  And—which is more—you'll be a man, my son!

Rudyard Kipling

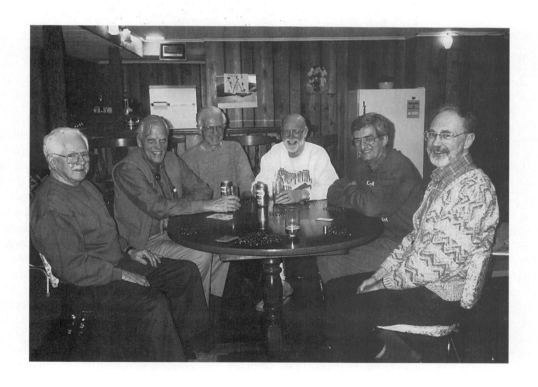

OBJECTIVES

At the conclusion of this chapter the student will be able to:

1. Define key terms listed.
2. Discuss the development of research on men's health and illness.
3. Discuss how changing gender relations influence the patterns of men's health and illness.
4. Identify major issues pertaining to men's health.
5. Describe selected theories of men's health and illness.
6. Identify connections between gender identity and health-related behaviors.
7. Discuss how men's health risks vary among different male groups.

KEY TERMS

Critical feminist theory	Gender order	Sex
Gender	Homophobia	Sex role theory
Gender identity	Masculinity	

Community health nurses usually find more widows in their service population than widowers. The educated public is also aware that men generally do not live as long as women. School nurses are often made painfully aware that adolescent males are prone to early death by suicide and automobile accidents. Public health educators are calling for early detection and prevention of testicular cancer and prostate cancer. Health care planners in some urban settings are likely to know that the life expectancy and health status of poor, inner-city, African-American men are lower than the male populations of some developing countries. AIDS advocates and educators recognize that, although women and heterosexuals are also at risk for HIV transmission, it is homosexual and bisexual men who are at highest risk for contagion. Nurses and physicians in clinical settings sometimes encounter a tendency among male patients to exhibit a tough posture that fosters denial of the seriousness of an illness.

These observations suggest that certain aspects of men's health and illness differ from those of women. Why do gender differences exist in relation to morbidity and mortality? To what extent do biologic differences between the sexes contribute to men's greater susceptibility to certain forms of illness? How do elements of men's psychology, conformity to masculine stereotypes, and cultural practices shape men's health and illness? What aspects of masculinity are conducive to health? This chapter presents research findings, discussions, and a conceptual framework that will help answer these and other questions about men's health. Readers will explore how gender identity and the **gender order** influence the patterning of men's health risks, the ways men perceive and use their bodies, and men's psychosocial adjustments to illness itself.

Some definitions need to be clarified before discussing how gender influences men's health and illness. Whereas **sex** refers to biologic aspects of a person's physical and genetic identity, **gender** refers to expectations and behaviors that individuals learn about femininity and masculinity. **Gender identity** can be understood as a person's inner sense of himself or herself as being womanly, manly, feminine, or masculine. In this chapter, gender identity is seen as an outgrowth of a historically changing pattern of relations between men and women and cultural definitions of masculinity and femininity. In this context, gender identity is better understood as a process than as a "thing" that people "have" (Messner & Sabo, 1990). We learn our gender identities from others in varying social, cultural, and historical contexts and, as we move from one stage of life to another, we make decisions about accepting or rejecting a wide array of cultural scripts for masculinity and femininity that supply direction, role models, props, motivations, rewards, and values (Sabo, 1994a; West & Zimmerman, 1987). The scripting of masculinity, as we see in this chapter, contributes to men's health and illness.

MEN'S HEALTH AND THE STUDY OF GENDER

Beginning in the 1960s, initial thinking about gender and health issues was grounded in the sociocultural model that challenged the prevailing biologic determinism and reductionism of the traditional biomedical model. Critics of the biomedical model cited its mechanistic approach, the overemphasis on biochemical processes, and overly simplistic explanations that attribute disease to one or two specific etiologic factors. Proponents of the sociocultural model, in contrast, argued that health and illness are best understood primarily in light of cultural values and practices, social conditions, and human emotion and perception. Holistic conceptions of health and illness have been elaborated by nursing theorists such as Newman, Parse, and Rogers.

The development of the sociocultural model during the 1960s set the conceptual stage for rethinking health and illness in light of gender. At first, researchers followed a basic "add and stir" approach, which treated gender as just another demographic variable for identifying health patterns and risk factors. The additive approach

proved useful in epidemiologic research that uncovered differential rates of illness between males and females or across male populations subgrouped by domain sociological variables such as race, ethnicity, socioeconomic status, or residential area. For example, descriptive research findings revealed that men experience more life-threatening diseases and die younger than women, women experience more non–life-threatening illnesses and live longer than men; women also see doctors more frequently than men. By the late 1970s, gender had become accepted as a standard demographic variable to be included in epidemiologic research. A growing body of research findings made it evident that variations in women's and men's health could not be adequately accounted for by biomedical explanations alone. It was also increasingly evident that sociocultural explanations of health and illness were not complete unless gender was taken into account.

During the 1970s and 1980s, researchers developed more comprehensive theoretical approaches to understanding linkages between gender and health issues. Many of the advances in theory and research on gender and health were fostered by the women's health movement and the growth of feminist scholarship. The knowledge and spirit generated by the women's health movement is illustrated by the work of the Boston Women's Health Collective. Their book, *Our Bodies, Ourselves: A Book by and for Women,* first published in 1969, entreated women to learn more about their bodies, medical practices and beliefs, and the workings of the medical system. The authors emphasized a holistic approach, preventive strategies for maintaining health, self-help, and a woman-centered critique of the male-dominated healthcare delivery system. (For latest edition, see Boston Women's Health Collective, 1993.)

Academic researchers studied different ways that gender socialization influenced perceptions of illness and adjustments to death. Sex discrimination in the healthcare delivery system and sex inequality in the health professions were documented. Feminist historians documented the oppression of women healers by the male-dominated clergy and physicians during the Middle

Ages (Ehrenreich, 1989), while feminist philosophers of science argued that medical science was tainted by patriarchal and male-centered biases (Daly, 1978). Sexism and structured sex inequality were believed to lead to the misdiagnosis and maltreatment of women (Cooperstock, 1971; Scully & Bart, 1981). By the mid-1980s, the growing importance of gender in understanding patterns of health and illness was an undeniable presence in epidemiology, medical sociology, and interdisciplinary studies of psychosocial aspects of illness (Stillion, 1986).

The Emerging Focus on Men's Health

One limitation of most of this pioneering scholarly work was that until only recently, researchers tended to equate the study of gender and health to studies of women's health and illness. While women were in the research spotlight, men remained backstage. Even men who were affiliated with the American "men's movement," which emerged in the early 1970s, were slow to cultivate awareness around men's physical health issues. There were not tens of thousands of men signing up to join the men's movement in the early 1970s. The first national conference of the men's movement was held in the summer of 1973 in Louisville, Kentucky, and annual "men and masculinity" conferences have occurred since then. The 1980s saw the growth of men's movements in the United States. The followers of Robert Bly's "mythopoetic men's movement," for example, use chants and drumming to help men get in touch with the cultural roots of masculinity. The National Organization for Men against Sexism (NOMAS) struggles against sexism and explores gender issues as varied as men's violence against women, men and spirituality, reproductive rights, men and pornography, homophobia, bisexuality and gay rights, and men's health.

Some of the early work on men and masculinity by Marc Feigen-Fasteau (1974) and Warren Farrell (1975) did make connections between conformity to traditional masculinity and men's emotional and physical health. In 1980, physician Sam Julty published *Men's Bodies, Men's Selves,* which pulled together a biomedical tour of male physiology and medical hygienic concerns with basic commentary on masculine psychology. Others focused on men's sexual and emotional health. For example, Michael Castleman (1980) couched his therapeutic suggestions for men to transform their sexual conduct and experiences within a critique of traditional masculinity. In the 1980s, scrutiny of men's health issues got a boost from scholarly dialogue under areas variously dubbed the *study of men and masculinity, men's critique of gender,* or the *new men's studies* (Brod, 1987; Kimmel & Messner, 1994).

Scholarly and public interest in men's health have increased in the 1990s. Sabo and Gordon (in press) have called the emerging research and writing on men's health and illness *men's health studies.* Magazines such as *Men's Health* and *Men's Fitness* are selling and a variety of news/documentary television shows have begun to focus on men's health issues.

In summary, scholars and researchers have been slow to study connections between gender and men's health and illness. The growing influence of the sociocultural model in mainline social science, the development of holistic conceptions of health in nursing theory, feminist theory, and research, and the emergence of men's health studies have helped to foster new ways of looking at men's health issues.

MEN'S OVERALL HEALTH STATUS

When British sociologist Ashley Montagu put forth the thesis in 1953 that women were naturally superior to men, he shook up the prevailing chauvinistic beliefs that men were stronger, smarter, and better than women. His argument was partly based on epidemiologic data that males are more vulnerable to mortality than females from before birth and throughout the life span.

Mortality

From the time of conception, men are more likely to succumb to prenatal and neonatal death than females. Men's chances of dying during the prenatal stage of development are about 12% greater than females and, during the neonatal (newborn) stage, 130% greater than females. A number of neonatal disorders are common to males but not females, for example, bacterial infections, respiratory illness, digestive diseases,

TABLE 16-1 Infant mortality rate* for males and females

Year	Both sexes	Males	Females
1940	47.0	52.5	41.3
1950	29.2	32.8	25.5
1960	26.0	29.3	22.6
1970	20.0	22.4	17.5
1980	12.6	13.9	11.2
1989	9.8	10.8	8.8

* Rates are for infant (under 1 year) deaths per 1000 live births for all races.
Adapted from *Monthly Vital Statistics Report,* Vol. 40, No. 8, Supplement 2, January 7, 1992, p. 41.

and some circulatory disorders of the aorta and pulmonary artery. Table 16-1 compares male and female infant mortality rates across time. Although the infant mortality rate decreases over time, the persistence of the higher rates for males suggests that biologic factors may be operating. Table 16-2 shows that males have higher mortality rates than females per 100,000 in every age category from under 1 year through over 85 years. Table 16-3 presents data on the 10 leading causes of death in the United States in 1989. Male mortality rates are higher than female rates in every category except for diabetes.

Females have greater life expectancy than males in the United States, Canada, and postindustrial societies (Verbrugge & Wingard, 1987; Waldron, 1986). This fact suggests a female biologic advantage, but a closer analysis of changing trends in the gap between women's and men's life expectancy indicates that social and cultural factors related to lifestyle, gender identity, and behavior are operating as well. Life expectancy among American females is about 78.3 years but is 71.3 years for American males (National Center for Health Statistics, 1990). As Waldron's (in

TABLE 16-2 Death rates by age and sex: 1960-1991

Age	Sexes	1960	1970	1980	1990	1991
Under 1 year:	Male	3,059.3	2,410.0	1,428.5	1,037.5	1,007.2
	Female	2,321.3	1,863.7	1,141.7	831.2	790.5
1-4 years:	Male	119.5	93.2	72.6	48.7	48.9
	Female	98.4	75.4	54.7	39.4	44.5
5-14 years:	Male	55.7	50.5	36.7	29.1	28.8
	Female	37.3	31.8	24.2	18.8	19.0
15-24 years:	Male	152.1	188.5	172.3	156.1	160.8
	Female	61.3	68.1	57.5	50.8	52.2
25-34 years:	Male	187.9	215.3	196.1	205.6	201.1
	Female	106.6	101.6	75.9	73.4	73.6
35-44 years:	Male	372.8	402.6	299.2	306.1	311.3
	Female	229.4	231.1	159.3	138.1	135.8
45-54 years:	Male	992.2	958.5	767.3	600.9	598.2
	Female	526.7	517.2	412.9	332.6	325.6
55-64 years:	Male	2,309.5	2,282.7	1,815.1	1,507.5	1,503.6
	Female	1,196.4	1,098.9	934.3	877.5	854.7
65-74 years:	Male	4,914.4	4,873.8	4,105.2	3,358.5	3,307.3
	Female	2,871.8	2,579.7	2,144.7	2,002.1	1,971.7
75-84 years:	Male	10,178.4	10,010.2	8,816.7	7,950.2	7,663.1
	Female	7,633.1	6,677.6	5,440.1	4,941.7	4,862.2
Over 85 years:	Male	21,286.3	17,821.5	18,801.1	17,521.6	17,150.9
	Female	19,008.4	15,518.0	14,746.9	13,727.5	13,328.4

Adapted from *Monthly Vital Statistics Report,* Vol 40, No. 13, September 30, 1992.

TABLE 16-3   Leading causes of death for males aged 15 to 34 years: United States, 1991

Cause	No. deaths	Percentage (%)
Unintentional injury	23,108	32
Homicide	13,122	18
Suicide	9,434	13
HIV infection	8,661	12
Cancer	3,699	5
Other	13,234	19
		100*

* Percentages do not add up to 100 due to rounding.
Adapted from *Morbidity and Mortality Weekly Report,* Vol. 43, No. 40, October 4, 1994.

press) analysis of shifting mortality patterns between the sexes during the twentieth century shows, however, women's relative advantage in life expectancy was rather small at the beginning of the twentieth century. During the mid-twentieth century, female mortality declined more rapidly than male mortality, thereby increasing the gender gap in life expectancy. Whereas women benefitted from the decreased maternal mortality, the mid-century trend toward a lowering of men's life expectancy was slowed by increasing mortality from coronary heart disease and lung cancer that were, in turn, mainly a result of higher rates of cigarette smoking among males.

The most recent trends show that differences between women's and men's mortality decreased during the 1980s, that is, female life expectancy was 7.9 years greater than males in 1979 and 6.9 years in 1989 (National Center for Health Statistics, 1992). Waldron explains that some changes in behavioral patterns between the sexes, such as increased smoking among women, have narrowed the gap between men's formerly higher mortality rates from lung cancer, chronic obstructive pulmonary disease, and ischemic heart disease. In summary, it appears that both biologic and sociocultural factors are involved with shaping patterns of men's and women's mortality. In fact, Waldron (1976) suggests that gender-related behaviors rather than strictly biogenic factors ac-

count for about three fourths of the variation in men's early mortality.

Morbidity

While females generally outlive males, females report higher morbidity rates even after controlling for maternity. National health surveys show that with the exception of injuries, females experience acute illnesses such as respiratory conditions, infective and parasitic conditions, and digestive system disorders at higher rates than males do (Givens, 1979; Cypress, 1981; Dawson & Adams, 1987). Men's higher injury rates are partly a result of gender differences in socialization and lifestyle, for example, learning to prove manhood through recklessness, involvement in contact sports, working in risky blue-collar occupations.

Females are generally more likely than males to experience chronic conditions such as anemia, chronic enteritis and colitis, migraine headaches, arthritis, diabetes, and thyroid disease. However, males are more prone to develop chronic illnesses such as coronary heart disease, emphysema, and gout. Whereas chronic conditions do not ordinarily cause death, they often limit activity or cause disability.

After noting gender differences in morbidity, Cockerham (1995) asks whether women really do experience more illness than men, or whether it could be that women are more sensitive to bodily sensations than men or that men are not as prone as women to report symptoms and seek medical care. He concludes that the best evidence indicates that the overall differences in morbidity are real and, further, that they result from a mixture of biological, psychological, and social influences (p. 42).

THEORIES OF MEN'S HEALTH AND ILLNESS

Efforts to explore how gender influences men's health derive from the sociocultural model and gender theory that underpin interdisciplinary studies of health and illness. Theories of gender help to explain men's health and illness in several ways.

Gender, Nature, and Nurture

The nature versus nurture debate has infused much thinking about differences in gender identity and behavior. Biologistic thinkers have argued that gender differences are "natural" in origin, deriving from instinctual, hormonal, morphologic, neurologic, or phylogenetic endowments. Proponents of the nurture thesis, in contrast, contend that gender differences are learned through socialization, social conditioning, or cultural adaptation. By developing an integrated theoretical view, some researchers point toward the border crossings between biogenetic and sociocultural explanations of variations in women's and men's health. While recognizing women's biologic propensity for greater life expectancy, for example, Waldron (1986) shows how trends toward decreased alcohol consumption during the 1980s were more marked among females than males and, consequently, were responsible for increases in men's mortality from chronic liver disease and cirrhosis.

Sex Role Theory

Sex role theory calls attention to the lethal aspects of the male role. In the words of Harrison, Chin, and Ficarrotto (1992, p. 282),

It is time that men especially begin to comprehend that the price paid for belief in the male role is shorter life expectancy. The male sex-role will become less hazardous to our health only insofar as it ceases to be defined as opposite to the female role, and comes to be defined as one genuinely human way to live.

Sex role theorists generally see **masculinity** as an inner, psychic, process that is tied to an outer web of sex roles and gender expectations.

FOUR MAJOR COMPONENTS OF THE TRADITIONAL MALE ROLE

1. No Sissy Stuff: the need to be different from women.
2. The Big Wheel: the need to be superior to others.
3. The Sturdy Oak: the need to be independent and self-reliant.
4. Give 'Em Hell: the need to be more powerful than others, through violence if necessary.

From "The male sex role" by R. Brannon, 1976, in *The forty-nine percent majority*, (pp 1-45) by D.S. David & R. Brannon (Eds.). Reading, MA: Addison-Wesley.

Gender socialization influences the extent to which boys adopt "masculine" behaviors that, in turn, can affect their susceptibility to illness or accidental deaths. A "give 'em hell" approach to life can lead to hard drinking and fast driving that account for about half of male adolescent deaths. That some men feel the need to be a sturdy oak and to avoid any signs of feminine dependency may contribute to the denial of symptoms and reluctance to visit physicians (see box below).

Critical Feminist Perspectives

Critical feminist theory recognizes that gender identity "develops and persists as a social, economic, and political category" (Anderson, 1988, p. 320). Many of the role expectations and psychological traits attached to masculinity in the current gender order such as aggressiveness, ambition, success-striving, virility, asceticism, and competitiveness are intricately tied to men's preoccupation with power over others and attempts to impose their definitions of reality on others.

Social scientists have long observed that social inequality influences the types and patterns of health and illness. Freund (1982) contends that power is the central feature of social organization that is related to differences in health. Health is thus conceptualized as an important and complex component of social inequality. The quality of health is viewed as an inherently valuable resource that is unequally distributed in various social hierarchies such as economic, political, racial, age, and gender hierarchies.

Health can also be understood as an important social resource for attaining and maintaining status in social hierarchies (Frank, 1991). Those at the bottom of the American class hierarchy, for example, have the highest rates of disease and disability, which, in turn, erodes their capacity to compete within the larger economy (Dutton, 1989). Powerful groups can attribute inferior health to less powerful groups as a justification for their oppression: the diagnosis of upper-class women as hysterical by the male-dominated medical profession during the nineteenth century enhanced men's patriarchal status and authority in the family and society; the labeling of prostitutes as criminals and carriers of sexually transmitted disease heightens their political and economic marginalization in relation to middle-class women or men (Ehrenreich, 1989).

Critical feminist analyses build on the premise that social inequality and power struggles profoundly inform gender relations and health outcomes. In addition to sex role theory's focus on gender identity, socialization, and conformity to role expectations, critical feminist thinkers emphasize that power differences shape relationships between men and women, women and women, and men and men. They also contend that gender identity and behavior are not simply imposed on individuals by socialization, but that individuals actively participate in the construction of their gender identity and behavior. Gender identity is actively worked out, revamped, and maintained by individuals who are immersed in socially and historically constructed webs of power relations. Sabo (1990), for example, found that men's persistent denial after a wife's mastectomy tended to bring back or conserve the old, pre-mastectomy relationship and, in effect, worked against a woman's urgings for interpersonal and marital change.

An integration of biomedical explanations, sex role theory, and critical feminist perspectives can help explain the complexities pervading men's health and illness. Just as there are differences between men's and women's health, variations also exist across subgroups of men.

MASCULINITIES AND MEN'S HEALTH

There is no such thing as masculinity; there are only masculinities (Sabo & Gordon, in press). A limitation of early gender theory was its "categoricalism" or its treatment of all men as a single, large category in relation to all women (Connell, 1987). The fact is, however, that all men are not alike, nor do all male groups share the same stakes in the gender order. At any given moment, there are competing masculinities — some dominant, some marginalized, and some stigmatized — each with their respective structural, psychosocial, and cultural moorings. Community health nurses need to recognize and assess the substantial differences between the health options of homeless men, working-class men, underclass men, homosexual men, men with AIDS, prison inmates, men of color, and their comparatively ad-

vantaged middle- and upper-class, white, professional male counterparts. Similarly, they must be aware that a wide range of individual differences exist between the ways that men and women act out femininity and masculinity in their everyday lives. Health profiles of several male groups are discussed next.

Adolescent Males

Pleck, Sonenstein, and Ku (1992) applied critical feminist perspectives to their research on problem behaviors and health among adolescent males. A national survey of adolescent, never-married males aged 15 to 19 years were interviewed in 1980 and 1988. Hypothesis tests were geared to assessing whether "masculine ideology," which measured the presence of traditional male role attitudes, put boys at risk with an array of problem behaviors. The researchers found a significant independent association with seven of ten problem behaviors. Specifically, traditionally masculine attitudes were associated with being suspended from school, drinking and use of street drugs, frequency of being picked up by the police, being sexually active, the number of heterosexual partners in the last year, and tricking or forcing someone into having sex. These kinds of behaviors, which are in part expressions of the pursuit of traditional masculinity, elevate boys' risk for sexually transmitted diseases, HIV transmission, and early death by accident or homicide. At the same time, however, these same behaviors can also encourage victimization of women through men's violence, sexual assault, unwanted teenage pregnancy, and sexually transmitted diseases.

Adolescence is a phase of accelerated physiologic development, and community health nurses are aware of the importance of good nutrition. Obesity puts adults at risk for a variety of diseases such as coronary heart disease, diabetes mellitus, joint disease, and certain cancers. Obese adolescents are also likely to become obese adults, thus elevating long-term risk for illness. National Health and Nutrition Examination Surveys show that obesity among adolescents increased by 6% between 1976 and 1980, and 1988 and 1991. While 22% of females 12 to 18 years old were overweight between 1988 and 1991,

20% of males were so (*Morbidity and Mortality Weekly Report,* 1994b).

Males are also a majority of the estimated 1.3 million teenagers who run away from home each year in the United States. For both boys and girls, living on the streets raises the risks for poor nutrition, homicide, alcoholism, drug abuse, and AIDS. Young adults in their 20s constitute about 20% of new AIDS cases and, when the lengthy latency period is calculated, it is evident that they are being infected in their teenage years. Runaways are also more likely to be victims of crime and sexual exploitation (Hull, 1994).

Men of Color

Patterns of health and illness among men of color can be partly understood against the historical and social context of economic inequality. Generally, because African Americans, Hispanics, and Native Americans are disproportionately poor, they are more likely to work in low-paying and dangerous occupations, live in polluted environments, be exposed to toxic substances, experience the threat and reality of crime, and worry about meeting basic needs. Cultural barriers can also complicate their access to available health care. Poverty is correlated with lower educational attainment, which, in turn, mitigates against adoption of preventive health behaviors.

The neglect of the public health in the United States is particularly pronounced in relation to African Americans (Polych & Sabo, in press). For example, in Harlem, where 96% of the inhabitants are African-American and 41% live below the poverty line, the survival curve beyond the age of 40 years for men is lower than that for men living in Bangladesh (McCord & Freeman, 1990). The probability for African-American men to die between 15 and 60 years of age is 30%, a figure in excess of that for men in such impoverished nations as Gambia, India, and El Salvador (Polych & Sabo, in press).

Although African-American men have higher rates of alcoholism, infectious diseases, and drug-related conditions, for example, they are less likely to receive health care and, when they do, they are more likely to receive inferior care (Gibbs, 1988; Bullard, 1992; Staples, 1995). The failure to meet the health needs of minority chil-

---

YOUNG AFRICAN-AMERICAN MALES: AN "ENDANGERED SPECIES"

- The number of young African-American male homicide victims in 1977 (*N* = 5734) was higher than the number killed in the Vietnam War between 1963 and 1972 (*N* = 5640) (Gibbs, 1988:258).
- Homicide is the leading cause of death among young African-American males. The probability of a Black male dying from homicide is about the same as a White male dying from accidents (Reed, 1991).
- More than 36% of urban African-American males are drug and alcohol abusers (Staples, 1995).
- In 1993 the AIDS rate for African-American males aged 13 years and older was almost five times higher than the rate for Caucasian males. (*Morbidity and Mortality Weekly Report,* 1994b).

---

dren escalates the cost of care incurred later in life. A longitudinal study of men enlisted in the Navy who averaged age 23 years showed that African-American men had higher rates of hospitalizations than Asian Americans, Caucasians, Native Americans, and Malyasians (Hoiberg, Berard, & Ernst, 1981). The researchers explained that the higher rates of hospitalization for African-American males were partly because they had not received comparable medical care as children and adolescents, thus increasing longer-range risk for illness as young adults. Statistics like those in the box above led Gibbs (1988) to describe young African-American males as an "endangered species."

As American and Canadian societies become more racially and ethnically diverse, increasing research attention is being focused on other groups such as Asians, Hispanics, Pacific-Islanders, and Native populations. Researchers are generating information that can aid community health nurses in assessing and treating diverse racial and ethnic groups (see the box on page 354 for an example of this type of information).

Like many other racial and ethnic groups, the health problems facing Native Americans and Native Canadians are correlates of poverty and so-

---

HEALTH RELATED FACTS ABOUT NATIVE AMERICANS AND NATIVE CANADIANS

- Alcohol is the number one killer of Native Americans between the ages of 14 and 44 years (May, 1986); 42% of Native American male adolescents are problem drinkers compared with 34% of same-age Caucasian males (Lamarine, 1988). Native Americans (10 to 18 years of age) comprise 34% of inpatient admissions to adolescent detoxification programs (Moore, 1988).
- Compared to the "all race" population, Native American youth exhibit more serious problems in the areas of depression, suicide, anxiety, substance use, and general health status (Blum et al., 1992). The rates of morbidity, mortality from injury, and AIDS are also higher (Sugarman, Soderberg, Gordon, & Rivera, 1993; Metler, Conway, & Stehn-Green, 1991).

---

cial marginalization such as dropping out of school, a sense of hopelessness, the experience of prejudice, poor nutrition, and lack of regular health care. Community health nurses need to be attuned to the potential interplay between gender, race, ethnicity, cultural differences, and economic conditions when working with racial and ethnic minorities.

Homosexual and Bisexual Men

Homosexual and bisexual men are estimated to be anywhere from 5% to 10% of the male population. In the past, homosexual men have been viewed as evil, sinful, sick, emotionally immature, and socially undesirable. Health professionals and the wider public have generally harbored mixed feelings and negative attitudes toward homosexual and bisexual men. This overall reaction to the sexual orientation of homosexuals is now referred to as **homophobia,** or the irrational fear or hatred of homosexual men, lesbians, or bisexuals. While the increased openness about sexuality and homosexuality since the 1960s has helped erode myths about homosexual men, mixed feelings persist among heterosexual (or straight) persons. For example, a poll by *U.S. News and World*

Report (July 5, 1993) reveals the presence of mixed feelings about gay rights and issues. While 65% of the 1000 American voters polled indicated they believed in equal rights for homosexuals, most regarded homosexuality as a lifestyle choice, and half opposed extending civil-rights laws to include homosexual men and lesbians. Fifty-three percent said they actually knew a homosexual man or a lesbian, and that this relationship made them feel better about homosexuals in general. Still, 60% opposed "legal partnerships" for homosexuals, and 70% indicated that homosexual men and lesbians should not be allowed to adopt children.

Homosexual men's identity, their lifestyles, and the social responses to homosexuality can affect the health of homosexual and bisexual men. Stigmatization and marginalization, for example, may lead to emotional confusion and suicide among homosexual male adolescents. For homosexual and bisexual men who are "in the closet" (*i.e.,* their homosexual sexual preferences are kept secret), anxiety and stress can tax emotional and physical health. When seeking medical services, homosexual and bisexual men must often cope with the homophobia of health care workers or deal with the threat of losing health care insurance if their sexual orientation is made known. By learning more about the myths and realities surrounding homosexuality, community health nurses will be more sensitive to the needs of homosexual and bisexual patients.

Whether they are heterosexual or homosexual, men tend to have more sexual contacts than women do, which heightens men's risk for STDs. Men's sexual attitudes and behaviors are closely tied to the way masculinity has been socially constructed. For example, men are taught to suppress their emotions, which can lead to a separation of sex from feeling. Traditionally, men are also encouraged to be daring, which can lead to risky sexual decisions. In addition, contrary to common myths about homosexual male effeminacy, masculinity also plays a powerful role in shaping homosexual and bisexual men's identity and behavior. To the extent that traditional masculinity informs sexual activity of men, masculinity can be a barrier to safer sexual behavior among men. This insight led Kimmel and Levine

(1989, p. 352) to assert that to educate men about safe sex means to confront the issues of masculinity. In addition to practicing abstinence and safer sex as preventive strategies, they argue that another measure of risk reduction would be to challenge traditional beliefs about masculinity.

Men who have sex with men remain the largest risk group for HIV transmission. For homosexual and bisexual men who are infected by the HIV virus, the personal burden of living with an AIDS diagnosis is made heavier by the stigma associated with homosexuality. The cultural meanings associated with AIDS can also filter into gender and sexual identities. Tewksbury (1995) examined the psychosexual adjustments of homosexual men to being HIV positive. His analysis of interviews with 45 HIV positive homosexual men showed how masculinity, sexuality, stigmatization, and interpersonal commitment mesh in the decision making around risky sexual behavior. Most of the men practiced celibacy to prevent others from contracting the disease, others practiced safe sex, and a few went on having unprotected sex.

Prison Inmates

There are 1.4 million men who are imprisoned in American jails and prisons. The United States has the highest rate of incarceration of any nation in the world (426/100,000) (American College of Physicians, 1992), followed by South Africa and the Soviet Union (Mauer, 1992). Racial and ethnic minorities are overrepresented among those behind bars. Black and Hispanic males, for example, constitute 85% of prisoners in the New York State prison system (Green, 1991). The estimated cost of incarceration for the United States is about $16 billion per year.

The prison system acts as a pocket of risk, within which men already at greater risk of a pre-existing AIDS infection, because of prison conditions are yet again exposed to heightened risk of contracting HIV (Toepell, 1992) or other infections such as tuberculosis (TB) (Bellin, Fletcher, & Safyer, 1993) or hepatitis. The corrections system is part of an institutional chain that facilitates transmission of HIV and other infections in certain North American populations, particularly among poor, inner-city, minority males. Prisoners are burdened not only by social disadvantage but also by high rates of physical illness, mental disorder, and substance use that jeopardize their health (Editor, *Lancet*, 1991).

AIDS prevalence is markedly higher among state and federal inmates than in the general United States population, with a known aggregate rate in 1992 of 202/100,000 (Brewer & Derrickson, 1992) compared with a total population prevalence of 14.65/100,000 (American College of Physicians, 1992). The cumulative total of American prisoners with AIDS in 1989 was estimated to be 5411, a 72% increase over the previous year (Belbot & del Carmen, 1991). The total number of AIDS cases reported in U.S. corrections facilities as of 1993 was 11,565 (a minimum estimate of the true cumulative incidence among U.S. inmates) (Hammett, cited in Expert Committee on AIDS and Prisons, 1994). In New York state alone, at least 10,000 of the state's 55,000 prisoners are believed to be infected (Prisoners with AIDS/HIV Support Action Network, 1992). In Canadian federal penitentiaries, it is believed that 1 in 20 inmates is HIV infected (Hankins, cited in Expert Committee on AIDS and Prison, 1994). The disproportionate rate of HIV/AIDS in prison is believed to be a result of the emphasis on incarceration as a strategy in the war on drugs (Polych & Sabo, in press).

HIV is primarily transmitted between adults by unprotected penetrative sex, or needle sharing without some sort of sterilization, with an infected partner. Sexual contacts between prisoners occur mainly through consensual unions and secondarily through sexual assault and rape (Vaid, cited in The Expert Committee on AIDS and Prisons, 1994). The amount of IV drug use behind prison walls is unknown, although it is known to be prevalent, and the scarcity of needles often leads to needle and sharps sharing (Prisoners with AIDS/HIV Support Action Network, 1992).

The failure to provide comprehensive health education and treatment interventions in prisons is not only putting more inmates at risk for HIV infections but also the public at large. Prisons are not hermetically sealed enclaves set apart from the community, but an integral part of society

(Editor, *Lancet,* 1991). Each year, an estimated 22 million admissions and discharges occur in correctional facilities in the United States. In 1989, prisons in the United States admitted 467,227 persons and discharged 386,228 (American College of Physicians, 1992). The average age of inmates admitted to prison in 1989 was 29.6 years, with 75% between 18 and 34 years; 94.3% were male. These former inmates return to their communities after having served an average of 18 months inside (Dubler & Sidel, 1989). Within 3 years, 62.5% will be rearrested and jailed. Recidivism is highest among poor African-American and Hispanic men. The extent to which the drug-related social practices and sexual activities of released and/or paroled inmates who are HIV positive are putting others at risk on return to their communities is unresearched and unknown.

The World Health Organization has observed that the rehabilitative and therapeutic aspects of prisons are not sufficiently used. Community health nurses need to press for comprehensive health care interventions to deal with the unique health needs of prisoners as well as their communities of origin. Just as prison acts as a pocket of risk for persons already exposed to greater health risks while they are in their communities, prison can also act as a pocket of opportunity for interventions (Polych, 1992).

Male Athletes

Injury is everywhere in sport. It is evident in the lives and bodies of athletes who regularly experience bruises, torn ligaments, broken bones, aches, lacerations, muscle tears, and so forth (see Figure 16-1). For example, there are about 300,000 football-related injuries per year that require treatment in hospital emergency rooms (Miedzian, 1991). Critics of violent contact sports claim that athletes are paying too high a physical price for their participation. George D. Lundberg (1994), editor of the *Journal of the American Medical Association,* has called for a ban on boxing in the Olympics and in the United States military. His editorial entreaty, while based on clinical evidence of neurologic harm from boxing, is also couched in a wider critique of the exploitative economics of the sport.

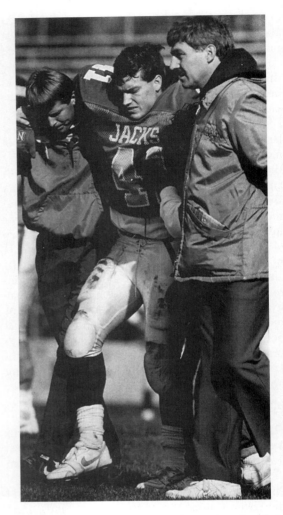

FIGURE 16-1 Many traditional male sports, such as football, result in painful and sometimes disabling injuries. *From* Athletic injury assessment *(ed. 3) by J.M. Booher & G.A. Thibodeau, 1994, St. Louis: Mosby. Copyright 1994 by Mosby-Year Book, Inc.*

Injuries are basically unavoidable in sports, but in traditional men's sports, there has been a tendency to glorify pain and injury, to inflict injury on others, and to sacrifice one's body in order to "win at all costs." The "no pain, no gain" philosophy, which is rooted in traditional cultural equations between masculinity and sports, can jeopardize the health of athletes who conform to its ethos (Sabo, 1994b).

The connections between sport, masculinity,

and health are evident in Klein's (1993) study of bodybuilders who use anabolic steroids, over-train, and engage in extreme dietary practices. He spent years as an ethnographic researcher in the muscled world of the bodybuilding subculture, where masculinity is equated to maximum mus-cularity and men's strivings for bigness and phys-ical strength hide emotional insecurity and low self-esteem. The links between masculinity and muscle have been embodied in cult heroes such as Joe Weider, Charles Atlas, Arnold Schwartzenegger, and Sylvester Stallone, who have served as male role models for generations of American boys and men. Klein exposes a tragic irony in American culture, namely, that the powerful male athlete, a symbol of strength and health, has often sacrificed his health in pursuit of ideal masculinity (Messner & Sabo, 1994).

A nationwide survey of American male high school seniors found that 6.6% used or had used anabolic steroids. About two thirds of this group were athletes (Buckley et al., 1988). Anabolic steroid use has been linked to health risks such as liver disease, kidney problems, atrophy of the testicles, elevated risk for injury, and premature skeletal maturation.

In many traditional men's sports such as rugby, football, wrestling, and boxing, the bodies of many athletes end up broken, battered, drugged, and in varying states of chronic pain. As girls and women increasingly enter the athletic realm, it remains to be seen whether they will conform to traditionally masculine values and practices that harm the body or create more healthful sportive practices. Nurses can play watchdog and preventive roles by monitoring the safety of athletic programs in their schools and communities. They can also promote athletic and fitness practices that call for fair play, health, and fitness rather than denial of pain and win-ning at all costs (Messner & Sabo, 1994).

MEN'S HEALTH ISSUES

As community health nurses become more at-tuned to gender differences in health, they can begin to focus assessment, treatment, and preven-tion on meeting the needs of both sexes. Next, a variety of issues and concerns that directly affect men's lives are discussed.

Testicular Cancer

The epidemiologic data on testicular cancer are sobering. Although relatively rare in the general population, it is the fourth most common cause of death among 15- to 35-year-old males, account-ing for 14% of all cancer deaths for this age group. It is the most common form of cancer af-fecting 20- to 34-year-old white males. The inci-dence of testicular cancer is increasing, and about 6100 new American cases were diagnosed in 1991 (American Cancer Society, 1991). If de-tected early, the cure rate is high, while delayed diagnosis is life-threatening. Therefore, regular testicular self-examination (TSE) is a potentially effective preventive means for insuring early de-tection and successful treatment. Regretfully, however, most physicians do not teach TSE tech-niques (Rudolf & Quinn, 1988).

Denial may influence men's perceptions of testicular cancer and TSE (Blesch, 1986). Studies show that most males are not aware of testicular cancer and even among those who are aware, many are reluctant to examine their testicles as a preventive measure. Even when symptoms are recognized, men sometimes postpone seeking treatment. Moreover, men who are taught TSE are often initially receptive, but the practice of TSE decreases over time. Men's resistance to TSE has been linked to awkwardness about touching themselves, associating touching genitals with homosexuality or masturbation, or the idea that TSE is not a manly behavior. And finally, men's in-dividual reluctance to discuss testicular cancer partly derives from the widespread cultural si-lence that envelopes it. The penis is a cultural symbol of male power, authority, and sexual dom-ination. Its symbolic efficacy in traditional, male-dominated gender relations, therefore, would be eroded or neutralized by the realities of testicular cancer.

Readers might make a comparison between cultural silences around testicular cancer and that of breast cancer. Both the penis and breast have sexual and gendered meanings associated with them that pervade cultural notions of mas-culinity and femininity, respectively. It was not until the early 1970s, when prominent women like American vice-presidential spouse Happy Rockefeller and actress Mary Tyler Moore openly discussed their breast cancer and mastectomy, that cultural silences were broken. In contrast, no male public figures have stepped forward to discuss their experiences with testicular cancer.

Diseases of the Prostate

Middle-aged and elderly men are likely to develop medical problems with the prostate gland. Some men may experience benign prostatic hyperplasia, an enlargement of the prostate gland that is associated with symptoms such as dribbling after urination, frequent urination, or incontinence. Others may develop infections (prostatitis) or malignant prostatic hyperplasia (prostate cancer). Prostate cancer is the third leading cause of death from cancer in men, accounting for 15.7 deaths per 100,000 population in 1989. Prostate cancer is now more common than lung cancer (Martin, 1990). This cancer develops in 1 in 10 men by age 85 years, with African-American males showing a higher prevalence rate than their Caucasian counterparts (Greco & Blank, 1993).

Treatments for prostate problems depend on the specific diagnosis and may range from medication to radiation and surgery. As is the case with testicular cancer, survival from prostate cancer is enhanced by early detection. Raising men's awareness about the health risks associated with the prostate gland, therefore, may prevent unnecessary morbidity and mortality. Community nurses should advise middle-aged and older males to undergo annual digital rectal examinations and a blood test for Prostate Specific Antigen (SPA).

Finally, more invasive surgical treatments for prostate cancer can produce incontinence and impotence. However, there is no systematic research on men's psychosocial reactions and adjustment to sexual dysfunction associated with treatments for prostate cancer. Community nurses should be alert to possible interpersonal problems, sexual concerns, and feelings of masculine adequacy that may exist among some men facing prostate cancer.

Alcohol Abuse

While social and medical problems stemming from alcohol abuse involve both sexes, males constitute the largest segment of alcohol abusers. Some researchers have begun exploring the connections between the influence of the traditional male role on alcohol abuse. Isenhart and Silversmith (1994) show how, in a variety of occupational contexts, expectations surrounding masculinity encourage heavy drinking while working or socializing during after-work or off-duty hours. Some predominantly male occupational groups such as longshoremen (Hitz, 1973), salesmen (Cosper, 1979), and the military (Pursch, 1976) are known to engage in high rates of alcohol consumption.

Findings from a Harvard School of Public Health (Wechsler et al., 1994) survey of 17,600 students at 140 colleges found that 44% engaged in "binge drinking," defined as drinking five drinks in rapid succession for males and four drinks for females. Males were more likely to report binge drinking during the past two weeks than females (50% and 39%, respectively). Sixty percent of the males who binge-drank three or more times in the past 2 weeks reported driving after drinking, compared with 49% of their female counterparts, thus increasing risk for accidental injury and death. Compared with non-binge drinkers, binge drinkers were seven times more likely to engage in unprotected sex, thus elevating the risk for unwanted pregnancy and sexually transmitted disease.

Alcohol-related automobile accidents are the top cause of death among 16- to 24-year-olds, especially among males (Henderson & Anderson, 1989). For all males, the age-adjusted death rate from automobile accidents in 1991 was 26.2/100,000 for African-American males and 24.2/100,000 for Caucasian males, 2.5 and 3.0 times higher than for Caucasian and African-American females, respectively (*Mortality and Morbidity Weekly Report*, 1994d). The number of automobile fatalities among male adolescents that result from a mixture of alcohol abuse and masculine daring is unknown.

The efforts of community health nurses to promote sobriety among male adolescents and responsible drinking among adult males are complicated by cultural equations between manhood and alcohol consumption. Mass media plays a role in sensationalizing and glorifying links between alcohol and male bravado. Postman, Nystrom, Strate, & Weingartner (1987) studied the thematic content of 40 beer commercials and identified a variety of stereotypical portrayals of the male role that were used to promote beer drinking: reward for a job well done; manly activities that feature strength, risk, and daring; male friendship and espirit de corps; and romantic success with women. The researchers estimate that between the ages of 2 and 18 years, children view about 100,000 beer commercials.

HIV/AIDS

HIV infection became a leading cause of death among males in the 1980s. Among men aged 25 to 44 years in 1990, HIV infection was the second leading cause of death (and the sixth leading cause of death among same-age women) (*Morbidity and Mortality Weekly Report,* 1993a). Among reported cases of AIDS for adolescent and adult men in 1992, 60% were men who had sex with other men, 21% were intravenous drug users, 4% were exposed through heterosexual sexual contact, 6% were men who had sex with men and injected drugs, and 1% were transfusion recipients. Among the cases of AIDS among adolescent and adult women in 1992, 45% were intravenous drug users, 39% were infected through heterosexual sexual contact, and 4% were transfusion recipients (*Morbidity and Mortality Weekly Report,* 1993b).

Because most AIDS cases have been among men who have sex with other men, perceptions of the epidemic and its victims have been tainted by sexual attitudes. In North American cultures, the stigma associated with AIDS is fused with the stigma linked to homosexuality. Feelings about men with AIDS can be mixed and complicated by homophobia.

Thoughts and feelings about men with AIDS are also influenced by attitudes toward race, ethnicity, drug abuse, and social marginality. Data from the Centers for Disease Control and Prevention (CDC) show, for example, that men of color aged 13 years and older were 51% ($N = 45,039$) of the 89,165 AIDS cases reported in 1993. Women of color represented 71% of the cases reported among females aged 13 years and older (*Morbidity and Mortality Weekly Report,*

1994b). The high rate of AIDS among racial and ethnic minorities has kindled racial prejudices in some minds, and AIDS is sometimes seen as a "minority disease." Nurses must understand, however, that whereas African-American or Hispanic males may be at greater risk of contracting HIV/AIDS, just as yellow fingers do not cause lung disease, it is not their race or ethnicity that confers risk, but the behaviors they engage in and the social circumstances of their lives.

Perceptions of HIV/AIDS can also be influenced by attitudes toward poverty and poor people. HIV infection is linked to economic problems that include community disintegration, unemployment, homelessness, eroding urban tax bases, mental illness, substance use, and criminalization (Wallace, 1991). For example, males constitute the majority of homeless persons. Poverty and homelessness overlap with drug addiction, which, in turn, is linked to HIV infection. Of persons hospitalized with HIV in New York City, 9% to 18% have been found to be homeless (Torres et al., 1990). Of homeless men tested for HIV at a New York City shelter, 62% of those who took the test were seropositive (Ron & Rogers, 1989). Among runaway or homeless youth in New York City, 7% tested positive for HIV, while this rate rose to 15% among the 19- and 20-year-olds. Of homeless men in Baltimore, 85% admitted to substance use problems (Weinreb & Bassuk, 1990). Nurses need to be aware that the social and moral attitudes they harbor toward the poor and drug users can also muddy their perceptions and treatment of men with AIDS.

Finally, community health nurses need to learn more about how HIV positive men think, feel, and behave, especially in terms of behaviors that are key vehicles for the transmission of the HIV virus such as unsafe sex and intravenous drug use. Survey researchers are providing useful information about how men's sexual practices, attitudes, and risk behaviors are linked to the growing AIDS epidemic (Toronto Department of Health, 1991). Interview studies of men with AIDS are also helping to produce a subtler understanding of human sexual behavior, where irrationality, physical urges, and complex gender identity dynamics play such a crucial role in shaping behavior and perception.

Suicide

The suicide rates for both African-American and Caucasian males increased between 1970 and 1989 while female rates were decreasing. Indeed, males are more likely than females to commit suicide from middle childhood until old age (Stillion, 1995, 1985). Compared with females, males typically deploy more violent means of attempting suicide (*e.g.,* guns or hanging versus pills) and are more likely to complete the act. Men's selection of more violent methods to kill themselves is consistent with traditionally masculine behavior (Stillion, White, McDowell, & Edwards, 1989).

Canetto (1995) interviewed male survivors of suicide attempts to better understand sex differences in suicidal behavior. While she recognizes that men's psychosocial reactions and adjustments to nonfatal suicide vary by race, ethnicity, socioeconomic status, and age, she also finds that gender identity is an important factor in men's experiences. Suicide data show that men attempt suicide less often than women but are more likely to die than women. Canetto (1995) indicates that men's comparative "success" rate points toward a tragic irony in that, consistent with gender stereotypes, men's failure even at suicide undercuts the cultural mandate that men are supposed to succeed at everything. A lack of embroilment in traditionally masculine expectations, she suggests, may actually increase the likelihood of surviving a suicide attempt for some men.

Elderly males in North America commit suicide significantly more often than elderly females. Whereas Caucasian women's lethal suicide rate peaks at age 50 years, Caucasian men 60 years old and older have the highest rate of lethal suicide, even surpassing the rate for young males (Manton, Blazer, & Woodbury, 1987). Canetto (1992, p. 92) argues that elderly men's higher suicide mortality is chiefly due to gender differences in coping. She writes,

. . . older women may have more flexible and diverse ways of coping than older men. Compared to older men, older women may be more willing and capable of adopting different coping strategies — "passive" or "active," "connected" or "independent" — depending on the situation.

She attributes men's limited coping abilities to gender socialization and development.

Violence

Men's violence is a major public health problem. The traditional masculine stereotype calls on males to be aggressive and tough. Anger is a by-product of aggression and toughness and, ultimately, part of the inner terrain of traditional masculinity (Sabo, 1993). Images of angry young men are compelling vehicles used by some males to separate themselves from women and to measure their status in regard to other males. Men's anger and violence derive, in part, from sex inequality. Men use threats and application of violence to maintain their political and economic advantage over women and lower-status men. Male socialization reflects and reinforces these larger patterns of domination.

Homicide is the second leading cause of death among 15- to 19-year-old males. Males aged 15 to 34 years were almost half (49%, $N = 13,122$) of homicide victims in the United States in 1991. The homicide rate for this age group increased by 50% from 1985 to 1991 (*Morbidity and Mortality Weekly Report,* 1994c).

Women are especially victimized by men's anger and violence in the form of stranger rape, acquaintance rape, wife-beating, assault, sexual harassment on the job, and verbal harassment (Thorne-Finch, 1992). That the reality and potential of men's violence affects women's mental and physical health is safely assumed. Community health nurses must also recognize, however, that men's violence also exacts a toll on men themselves in the forms of fighting, gang clashes, hazing, gay-bashing, intentional infliction of injury, homicide, suicide, and organized warfare. There is paleontologic evidence that the institutions of war and patriarchy emerged during the same phase of social evolution about 12,000 to 14,000 years ago (Eisler, 1988). War has always been a predominantly male activity (Connell, 1992). It is ironic that the modern nursing profession was birthed by the nurturing and caring hands of Florence Nightingale on the battlefields of the Franco-Prussian war. Male victims of men's violence require assessment and treatment, while male victimizers need to be referred to police, social services, and/or rehabilitation.

Finally, although there may be some biologic impetus for men's higher levels of aggression compared with women, we also know that male aggression varies a great deal across cultures, individuals, and historical settings. To the extent that masculinity is culturally defined and malleable, therefore, health promoters can encourage the development of more cooperative, peaceful, and empathic forms of masculinity.

Coronary Heart Disease

There are no simple explanations of how gender contributes to the development of coronary heart disease (CHD) in men. To begin with, as men's and women's roles, psychologies, and lifestyles in the family and workplace continue to change, so also do their respective risks for CHD. Second, gender identity and gender roles not only appear to elevate risk for CHD, but they also influence men's personal reactions and adjustments to heart disease once it occurs. And finally, recent research shows that gender bias may be shaping the ways that health care professionals perceive, diagnose, and treat men and women presenting with symptoms of CHD.

Because CHD is the leading cause of death among males and the bulk of medical research on CHD has been done on males, heart disease is often regarded as a "man's disease." Indeed, the incidence of CHD among men has been about twice that of women, although rates are more comparable at age 70 years (Kannel, Hjortland, McNamara, & Gordon, 1976). Heart disease is also more prevalent among African-American and Native American males than their Caucasian counterparts (Cockerham, 1995). Biologic risk factors do not account for the differential rates of CHD between the sexes, and a number of psychosocial factors are believed to be operating. It may be that men's higher rates of CHD to the aggressive and independent ways they cope with stress. Harrison, Chin, and Ficarrotto (1992) suspect that smoking and coronary prone behaviors linked to the Type A personality account for men's greater risk for CHD mortality. Helgeson (1995) notes that Type A behavior that closely corresponds with negative masculine personality traits such as competitiveness, hostility, and suppression of emotion is tied to men's risk for CHD. In addition, her research shows that once men are diagnosed and treated for CHD, their adjustment and survival is influenced by two factors related to the male role: (1) avoidance of intimate social relationships and the semblances of "feminine" dependency; and (2) tendencies among men to deny symptoms and eschew preventive health behaviors.

In summary, gender is playing an important role in the development of CHD among males and their psychosocial adjustments to illness when it does occur. However, the notion of CHD as a "man's disease" can be misleading in two important ways. First, although it rightfully calls attention to the fact that men's mortality from CHD exceeds that of women, it also hides the fact that CHD is also a leading cause of death among females, particularly elderly females (Micevski, 1995). Second, the idea of a "man's disease" draws on a biomedical conception of illness as an innate, biologic phenomenon, thus deemphasizing the influence of psychosocial and cultural factors in shaping not only health and illness, but gender identity and behavior as well.

Chapter Highlights

- Males are at higher risk at every developmental stage for morbidity and mortality than females are. The reasons are not clear.

- Gender identity can be understood as a person's inner sense of himself or herself as being womanly, or manly; feminine, or masculine.

- The variations in women's and men's health cannot be adequately accounted for by biomedical explanations alone.

- An integration of biomedical explanations, sex role theory, and critical feminist perspectives can help explain the complexities pervading men's health and illness.

- Expressions of the pursuit of traditional masculinity elevate an adolescent male's risk for sexually transmitted diseases, HIV transmission, and early death by accident or suicide.

- Primary prevention should be focused on African-American males in the United States where the survival curve for this high-risk group beyond the age of 40 years is lower than that of men in Bangladesh.

- Homosexual men's identity, their lifestyles, and the social response to homosexuality can affect the health of homosexual and bisexual men.

- The failure to provide comprehensive health education and treatment in prisons puts inmates at risk for the spread of HIV infection.

- Males who equate masculinity with sports may use steriods, overtrain, and use dietary practices to achieve impossible goals.

- One in ten men develops prostate cancer by age 85 years. Early detection is extremely important.

- Males are more likely than females to commit suicide from middle childhood to old age.

- Men's anger and violence derive, in part, from sex inequality. Men use threats and application of violence to maintain their political and economic advantage over women and lower-status men.

- Gender plays an important role in the development of coronary heart disease in men.

 ## CRITICAL THINKING EXERCISE

1. Assume that you are asked to prepare a half-hour presentation for college males that focuses on the health risks of young men. Form a small group of three to four nursing students and identify five key messages or clusters of information that you would include in your presentation.

2. You have just been appointed the highest-ranking public health official in your state or province. You decide to develop two educational initiatives that aim to enhance men's health. What two public health priorities would you identify to maximize prevention of mortality and morbidity among males?

REFERENCES

American Cancer Society. (1991). *Cancer facts and figures—1991.* Atlanta, GA: American Cancer Society.

American College of Physicians. (1992). The crisis in correctional health care: The impact of the national drug control strategy on correctional health services. *Annals of Internal Medicine, 117*(1), 71-77.

Anderson, M.L. (1988). *Thinking about women: Sociological perspectives on sex and gender.* New York: Macmillan.

Bard, M., & Sutherland, C. (1955). Psychological impact of cancer and its treatment. *Cancer, 8,* 656-677.

Belbot, B.A., & del Carmen R.B. (1991). AIDS in prison: Legal issues. *Crime and Delinquency, 31*(1), 135-153.

Bellin, E.Y., Fletcher, D.D., & Safyer, S.M. (1993). Association of tuberculosis infection with increased time in or admission to the New York City jail system. *Journal of the American Medical Association, 269*(17), 2228-2231.

Berman, A.L., & Hays, J.E. (1973). Relation between death, anxiety, belief in afterlife and locus of control. *Journal of Consulting and Clinical Psychology, 41,* 318-24.

Blesch, K. (1986). Health beliefs about testicular cancer and self-examination among professional men. *Oncology Nursing Forum, 13*(1), 29-33.

Blum, R., Harman, B., Harris, L., Bergeissen, L., & Restrick, M. (1992). American Indian-Alaska native youth health. *Journal of the American Medical Association, 267*(12), 1637-44.

Boston Women's Health Collective. (1993). *The new our bodies, ourselves.* New York: Simon & Schuster.

Brannon, R. (1976). The male sex role. In D.S. David, & R. Brannon (Eds.). *The forty-nine percent majority*. Reading, MA: Addison-Wesley.

Brewer, T.F., & Derrickson, J. (1992). AIDS in prison: A review of epidemiology and preventive policy. *AIDS, 6*(7), 623-628.

Brod, H., (Ed.). (1987). *The making of masculinities: The new men's studies* Boston: Allen & Unwin.

Buckley, W.E., Yesalis, C.E., Friedl, K.E., Anderson, W.A., Streit, A.L., & Wright, J.E. (1988). Estimated prevalence of anabolic steroid use among male high school seniors. *Journal of the American Medical Association, 260*(23), 3441-46.

Bullard, R.D. (1992). Urban infrastructure: Social, environmental, and health risks to African-Americans, pp. 183-196. In B.J. Tidwell (Ed.). *The state of black America, 1992*. New York: National Urban League.

Canetto, S.S. (1995). Men who survive a suicidal act: Successful coping or failed masculinity? In D. Sabo & D. Gordon (Eds.). *Men's health and illness*. Newbury Park, CA: Sage.

Canetto, S.S. (1992). Gender and suicide in the elderly. *Suicide and Life-Threatening Behavior, 22*(1), 80-97.

Castleman, M. (1980). Sexual solutions: An informal guide. New York: Simon and Schuster.

Cockerham, W.C. (1995). *Medical sociology.* Englewood Cliffs, NJ: Prentice-Hall.

Connell, R.W. (1987). *Gender and power.* Stanford: Stanford University Press.

Connell, R.W. (1992). Masculinity, violence, and war. In M. Kimmel, & M. Messner (Eds.). *Men's lives* (pp. 176-183). New York: Macmillan.

Cooperstock R. (1971). Sex differences in the use of mood-altering drugs: An explanatory model. *Journal of Health and Social Behavior, 12*, 238-244.

Cosper, R. (1979). Drinking as conformity: A critique of sociological literature on occupational differences in drinking. *Journal of Studies on Alcoholism, 40*, 868-891.

Cypress, B. (1981). Patients' reasons for visiting physicians: National ambulatory medical care survey, U.S. 1977-78. DHHS Publication No. (PHS) 82-1717, Series 13, No. 56. Hyattsville, MD: National Center for Health Statistics, December, 1981.

Daly, M. (1978). *Gyn-ecology: The metaethics of radical feminism.* Boston: Beacon Press.

Dawson, D.A., & Adams, P.F. (1987). Current estimates from the national health interview survey: U.S., 1986. Vital Health Statistics Series, Series 10, No. 164. DHHS Publication No. (PHS) 87-1592, Public Health Service, Washington, D.C., U.S. Government Printing Office.

Dubler, N.N., & Sidel, V.W. (1989). On research on HIV infection and AIDS in correctional institutions. *The Milbank Quarterly, 67*(1-2), 81-94.

Dutton, D. (1986). Financial, organizational, and professional factors affecting health care utilization. *Social Science and Medicine, 23*(7), 721-735.

Editor. (1991, March 16). Health care for prisoners: Implica-

tions of "Kalk's refusal," *Lancet, 337*, 647-648.

Ehrenreich, B., & English, D. (1979). *For her own good: 150 years of expert's advice to women.* New York: Anchor Books.

Eisler, R. (1988). *The Chalice and the blade: Our history, Our future.* San Francisco: Harper San Francisco.

Expert Committee on AIDS and Prison. (1994). *HIV/AIDS in prisons: Summary report and recommendations to the Expert Committee on AIDS and Prisons* (Ministry of Supply and Services Canada Catalogue No. JS82-68/2-1994). Ottawa, Ontario, Canada: Correctional Service of Canada.

Farrell, M., & Rosenberg, S.D. (1981). *Men at midlife.* Dover, MA: Auburn House.

Farrell, W. (1975). *The liberated man: Beyond masculinity.* New York: Random House.

Feigen-Fasteau, M. (1974). *The male machine.* New York: McGraw-Hill.

Frank, A. (1991). For a sociology of the body: An analytical review, pp. 36-102. In M. Featherstone, M. Hepworth, & B. Turner (Eds.). *The body: Social process and cultural theory.* London: Sage.

Freund, P. (1982). *The civilized body: Social domination, control and health.* Philadelphia: Temple University Press.

Gibbs, J.T. (Ed.). (1988). *Young, black, and male in America: An endangered species.* Dover, MA: Auburn House.

Givens, J. (1979). Current estimates from the health interview survey: U.S. 1978. DHHS Publication No. (PHS) 80-1551, Series 10, No. 130. Hyattsville, MD: Office of Health Research Statistics.

Gould, R.L. (1972). The phases of adult life: A study in developmental psychology. *American Journal of Psychiatry, 129*, 521-531.

Grandstaff, N.W. (1976). The impact of breast cancer on the family. In J.M. Vaeth (Ed.). *Breast cancer: Its impacts on the patient, family, and community* (pp. 146-156). New York: S. Karger.

Greco, K.E., & Blank, B. (1993). Prostate-specific antigen: The new early detection test for prostate cancer. *Nurse Practitioner, 18*(5), 30-38.

Green, A.P. (1991). Blacks unheard. pp. 6-7. *Update (Winter), New York State Coalition for Criminal Justice.*

Hankins, C.A., Laberge, C., Lapointe, N., Lai Tung, M.T., Racine, L., & O'Shaughnessy, M. (1990). HIV infection among Quebec women giving birth to live infants. *Canadian Medical Association Journal, 143*(9), 885-893.

Harrison, J., Chin, J., & Ficarrotto, T. (1992). Warning: Masculinity may be dangerous to your health. In M.S. Kimmel, & M.A. Messner (Eds.). *Men's lives* (pp. 271-285). New York: Macmillan.

Helgeson, V.S. (in press). Masculinity, men's roles, and coronary heart disease. In D. Sabo, & D. Gordon (Eds.). *Men's health and illness*. Newbury Park, CA: Sage.

Henderson, D.C., & Anderson, S.C. (1989). Adolescents and chemical dependency. *Social Work in Health Care, 14*(1), 87-105.

Hitz, D. (1973). Drunken sailors and others: Drinking problems in specific occupations. *Quarterly Journal of Studies on Alcohol, 34,* 496-505.

Hoiberg, A., Bernard, S., & Ernst, J. (1981). Racial differences in hospitalization rates among navy enlisted men. *Public Health Report, March-April, 96*(2), 121-127.

Hull, J.D. (1994). Running scared. *Time* (November 21), *144*(2), 93-99.

Isenhart, C.E., & Silversmith, D.J. (1994). The influence of the traditional male role on alcohol abuse and the therapeutic process. *Journal of Men's Studies, 3*(2), 127-135.

Julty, S. (1980). *Men's bodies, men's selves.* New York: Delta.

Kannel, W.B., Hjortland, M.C., McNamara, P.M., & Gordon, T. (1976). Menopause and the risk of cardiovascular disease. *Annals of Internal Medicine, 85,* 447-452.

Kimmel, M.S., & Levine, M.P. (1994). Men and AIDS. In M.S. Kimmel, & M.P. Levine (Eds.). *Men's lives* (pp. 318-329). New York: Macmillan.

Kimmel, M., & Messner, M. (Eds.). (1994). *Men's lives.* New York: Macmillan.

Klein, A. (1993). *Little big men: Bodybuilding subculture and gender construction.* Albany: SUNY Press.

Lamarine, R. (1988). Alcohol abuse among Native Americans. *Journal of Community Health, 13*(3), 143-153.

Levinson, D.J., Darrow, C.M., Klein, E.G., Levinson, M.H., & McKee, B. (1974). The psychosocial development of men in early adulthood and the midlife transition. In D.F. Ricks, A. Thomas, & M. Rof (Eds.). *Life history research in psychopathology* (Vol. 3). Minneapolis: University of Minnesota Press.

Lundberg, G.D. (1994). Let's stop boxing in the Olympics and the United States military. *Journal of the American Medical Association,* 271(22), 1790.

Manton, K.G., Blazer, D.G., & Woodbury, M.A. (1987). Suicide in middle age and later life: Sex and race specific life table and cohort analyses. *Journal of Gerontology, 42,* 219-227.

Marcus, A.C., & Siegel, J.M. (1982). Sex differences in reports of illness and disability: A preliminary test of the "fixed-role" obligations hypothesis. *Journal of Health and Social Behavior, 22,* 174-182.

Martin, J. (1990). Male cancer awareness: Impact of an employee education program. *Oncology Nursing Forum, 17*(1), 59-64.

Mauer, M. (1992). Men in American prisons: Trends, causes, and issues. *Men's Studies Review, 9*(1), 10-12. (A special issue on Men in Prison, edited by Don Sabo and Willie London.)

May, P. (1986). Alcohol and drug misuse prevention programs for American Indians: Needs and opportunities. *Journal of Studies of Alcohol, 47*(3), 187-195.

McCord, C., & Freeman, H.P. (1990). Excess mortality in Harlem. *New England Journal of Medicine, 322*(22), 1606-1607.

Messner, M.A., & Sabo, D. (1994). *Sex, violence, and power in sports: Rethinking masculinity.* Freedom, CA: Crossing Press.

Messner, M.A., & Sabo, D. (1990). *Sport, men, and the gender order: Critical feminist perspectives.* Champaign, IL: Human Kinetics Publishers.

Metler, R., Conway, G., & Stehr-Green, J. (1991). AIDS surveillance among American Indians and Alaska natives. *American Journal of Public Health, 81*(11), 1469-1471.

Metze, E. (1978). Couples and mastectomy. In P.C. Brand, & P.A. van Keep (Eds.). *Breast cancer: Psychological aspects of early detection and treatment* (pp. 25-31). Baltimore: University Park Press.

Micevski, V. (1995). Gender bias: The treatment of women with chest pain. Unpublished manuscript, D´Youville College, Division of Nursing.

Miedzian, M. (1991). *Boys will be boys: Breaking the link between masculinity and violence.* New York: Doubleday.

Moore, D. (1988). Reducing alcohol and other drug use among Native American youth. *Alcohol Drug Abuse and Mental Health, 15*(6), 2-3.

Montagu, A. (1953). *The natural superiority of women.* New York: MacMillan.

Morbidity and Mortality Weekly Report. (1993a). Update: Mortality attributable to HIV infection/AIDS among persons aged 25-44 years — United States, 1990-91, *42*(25), 481-486.

Morbidity and Mortality Weekly Report. (1993b). Summary of Notifiable Diseases — United States, 1992, *41*(55).

Morbidity and Mortality Weekly Report. (1994a). Prevalence of overweight among adolescents — United States, 1988-91, *43*(44), 818-819.

Morbidity and Mortality Weekly Report. (1994b). AIDS among racial/ethnic minorities — United States, 1993, *43*(35), 644-651.

Morbidity and Mortality Weekly Report. (1994c). Homicides among 15-19 year-old males — United States, 1963-1991 *43*(40), 725-728.

Morbidity and Mortality Weekly Report. (1994d). Deaths resulting from firearm- and motor-vehicle-related injuries — United States 1968-1991, *43*(3), 37-42.

National Center for Health Statistics. (1990). *Health, United States, 1989.* Hyattsville, MD: Public Health Service.

National Center for Health Statistics. (1992). Advance report of final mortality statistics, 1989. *Monthly Vital Statistics Report, 40*(8) [suppl 2] (DHHS Publication No. (PHS) 92-1120).

Pleck, J., Sonenstein, F.L., & Ku, L.C. (1992). In R. Ketterlinus, & M.E. Lamb (Eds.). *Adolescent problem behaviors.* Hillsdale, NJ: Lawrence Erlbaum Associates.

Polych, C. (1992). Punishment within punishment: The AIDS epidemic in North American prisons. *Men's Studies Review, 9*(1), 13-17.

Polych, C., & Sabo, D. (in press). Gender politics, pain, and illness: The AIDS epidemic in North American prisons. In D. Sabo, & D. Gordon (Eds.). *Men's health and illness.* Newbury Park, CA: Sage.

Postman, N., Nystrom, C., Strate, L., & Weingartner, C. (1987). *Myths, men and beer: An analysis of beer commercials on broadcast television, 1987.* Falls Church, VA: Foundation for Traffic Safety.

Prisoners with AIDS/HIV Support Action Network. (1992). *HIV/AIDS in prison systems: A comprehensive strategy.* (Brief to the Minister of Correctional Services and the Minister of Health). Toronto, Ontario, Canada: Prisoners with AIDS/HIV Support Action Network.

Pursch, J.A. (1976). From quonset hut to navel hospital: The story of an alcoholism rehabilitation service. *Journal of Studies on Alcohol, 37,* 1655-66.

Reed, W.L. (1991). Trends in homicide among African Americans. *Trotter Institute Review, 5,* 11-16.

Ron, A., & Rogers, D.E. (1989). AIDS in New York City: The role of intravenous drug users. *Bulletin of the New York Academy of Medicine, 65*(7), 787-900.

Rudolf, V., & Quinn, K. (1988). The practice of TSE among college men: Effectiveness of an educational program. *Oncology Nursing Forum, 15*(1), 45-48.

Sabo, D. (1994a). Doing time doing masculinity: Sports and prison. In M.A. Messner & D. Sabo (Eds.). *Sex, violence, and power in sports: Rethinking masculinity* (pp. 161-170). Freedom, CA: Crossing Press.

Sabo, D. (1994b). The body politics of sports injury: Culture, power, and the pain principle. Paper presented at the annual meeting of the National Athletic Trainers Association, Dallas, June 6, 1994.

Sabo, D. (1990). Men, death anxiety, and denial: Critical feminist interpretations of adjustments to mastectomy. In E.J. Clark, J.M. Fritz, & P.P. Rieker (Eds.). *Clinical sociological perspectives on illness and loss: The linkage of theory and practice* (pp. 71-84). Philadelphia: Charles Press.

Sabo, D., Brown, J., & Smith, K. (1986). The male role and mastectomy: Support groups and men's adjustment. *Journal of Psychosocial Oncology, 3*(2), 19-31.

Scully, D., & Bart, P. (1981). A funny thing happened on the way to the orifice: Women in gynecology textbooks. In P. Conrad & R. Kern (Eds.). *The sociology of health and illness: Critical perspectives.* New York: St. Martins.

Staples, R. (in press). Health and illness among African-American males. In D. Sabo, & D. Gordon (Eds.). *Men's health and illness.* Newbury Park, CA: Sage.

Stillion, J. (1995). Premature death among males: Rethinking links between masculinity and health. In D. Sabo, & D. Gordon (Eds.). *Men's health and illness.* Newbury Park, CA: Sage.

Stillion, J. (1985). *Death and the sexes: An examination of differential longevity, attitudes, behaviors, and coping skills.* New York: Hemisphere.

Stillion, J.M., White, H., McDowell, E.E., & Edwards, P. (1989). Ageism and sexism in suicide attitudes. *Death Studies, 13,* 247-261.

Sugarman, J., Soderberg, R., Gordon, J., & Rivera, F. (1993). Racial misclassification of American Indians: Its effects on injury rates in Oregon, 1989-1990. *American Journal of Public Health, 83*(5), 681-684.

Thorne-Finch, R. (1992). *Ending the silence: The origins and treatment of male violence against women.* Toronto: University of Toronto Press.

Toepell, A.R. (1992). *Prisoners and AIDS: AIDS education needs assessment.* Toronto, Ontario, Canada: John Howard Society of Metropolitan Toronto.

Toronto Department of Health. (1991). *Men's Survey '90, AIDS. Knowledge, attitudes, behaviours: A study of gay and bisexual men in Toronto (1991).* Toronto, Ontario: The City of Toronto Department of Public Health and the Toronto Lesbian and Gay Community Appeal.

Torres, R.A., Mani, S., Altholz, J., & Brickner, P.W. (1990). HIV infection among homeless men in a New York City shelter. *Archives of Internal Medicine, 150,* 2030-2036.

Vaillant, G.E., & McArthur, C.C. (1972). Natural history of male psychological health: The adult life cycle from eighteen to fifty. *Seminars in Psychiatry, 4,* 415-427.

Verbrugge, L.M., & Wingard, D.L. (1987). Sex differentials in health and mortality. *Women Health, 12,* 103-145.

Waldron, I. (in press). Contributions of changing gender differences in behavior and social roles to changing gender differences in mortality. In D. Sabo & D. Gordon (Eds.). *Men's health and illness.* Newbury Park, CA: Sage.

Waldron, I. (1986). What do we know about sex differences in mortality? *Population Bulletin of the U.N., No. 18-1985* (pp. 59-76).

Waldron, I. (1976). Why do women live longer than men? *Journal of Human Stress, 2,* 1-13.

Wallace, R. (1991). Traveling waves of HIV infection on a low dimensional "socio-geographic" network. *Social Science Medicine, 32*(7), 847-852.

Wechler, H., Davenport, A., Dowdall, G., Moeykens, B., & Castillo, S. (1994). Health and behavioral consequences of binge drinking in college: A national survey of students at 140 campuses. *Journal of the American Medical Association, 272*(21), 1672-1677.

Weinreb, L.F., & Bassuk, E.L. (1990). Substance abuse: A growing problem among homeless families. *Family and Community Health 13*(1), 55-64.

West, Z., & Zimmerman, D.H. (1987). Doing gender. *Gender and Society, 1*(2), 125-151.

17

CARING FOR OLDER ADULTS

Joan M. Cookfair

To everything there is a season,

and a time for every purpose under heaven.

Ecclesiastes 3:8

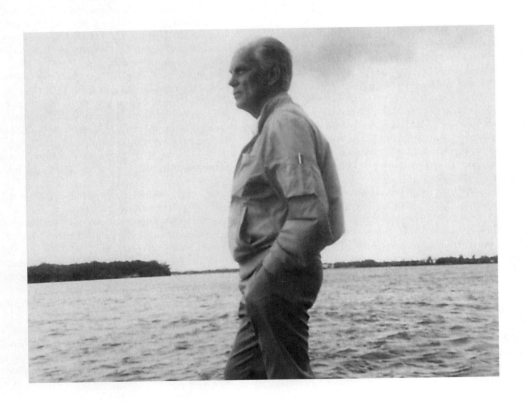

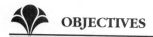

OBJECTIVES

At the conclusion of this chapter the student will be able to:

1. Define the key terms listed.
2. Describe the characteristics of the elderly population.
3. Describe selected theories of biologic aging.
4. Describe selected psychosocial theories of aging.
5. Describe normal physical and cognitive changes that occur with the aging process.
6. Discuss primary, secondary, and tertiary interventions to prevent physical disabilities that may occur as a result of the aging process.
7. Describe some health problems that are common to the aging population.
8. Identify selected community resources available to the aging population.
9. Discuss common health problems of the frail elderly.
10. Discuss the role of the nurse with the frail elderly.
11. Discuss spiritual nursing as it relates to the elderly.

KEY TERMS

Activity theory
Auto immune theory
Continuity theory
Disengagement theory
Error and fidelity theory
Examination stage

Frail elderly
Late maturity
Life course theories
Neuroendocrine theory
Presbycusis

Presbyopia
Social competence and
   breakdown theory
Somatic mutation theory
Spiritual nursing

Late maturity is a phase of life that begins at about 65 years of age and continues until death. Typically it includes the retirement years and may involve a period of infirmity and dependence. More people are living to later maturity in this decade than in decades past. This is due, in part, to improved sanitation, better nutrition, fewer deaths from infectious disease, and improved technology. Table 17-1 illustrates the increase in the older population since 1900 and the projected increase through 2050. The older population is expected to increase most rapidly between the years 2010 and 2030 when the children of the baby boom (those born between

1946 and 1964) reach 65 years of age. Figure 17-1 demonstrates the projected demographic trends for the elderly (U.S. Bureau of the Census, 1984). This projection emphasizes the need to plan for the care of the elderly in the coming decades.

THE AGING PROCESS

The causes of biologic aging have never been proved, although there are several theories that attempt to explain it.

The **error and fidelity theory** defines fidelity as the faithful production of the correct proteins from the point of gene transcription and translation of the RNA into the amino acids of

TABLE 17-1 Actual and projected growth of the older population, 1900-2050

Year	Total population all ages	55 to 64 years Number*	%	65 to 74 years Number*	%	75 to 84 years Number*	%	85 years and over Number*	%	65 years and over Number*	%
1900	76,303	4,009	5.3	2,189	2.9	772	1.0	123	0.2	3,084	4.0
1910	91,972	5,054	5.5	2,793	3.0	989	1.1	167	0.2	3,950	4.3
1920	105,711	6,532	6.2	3,464	3.3	1,259	1.2	210	0.2	4,933	4.7
1930	122,775	8,397	6.8	4,721	3.8	1,641	1.3	272	0.2	6,634	5.4
1940	131,669	10,572	8.0	6,375	4.8	2,278	1.7	365	0.3	9,019	6.8
1950	150,967	13,295	8.8	8,415	5.6	3,278	2.2	577	0.4	12,270	8.1
1960	179,323	15,572	8.7	10,997	6.1	4,633	2.6	929	0.5	16,560	9.2
1970	203,302	18,608	9.2	12,447	6.1	6,124	3.0	1,409	0.7	19,980	9.8
1980	226,505	21,700	9.6	15,578	6.9	7,727	3.4	2,240	1.0	25,544	11.3
1990	249,657	21,051	8.4	18,035	7.2	10,349	4.1	3,313	1.3	31,697	12.7
2000	267,955	23,767	8.9	17,677	6.6	12,318	4.6	4,926	1.8	34,921	13.0
2010	283,238	34,848	12.3	20,318	7.2	12,326	4.4	6,551	2.3	39,195	13.8
2020	296,597	40,298	13.6	29,855	10.1	14,486	4.9	7,081	2.4	51,422	17.3
2030	304,807	34,025	11.2	34,535	11.3	21,434	7.0	8,612	2.8	64,581	21.2
2040	308,559	34,717	11.3	29,272	9.5	24,882	8.1	12,834	4.2	66,988	21.7
2050	309,488	37,327	12.1	30,114	9.7	21,263	6.9	16,034	5.2	67,411	21.8

From U.S. Bureau of the Census, Decennial Censuses of Population (for 1900–1980). U.S. Bureau of the Census, Projections of the Population of the United States, by Age, Sex, and Race: 1983 to 2080. Current Population Reports, Series P-25, No. 952, May 1984 (for 1990–2050). Projections are middle series.
* Numbers in thousands

the cellular structure. As the ability to accurately transfer messages decreases, errors occur that may result in the production of altered proteins. Proliferation of the errors over time results in a progressive deterioration of the cells and ultimately, in death (Burke & Walsh, 1992).

The **somatic mutation theory** suggests that cumulative exposure to background radiation will gradually result in cell mutations and eventual death (Cristofalo, 1988).

The **neuroendocrine theory** views aging as the gradual deterioration of neurons and hormones. This deterioration may adversely affect the body systems (Cristofalo, 1988).

The immune system not only protects the body from infection, but from atypical mutant cells that may invade the body. The immune system of the older adult may not be able to produce an adequate supply of antibodies or phagocytic cells to destroy the mutant cells. The **autoimmune theory** proposes that aging results when impaired antibodies react with normal cells of the body and kill the normal cells. Thus the body begins to deteriorate in multiple ways (Florini, 1981).

Other biologic theories include the effects of temperature, nutrient deprivation, the wear and tear theory, and the idea that one cell or type of tissue is a kind of biologic clock (Burke & Walsh, 1992). No theory has been proved as the cause of aging, although all of them seem to contribute to the reasons for the aging process. We do know that there are several characteristics of aging (see box on p.370).

Some of the myths that continue to exist regarding aging include the following:

1. Older persons have memory loss. Memory loss is rarely a consequence of aging, although the stress of the aging process may make it difficult to focus cognitively.

2. The older adult is not productive. Forced retirement and loss of control of his or her life may cause the older adult to suffer loss of self-esteem.

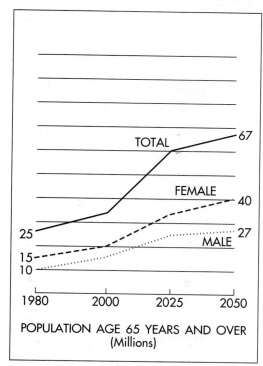

POPULATION AGE 65 YEARS AND OVER
(Millions)

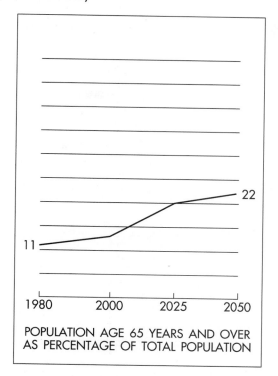

POPULATION AGE 65 YEARS AND OVER
AS PERCENTAGE OF TOTAL POPULATION

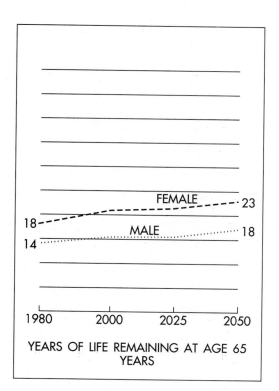

YEARS OF LIFE REMAINING AT AGE 65
YEARS

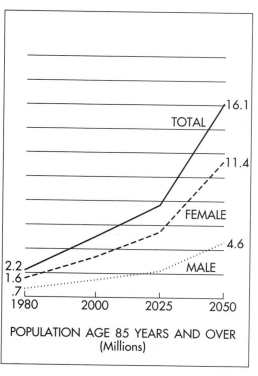

POPULATION AGE 85 YEARS AND OVER
(Millions)

FIGURE 17-1 Projected demographic trends for the elderly, 1980–2050. (From US Bureau of the Census.)

Continued

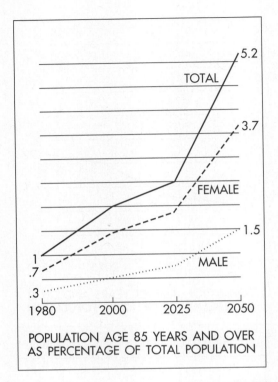

POPULATION AGE 85 YEARS AND OVER
AS PERCENTAGE OF TOTAL POPULATION

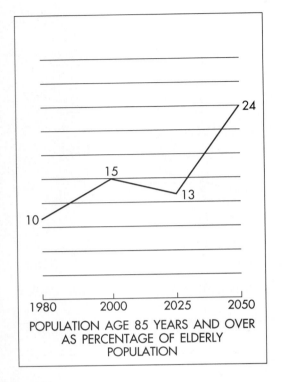

POPULATION AGE 85 YEARS AND OVER
AS PERCENTAGE OF ELDERLY
POPULATION

FIGURE 17-1 cont'd.

CHARACTERISTICS OF AGING

- There is increased mortality with age.
- There are changes in the chemical composition of the body with age. There is a decrease in lean body mass and an increase in fat. There is an increase in lipofusion pigment in certain tissues and increased cross-linking in matrix molecules.
- There is a broad spectrum of progressive deteriorative body changes.
- There is a reduced ability to respond adaptively to environmental changes.
- There is a well-documented but poorly understood increased vulnerability to disease with age.

From "An Overview of the Theories of Biological Aging" (p. 120) by V. Cristofalo, 1988. In J. Birren & V. Bengston (Eds.). *Emergent Theories of Aging,* New York: Springer Publishing. Adapted by permission.

The individual who continues to be involved in the workforce or finds other roles to maintain self-esteem continues to be productive unless illness or fragility make it impossible.

3. Many older persons are resistant to change. Most likely an older person who is resistant to change has always been that way (Clark, 1992). There are several psychosocial theories that attempt to explain the things that do happen to the aging adult.

PSYCHOSOCIAL THEORIES OF AGING

Aging is defined as "the transformation of the human organism after the age of physical maturity — that is, optimum age of reproduction — so that the probability of survival constantly decreases and there are regular transformations in appearance, behavior, experience, and social roles" (Birren & Bengston, 1988, p. 160). There are several theories that attempt to define the ag-

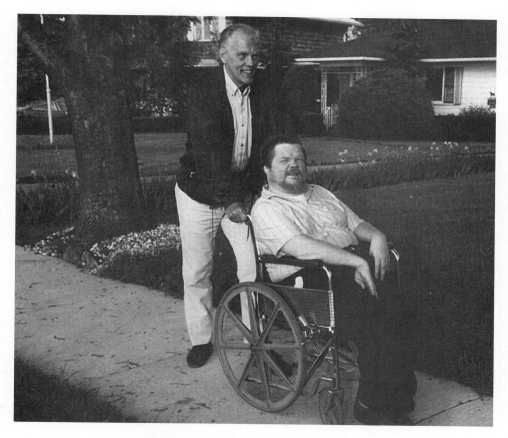

FIGURE 17-2 The older adult doing volunteer work.

ing process in terms of psychologic and environmental influences.

The **disengagement theory** proposes that older adults gradually withdraw from the roles they occupied in middle age, and that this withdrawal is beneficial both to themselves and younger people in that society (Cummings & Henry, 1961).

The **activity theory** includes the suggestion that to maintain a positive sense of self, older adults must substitute new roles for those lost as a result of aging. Figure 17-2 shows a retired adult doing volunteer work. This type of activity is a desired one if at all possible.

Life course theories include the work of Erik Erikson (1959). He viewed maturity as a developmental stage that could not be completed

successfully until previous stages had been concluded.

The crucial task of later adulthood is to evaluate one's life and affirm that the life has been positive. This affirmation reinforces integrity of the personality instead of anxiety and despair. The theory has been criticized as being overly simplistic because it does not address the many dilemmas and crises through which the elderly proceed (Burke & Walsh, 1992).

Robert Havighurst (1975) calls later maturity the **examination stage** and maintains that the elderly adult must accomplish the following tasks:

- Decide where and how to live remaining years.

- Continue supportive, close relationships with spouse or significant others (including sexual activity).
- Find a satisfactory and safe living space.
- Adjust living standards.
- Maintain maximum level of health.
- Maintain contact with children, grandchildren, and other relatives.
- Maintain interest in people and in events, such as civic affairs.
- Pursue new interests and maintain earlier ones.
- Find meaning in life after retirement.
- Work out a philosophy.
- Adjust to death of spouse and other loved ones.

The **continuity theory** suggests that maturing adults try to assess the here-and-now as it relates to their memories of the past. Strategies are implemented that are consistent with remembered patterns of coping. Change comes about as a result of the persons reflecting on past experience and setting goals for the future (Burke & Walsh, 1992).

The **social competence and breakdown theory** points out that a negative spiral of feedback can occur if an individual experiences a health-related crisis, is labeled as dependent by the social environment, becomes unable to perform tasks that were previously a part of his or her life, or develops a self-concept of incompetence. Kuypers and Bengston (1973) suggest that the spiraling breakdown can be reversed by what they call social reconstruction syndrome. They recommend improving environmental supports and fostering a sense of competency in the individual.

Other psychosocial theories of aging include the subculture theory, which points out the fact that the older adults in the United States and Canada have the opportunity to associate with a subculture through such organizations as the American Association of Retired Persons, the Gray Panthers, and others. This subculture cuts across gender, race, and class so that the elderly can develop their own identity.

The exchange theory points out that the elderly withdraw from social interaction because they have fewer resources (Homans, 1961).

A PSYCHOANALYTIC THEORY OF AGING

Carl Jung (1971, p. 17) says about aging, "We cannot live the afternoon of life according to life's morning; for what was great in the morning will be little at evening and what in the morning was true will at evening have become a lie". Jung reports that, although many persons reach old age with unsatisfied life goals, it is unwise to look back. It is essential to find a goal for the future. He suggests that in the later years, individuals need to spend time in reflection to find a meaning and purpose in life that makes it possible to accept approaching death: "An old man who cannot bid farewell to life appears as sickly and feeble as the young man who cannot embrace it" (Jung, 1971, p. 20).

Any of the theories may be useful when attempting to explain why an older adult reacts in certain ways under certain conditions. It is important to remember that none of the theories have been proved and many are not applicable in all situations, across cultures, or for each client with which the nurse comes in contact. These theories only seek to help us understand.

NORMAL PHYSICAL CHANGES

The older adult gradually experiences normal physical changes. Skin turgor decreases because the sebaceous glands, which normally lubricate the skin with oil, become less active. The skin becomes drier. Irregular areas of dark pigmentation, commonly called age spots, appear on the skin (Eliopoulos, 1990; Murray & Zentner, 1993).

The face changes in appearance. Wrinkles appear, which are caused by the repeated stress of smiling or frowning and the pull of gravity.

There are changes inside the mouth that may require attention. Periodontal disease in older adults may predispose them to loss of teeth. Dentures can subtly alter a person's appearance. Ill-fitting dentures can be very uncomfortable and interfere with adequate nutrition and speech (Eliopoulos, 1990; Murray & Zentner, 1993).

There is a gradual loss of hair and hair color. Melanin production in the hair follicle diminishes (Eliopoulos, 1990; Murray & Zentner, 1993).

Older adults experience an increasing loss of muscle strength and endurance. Muscle cells atrophy, and lean muscle mass is lost, thereby making bony prominences more pronounced. Intervertebral spaces narrow, resulting in shortening of the trunk. Planned physical activity and proper nutrition can slow the process.

Nervous system changes accompany the aging process. Older adults, particularly those over 80 years of age, may have altered sensory response so that nerve transmission is delayed and sensory thresholds increase. Thus, the older adult may be slower to make decisions, have slower voluntary movements, and may be less responsive to pain than a younger person. The older adult may have decreased equilibrium and coordination (Hogstel, 1981; Murray & Zentner, 1993).

There are some changes in vision that occur with aging. Lacrimal glands produce fewer tears; the lens thickens and **presbyopia,** an impaired ability of the lens to change shape for near vision, occurs.

Hearing loss may occur because of changes in the organ of Corti. Approximately 13% of adults over 65 years of age experience **presbycusis,** which is a progressive loss of hearing (Eliopoulos, 1990; Murray & Zentner, 1993).

The cardiovascular system may change as the vessel membranes thicken and cardiac output decreases. The older adult must learn to adapt to less strenuous exercise; for example, brisk walking may be more appropriate than jogging. Peripheral vascular changes may include venous stasis and varicose veins, and pedal pulses may be weaker.

Changes in the respiratory system that result from aging affect both internal and external breathing. There is a gradual decline in the structure and function of the respiratory muscles (Eliopoulos, 1990; Murray & Zentner, 1993).

There is a loss of nephron units in the kidneys, which causes a decrease in the filtration rate. Excretion of toxic substances occurs more slowly than in a younger adult. There is also a slowing of peristalsis in the intestinal tract because of fewer stimuli from the autonomic nervous system. The older adult should be encouraged to increase fluid intake and to exercise daily to stimulate kidney filtration. High-fiber foods and exercise may stimulate peristalsis.

The aging man continues to produce testosterone. There is, however, a gradual decline in sexual vigor, muscle strength, and sperm production. The ability of women to continue experiencing pleasurable sexual activity remains, although there is a thinning of the vaginal wall that may make penetration difficult and less satisfying to both partners.

Aging depresses immunity in a general way. Older adults who learn to adapt to the normal changes of aging stay healthy and lead productive lives. Proper nutrition, adequate rest and sleep, planned exercise and activity, and lack of emotional stress assist the older adult to remain healthy.

NORMAL COGNITIVE CHANGES

Cognitive changes depend on many factors; however, the innate mental acuity of the individual does not change. An intelligent 7-year-old will remain an intelligent person at the age of 70 years if illness does not intervene. Sociocultural influences, life role, adaptability, and motivation all affect cognition. Wisdom and experience unite in the healthy elderly person, so that some persons may demonstrate crystalized cognition and the ability to perceive relationships, engage in formal abstraction, and understand the ramifications of intellectual and cultural complexities. Some older persons may experience difficulty with immediate recall of new learning because of delayed sensory input, but the accumulated learning of a lifetime will compensate (Murray & Zentner, 1993). Table 17-2 describes prevention at primary, secondary, and tertiary levels for disease or disability in older adults.

HEALTH PROMOTION IN THE SENIOR CITIZEN CENTER

The older retired adult who remains healthy may function as well as ever and may enjoy the freedom to pursue interests and hobbies rather than full-time employment. The person who becomes less mobile may benefit from community support services such as Meals on Wheels, transportation services, shopping aides, and telephone reassurance programs. Senior citizen centers may provide social outlets, warm meals, and referral services to all citizens who seek them. A useful service to those who need assistance is the adult day-care center, which can meet the unique

Text continues on p. 377

TABLE 17-2 Prevention of Disability in the Older Adult

Physical disabilities associated with the natural aging process	Primary prevention	Secondary prevention	Tertiary prevention
Hearing Presbycusis: loss of auditory acuity associated with age	Encourage avoidance of excessive noise.	Recommend auditory check if the individual complains of difficulty hearing or if the individual seems inattentive or is giving inappropriate responses to verbal cues.	Encourage examination by otologist to identify possible medical reasons for hearing loss; then recommend client go to an audiologist for evaluation. Counsel client and family in communication techniques; for example, to speak slowly and clearly, not louder; face the person to facilitate lip reading; use nonverbal cues when possible (e.g., smiles and waves); write messages and avoid fatigue and environmental distractions; encourage use of hearing aid if helpful.
Taste and smell Loss of ability to enjoy food because of decrease in threshold for taste and smell	Encourage a well-balanced diet and pleasant surroundings during mealtimes.	Recommend listing foods eaten during 24-hour period to determine balanced nutrition.	Encourage vitamin food supplements if well-balanced diet is not adhered to; suggest condiments other than salt to enhance taste of food. Recommend homemaker or family assistance for older adult eating poorly.
Touch Decrease in tactile sensation	Encourage avoidance of sudden, unexpected changes in body position in space.	Encourage use of cane for extra balance if necessary.	Encourage the individual to allow time before changing position (e.g., sitting to standing); incorporate sensory stimulation in all aspects of rehabilitation program.

TABLE 17-2   Prevention of Disability in the Older Adult   cont'd

Physical disabilities associated with the natural aging process	Primary prevention	Secondary prevention	Tertiary prevention
Vision			
Presbyopia (old sight): associated with aging; lens loses ability to accommodate to near and far vision	Encourage regular eye examinations, general check using Snellen eye chart for acuity, general check for peripheral vision; refer for eye examination if necessary.	Recommend wearing bifocals as needed to prevent accidents and mistakes; recommend strong reading glasses to prevent fatigue and disengagement.	Recommend cessation of driving if vision level is less than 20/40; recommend magnifying glasses for reading, adequate glare-reduction lighting, use of large print, and more auditory cues.
Possibility of glaucoma: caused by high intraocular pressure; insidious onset	Encourage regular eye examinations that include screening for glaucoma.	Refer for treatment if glaucoma is detected.	Encourage use of prescribed medication; assist with activities of daily living, transportation, and recreation if blindness occurs.
Cataracts: caused by a degenerative opacity of lens of eye, which results in obstruction of light rays to retina	Encourage regular eye examinations.	Recommend surgical intervention if needed.	Encourage cataract lenses, possibly contact lenses; educate to adapt to difficulty in focusing and aphakia (lack of focusing ability) and to compensate for lack of depth perception.
Muskuloskeletal			
Decreased skeletal bone mass because of decreased intestinal absorption of calcium; more common in women than in men	Encourage supplemental calcium and hormone therapy for postmenopausal women; recommend at least two glasses of milk/day in diet.	Recommend oral daily supplement of vitamin D and calcium; refer to physician for follow-up therapy; counsel to avoid falls and excessive weight bearing.	Recommend hyperextension exercises to strengthen flabby muscles and avoid heavy lifting or accidental falls if osteoporosis is present; counsel in use of orthopedic support walkers, analgesics, heat, and massage.
Muscles: progressive loss of muscular strength because of changes in collagen fibers, less flexibility	Encourage daily exercise, walking, rotating hips, straightening legs, and rotating arms and shoulders.	Provide slow, prolonged stretching exercises.	Recommend continuing exercises in a home care program to encourage functional motion; assist with activities of daily living if function is lost or limited.

Continued

T A B L E 17-2   Prevention of Disability in the Older Adult   cont'd

Physical disabilities associated with the natural aging process	Primary prevention	Secondary prevention	Tertiary prevention
Joints: decrease in cartilage so that bone makes direct contact with bone and can result in degenerative arthritis	Encourage adherence to moderate exercise program to prevent stiffening of joints; ensure adequate rest and avoidance of extreme cold.	Encourage rest of affected joint, analgesics as ordered; recommend adherence to prescribed exercise; encourage weight reduction if appropriate.	Encourage warm soaks, analgesics if necessary, rest, and medical assistance; instruct in the use of canes and walkers; rehabilitate after hip replacement if necessary.
Skin, hair, and toes: wrinkling of skin and graying of hair because the cell layers of the epidermis are thinning	Encourage staying out of the sun because the sun speeds up the aging process; use sun screen when it is necessary to be outside.	Encourage use of moisturizing cream if psoriatic patches begin to appear.	Avoid trauma that may result in senile purpura and lead to skin infection; apply dressings and antiseptics as needed.
Graying of hair because of a reduction in melanin			
Rate of nail growth decreases and causes thickening nails	Encourage soaking before cutting nails to prevent injury.	Refer to podiatrist.	
Immunity			
Depressed as part of the aging process	Encourage annual influenza and pneumonia vaccines and avoidance of stress, cold, and chills; maintain prudent nutrition; wear appropriate clothing and avoid exposure to viral infection.	Monitor changes in health status; refer for early medical treatment.	Encourage adherence to prescribed regime; assist in client recovery or adaption to chronic illness.
Nervous System			
Loss of neurons in frontal lobe; decreased availability of neurotransmitters	Encourage stress management, adequate rest, structured environment.	Monitor changes in mental status.	Refer for medical examination if changes occur, assist with activities of daily living and medical regimen.
Sexuality			
Men, penile erection takes longer; women, loss of vaginal lubrication.	Give information to older adults about the cause of the problem.	Encourage use of vaginal lubrication.	Refer for professional counseling if the problems become upsetting to clients.

needs of the older age group in the community in a number of ways. It is primarily a social center that plans events and activities designed to capture the interest of the senior citizen and to stimulate social interaction. In addition, programs for health promotion may be facilitated.

In the community setting, the adult day-care center and the senior citizen center may assist the older adult in meeting physical and social needs. A community health nurse who is either on site or on call can monitor and guide the health care of the clients at the centers. The day-care center or senior citizen center may arrange regularly scheduled blood pressure clinics and physical assessment clinics to gather baseline information and to screen for potential or actual health problems. The nurse can answer questions regarding medical diagnoses and medications ordered by physicians that may alarm, confuse, or cause anxiety for the older adult. In addition, information concerning current news items such as cholesterol and diet management

can be made available. Subtle changes in the overall health status of the senior citizen can be detected, and proper action can be taken when signs of a potential problem appear. In this case the nurse can make referrals to appropriate health professionals and community resources.

State funding in the form of grants has been made available in some areas to support these centers. This financial aid attests to the invaluable services in the areas of social interaction and health promotion the centers offer mature adults in the community.

Similar services may be provided by various community services and agencies such as the local YMCA or Jewish Community Center. Nurses should become familiar with the available resources in their area and refer clients as appropriate.

THE FRAIL ELDERLY

The **frail elderly** are persons who are usually but not always over the age of 75 who have

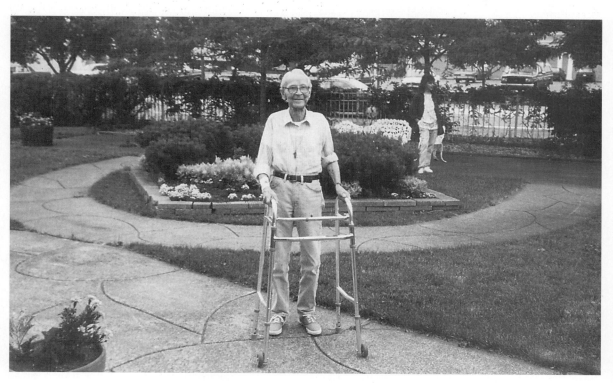

FIGURE 17-3 An older adult (age 90 + years) can enjoy a garden with the help of a walker to stabilize balance.

health problems, limited income, and a lack of social resources (Burke & Walsh, 1992). This group has special problems the younger mature adult may not have. They present a unique and difficult challenge (Figure 17-3).

Common Health Problems of the Frail Elderly

Coronary artery disease. Coronary artery disease is the leading cause of death for individuals over 65 years of age (Figure 17-4). In the frail elderly, who may be sedentary or bedridden, symptoms may be minimal even though there is a pathologic condition. An infection or excessive stress may trigger a major attack. For those persons who have symptoms, such as angina or hypertension, careful monitoring of vital signs and supervision of medical regimes can be very helpful. The possibility of cerebral vascular accidents or transient ischemic attacks is 10 times greater in persons 75 to 85 years of age than in the younger mature persons. Education and encouragement regarding the value of compliance with prescribed therapies can be of great value to the older mature persons. The incidence of congestive heart failure, arrythmias, and conduction disorders also increases with age. Community health nurses should be sensitive to any change in vital signs, such as a rise in blood pressure, a rapid pulse, or an arrythmia. Any of these may be a symptom of impending cardiac crisis (Burke & Walsh, 1992).

Peripheral vascular disease. Some of the frail elderly may experience leg pain when walking. It is often relieved by rest. This pain may occur from mild narrowing of the arteries. Pain that is not relieved by rest may necessitate medical follow-up. Severe compromised circulation could lead to ulceration, gangrene, infection, and even possible loss of a limb. Nurses should be able to recognize "the 6 Ps": pallor, pain, pulselessness, paresthesia, paralysis, and polar (cold). Any of these may indicate the need for immediate medical referral (Lewis, 1990).

Another circulatory problem of the frail elderly may be varicose veins. The use of support hose can alleviate much of the discomfort caused by vericose veins. Chronic venous insufficiency may result in lower leg edema, aching in the calves of the legs, or redness in a localized area. Any of these symptoms should be referred for evaluation of possible thrombophlebitis.

Cancer. Cancer is the second leading cause of death among the elderly. In men over 65 years of age, prostate cancer is the most common. Gastrointestinal cancer ranks second. For women in this age group, breast cancer is first and gastrointestinal cancer is second (Lewis, 1990). Changes in the immune system might account for the prevalence of these cancers (see auto immune theory, p.368). The incidence of multiple cancers may occur in the same person because of the inability of the older person's immune system to destroy mutant cells. Persons who have a history of cancer should be encouraged to have frequent examinations.

Other cancers that may affect the elderly include lung cancer, head and neck cancer, multiple myeloma, non-Hodgkins lymphoma, colon cancer, and skin cancer.

Chronic lung disease. Chronic lung disease is present in many of the frail elderly and can lead to serious health problems. Emphysema, bronchoconstriction, bronchitis, or asthma may be present. Asthma can be precipitated by upper respiratory infection, exposure, or pollutants. Actually, the presence of any of these may lead to a fatality if the person is infected with a viral or bacterial upper-respiratory infection. Persons over 65 years of age should be encouraged to get yearly immunizations for influenza and pneumonia. Any upper-respiratory infection should be treated aggressively.

Diabetes mellitus. Diabetes mellitus should be suspected if an older client complains of polidipsia, polyurea, frequent infections, or numbness and tingling of the extremities. The condition is the most common disorder of persons over 85 years of age, affecting one out of four (Burke & Walsh, 1992). An elderly person with diabetes has an increased risk for cataracts and is at high risk for retinopathy. Impaired vision may necessitate long-term health supervision for the diabetic older person living at home.

Osteoporosis. Osteoporosis, a decrease in bone tissue mass, is found in one fourth of all white women in the United States who are past menopause. Men older than 80 years of age are

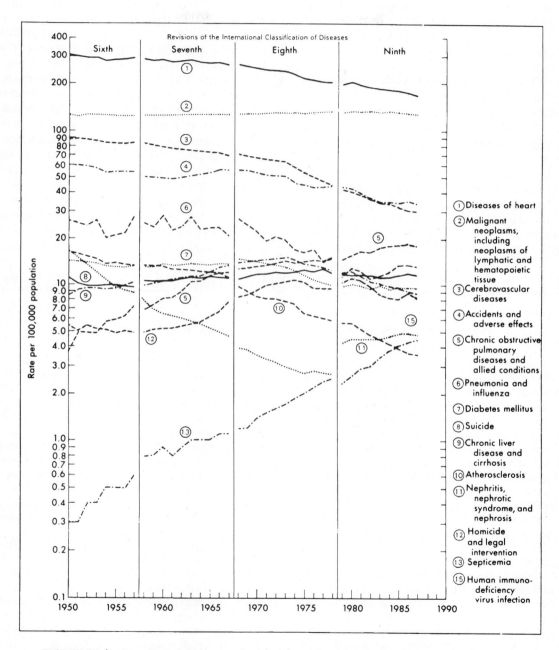

FIGURE 17-4 Age-adjusted death rates for 14 of the 15 leading causes of death in the United States, 1950 to 1990. *(From* Monthly Vital Statistics Report *by the National Center for Health Statistics [DHHS 38 (5)], September 26, 1989, Washington, DC: U.S. Government Printing Office.)*

also at risk for this problem, which predisposes the person to bone fractures in the affected areas. There are indications that an increase in calcium in the diet may help prevent osteoporosis. Persons with this disorder are at high risk for fractures and subsequent immobility.

Benign prostatic hypertrophy. Aging men frequently experience a condition called benign prostatic hypertrophy. This enlargement of the prostate gland is easily corrected by surgical intervention. Failure to intervene can lead to urinary retention and severe distress.

Neurologic diseases. A number of neurologic diseases may cause disability in later maturity. Parkinson's disease is a progressive degenerative disorder that can be highly debilitating. A client with this disease must be carefully monitored. Alzheimer's disease is also a progressive

degenerative disorder. A client with Alzheimer's disease needs in-depth monitoring. In addition, extensive family therapy is required to help family members deal with the resulting multiple problems. Pernicious anemia occurs because of a lack of intrinsic factor that is essential for the absorption of vitamin B_{12}. A client with pernicious anemia may require supplemental B_{12} injections on a routine basis. Lymphatic leukemia, which is a neoplasm of blood-forming tissues, is a severe health hazard that may occur in late maturity.

Skin disorders. Skin disorders can be troublesome for the elderly. Pruritis and itching caused by dryness can be relieved by the use of lotions. Senile purpura, caused by a loss of subcutaneous tissue, can be minimized if the person is careful to avoid injury. Benign and malignant skin lesions are lessened by the avoidance of direct

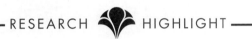

RESEARCH HIGHLIGHT

Bone Mineral Density and Factors Associated with Menopause

A study on osteoporosis was conducted in a community-based sample of 555 upper-middle-class Caucasian women between the ages of 60 and 89 years who had been postmenopausal for at least 5 years. During structured interviews, participants provided histories related to their use of tobacco, contraceptives and noncontraceptives (estrogen), medications (thiazide); and to their menstruation and reproductivity. Precision errors were provided for the scanners (absorptiometry) used to measure bone density at four anatomic sites (ultradistal wrist, midshaft radius, lumbar spine, and hip) to determine the association of age at menopause and number of reproductive years (years between menarche and menopause) with bone mineral density in women who had either experienced natural menopause (n = 391) or hysterectomy with bilateral oophorectomy (n = 164). Multiple, separate two-tailed analyses of these two groups, whose composite mean of 48 served to distinguish between early and late menopause categories, included control for potential confounding covariates. While comparisons were achieved between

three distinct age groups (60 to 69 years, 70 to 79 years, 80 to 89 years), analyses for the number of reproductive years ($\overline{X}$ 35) were confined to the women who experienced natural menopause.

The major results of this study were as follows: (1) In every analysis, there was a significant and positive association between age at menopause and bone mineral density, (2) number of reproductive years had significant positive associations with bone mineral density at all sites, and (3) at every site, total number of reproductive years explained more of the variance in bone mineral density than did either age at menarche or age at menopause.

The investigators report that their study was the first to reveal an increase with reproductive years in bone mineral density at all four sites, and to compare this association with other reproductive variances. Because osteoporosis is greater in elderly women who report early menopause or fewer reproductive years, consideration might be given to the inclusion of longevity of reproductivity in the assessment of the elderly to detect women at risk and to provide earlier therapeutic intervention.

From "Early Menopause, Number of Reproductive Years, and Bone Mineral Density in Postmenopausal Women" by D. Knitz-Silverstein and E. Barrett-Connor, 1993, *American Journal of Public Health, 83*(7), 983-988.

TABLE 17-3 Mean Heights and Weights and Recommended Energy Intakes for Adults

Gender	Age (years)	Weight (kg)	Weight (lb)	Height (cm)	Height (in)	Energy needs (with range) (kcal)
Male	23-50	70	154	178	70	2700 (2300-3100)
	51-75	70	154	178	70	2400 (2000-2800)
	76+	70	154	178	70	2050 (1650-2450)
Female	23-50	55	120	163	64	2000 (1600-2400)
	51-75	55	120	163	64	1800 (1400-2200)
	76+	55	120	163	64	1600 (1200-2000)

Adapted from *Recommended Dietary Allowances* (9th ed.). Food and Nutrition Board, Committee on Dietary Allowances, 1980, Washington, DC: National Academy of Sciences.

sunlight. The fragile elderly should be made aware that chronic open sores, thickened scaly areas, and draining lesions could be symptoms of a serious health problem (Burke & Walsh, 1992).

Nutrition. Adequate nutrition can be difficult for the elderly to maintain. Often, decreased mobility will lead to obesity, and chronic disease may lead to malnutrition. The nurse should weighing the person to determine whether he or she is within normal limits for his or her age and height. This procedure will serve as a baseline (see Table 17-3). If there seems to be a problem, a 24-hour dietary recall may enable the nurse to determine whether there is an adequate caloric intake as well as the appropriateness of the foods the person is ingesting. The recommended caloric intake for women over 75 is 1600 calories. For men it is 2050 calories. Older adults must still have a diet that includes calcium, iron, and vitamins A, C, and B. It is also important that some fiber be included (Clark, 1992).

Safety. "Safety can be defined as freedom from danger. Another phrase that is used to denote safety is protection from hazards" (Burke & Walsh, 1992, p. 407). Safety is a big issue for the frail elderly.

Accidents and adverse drug reactions are serious problems for this age group. For example, the rate of unintentional injury increases with each age increment. It is the fifth leading cause of death for those over 85 (Lambert & Sattin, 1988). Stairs in the home become difficult to climb for some older persons. Uncertain balance, as a re-sult of either some types of drugs or transient ischemic attacks, can precipitate an episode resulting in injury. When the elderly are assessed at home, the nurse should always be aware of the possible risk of the person slipping or falling. It is important to note any physical disabilities, cognitive and sensory impairments, environmental hazards, and any history of falling. The box below describes some of the environmental hazards.

Falls are especially dangerous to elderly women, who may have osteoporosis. Both men and women should be given information con-

---

ENVIRONMENTAL HAZARDS TO THE ELDERLY

- Poorly lighted stairs
- Stairs without bannisters
- Absence of a grab bar in the tub
- Glare in the hallway
- Absence of workable smoke alarm
- Poorly placed extension cords
- Throw rugs
- Clutter
- Inappropriate footwear or long clothing
- High beds
- Restraints and protective devices

From *Gerontological Nursing* (p. 410) by M. Burke & M. Walsh, 1992, St. Louis: Mosby.

cerning environmental risk factors and the side effects of some medications they are taking.

Depression. Depression is a common health problem for the frail elderly. Depression may be defined as feelings of sadness, despair, and discouragement resulting from some personal loss or tragedy (Glanze, Anderson, & Anderson, 1990). Growing older necessitates having to deal with multiple losses. Friends and spouses may die. Some folks may outlive their children. Family members may relocate. One's economic position may result in an inability to live according to a former lifestyle. Physical disabilities may result in pain and immobility. The losses become cumulative, and the gains diminish. Elderly who have had a lifetime of chronic depression may be un-

able to cope at all. When assessing the health state of an older person, nurses must include the possibility of chronic depression. Some of the symptoms to look for include the following:

- The elderly person looking sad and hopeless and feeling depressed most of the time
- Markedly diminished interest or pleasure in all or most activities shown through apathy or withdrawal
- Significant weight loss or gain
- Insomnia (difficulty sleeping) or hyperinsomnia (sleeping too much)
- Fatigue or loss of energy
- Feelings of worthlessness, low self-esteem, or inappropriate guilt

---

RESEARCH HIGHLIGHT

Suicide in the Elderly

Eighteen elderly (ages 67 to 74 years), Caucasian, self-sufficient, independent urbanites from three communities, 16 of whom were women, voluntarily participated in a study that elicited their perceptions of suicide. Before the audiotaped indepth interviews, the nondepressed participants, as determined by the Beck Depression Inventory or their psychiatrist or psychiatric mental health nurse specialists, were told that suicide was a major problem for the elderly and that health care providers have limited understanding of the causes or how to intervene. The participants were told that their input would help health care providers to better understand suicide in the elderly.

The grounded theory approach was used to analyze the transcribed data, and maintenance of control was the rubric that served to encompass the emergent concepts of participating in timing of death and accepting suicide as an alternative. These concepts furnished information related to deterrents, specific risk factors, and causality. Responding to suicidal ideation, a third concept, was included because it provided data about how the elderly desired health care professionals to respond to them. Participants' views included actual commentaries

to substantiate the descriptions provided for each concept.

Because the investigators are continuing to gather and analyze data, they caution that the provision of broader categories is premature. However, they did indicate that there is evidence throughout their data that the elderly are concerned about maintaining individual control over their own life and death situations. Suggestions for further research were related to the findings (deterrents, risk factors, life-circumstances). The suggestions included longitudinal studies that examined the relationship between the passage of time and the elderly's perception of suicide. Emphasis was given to the relationship between depression and suicide since at the experiential level, they were inextricably intertwined.

Implications for nursing include anticipatory guidance associated with societal changes (living wills and advanced directives), advanced medical technology, and coping strategies. It also requires both the sensitivity required to pursue problem resolution to provide some hope and control and the willingness to discuss dying with the elderly.

From "Suicide in the elderly: Staying in Control" by M.M. Courage, K.L. Godbey, D.A. Ingram, L.L. Schramn, & E. Hale, 1993, *Journal of Psychosocial Nursing and Mental Health Services, 31*(7), 26-33.

- Diminished ability to think or concentrate, or difficulty making decisions
- Psychomotor agitation (excessive activity that is usually nonproductive) or retardation
- Recurrent thoughts of death or a suicide attempt (Burke & Walsh, 1992, p. 372)

It is especially important to intervene quickly if the client is male because elderly males are at a higher risk for suicide than any other group (21.6 per 100,000 for those 65 years old or older, compared with 12.8 per 100,000 for the population as a total group. The suicide rate for males over the age of 85 years is 71.9 per 100,000). The suicide rate for women is only 7.5 per 100,000 in this age group (National Center for Health Statistics, 1990). The nurse who works with the depressed client, whether one-on-one or in a group, must listen carefully, convey an attitude of caring without being solicitous, reinforce feelings of self-esteem, and refer for psychologic intervention if the depression seems to become unmanageable.

Group work may include the sharing of memories, which can assist the person to bond with other members of his or her age group through reminiscing. This may facilitate a resocialization for depressed clients and an acceptance of each other. Many older adults feel isolated when family and friends are gone. One elderly gentleman said, "There's no one left who remembers." Reminiscing may also assist in a life review that helps the person to raise self-esteem which, in turn, will favorably influence the intrapsychic climate (Blackman, 1980). There are clearly several ways a nurse may assist a depressed elderly person to reconnect and find meaning in life. Listening, having a caring attitude, encouraging and facilitating some socialization, and referring the elderly person to a professional counselor if the depression becomes overwhelming or there are thoughts of suicide are some of the ways a nurse can assist.

Cognitive changes. With age, the following physical changes occur in the brain: loss of brain volume and weight, loss of protein, decrease in lipids, and changes in the neurotransmitters. How these changes affect the cognitive ability of the frail elderly person is not clear. There is research to support the fact that, by the age of 70 years, there is a decline in the ability to think in abstract terms. The ability to memorize and recall new information is lessened in some individuals. Some persons, however, show no decline in cognition up to their 80s or beyond. Healthy elderly persons continue to function much as they did when they were in their late 50s (Burke & Walsh, 1992). However, there are some cognitive disorders that manifest themselves in some elderly persons.

Organic disorders that happen because of changes in the neurons, circulatory problems, and other physical phenomenon are the most common cognitive disorders that affect the elderly. These organic disorders are generally classified as dementia and may lead to total dependence. It is usually irreversible and often is the cause for institutionalization.

Alzheimer's disease is the most common cause for dementia. It is insidious and develops over years. Cognitive ability decreases gradually. There may be rapid mood changes and wandering behavior. There may be interrupted sleep patterns and impulsivity. As the disease progresses, the individual may become totally disoriented, incontinent, and unable to function. Persons with this disability who remain at home require so much care and supervision that the community health nurse should include the caregiver in the plan of care. Plans for respite services, help with personal care of the client, and assistance with regard to institutionalization of the client if it becomes necessary, should be arranged.

Circulatory problems caused by cerebral vascular accidents or emboli may result in some dementia. Usually, persons with this disorder can be helped by nursing intervention that includes some reality orientation and a planned, structured environment.

Other physical phenomenon that may contribute to dementia are Parkinson's disease, side effects from prescribed medications, and chronic alcoholism (Korsakoff's syndrome) (Burke & Walsh, 1992).

Confused states that are transient and self-limiting may be precipitated by surgical procedures, hospitalization, and extreme stress. The elderly person who is carefully supported during this period will almost always fully recover. Care should be taken not to label an individual as having dementia when an episode of confusion has been precipitated by a stressful event.

SPIRITUAL NURSING CARE

It should be remembered that adults in later maturity are coping with the knowledge that they are moving toward the part of the life cycle that

is a mystery. To some this is viewed as an end to being and to others as a peaceful journey. To all persons it is unknown. **Spiritual nursing** care of the elderly client includes listening to concerns, providing an opportunity to talk about death, and assisting in summing up or reminiscing about his or her life, if he or she cares to do so. An individual with a strongly developed religious life may enjoy quoting familiar Bible pas-

---

SELECTED NURSING DIAGNOSES RELATED TO PERSON IN LATER MATURITY*

Pattern 1: exchanging

Altered nutrition: more than body requirements
Altered nutrition: less than body requirements
Hypothermia
Hyperthermia
Stress incontinence
Potential for injury
Potential for trauma
Potential for disuse syndrome
Potential impaired skin integrity

Pattern 2: communicating

Impaired verbal communication

Pattern 3: relating

Impaired social interaction
Social isolation
Altered role performance
Sexual dysfunction
Altered family processes
Altered sexuality patterns

Pattern 4: valuing

Spiritual distress

Pattern 5: choosing

Ineffective individual coping
Impaired adjustment
Defensive coping
Ineffective denial
Ineffective family coping: disabling
Ineffective family coping: compromised
Family coping: potential for growth
Decisional conflict
Health seeking behaviors

Pattern 6: moving

Impaired physical mobility
Fatigue
Potential activity intolerance
Sleep pattern disturbance
Diversional activity deficit
Impaired home maintenance management
Altered health maintenance
Bathing/hygiene self-care deficit
Dressing/grooming self-care deficit

Pattern 7: perceiving

Body image disturbance
Self esteem disturbance
Chronic low self esteem
Situational low self esteem
Sensory/perceptual alterations
Unilateral neglect
Hopelessness
Powerlessness

Pattern 8: knowing

Knowledge deficit
Altered thought processes

Pattern 9: feeling

Pain
Chronic pain
Dysfunctional grieving
Anticipatory grieving
Post-trauma response
Anxiety
Fear

* Other of the NANDA diagnoses related to physiologic phenomena are applicable to the ill individual in this group.
From "NANDA Approved Nursing Diagnostic Categories" by North American Nursing Diagnosis Association, Summer 1988, *Nursing Diagnosis Newsletter, 15*(1), pp. 1-3. Copyright 1988 by NANDA. Reprinted by permission.

sages and praying. If the religious grounding of the person is unfamiliar to the nurse, referral to an appropriate pastoral source may be very important. It may be even more urgent for persons who regard death as an end to being to discuss anxieties and concerns either about themselves or others at this point in their lives. Anxieties of a practical nature are easier to deal with than are anxieties about approaching death. These concerns are best handled with compassion, a nonjudgmental approach, patience, and an honest interest in the client's welfare, thoughts, feelings, and opinions (Carroll, 1985).

The box on p. 384 lists selected nursing diagnoses that were approved by the North American Nursing Diagnosis Association (NANDA)

(1988) that could relate to persons in later maturity who were experiencing health problems or anxieties or both.

Permanent cognitive changes may result from organic changes in the brain. These should be differentiated from temporary episodes of confusion brought about by external events. Advocacy for the elderly includes protection from abuse and preservation of quality of life. Spiritual nursing care includes listening to concerns, perhaps providing an opportunity to talk about death, and assisting in summing up or reminiscing about life.

SOCIAL CONCERNS FOR THE ELDERLY

Elder abuse happens too often in the United States and Canada. It may be physical or psycho-

TABLE 17-4   Nursing Care Plan

Nursing diagnosis	Goal	Plan/intervention	Evaluation
Knowledge deficit about the administration of diabetes medication and testing blood sugars (glucose)	Within 3 weeks the client's daughter will be able to administer insulin and test blood glucose.	Nurse to visit daily to teach daughter to administer insulin and test blood glucose.	Within 3 weeks the daughter will be administering insulin and testing blood glucose daily.
Altered nutrition related to lack of knowledge about diabetic diet	Client, daughter will understand importance of maintaining diabetic diet.	Nurse to teach client, daughter appropriate dietary management.	Client will be maintained on a diabetic diet.
Knowledge deficit concerning failing sight	Client, daughter will understand need for frequent checkups and safety in the home.	Nurse to teach client, daughter importance of safety in the home and need for frequent examinations.	Safety hazards in the home are removed. Client visits ophthalmologist when appointments are scheduled.
Impaired home maintenance management of transient ischemic attacks, confusion, dizziness	A personal care aide will be placed for activities of daily living assistance and moderate exercise.	Nurse to supervise personal care aide and write up plan of care.	Personal care aides will be placed on a 24-hour basis. Nurse to supervise weekly.
Self-esteem disturbance	Client will understand the need for assistance and support to maintain her in her home.	Nurse to counsel client concerning the importance of a positive adjustment to her medication, diet, exercise, and safety.	The client will not become depressed about her supervision in the home.

On an ongoing, long-term basis, the nurse will make weekly visits to monitor blood sugars and blood pressure, and supervise personal care aides. The client system must include the client's daughter in the ongoing assessment to give her relief from her mother's care when necessary and provide support and encouragement.

■ CASE STUDY

Mrs. Rosario, an 82-year-old widow, was referred to a home health agency by a hospital discharge planner. Her physician had requested health teaching and supervision. Her referral included the information that she was a newly diagnosed insulin-dependent diabetic. She was hypertensive and had mild retinopathy. She also had periods of dizziness and confusion related to transient ischemic attacks.

A home visit was made the morning after her discharge. After testing Mrs. Rosario's blood glucose with a glucometer and finding it to be 170, the nurse injected her with insulin and assisted her with eating breakfast. An assessment revealed this information: Mrs. Rosario's vital signs were as follows: temperature, 98.6°; pulse, 80; respirations, 20; blood pressure 160/90. She was oriented and alert and said she was happy to be home. The home was modest, but well kept and in a pleasant neighborhood. Mrs. Rosario had lived there for 50 years and wished to remain at home as long as doing so was not a burden to anyone. A daughter lived nearby and visited daily. Mrs. Rosario had a son in another city who called frequently, and a total of six grandchildren.

Mrs. Rosario had immigrated to the United States when she was 19 and spoke English with a strong Italian accent. She was, at this time in her life, a widow. Her income consisted of her husband's social security checks, a small retirement annuity, and some private funds from a family inheritance. She had Medicare A and B.

While writing Mrs. Rosario's care plan, the nurse was aware that this formerly active, healthy woman was progressing toward a difficult period in her life when her retinopathy would perhaps cause blindness. Her hypertension could precipitate transient ischemic attacks that could cause dizziness and possible falls. The diabetes placed her at high risk for infections, neuropathies, and kidney infections. Her frequent confusion could lead to an altered mental state. The nurse arranged with the client's daughter to meet at the home the following day. The daughter had expressed a willingness to assist with her mother's care.

The following day, the nurse attempted to assess the following:

1. What do the patient and the daughter know about diabetes?

2. What do they understand about diet and appropriate nutrition?

3. Do they understand that some exercise is a good idea?

4. Is the daughter willing and able to inject her mother with the insulin?

5. Do they understand that the retinopathy must be carefully monitored and could be progressive?

6. Are they both aware of the dangers inherent in the transient ischemic attacks?

7. How committed are they to keeping Mrs. Rosario in the home?

The care plan in Table 17-4 was made as a result of the interview.

---

logic. It may involve neglect or even financial abuse such as misappropriation of funds. Nurses need to be sensitive to the possibility that this may occur in the home. If caretakers are overly stressed, alcoholic, or exhausted, abuse is more likely to be a problem (Albrecht & Swanson, 1993). Most states and provinces have laws against elder abuse. The code for nurses mandates that nurses take action when health care or the safety of the client is jeopardized (see Chapter 31).

Quality of life issues are becoming more urgent as the population ages. Nurses who work with families in the home may be assisting relatives to make choices having to do with declaring a relative incompetent, honoring a living will, and appropriate time and manner to institutionalize. It is an awesome responsibility to assist families with these decisions. Advocacy and advice must be given as objectively as possible and with an awareness of the need for beneficence (see Chapter 31).

Chapter Highlights

- The adult in later maturity can enjoy good health and an active life. There are several theories about biologic and psychologic aging.

- Biologic theories of aging include the error and fidelity theory, the somatic mutation theory, the neurotransmitter theory, and the auto immune theory.

- Psychosocial theories of aging include the disengagement theory, the activity theory, and the continuity theory.

- Physical and cognitive changes are normal with aging. Prevention at primary, secondary, and tertiary levels can help prevent disability as these changes occur.

- According to Erikson, developmental tasks of aging include developing a feeling that one's life has not been meaningless. Havighurst calls later maturity the examination stage, and Jung recommends that older people spend time in reflection.

- Mature adults face common health problems. Periodic physical assessment can identify some developing problems before they become disabling. Prevention can occur at primary, secondary, and tertiary levels.

- Of the several community resources for adults in later maturity, some of the most pleasurable are the senior center and the adult day-care center.

- The frail elderly persons have a number of common health problems nurses must be aware of. It is important to assess safety and nutrition. Advocacy should include prevention of abuse, assessment of the quality of life, and concern about caretakers.

 CRITICAL THINKING EXERCISE

An elderly gentleman, age 92 years, has been admitted to an adult residence because of repeated falling episodes in his home. The home health nurse monitoring his blood pressure discovers he is depressed. The nurse decides to try remenicense therapy to get him to talk about his past experiences.

1. Why might this assist the gentleman to adjust to his present surroundings?
2. Considering his developmental stage, what kinds of activities might lead him to a better adjustment to his surroundings?

REFERENCES

Albrecht, M., & Swanson, J. (1993). *Community health nursing: Promoting the health of aggregates.* Philadelphia: W.B. Saunders.

Birren, J., & Bengston, V. (1988). *Emergent theories of aging.* New York: Springer.

Blackman, J.C. (1980). Group work in the community: Experiences with reminiscence. In I. Burnside (Ed.). *Psychosocial care of the aged* (pp. 126-144). New York: McGraw-Hill.

Brookbank, J.W. (1990). *The biology of aging.* New York: Harper & Row.

Burke, M., & Walsh, M. (1992). *Gerontologic nursing care of the frail elderly.* St. Louis: Mosby.

Burnside, I. (1980). *Psychosocial nursing care of the aged* (2nd ed.). New York: McGraw-Hill.

Carroll, D. (1985). *Living with dying.* New York: McGraw-Hill.

Clark, M.J. (1992). *Nursing in the community.* Norwalk, CT: Appleton & Lange.

Cristofalo, V.J. (1988). An overview of the theories of biological aging. In J. Birren, & V. Bengston (Eds.). *Emergent theories of nursing* (pp. 118-127). New York: Springer.

Cummings, E., & Henry, W.E. (1961). *Growing old: The process of disengagement.* New York: Basic Books.

Eliopoulos, C. (1990). *Gerontological nursing* (3rd ed.). Philadelphia: J.B. Lippincott.

Erikson, E. (1959). *Identity and the life cycle, selected papers.* New York: International University Press.

Florini, J.R. (1981). *Handbook of biochemistry in aging.* Boca Raton, FL: CRC Press.

Glanze, W., Anderson, K., & Anderson, L. (Eds.). (1990). *Mosby's medical nursing and allied health dictionary.* St. Louis: Mosby.

Havighurst, R. (1975). A social psychological perspective on aging. In W.S. Sze (Ed.). *Human life cycle.* New York: Aronson.

Hochschild, A.R. (1975). Disengagement theory: A critique and proposal. *American Sociological Review, 40,* 553-569.

Hogstel, M. (1981). *Nursing care of the older adult.* New York: Wiley & Sons.

Homans, G.C. (1961). *Social behavior: Its elementary forms.* New York: Harcourt, Brace, Jovanovich.

Jung, C. (1971). The stages of life. In J. Campbell (Ed.). *The*

Kuypers, J.A, & Bengston, V.L. (1973). Social breakdown and competence: A model of normal aging. *Human Development, 16,* 181-201.

Lambert, D., & Sattin, R. (1988). Deaths from falls, 1978-1984. *Division of Injury, Epidemiology and Control, Center for Environmental Health and Injury Control, 37*(SS-1), 21-26.

Lewis, C.B. (1990). *Aging, the health care challenge* (2nd ed.). Philadelphia: Davis.

Murray, R., & Zentner, J. (1993). *Nursing assessment and health promotion strategies through the life span* (5th ed.). Norwalk, CT: Appleton & Lange.

National Center for Health Statistics. (1990). *Health, United States, 1989.* Hyattsville, MD: U.S. Public Health Service.

North American Nursing Diagnosis Association. (1988). NANDA approved nursing diagnostic categories. *Nursing Diagnosis Newsletter, 15*(1), 1-3.

U.S. Bureau of the Census. (1984, May). Series P-25, No. 952.

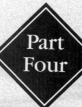

Part Four

Caring for the Family in the Community

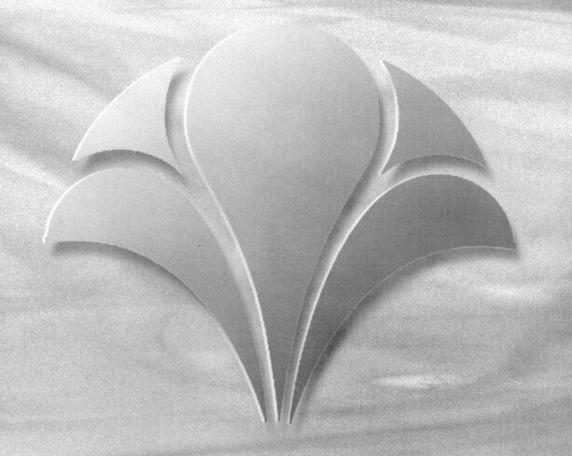

A nurse who practices within a family unit must frequently involve the entire family in a plan of care. Understanding family coping mechanisms may assist the nurse in creating an effective plan.

Chapter 18 describes various types of families and focuses on functional families. These are families with adaptive coping styles that normally operate at a high level of wellness. This is not to say that situational crises do not occur. However, they are dealt with in a way that maintains the family as a system and brings about the best possible resolution. The chapter also points out some of the changes that are occurring in today's family structure. More women are in the work force; modern technology and an aging population are subtly influencing family life. Assessment tools for planning family care are also provided.

Chapter 19 describes the characteristics of families who are at risk for, or who have developed, dysfunctional behavior. The effect of multiple stressors on families such as these is discussed. The role of the nurse in enabling dysfunctional families to move toward wellness is complex and may require self-analysis on the part of the nurse before beginning such assistance.

Just as wellness in an individual can affect an entire family, the wellness of a family can affect an entire community. A nurse practicing in a community may be able to raise the level of wellness in an entire community by raising the level of wellness in just one family.

18

THE FAMILY AS A UNIT OF SERVICE

Sandra L. Termini

The family of the future may neither vanish nor enter upon a new golden age. It may break up and shatter, only to come together again in weird and novel ways.

Alvin Toffler

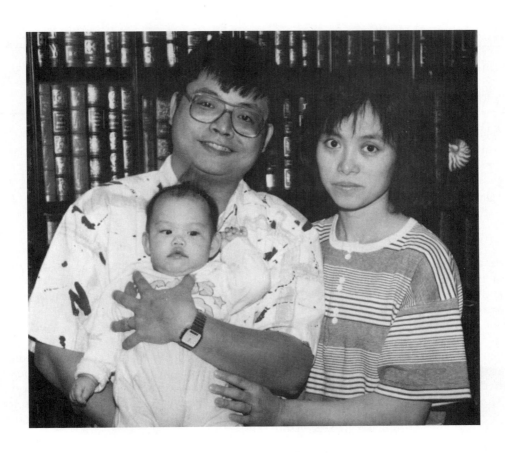

OBJECTIVES

At the conclusion of this chapter the student will be able to:

1. Define the key terms listed.
2. Identify five types of families.
3. Describe evolving family structures.
4. Describe role behavior within the family unit.
5. Explain communication theory.
6. Describe crisis theory.
7. Define the functional family.
8. Describe adaptive family coping patterns.
9. List three conceptual frameworks that can be used to understand the family unit.
10. Use a systems framework to identify the interactive aspect of the individual's and the family's level of wellness.
11. Use the nursing process to raise the level of wellness in a family.
12. Use a systems framework to identify the interaction between the family's and the community's level of wellness.

KEY TERMS

Blended family	Family	Maturational crises
Communication	Family developmental tasks	Nuclear family
Crisis theory	Family life cycle	Nuclear family dyad
Ecomap	Genogram	Single-parent family
Extended family	Kin network family	Situational crises

A thorough understanding of the family is essential to the practice of professional nursing. Even in the early 1900s, community health nurses recognized the importance of planning care for the family. In instances in which one person had a health problem, the entire family was involved in setting priorities and planning and giving care. Nurses have long recognized that the family's health values, beliefs, and practices influence the health status of its individual members.

Providing care in the client's home rather than in a hospital or a clinic gives the nurse a totally different perspective and presents a more accu-rate picture of the individual as part of a family and a community system. Home nursing care takes place in the client's territory, and health care planning responsibilities are shared equally by the health care provider and the client family system.

In this chapter the definition of family in contemporary society is reviewed, various types of families are described, several conceptual frameworks for studying the family are discussed, and the process of providing nursing care for the family as a unit is examined.

Knowledge of theory provides only part of a

nurse's preparation in planning family care. Nurses must also consider their own personal family experiences and background because these experiences help form the perceptual field through which nurses view other families. Understanding one's own culture and values helps a nurse both to respect and to be more objective in evaluating families with differing lifestyles.

WHAT IS A FAMILY?

Various intellectual disciplines have developed their own definitions of **family.** Each is based on the particular emphasis of that field. Biologic definitions of family describe mating, reproduction, and descent, and do not emphasize psychosocial aspects of partnering or parenting. Sociologists view the family as a social group usually related by blood or contract. Legal definitions of family consider the phenomena of marriage, divorce or separation, and adoption, and how they create nonbiologic family configurations. These are only a few examples of the differing focuses of various disciplines.

Common to all definitions of family are that families comprise more than one person, with at least one adult, and that these persons are related to one another by blood or social contract. It is very important to remember that the structure and form of the family are dynamic and ever changing. Anthropologists acknowledge that some form of family is found in every culture. Historical references to family forms are found in folklore and in ancient written manuscripts such as the Old Testament of the Bible. Scientists are not in complete agreement regarding a clear path of evolution from primitive human life forms to the contemporary family. The significant fact is that the concept of family has existed in some form since the beginning of time and has survived centuries of change, disruption, and technological growth.

TYPES OF FAMILIES

Typical family structures vary from culture to culture. Even within one culture the family structure is constantly changing and evolving into new forms (Friedman, 1992; Hymovich and Chamberlin, 1980; Sussman, 1971). The more common types of families are described here.

The **nuclear family** consists of husband and wife with one or more children. Although this family type is the idealized or perceived "typical" family, it represented only 38% of American families in 1985 (National Data Bank, 1986) (Figure 18-1).

The **nuclear family dyad** is the term applied to the increasing number of adult couples who choose to remain childless, or to "empty nesters" whose children have grown and left home.

The **single-parent family** consists of only one parent with one or more children, which is an arrangement resulting from divorce, separation, abandonment, death, or a never-married parent.

The single adult living alone does not fit the strict definition of a family, which is comprised of more than one person, but may be viewed as part of a family modified as a result of divorce, abandonment, death, or the choice to live alone. This person may still function as a part of his or her original birth family, which is also known as the family of orientation.

The three-generation or **extended family** can encompass any combination of the nuclear, dyad, single parent, or single adult. At one time it was common in Western cultures for several generations of a family to share a home. With the advent of modern technology, communication networks, and transportation systems, nuclear families are more likely to be geographically mobile. Relatively frequent career-related moves around the state or country have contributed to the separation and fragmentation of the extended family system.

The **kin network family** includes nuclear families or unmarried members living in close proximity of one another and working together in a reciprocal system of exchange of goods and services. This family form has probably arisen to provide the support network once found in extended families.

THE EVOLVING FAMILY STRUCTURE

Life in the United States has changed dramatically in the last several decades. As Americans struggle to keep up with technological developments that alter virtually every aspect of daily life, new family structures emerge to meet the

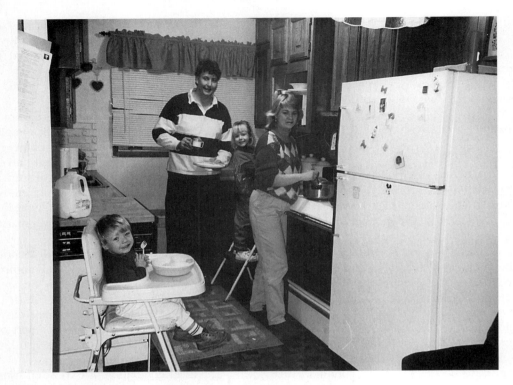

FIGURE 18-1   In the modern nuclear family both parents often work. The pace is hectic; everyone helps.

needs of a new day. Economic changes have contributed to an increasing number of women in the work force. In 1960, 27.7% of married women between the ages of 25 and 34 years were in the work force. In 1990, 73% of married women in the same age-group worked outside the home. In 1960, 18% of working women had children under the age of 6 years. This number increased to 59.9% in 1991 (U.S. Department of Commerce, 1992).

Concurrent with these changes were the advent and development of effective methods of family planning. The ability to exert some control over women's reproductive functions has resulted in smaller families and has allowed families greater capability to make dual career choices. As more women have developed and continued their careers, family members gradually have had to adapt and change their definitions of sharing household responsibilities (Lewis, 1984). Modern-day pursuits of a comfort-

able lifestyle, coupled with the expectation that the small nuclear family should meet all the needs of its members for nurturance, affection, and survival, place the family under extraordinary pressure.

Various evolving family structures have resulted from these social changes (Hymovich & Bernard, 1973; Sussman, 1971). The unmarried parent with child family consists of an unmarried adult and one or more children who are either biologically produced, or adopted by an unmarried adult.

The unmarried couple with child family is one in which the adult couple shares emotional bonds without the legal sanction of marriage. The couple may abide by some form of social contract and may or may not have children.

Same sex families consist of two men or two women living together, who are usually bound by some form of social contract. The couple may or may not have children by adoption or by previous or alternative reproductive arrangements. Their relationship may or may not include a sexual relationship.

A cohabiting retired couple is an unmarried retired couple living together without legal sanctions. Often this is because of economic necessity; that is, retirement or Social Security benefits can be lost or negatively affected by marriage.

The **blended family** or stepfamily has evolved as a family form concurrent with the rising divorce rate. This family group results when one or both adults who have been part of a previous family join together to form a new family, which may include children by these previous families or relationships.

ROLES WITHIN THE FAMILY

Within any social group, persons assume responsibilities for various tasks that are defined in terms of a certain role; for example, parent, breadwinner, student, and son or daughter. An individual's understanding of a given role or role expectations governs how he or she expects to interact with others regarding certain issues or tasks. For example, a parental role expectation may include control of a child's bedtime and the assumption that the child will comply with the designated time. Obviously expectations are not always met in the course of daily living.

Roles are learned primarily during childhood by examples set by adults, authorities at school, and the media. When two individuals from separate family systems merge to begin their own family, each brings along personal role expectations based on previous experiences. A young woman who was brought up in a traditional home may expect her role to be that of housewife and mother, as was her mother's. If her husband is the product of a two-career family, he may expect his wife to assume a career role, as his mother did. As the two learn more about each other, ideally they develop a new set of roles, based not totally on previous family experiences but established according to the particular needs of their new relationship.

Each change or crisis in the couple's (family's) life and movement through each developmental stage require the family to adapt and perhaps renegotiate various roles to maintain its equilibrium. The career woman who returned to work after the birth of her first child may find that having her second or third child necessitates stepping out of the career role at least temporarily to assume a full-time mothering role. Her partner may be willing to assume some of the caretaking responsibilities associated with child-bearing and homemaking, as well as maintaining the breadwinner role. Some families negotiate ways for both parents to share both roles equally. Others decide to maintain the woman as breadwinner and have her partner assume the homemaker/primary parent roles.

The more flexibility individuals can attain in their role expectations, the better able they are to adapt in times of crisis. The ability to adapt and adjust family roles and responsibilities is what ensures that each member's needs are met. For example, when a family member becomes ill or disabled, a void may be created in the usual functioning of the family. In a functional family, other family members are able to adapt and change their roles and expectations so they can assume the responsibilities that belonged to the disabled member. This shifting and sharing of responsibilities enables necessary family processes to continue.

THE FUNCTIONAL FAMILY

Each family is a dynamic, constantly changing system whose individual members interact with one another and form a unit that is capable of interacting with the community. In the well-adjusted or functional family, each member interacts with others in a positive, facilitative manner that provides nurturance and support not obtained from the wider world. Ideally, each family member is a better person for having been part of that family. Experts in family studies have identified the following attributes as common to most well-adjusted functional families (Otto, 1963):

- Open, effective communication patterns
- Provision for basic physical, emotional, and spiritual needs
- Provision for security, support, and nurturance
- Responsiveness to individual family member's needs
- Equitable division of tasks and responsibilities, with flexibility in assigned roles

- Commitment to family unity
- Regular interaction among members
- Involvement in the community
- Competence in problem solving and crisis management

When assessing a family's state of health, the nurse determines how many of these attributes are manifested in the family's normal daily activities. It is of crucial importance to recognize that these functions and traits describe the ideal family and that only a small percentage of families are "ideal." Although very few families possess all the characteristics noted above, the more that are present, the more functional the family will be.

Each family must also be assessed with the understanding that what is usually described as normal, healthy family behavior actually may be unhealthy for some families. Conversely, behavior patterns that are identified as maladaptive in most families may serve a particular function in maintaining one family's health. For example, it might be considered healthy in a two-career family for all family members to share equal responsibility for household tasks rather than expect the woman to have a full-time career outside the home and also to assume complete responsibility for the household. In some families, however, the attitudes and beliefs regarding the importance of the man's role as breadwinner is strong, and household tasks may be perceived as "woman's work." This family may be better able to maintain its equilibrium or well-being by adhering to the traditional sex role-defined areas of responsibility and adjusting the wife's workload in some other way.

Family unity is another important characteristic of functional families. For the average family, this unity may mean spending time together and sharing common interests, hobbies, goals, and a common place of residence. Some families, however, seem to function well by building "space" into their family system with separate activities, recreation, or vacations. Sometimes career needs conflict, and couples actually may spend time working and living in different cities. At face value this "commuting" lifestyle may appear dysfunctional, but for some families it may in fact be satisfying and even essential to its survival. Just as individual persons are different from one another, so each family has its own patterns of interaction with one another and with the community. The nurse needs to see each family in its own light, using the criteria of healthy family functioning only as a guide and allowing for individuality and the complex diversities that are common in today's society.

ADAPTIVE FAMILY COPING PATTERNS
Crisis Theory

As families develop and grow through the life cycle, they are faced with normal periods of transition or biologic growth that require them to undergo new sets of behaviors and psychologic growth. These transitional periods are known as **maturational crises.** One example is forming a couple relationship, during which intimacy skills must be mastered. The birth of a first child, which requires parents to adapt to and accommodate the dependency of the new baby through parent-infant bonding and caretaking behaviors, is another maturational crisis. Other crises, which may threaten the family's physical, psychologic, and social integrity and that may cause some disequilibrium in the family system are known as **situational crises.** Some examples include the death of a loved one, loss of a job, accidental injuries, and even positive events such as buying a new house or winning the lottery. Crisis theory, which is based on the works of theorists and researchers (Caplan, 1964; Erikson, 1950; Lindemann, 1944), focuses on the concept of offering preventive mental and emotional health care.

As these examples suggest, a crisis is defined as an "upset in a steady state," when an individual or a family experiences tension that results from a problem the members cannot solve. Some results of the crisis are anxiety, inability to function, and emotional upset (Caplan, 1964). Occasionally the family's customary coping methods are ineffective in resolving the problem, and a period of disorganization occurs. Thus a positive focus during a crisis is important. The crisis should be considered both a problem and an opportunity because it may cause the family to become receptive to therapeutic care. Not all families are equally able to cope with crises. These critical periods require the family to be adaptable and flexible and to have strong coping skills. As the crises are weathered in a positive, constructive manner, the family's cohesiveness will improve. The community health nurse is in an excellent position to intervene to restore family equilibrium and prevent ill health. After identifying that the family is in actual or potential crisis, the nurse can take the following steps:

1. Help the family identify the problem leading to the crisis.

2. Help the family to identify its resources to assist in dealing with the problem.

3. Collaborate with the family to formulate and implement an action plan to alleviate the problem.

The family that has flexible role definitions copes much more readily with changes than does the family that rigidly defines what its members can or cannot do. Concern for an individual family member ensures that all are responsive to the one in need and that efforts will be directed toward care for that person while maintaining the needs of other family members.

Communication Theory

One of the most important elements of coping is the ability to communicate openly and clearly regarding problems. Good communication and problem-solving skills then become means to identify potential solutions. **Communication** can be described as the giving and receiving of information or messages. This exchange of information involves a complex process, which results in varying degrees of clarity. When a communication is clear, the receiver understands the message that has been given, and communication is said to be functional. When the receiver does not understand the message that has been given, that communication is described as dysfunctional (Hall & Weaver, 1985).

The community health nurse must be alert to the patterns of communication evident within the family being cared for. When inadequate or faulty communication between family members is identified, attempts are made by the nurse to clarify issues and needs amongst family members. If dysfunctional communication patterns are impeding family health and processes, it becomes important to refer the family or individual members to a community resource that can provide professional counseling.

CONCEPTUAL FRAMEWORKS FOR STUDYING THE FAMILY

Assessing and evaluating family health are extremely complex tasks. One method of systematic study of the family is through the use of various conceptual frameworks that have been developed for the purpose of scientific investigation by various disciplines. Some commonly used concepts for the study of the family are the developmental framework, the structural-functional framework, the symbolic-interactional framework, and the systems theory framework.

Developmental Framework

The developmental framework is one that is particularly suited to application in many different fields of investigation. This framework was developed in 1948 by Evelyn Duvall and Reuben Hill for use at the First White House Conference on Family Life (Duvall, 1977). It provided a method for social scientists to systematically study the family and to describe and share their findings. It continues to serve as a valuable and reliable method for predicting or anticipating a family's need for assistance or anticipatory guidance during various stages of the life cycle. It incorporates general systems theory in describing family changes or adaptations.

The family developmental framework is based on the predictability of family life experiences, which have been observed to follow a universal sequence across the family's life cycle (Duvall, 1977). To fully comprehend any individual or family, one must consider both the uniqueness of the person and the blend of the family members. Two main concepts are important: (1) **family life cycle,** which is that period beginning with the formation of the family and ending with the dissolution of the family through the death, separation, divorce, or physical relocation of its members; and (2) **family developmental tasks,** which are defined as responsibilities connected with each particular stage of family life. Developmental tasks need to be accomplished successfully for the family to continue to move successfully through the life cycle. According to Duvall, there are eight developmental stages.

Table 18-1 lists the developmental tasks associated with each stage of the family life cycle. The nurse who is planning care can assess the family's developmental stage, evaluate the family's attainment of the appropriate developmental tasks, and then assist the family in identifying possible ways to fulfill the appropriate tasks for that particular stage. Although this theory is extremely valuable in family assessment, it should be noted that Duvall considers the middle-class nuclear family to be the "normal" type of family. Her framework may be considered less relevant for application to the care of families that are not within the "middle" socioeconomic class definition, or for single-parent or blended families.

Structural-Functional Framework

This approach was developed by sociologists and anthropologists and focuses on the relationships between family systems and other social systems such as school, workplace, or the health-care delivery system. Attention also is paid to the inter-relationships of family members. Although this framework provides a strong reference for studying the relationships between family members and outside social organizations, it is inadequate in incorporating the processes and dynamics of social change.

Symbolic-Interactional Framework

This concept was developed within the fields of sociology and social psychology. It focuses on the interactions of family members as described by roles, decision-making processes, communication patterns, and conflict resolution. Although this framework provides a thorough view of the interior structure of the family, it does not include or consider the family's interactions with outside social systems.

Systems Theory Framework

This concept, which initially was developed by biologist Ludwig von Bertalanffy (1968), is used by many disciplines. It extends beyond the theory that the whole is made up of the sum of its parts, which are interdependent and interrelated, and that if change occurs in any one part of the

TABLE 18-1   Family life cycle

Family life cycle stages	Family development tasks
Marriage phase	Establishment of: relationship boundaries; roles; financial plans; home; relationships with friends, family members; parenthood plans
Childbearing family	Redefinition of marital relationship; taking on the role of parents; reevaluation of home space arrangements, career plans, financial plans
Preschool-child family	Providing for safety, security, and nurturance needs of child; coping with fatigue and lack of privacy; beginning socialization of child
School–aged-child family	Adjustment to separation from family; development of peer relationships by child; establishing educational goals; entering parent/child/teacher community
Teenager-family	Fostering autonomy while maintaining structure in adolescence; dealing with midlife career and personal issues; beginning concern with providing for grandparents
Launching phase	Assisting young–adult-aged children in establishing independent identities; redefinition of marital relationship as children leave home
Middle-aged family	Rebuilding couple identity; incorporation of new family members — spouses and grandchildren: caretaking of older generation
Elderly family	Adaptation to retirement; financial realignment; bereavement issues; dealing with loneliness; coping with health problems

Adapted from *Marriage and Family Development* (5th ed.) (p. 144) by E. Duvall, 1977, Philadelphia: J.B. Lippincott.

system, the other parts are affected and must regain balance (Brill, 1978). Systems theory, on the other hand, defines the whole as more than the sum of its parts. A system may receive input from outside and may put energy out into its environment, which is known as *output.* These energy exchanges create a change in the system and thus require adjustment of the system. Although this theory has broad applications, it can be applied to the family in the following manner. The family is a living system whose parts are its individual members, who are interrelated and interdependent. The patterns of interaction among its members affect each person. The family interacts with a larger system, the community, which also affects its well-being. Systems theory has been used (Ackerman, 1984) to describe how families adapt and change over time through information exchange and feedback processes among themselves and with the community.

In addition, systems theory provides a framework by which to explain that the whole of the family is affected by the interaction of its members and by the family's interaction with the community.

FAMILY HEALTH

Family health may be described and evaluated by means of the Neuman systems model. The family may be conceptualized as a system composed of individual members who are interrelated in such a fashion that a change in any one function sets off a series of changes in the other functions. When one family member becomes ill, other family members are expected to give assistance. The illness may alter work patterns and require restriction of previous plans. A long-term chronic illness may deplete the family financially and emotionally. If a breadwinner becomes disabled, his or her career may be jeopardized and there will be a loss of earnings. In most instances this change requires the rest of the family members to adapt or alter some aspect of their own lifestyles.

By contrast, if at least one family member subscribes to a healthy lifestyle, the example that is set by valuing the principles of health maintenance and health promotion can positively affect the family's health. If this person is one of the adult members who shares family caretaking, he or she may foster healthy nutrition, encourage exercise programs, set a good example for stress management, and provide for preventive medical or dental care. For example, wellness is more commonly experienced in families in which nutrition and exercise are valued and preventive medicine is practiced. Individuals who are members of families that do not value healthy lifestyle behaviors may not do so themselves. The opposite effect can be observed when one member of a family that does not value health adopts a wellness consciousness. It is not uncommon for one or more family members to be impressed enough by the outcome of a healthier lifestyle that they gradually alter their own attitudes and adopt healthier habits.

NURSING CARE OF THE FAMILY

Providing high-quality nursing care to the family involves the application of the same principles that are involved in caring for an individual client. The nursing process is the prescribed method because it is based on a scientific approach that involves the collection of data to make appropriate clinical judgments and to plan the care and identify interventions. Evaluation and reassessment are used to determine the effectiveness of the interventions and make necessary revisions or modification in care.

Assessment

Assessment of the family involves the use of the five senses to compile appropriate information that allows for the identification of actual or potential health problems, and the development of a plan to improve the level of wellness of the family. A thorough nursing assessment includes family history, family health assessment, and physical assessment. A variety of tools are available for recording the history, health, and physical assessments. To use an assessment tool in planning care, the nurse must be familiar with such concepts as family types, role theory, crisis theory, communication theory, and stages of development, all of which were described earlier in this chapter.

Genogram. One example of an assessment

— RESEARCH ♦ HIGHLIGHT —

Nurse Case Management from the Client's View

Sixteen subjects, 11 women and 5 men, ranging in age from 66 to 100, who either lived alone (11) or with a spouse or relative (5), consented to participate in a study that explored their perspectives of working with a nurse case manager. They had worked with 13 different nurse case managers and their interactions, though varied, spanned from 2 months to 2 years after hospital referral for either an acute episode or an exacerbation of a chronic long-term illness.

Initial participants, 9 of whom were under care, were identified as successful by nurse case managers. Characteristics of latter participants varied or they were viewed as not experiencing positive outcomes by nurse case management. Semistructured, open-ended interviews designed to elicit stories related to participants' experiences with nurse case managers were audiotaped and transcribed for coding and analysis. Persistent observation, triangulation of sources, peer debriefing, and member checks were strategies used within the design to credibly reflect the true state of human experience.

The results of this qualitative study, which focused on the process of care, identified participants' growth as insider-experts as constituting three intrapersonal and interpersonal phases: bonding, working, and changing, each of which affected the other. Descriptions of each phase were accompanied by actual transcripts to illustrate the affective, cognitive, and behavioral changes experienced by clients and their families as they interacted with nurse case managers who assisted them in their resumption and assumption of self-care activities. Nurse case managers were not only viewed as experts during intervention, but also as insiders. Clients felt known and cared about as individuals as they assumed responsibilities and managed to the extent that they also became insider-experts. While some clients no longer required the services of nurse case managers, others that did managed their care with greater independence and appropriate use of the health care system.

Suggestions for research extended across all settings and included implications for education and health care reform.

From "Nurse Case Management from the Client's View: Growing as Insider-Expert" by G.S. Lamb & J.E. Stempel, 1994, *Nursing Outlook, 42*(1), 7-13.

---

tool is the **genogram.** It has been used by health care professionals to gain a retrospective perception of a family system as it has developed over time (Figure 18-2). This tool is based on generalized information about the evolution of the family over one or more generations and can clearly depict the family structure. The format used for the genogram is a simple family tree structure. The data elicited by careful interviewing provide information on child-rearing practices; health-values, beliefs, and attitudes; social information; and traditions that can affect the family's health or well being.

The genogram in Figure 18-2 shows "family M". Larry M. has just returned home from the hospital after undergoing cardiac bypass surgery.

We can see that his birth family has a history of cardiac problems: his father died of a "heart attack." Also evident is the fact that the M. family shares an obesity problem. Shelly M., Larry's wife, is a full time homemaker and prides herself on being a good cook.

The completed genogram provided the nurse with a quick and easy way to obtain a family history. The development of this genogram helped Larry and Shelly to identify some of his cardiac risk factors, and consider the need for intervention.

The genogram may be used in conjunction with one or more other tools described in the following sections to develop a complete assessment.

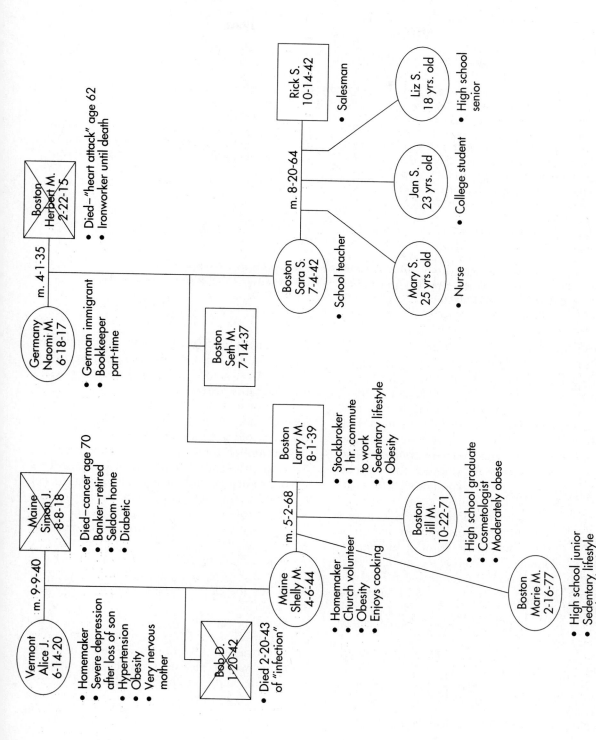

FIGURE 18-2 Genogram of the "M" family.

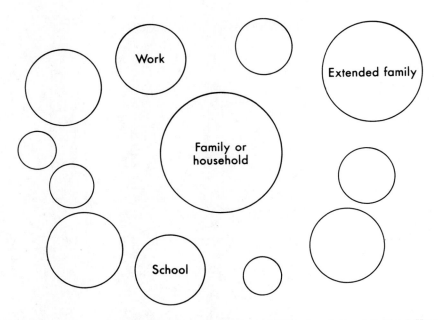

FIGURE 18-3 Ecomap. *From "Diagrammatic assessment of family relationships" by A. Hartman, 1978,* Social Casework, 59, 469. *Copyright 1978 by Family Service Association of America. Reprinted by permission.*

Ecomap. An **ecomap** (Figure 18-3) may be used to provide additional information regarding the family as a system and its interactions with other systems such as work, health care, school, extended family, friends, or recreation. This tool borrows from the science of ecology, which studies the delicate balance that exists in nature between living things and their environment. The ecomap explores the ways in which this balance may be maintained for the good of all (Hartman, 1978). The completed ecomap clearly illustrates all the important interaction patterns between the family and other systems, and the nature of the relationship and the direction of the energy flow, or resources. The completed ecomap (Figure 18-4) enables both the nurse and the couple shown in the genogram (Figure 18-2), Larry and Shelly, to identify areas in which they may seek help; for example, through friends, church, family, and neighbors.

Other assessment tools. Many community health-care providers develop their own assessment tools to be used alone or in conjunction with other standardized forms. Figure 18-5 depicts a family assessment tool that is comprehensive in nature. This tool includes items related to the family structure and resources, the physical and social environments, and family health, health practices, and lifestyle. These basic demographic and factual data give the nurse an overview of the family system.

The tool used for physical assessment can follow any problem-oriented format developed for client history and physical examination. In collecting the family's health history, the nurse looks for indicators of factors that might place family members at risk for health problems. For example, Sally B.'s father, grandfather, brother, and two paternal aunts suffered from alcoholism. Because this family history predisposes Sally herself to alcoholism, the nurse should carefully investigate this possibility.

Another example is that of Larry M. (from Figure 18-2), aged 54 years, whose father died of a myocardial infarction at age 62. The nurse certainly would include screening for signs of impending cardiovascular problems in Larry's physical assessment. A teaching plan for Larry

Text continues on p. 406

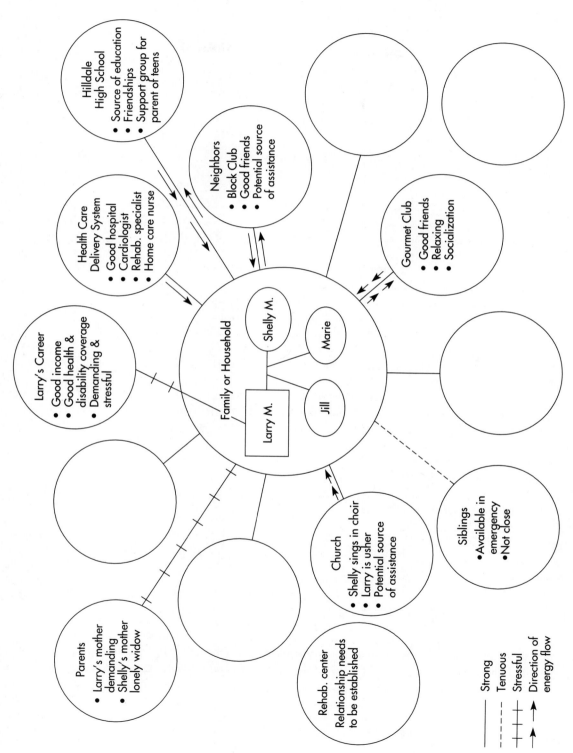

FIGURE 18-4 Ecomap showing the "M" family's systems of support.

Client name:	Case no. :
Client address:	Phone no. :

Reason for admission:

Family constellation:

Name	Relationship	Age

Social history:

Name	Ethnicity	Occupation	Income

Neighborhood data: Affluent _____ Moderate _____ Poverty _____
Adequate utilities: Yes _____ No _____
Neighbors: Friendly _____ Noncommittal _____ Hostile _____
Transportation: Convenient _____ Accessible _____ Not available _____
Health care facilities accessible: Yes _____ No _____

Family health care data:
Present family illnesses (list) _____

Past action taken when family member ill _____
_____
_____

Family dynamics:
Role of each member _____

Leadership: Patriarchal _____ Matriarchal _____ Egalitarian _____ Democratic _____
Communication style: Open _____ Closed _____ Direct _____ Indirect _____
Values system: Family _____ Religion _____ Materialism _____ Ethnic beliefs _____ Health _____
Health beliefs: Myths _____ Old wives' tales _____ Cultural beliefs _____ Fact _____
Family priorities: _____

FIGURE 18-5 Comprehensive family assessment tool and care plan.

Family coping skills:

	Adequate skills	Needs assistance
Communication patterns: Express thoughts and feelings with one another		
Emotional support: Encourage and care about one another		
Community interaction: Involved in community activities, maintain friendships		
Accepting help: Able to tap resources when needed		
Flexibility of roles: Able to adjust responsibilities in change or crisis		
Crisis management: Draws family together, viewed as a growth experience		

Family wellness behaviors:

	Acceptable habits	Needs improvement
Nutritional status		
Exercise program		
Alcohol consumption		
Drug habits		
Smoking		
Sleep patterns		
Stress management		
Practices preventive health care		

Risk factors identified: _____

_____

_____

Notes _____

_____

_____

_____

Signature _____

Home Care Nurse

FIGURE 18-5, Cont'd.

would include an evaluation of his dietary and nutritional habits, and a plan for healthy eating developed collaboratively with Larry and his wife. Larry, the nurse, and the physician would begin developing a safe plan for exercise, stress management, and realistic dietary strategies.

Finally, Mary W. is a 45-year-old woman with a history of gestational diabetes during her last two pregnancies. Although Mary presently does not display any overt symptoms of diabetes, it is known that adult-onset diabetes often develops later in life in women with a history of gestational diabetes. Therefore, screening for diabetes will be an important component of Mary's physical assessment. Family teaching will include alerting Mary and her family to the importance of watching for signs of diabetes such as unexplained weight loss, excessive thirst, extreme hunger, and frequent urination. Mary will be encouraged to contact her physician at the earliest sign of any of these symptoms.

In addition to physical assessment of the individual members, assessment of a family's level of health also includes identification of lifestyle behaviors, such as nutritional and exercise patterns, preventive health care, stress management, and identification of risk factors. It may be possible to focus on one member of a family who has an altered health state, or it may be necessary to develop a plan of care that includes all family members because in some way the illness of one member affects each of them.

Nursing Diagnosis

After completing the assessment phase of family care, the nurse will be able to identify family strengths and determine the existence of any actual or potential health problems. These factors will be developed into statements called *nursing diagnoses*. A nursing diagnosis contains both a statement of the problem, and it's etiology.

In a review of Sally B's assessment, the following nursing diagnosis might be formulated: "potential for alcohol dependency related to knowledge deficit." Larry M. is a 245-pound and 5'10"

tall male, who describes a diet high in saturated fats and sugar. The appropriate nursing diagnosis for Larry might be "altered nutrition: more than body requirements."

Planning

The nurse and family work together collaboratively to develop a list of goals, strategies, and expected outcomes. The family prioritizes its identified needs, and a plan of care begins with the formulation of interventions or actions.

One of the most important roles of the community health nurse is to serve as a resource person and a liason between the family and individual and the community. The nurse's awareness of various resources available, and the ability to match these resources with the family's needs, facilitate the development and implementation of an effective care plan. Referral of a family to a counseling agency, knowing where to call to arrange transportation for an elderly client, or providing information regarding health promotion training opportunities are good examples of duties performed by the community health nurse.

With regard to Larry M., the family's concern for his well being might lead to the identification of the goals that Larry and the rest of the family will reduce their total intake of fat and that Larry will restrict his caloric intake to reduce his weight. The nurse uses principles of health teaching to educate the family about a nutrition plan. The family then determines what menu and food preparation plan will fit with their lifestyle and preferences.

Implementation

Once goals and actual or potential problems are identified and then prioritized by the family, the nurse and family define appropriate measures or actions to rectify the problems. These measures are known as *interventions*. Implementation of the interventions involves the actual execution of the nursing care or client self-care regimen. Interventions may involve administering a prescribed medical treatment or medication, providing comfort measures, giving physical care, or providing health teaching or counseling.

Both Sally B. and Larry M. in our previous examples are prime candidates for interventions that are based on health teaching and counseling. Another example of an intervention is the use of positioning to enhance the comfort level of a new mother after childbirth.

Evaluation and Reassessment

To determine the effectiveness of the nursing interventions in alleviating or preventing any given client problem, a regular system of patient observation, interview, and reassessment must be undertaken. This process identifies the problem as remedied, improved, unchanged, or worsened from previous findings. Problems that are remedied are removed from the problem list. Problems that show improvement may warrant continuation of the interventions. Problems that are unimproved or have worsened may require a modification in the plan of care.

THE FAMILY/COMMUNITY SYSTEM

The interrelationship between the health of the family and the health of the community was recognized by the American Public Health Association (APHA) in 1980 when it described the role of public health nurses in terms of working with families toward the goal of improving the health of the community (APHA, 1980).

Levels of wellness of individuals, families, and communities are directly or indirectly interrelated. The family serves as a moderator between the wellness of its individual members and the wellness of the community (Dunn, 1967). The healthy or functional family contributes to the community by preparing its members to function productively in societal roles in the workplace, in school, or in their own families. Communities with many unhealthy families will suffer ill effects because these families are less able to fulfill societal roles and they place demands on the community's health care delivery systems (Stanhope & Lancaster, 1992).

The systems theory can be used to describe this relationship between the family and the community. The family is described as a dynamic system made up of smaller parts, which are its individual members. The family system is also conceptualized as a subsystem of a larger system, the community.

General systems theory can be used to define the family as an open system; that is, a system that exchanges energy with its environment. The family performs certain functions that result in the output of energy into the community. For example, the reproduction and socialization of new family members contributes new persons to the community.

Any contributions a family makes to community function may be considered outputs of energy into the community system. Volunteer work performed for community organizations and the contribution of valuable skills in the workplace serve as positive examples of contributions. Sometimes the family's output is negative in nature, such as a situation in which a family member's actions result in crime or personal injury to other community members.

Services provided by the community act as energy input into the family system. The adequacy of community functions or services such as security (fire and police protection), the availability of health care providers (hospitals, clinics, and doctors' offices), transportation systems, and educational institutions may determine the level of health or wellness of the community's families. In a community in which health care facilities are too few or inaccessible because of distance from public transportation, families may be unable to secure adequate primary or tertiary health care. The lack of preventive care and adequate rehabilitation services to segments of the community population impedes the family's ability to attain optimal wellness. When large segments of a community's families experience impaired health, the community as a whole may suffer. Nursing care provided to the family to enhance its health status serves to increase the level of wellness of the entire community.

■ CASE STUDY

Larry M. is a 54-year-old white male who has just been discharged from the hospital following bypass surgery necessitated by a myocardial infarction that was caused by severe coronary artery disease. A follow-up home visit by the community health nurse is scheduled on postoperative day 7, the day after Larry's hospital discharge.

The purpose of the visit is the evaluation of Larry's postoperative status, evaluation and reinforcement of the implementation of the postoperative care plan for the medication regime and activity level, follow-up physician's office visit, and initiation of rehabilitation therapy.

In addition, the nurse will evaluate the level of functioning of the family during this situational crisis, and will alert to any signs of inadequate coping mechanisms.

Larry's health history indicates that he has been generally healthy without any previous chronic or life-threatening illnesses. He describes a sedentary lifestyle, a high-powered professional career, and a diet high in calories and saturated fat. Before his recent illness, Larry smoked 1.5 packs of cigarettes per day. He has stopped smoking since his hospitalization and intends to continue not smoking. Larry's family history indicates that his father died at age 62 of a "heart attack." His mother is alive and well at 76 years of age, but has hypertension. Larry's wife, Shelly, appears moderately obese, as do his two daughters, ages 17 and 23 years. Shelly is a full-time homemaker who prides herself at being an excellent cook. She enjoys preparing traditional foods she ate as a child, using sauces with lots of butter and cheese. The family's interests include church activities, watching movies, and participation in a gourmet cooking club.

The nurse's initial assessment of Larry indicates that he is a 5′10″ tall, 245-pound white male. His blood pressure is 172/90, pulse is 92, and temperature is 99.2. All incisional sites appear clean and dry. Larry describes his activity level as limited. He ambulates only very short distances and sits in a chair briefly. He states he is still feeling tired and slightly short of breath upon exertion.

Larry's discharge instruction sheet indicates that his medication regime includes ASA 325 mg QD; dipyridamole 50 mg TID; a vasodilator that increases collateral circulation to the heart wall; and Digoxin, .25 mg QD, to increase the force of myocardial contraction and the electrophysiologic action of the heart. Larry should ambulate hourly, building up to 5-minute walks by postoperative day 14. He should watch for any weight gain of more than two pounds, which might indicate a compromise in cardiac function. His prescribed nutritional plan is low in saturated fat, with a mild sodium restriction, which means no added salt in food preparation or at the table. Larry is to return to his physician for an office visit on postoperative day 10, and begin rehabilitation therapy the next day.

In reviewing this plan of care, the nurse identifies several problems. Larry has not been taking his medications as ordered. He states that he is "not a pill taker," and has trouble remembering. His reluctance to ambulate seems to be related to anxiety about his cardiac condition. Shelly has developed a chart to keep track of Larry's daily weight, and both are aware of the significance of this monitoring.

On reviewing the nutrition plan, the nurse finds knowledge deficits in both Larry's and Shelly's knowledge at the implementation level. There is also some resistance by the whole family about whether they will enjoy this "new way of eating."

Larry and Shelly are aware of the dates for Larry's doctor visit and the schedule for Larry's rehabilitation therapy. Both seem to comprehend the importance of these events in Larry's recovery.

During the course of the visit, the nurse notes the tension apparent amongst the family members. She discusses with them the role adjustments they are experiencing, and allows Shelly to vent her anxiety regarding the change in the family roles and responsibilities, Larry's health, and the financial considerations of his illness. Shelly admits to being exhausted, stating that she has not slept well since Larry became ill.

Together, the nurse and family develop the following list of identified strengths and problems or nursing diagnoses.

Case Study continued on p. 410

TABLE 18-2   Family nursing care plan

Assessment	Nursing diagnosis	Goal	Plan/interventions	Evaluation
Physical findings	High risk for disuse syndrome related to post-op immobility	Promote appropriate post-op activity level	Instruct Larry re: appropriate activity level	Instruction provided
	Altered nutrition: more than body requirements related to knowledge deficit	Promote weight reduction and reduce cardiovascular risk factors by dietary modification	Evaluate comprehension & recall of prescribed nutrition plan	Knowledge deficit identified
			Review dietary plan with Larry & Shelly	Instruction/return demonstration provided
			Identify some actual food/menu plans	Menu plan developed for upcoming week
Behavioral patterns	Sleep pattern disturbance, Shelly, related to anxiety	Restore adequate sleep patterns, Shelly	Provide support regarding Larry's progress	Information provided
			Instruct in relaxation techniques	Instruction provided
			Refer to stress management classes in community	Referral made
			Counsel regarding "caretaker" role	Counseling provided
			Monitor for progress, possible referral for counseling	At present, progress is made, no need for referral
	High risk for cardiac impairment related to noncompliance with medication regime: ASA 325 mgm QD; Dipyridamine 50 mgm TID AC; Digoxin .25 mgm QD	Larry will comply with medication regime	Health-motivate through instruction as to purpose and function of meds	Instruction provided
			Repeat medication instructions	Medication schedule cards posted on refrigerator
Family interactions	Altered family processes related to situational crisis of Larry's illness	Enhance necessary coping mechanisms of the family	Instruct Shelly as to stress of caretaker role	Instruction given
			Health-counsel family as to normal post-op reactions of patient/ family members in situations of life-threatening illness	Health counseling provided
			Encourage family members to vent & share their anxieties and concerns re: disrupted family patterns	Active family discussion supported

Strengths

1. Larry is young and previously healthy.
2. No signs of postoperative complications are apparent.
3. The M. family is a close and caring family. The family members offer one another support.
4. Shelly has no outside career commitments at present, thereby enabling her to be available to assist Larry in his recovery.

Nursing Diagnoses

1. High risk for disuse syndrome related to postoperative immobility.

2. High risk for cardiac impairment related to noncompliance with medication regime.
3. Altered nutrition: more than body requires related to knowledge deficit in recommended nutritional plan.
4. Sleep pattern disturbance, Shelly, related to anxiety.
5. Altered family processes related to situational crisis.

Table 18-2 shows an example of another type of family care plan that is used by the nurse to formulate a plan of care for Larry and his family.

Chapter Highlights

- Although there are many definitions of a family, all include the following characteristics: families are composed of more than one person, they include at least one adult, and the persons are related to each other by blood or formal or informal social contract.

- Family structures are constantly changing. The nuclear family is perceived as the "typical" family but actually represents fewer than half of all American families.

- Members of families learn to assume various roles as children on the basis of examples set by parents, school authorities, and the media.

- Individuals from different family systems may have different and conflicting expectations of role behaviors. Characteristics common to functional families include effective communication patterns, provisions for members' physical and emotional needs, flexibility within roles, commitment to family unity, involvement in the community, and ability to solve problems.

- Community health nurses can use their knowledge of crisis theory to help families cope with both maturational and situational crises.

- An understanding of communication theory is important in assessing a family's ability to communicate openly and to solve problems.

- Conceptual frameworks useful for studying the family include the developmental framework, structural-functional approach, and the systems theory approach.

- The health of one family member affects the health of other family members.

- The community health nurse can use the nursing process to provide nursing care to the family unit.

- The genogram and ecomap are assessment tools that allow the nurse to gather information and assess family strengths and weaknesses.

- Healthy families contribute to the health of the community, whereas unhealthy families place demands on community resources and lower the community's overall health.

CRITICAL THINKING EXERCISE

Bob (42) and Tony (33) are a same-sex family who have been partners for 10 years. Tony has known that he is HIV positive for two years. Bob has never wanted to be tested. Tony becomes acutely ill with an upper respiratory infection. A visit to an emergency room confirms that he has *Pneumocystis Carrini*. Both men have previously been in denial about this possibility. Bob wants to contact Tony's parents. Tony is reluctant because his parents do not know that he is gay. Bob protests that he does not know his own HIV status and feels he may need some help in dealing with their present crisis. Bob's parents are deceased.

1. As a nurse wishing to assist them to deal with this crisis in a positive way, how will you help Bob and Tony identify the problem leading to this crisis?
2. How will you assist the family to find acceptable resources to help deal with the altered health state?
3. What blocks to communication may interfere with your therapeutic intervention with this family?

REFERENCES

Ackerman, N.J. (1984). *A theory of family systems.* New York: Gardiner Press Inc.

Aguilera, D.C., & Messick, J.M. (1990). *Crisis intervention theory and methodology* (6th ed.). St. Louis: Mosby.

American households: The 1990 census reveals dramatic changes in the American family—Here's what you need to know. *American Demographics 14*(suppl 24), July 1992.

American Public Health Association. (1980). *The definition and role of public health nursing in the delivery of health care.* Washington, DC: Author.

Bell, R.R. (1983). *Marriage and family interaction.* Homewood, IL: Dorsey.

Benner, P., & Pratt, K. (1991). Dialogues with excellence: Extending the community care. *American Journal of Nursing 91*, 58-59.

Bohannan, P. (1985). *All the happy families: Exploring the varieties of family life.* New York: McGraw-Hill.

Brill, N.K. (1978). *Working with people: The helping process.* Philadelphia: J.B. Lippincott.

Caplan, G. (1964). *Principles of prevention psychiatry.* New York and London: Basic Books, Inc.

Cheal, D. (1993). Unity and difference in families. *Journal of Family Issues, 14*(1), 5-19.

Clemen-Stone, S., Eigsti, D.G., & McGuire, S.L. (1994). *Comprehensive community health nursing* (4th ed.). St. Louis: Mosby.

Clements, I., & Roberto, F. (1983). *Family health: A theoretical approach to nursing care.* New York: Wiley & Sons.

Dunn, H.L. (1967). *High level wellness* (7th ed.). Arlington, VA: Beatty.

Duvall, E.M. (1977). *Marriage and family development* (5th ed.). Philadelphia: J.B. Lippincott.

Duvall, E.M., & Miller, B.C. (1985). *Marriage and family development* (6th ed.). New York: Harper & Row.

Erikson, E.H. (1950). *Childhood and society.* New York: W.W. Norton & Co.

Friedman, M.M. (1992). *Family nursing theory and assessment.* New York: Appleton-Century-Crofts.

Gellner, P., Landers, S., O'Rourke, D., & Schlegel, M. (1994). Community Health Nursing in the 1990's—Risky Business? *Holistic Nursing Practice, 8*(2), 15-21.

Glick, P.C. (1990). American families: As they are and were. *Sociology and Social Research, 74*(3), 139-145.

Glick, P.C. (1984). American household structure in transition. *Family Planning Prospective, 16*(5), 204-211.

Hall, J.E., & Weaver, B.R. (1985). *A systems approach to community health* (2nd ed.). Philadelphia: J.B. Lippincott.

Hartman, A. (1978). Diagrammatic assessment of family relationships. *Social Casework, 59,* 465-479.

Hymovich, D.P., & Bernard, M.U. (1973). *Family health care.* New York: McGraw-Hill.

Hymovich, D.P., & Chamberlin, R. (1980). *Child and family development.* New York: McGraw-Hill.

Lewis, G.L. (1984). Changes in women's role participation. In I. Frieze et al. (Eds.). *Women and sex roles: Social psychological perspective.* New York: Norton.

Lindemann, E. (1944). Symptomatology and management of acute grief. *American Journal of Psychiatry, 141,* 148.

Miller, J.R., & Janosik, E.H. (1980). *Family-focused care.* New York: McGraw-Hill.

Minuchin, S. (1974). *Families and family therapy.* Cambridge, MA: Harvard University Press.

Neuman, B. (1989). *The Neuman systems model* (2nd ed.). East Norwalk, CT: Appleton & Lange.

North American Nursing Diagnosis Association. (1992). *Nanda nursing diagnoses: Definition and classification 1992-1993.* Philadelphia: Author.

Nye, F.I., & Berardo, F.M. (Eds.). (1981). *Emerging conceptual frameworks in family analyses.* New York: Praeger.

Otto, H.E. (1963). *Criteria for assessing family strength. 2*(2):329-333, Baltimore: Waverly Press.

Pendagast, B.S., & Sherman, C.O. (1977). A guide to the genogram family systems training. *The Family 5,* 3-14.

Queen, S.A., & Haberstein, R.W. (1974). *The family in various cultures.* Philadelphia: J.B. Lippincott.

Reinhardt, A.M., & Quinn, M.D. (Eds.). (1973). *Family-centered community nursing: A sociocultural framework.* St. Louis: Mosby.

Scanzoni, J., & Marsiglio, W. (1993). New action theory. *Journal of Family Issues, 14*(3), 105-132.

Stanhope, M., & Lancaster, J. (1992). *Community health nursing: Process and practice for promoting health* (3rd ed.). St. Louis: Mosby.

Sussman, M. (1971). Family systems in the 1970s: Analysis, policies, programs. *Annals of the American Academy of Political and Social Science, 396,* 5-19.

Swanson, J.M. (1993). *Community health nursing: Promot-* *ing the health of aggregates.* Philadelphia: W.B. Saunders.

Thorne, B., & Yalom, M. (1982). *Rethinking the family: Some feminist questions.* New York: Longman.

Tinkham, C.W., Voorhees, E.F., & McCarthy, N.C. (1984). *Community health nursing: evolution and process in the family and community.* Norwalk, CT: Appleton-Century-Crofts.

Toffler, A. (1970). *Future shock.* New York: Bantam.

U.S. Department of Commerce, Bureau of the Census. (1988). *Statistical abstract of the United States.* Washington, D.C.: Bureau of the Census.

U.S. Department of Commerce, Bureau of the Census. (1986). *Statistical abstract of the United States.* Washington, D.C.: Bureau of the Census.

U.S. Department of Commerce, Bureau of the Census. (1992). *Statistical abstract of the United States.* Washington, D.C.: Bureau of the Census.

Visher, E., & Visher, J. (1979). *Step families: A guide to working with stepparents and stepchildren.* New York: Brunner/Mazel.

von Bertalanffy, L. (1968). *Organismic psychology and systems theory.* Worcester, MA: Clark University Press.

Walsh, F. (Ed.). (1982). *Normal family processes.* New York: Guilford.

Wright, L.M., & Leahy, M. (1984). *Nurses and families: A guide to family assessment and intervention.* Philadelphia: Davis.

19

THE FAMILY COPING WITH MULTIPLE STRESSORS

Janice Cooke Feigenbaum

Just as the individual consists of internal factors, so the family can be similarly viewed as one singular internal environment or system where each individual within helps define it by their interactions as they become a composite of total family relationship characteristics.

Betty Neuman

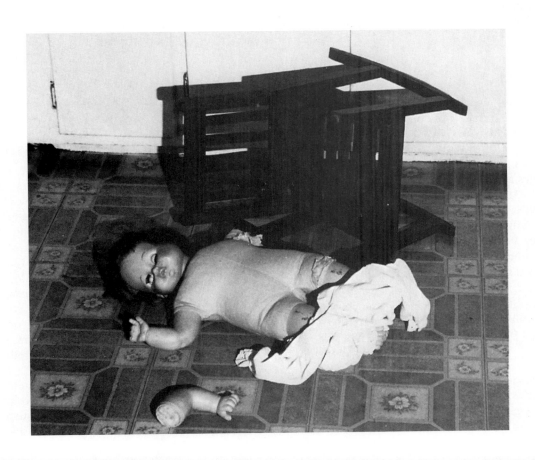

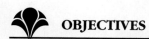

OBJECTIVES

At the conclusion of this chapter the student will be able to:

1. Define characteristics of the nursing diagnosis of altered family processes.
2. Recognize stressors confronting families with multiple stressors.
3. Describe the impact of coping with multiple stressors on the integrity of families, and the development of family members.
4. Describe the effects on a community of a high prevalence of families coping with multiple stressors.
5. Use the nursing process while caring for families coping with multiple stressors.

KEY TERMS

Altered family processes
Disengagement
Enabling
Enmeshment

Extrafamily stressors
Family violence
Ineffective family coping
Interfamily stressors

Intrafamily stressors
Regression
Scapegoating
Stressors

Families, especially ones experiencing the effects of multiple stressors, demonstrate a wide range of behaviors and levels of wellness. In effect, many of these behaviors will be almost opposite of those observed in healthy or functional families as discussed in Chapter 18. Currently, the North American Nursing Diagnosis Association (NANDA) is reviewing the diagnostic concepts and definition of the nursing diagnosis of "**Altered family processes**—addictive behavior (individual and family)." This phenomenon has tentatively been defined in the following way:

The state in which the psychosocial, spiritual and physiological functions of a family unit are chronically disorganized, leading to conflict, denial of problems, resistance to change, ineffective problem solving, and a series of self-perpetuating crises (Kim, McFarland, & McLane, 1993, p. 362).

These criteria imply that the levels of wellness of these families tend to be minimal because their energy levels will be depleted as they attempt to perpetuate a sense of system stability

and harmony within their created environment (Neuman, 1983; Reed, 1993).

CHARACTERISTICS OF FAMILIES WITH MULTIPLE STRESSORS

Families coping with multiple stressors feel so overwhelmed with the challenges of everyday life that they further tend to encourage dependency and learned helplessness among family members instead of encouraging each member to develop autonomy and individuality. If a member within the system attempts to develop these independent characteristics, the family usually responds negatively while it attempts to conserve energy. Thus, these families tend to be very rigid and authoritative toward their members. All are expected to conform totally with the family's system of rules and expectations.

The boundaries of the systems of families with altered processes tend to be quite rigid and impermeable. These closed systems are suspicious of people, objects, and knowledge outside their own boundaries. This means that the family may view the nurse in a suspicious manner.

Severe chronic health problems, such as substance abuse (especially alcoholism), mental illness, incest, and violence, frequently occur in dysfunctional families. Jack Weitzman described these families as ones in which "the most obvious defining characteristic is the presence of a serious symptom, often multiple symptoms, of long duration and high intensity" (Weitzman, 1985, p. 474). He further noted that "these are families greatly at risk for symptom production and further disintegration. They are highly volatile entities in which the basic building blocks of family life are badly damaged. . . . The ideas of members actually enjoying one another's presence, sharing in activities, and having fun is rare indeed" (p. 475).

Susan Meister (1984) suggested that a poor fit between the family's resources and the demands for them leads to an alteration in functioning, disorganization, and possibly dysfunction. She explained as follows:

When the family does well in achieving resource/demand fit, then it has a greater capacity to contribute to the members—who are also juggling personal resources and demands. Similarly, members achieving functional degrees of fit have greater capacity to contribute to family-level resource.

If the family is not able to "fit" resources to demands, then the family is less able to contribute to the efforts of its members as they face the individual requirements to "fit" resources and demands. Over time, members who are struggling to meet demands become less able to contribute to the family's processes or coping with demands. . . . It is the dysfunctional fit of resources and demands that bears directly upon family violence (1984, p. 67).

The terms *dysfunctional* and *disorganized* have frequently been used to label families who are attempting to cope with multiple stressors. The effect of these labels has often been an added stressor for these family systems. In light of this reality, the nurse is encouraged to avoid labelling a family, and instead focus on the family's perspective of its experiences.

It is difficult to estimate the percentage of families that are altered as a result of trying to cope with multiple stressors, because many of their problems and attempts to resolve them are hidden from health care and legal professionals. It is, however, possible to infer this number by considering statistics related to one problem frequently exhibited by dysfunctional families, namely alcoholism.

It is estimated one in every ten Americans is an alcohol abuser, and these individuals create serious problems for others: "on the average, (for) some four to six other persons, including mates, children, friends, employers, and even total strangers" (Carson, Butcher, & Coleman, 1988, p. 368). In the United States the effects of alcoholism include more than 50% of deaths and major injuries caused by automobile accidents, 50% of murders, 40% of assaults, 35% of rapes, and 30% of suicides. Further, "the financial drain imposed on the economy by alcoholism is estimated to be over $25 billion a year, in large part comprised of losses to industry from absenteeism, lowered work efficiency, and accidents" (Carson et al., p. 369).

Violence, including sexual abuse, is another ineffective and harmful family behavior. Its incidence is more difficult to confirm. It is estimated that annually, 3.8% (1.5 to 2 million) of American children between 3 and 17 years of age who live in homes with two parents, and 30% of married women, are victims of abuse within American families (Van Husselt, Morrison, Bellack, & Hersson, 1988, p. xi). In addition, wife abuse occurs more often than rape by a stranger, and child abuse is more prevalent than chickenpox (Campbell & Campbell, 1993).

Many women are physically abused during pregnancy. The actual rate of this phenomenon is unknown. Thus, there is a wide range of prevalence rates of the abuse of pregnant women, from 1 in 12 to 1 in 6 (Bohn & Parker, 1993, p. 156). Physical abuse of the mother during pregnancy has been identified as a factor in causing preterm deliveries and low-birth-weight infants (Bohn & Parker, 1993, p. 157).

These statistics show how the presence of large numbers of families with altered family processes within the community may create problems for all members of the society. The community health nurse, who frequently encounters these families, is in an ideal position to care for them, to act as their advocate, and in effect, to improve the health of the community at large.

Careful consideration of the criteria for the nursing diagnosis of altered family processes is mandatory. It is important for the nurse to recognize that a family should be diagnosed as altered only when it demonstrates behaviors related to this nursing diagnosis and not because the family does not fit the nurse's idea of a healthy family. That is, same sex family units, single-parent units, childless couples, dual-career families, blended families, and families receiving welfare are not altered or dysfunctional just because they exhibit characteristics different from the ideal image of a middle-class family of mother, father, and two or three children. In effect, a nuclear family, just as any of the others mentioned, may be an altered one if it demonstrates behaviors associated with this nursing diagnosis.

NURSING CONCERNS

It is important that nurses who work with families coping with multiple stressors develop an awareness of their own personal thoughts and feelings regarding each family's situations. Because these families are prone to experiencing hopelessness, worthlessness, powerlessness, and high levels of anxiety, the nurse may also begin to feel these emotions. In addition, the family may be suspicious of anyone who is not a member of its system and thus may respond to the nurse as a threat to its existence. This reaction frequently leads the family to reject the nurse's overtures of help. Thus the nurse may be prone to experiencing frustration, rejection, and uselessness.

The potential for violence among altered families may cause concern for personal safety, particularly among community health nurses as they make home visits, working in these environments alone and with minimal access to support in time of danger. If safety is a concern in a specific situation, two nurses can be assigned to work together with the family.

The nurse also needs to develop an awareness of the strengths and liabilities of his or her own present family system and family of origin. Knowledge of personal desires for change is im-

portant to prevent nurses from reacting to client family members as if they belonged to their own family system. Judith Nelsen highlighted this tendency as follows:

Practitioners having fantasies that they will tell off parents they see, tell children to shape up, coerce couples on the verge of divorce into reconciling, or otherwise do something likely to meet their own needs rather than clients' are not ready to see families. Such negative motivations need not persist if they are recognized and discussed, perhaps with a supervisor (Nelson, 1983, p. 56).

The nurse needs to acknowledge that negative feelings, as well as caring, concern, love, and a desire to help, are part of therapeutic relationships with individuals and families. Thus the occurrence of these negative emotions should not threaten the nurse's feeling of competence. Instead the nurse should recognize that identification of these reactions is the initial step in being able to cope with them so they do not interfere with the caring implementation of the nursing process. It is helpful before each visit to a family with altered processes or to one already diagnosed as such, for the nurse to ask the following questions:

- How do I feel about caring for this family today?
- What do I think about caring for this family today?
- How might these feelings and thoughts influence my abilities to care for this family today?
- How may I cope with these feelings and thoughts so I may effectively care for this family today?

ASSESSMENT

After coping with one's own stressors, the nurse begins to care for the family by implementing the nursing process: gathering data about the family by observing how members relate with each other, with the nurse, and with the home setting (Table 19-1). Both verbal and nonverbal behaviors provide information. The assessment process also involves identifying the family's strengths and its problems.

In light of Neuman's (1983) framework, the nurse assesses stressors in terms of their interre-

TABLE 19-1 Characteristics of families with altered processes

Stressors	Variables				
	Physiological	Psychological	Sociocultural	Developmental	Spiritual
Intrafamily	Physical neglect Malnutrition Physical/sexual abuse Hyperactivity Low energy level Lack of attention to symptoms Noncompliance with health care regimens Physical dependence on drugs	Lack of warmth Anger/hostility Depression Dysfunctional grief Hopelessness Helplessness Powerlessness Worthlessness Frustration Avoidance of feelings View of stressors as burden Desire to escape Guilt Dependence on drugs	Perpetuation of family myths Distortion of reality Rigid rules Lack of empa– thetic commun- ication Ineffective role patterns Lack of interde- pendence Scapegoating Enabling Lack of fit be- tween resources and demands	Insufficient knowl- edge of phases Unrealistic expec- tations Regression Learned helpless- ness	Rigid spiritual be- liefs Religious conflicts Overdependence on supreme be- ing
Interfamily	Avoidance of con- tact	Avoidance of con- tact	Suspicion of others Belief that no one can help Belief that no one cares Bitterness toward others	Lack of interde- pendence Fear of asking for help	Belief that situa- tions will only get worse Cynicism regard- ing motives of others
Extrafamily	Limited housing resources Lack of mobility	Fear of accepting help from agen- cies Fear of loss of control View of schools/ governmental agencies as inter- fering	Lack of money Unemployment	Avoidance of in- terdependence	Belief that helpers have failed Belief that nothing can help Rejection of sup- port groups Withdrawal from religious groups Lack of faith in the system

lationships of five variables (physiologic, psychologic, sociocultural, developmental, and spiritual).

Physiologic Variables

The nurse assesses the family for signs of physical health problems. Within these families, these problems may result from neglect, malnutrition, physical abuse, hyperactive behaviors, lack of at-

tention to symptoms of illness, and ineffectively coping with a treatment regimen for an illness. Betty Neuman suggested that the presence of a low energy level among family members indicates family instability inasmuch as the system's energy is focused on conflicts, emergencies, and survival (Neuman, 1983).

Substance abuse. The use of alcohol and

other chemical substances such as marijuana and cocaine should be investigated. Some family members coping with alcoholism or drug dependency or both may view this problem as the major stressor confronting the family. Other families may use these substances as they attempt to cope with other stressors in their lives.

The use of alcohol and other substances creates grave problems for the family because of the chemical properties of the substances ingested. These properties are related to the concepts of dependency and tolerance and cross-tolerance. Dependency develops as a person adapts to having the substance in his or her body. Two compo-

nents of dependency occur. One is physical dependency, which develops when physiologic symptoms, such as tremors, nausea, diaphoresis, and abdominal cramps, occur. The second is psychologic dependence, which refers to the compulsion and craving for the effects of the substance; that is, a feeling of self-esteem and well being. The implications of the psychoneurology of dependency are being delineated, and it appears that both physiologic and psychologic components are part of the same reaction of the body that is related to the activities of the neurotransmitters (Blum, 1991). What is most important for the nurse to acknowledge is that once

---

 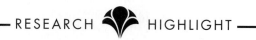

RESEARCH HIGHLIGHT

Physical and Sexual Abuse Among Runaways

This descriptive study, conducted over a 6-month period at a runaway shelter where youths were referred from a variety of local/district social service agencies and in a few instances, self-referral, had a two-fold purpose: (1) to describe runaway youths' self-reported experiences of physical/sexual abuse within the family structure, and (2) to identify patterns of alcohol and drug abuse among them. In face-to-face, open-ended interviews, a convenience sample of 78 youths (69 Caucasian, 9 African-American), ranging in age from 11 to 17, responded to questions from a clinical instrument that contained sensitive issues associated with the youths' current and past situations. Some questions remained unanswered because the youths had the option of excluding those that they considered intrusive. The handwritten notations from the interviews (which lasted approximately one and one half hours), were categorized and coded.

Results from 44 females (7 African-American), and 34 males (2 African-American), were displayed in tables that provided data related to their demographic characteristics, custody status, living arrangements before running away, significant other, alcohol/drug use, and experienced physical and sexual abuse. The youths sought refuge either on the

street or at the runaway shelter, because they experienced physical and/or sexual abuse within the family environment. The data also confirmed that conflict in the home was the greatest contributing factor to abuse. Drug and alcohol abuse alone or in combination with conflict in the home immediately followed home conflict in frequency. While one or more than one individual was identified as the abuser, the father was the most frequent perpetrator.

Beer and wine were the most frequently used forms of alcohol (44 of 71 respondents), and the reported age at first use ranged between 7 and 17 years. Liquor was the most frequently used form of alcohol among parents. Twenty-three of 71 youths indicated that they used drugs; the most frequent type of drug used was marijuana.

In their interactions with youths who have experienced physical/sexual abuse, health care workers must provide an environment conducive to systematic inquiry to gain an increased understanding of how conflicts and tensions within families lead to abuse, and to provide strategies for resolution. The authors suggest that the incidence of drug and alcohol abuse among all youths and their families should be extensively investigated.

From "Self-reported experiences of physical and sexual abuse among runaway youths" by J.K. Warren, F. Gary, & J. Moorhead. (1994). *Perspectives in Psychiatric Care, 30*(1), pp. 23-28.

the dependency has developed, the individual needs the effects of the chemical substance to feel a sense of normalcy. At this point, the substance controls the individual's and family's life instead of the person controlling the use of the drug.

This situation is complicated by the related physiologic processes of tolerance and cross-tolerance. When drug (including alcohol) tolerance and dependencies develop, the person requires larger amounts to prevent withdrawal symptoms and to feel "normal."

The individual also is at risk for problems associated with substance abuse, such as violence, employment difficulties, financial drain, and physical complications. These problems frequently confront these families again and again as a result of substance abuse. (Chemical dependence is discussed in greater detail in Chapter 23.)

It is important for the nurse to assess the extent to which each family member uses alcohol and other chemical substances. This requires the nurse to assess each person's nonverbal reactions as the individual answers questions related to the following three aspects of chemical dependency:

- Frequency: "How often do you drink alcohol?"
- Magnitude: "When you do drink, how much alcohol do you have?"
- Circumstances: "When do you usually drink alcohol?" "With whom do you usually drink alcohol?" "Under what circumstances do you usually drink alcohol?"

Family violence. Cues to abuse and violence within the family must be assessed. Within a family system, violence may be directed at any member by another and can include sexual acts, as well as other forms of physical aggression.

Family violence is a profound event that will affect each member of the system. A violent family is one in which all members are in pain. All are capable of hurting each other, all are learning that violence is an acceptable form of behavior, and all are at increased risk of resorting to the use of violence (Campbell & Campbell, 1993).

This reality means the cycle of violence will be perpetuated for another generation.

The problem of violence is difficult to define and approach. Table 19-2 lists the types of abuse found in families with altered processes. The fact that only physical, sexual, and incestuous abuse are beginning to be studied must be noted. Nevertheless, other forms of family abuse are important and should be considered as the nurse cares for a family.

Some theories that concern causative factors of family violence include a low level of frustration tolerance, a family's beliefs that crises should

TABLE 19-2 Types of family violence

Type	Characteristics
Physical	"Malnutrition and injuries such as bruises, welts, sprains, dislocation of extremities, lacerations"*
Psychologic	"Verbal assault, threat, fear, or isolation"*
Material	"Theft or misuse of money or property"*
Medical	"Withholding of required medication or aids" (e.g., false teeth, glasses, hearing aids)*
Sexual	"Any sexual activity between a child and an adult (or any individual significantly older than the child), whether by force or what may appear to be consent" (Kelley, 1985, p. 234)
Family	"At least one member is using physical force against another, resulting in physical and/or emotional destructive injury" (Campbell, 1984, p. 217)
Incest	"The occurrence of sexual relations between blood relatives, or two persons related to one another by some form of kinship tie" (Wilson & Kneisl, 1992, p. 535)
Violence	"Behavior by an individual that threatens or actually does harm or injury to people or property" (Wilson & Kneisl, 1988, p. 1176)

Information from "Assessing elder abuse: A study" by T. Fulmer & V. Cahill, 1984, *Journal of Gerontological Nursing, 10*(12), pp. 16-20.

* Fulmer and Cahill, 1984, pp. 17-18.

TABLE 19-3   Profile of the violent family

Identifying data	Child physical abuse		Child sexual abuse	
	Abuser	Victim	Abuser	Victim
Age	Mother, average age = 26; father, average age = 30; all ages	Most under 2 years; average age = 4 years; all ages	All ages; 21 to 30 years old most often; 11 to 20 years old next often	All ages; 6 to 9 years old at onset; 12 years old when disclosed; mean age = 7.9 years
Sex	Male and female; father more often than mother, but mother more violent	Not a factor	Male; accomplice sometimes female	Male and female; most reported cases are female (7 females to 1 male); in females, 63% are younger than 12 years old; in males, 64% are older than 12 years old
Relationship	Father or stepfather; not a stranger most often (e.g., babysitter or guardian)	Acquainted or known; oldest/youngest daughter or only child most often	Father more often than mother	Son/daughter or stepchild
Marital status	Married and living with spouse	Single	Married and living with spouse	Single
History of childhood physical/sexual abuse	60% of cases	Repeated multiple victimization or neglect	70% of cases	Repeated multiple victimization
Socioeconomic status (SES)	Evident at all SES levels; rate twice as high in reported cases of families under the poverty line ($5999) as in families of $20,000 + income		Evident in all SES levels; found cases most often lower SES	
Occupation	Reported cases most often skilled or semiskilled	Student	Found cases most often professional, skilled, or semiskilled	Student
Employment status	Unemployment not disproportionately prevalent; abuse twice as high if father is employed part time	Not employed	Employed; higher rate if part time or unemployed	Not employed
Race	Blacks and minorities inaccurately represented; all races		Same as abuser	Not a factor

From "Nursing intervention in family abuse and violence" by T. Foley & B. Grimes (pp. 930-933) in *Principles and Practice of Psychiatric Nursing* (3rd ed.), (1987), by G. W. Stuart & S. J. Sundeen (Eds.), St. Louis: Mosby.

TABLE 19-3 Profile of the violent family   cont'd

Spouse abuse		Sibling abuse		Elder abuse	
Male	Female	Abuser	Victim	Abuser	Victim
Often 17 to 30 years old at disclosure; all ages; seen in abuse of elders		All ages; most reported cases are 17 years old or less; rate decreases as age increases		40 to 60 years old	60 years old and older
Male and female; most reported cases have female victims		Male most often; higher incidence in all-male-sibling families	Male most often; higher incidence in all-male-sibling families	Female	Not a factor; more elder are female
Spouse or partner		Brother to brother as victim most often; brother to sister as victim next often		Son/daughter, relative, or caretaker	Parent of abuser most often
Married most often; living together next often		Single	Single	Married	Widowed
Most were subject to repeated victimization as children		Live in abusive/violent home; often victims of parent/guardian as well		Data not widely available; positive history in some cases	Positive history in some cases; repeated victimization
Evident at all SES levels; five times more common in families at or below poverty line than in families over $20,000 income in reported cases		Evident at all SES levels		Not a factor; evident at all SES levels; found cases mostly lower to middle class and found through health care systems	
Reported cases skilled or semiskilled most often		Childhood (or history of delinquency)		Professional or semiskilled	Not employed
Violence two or three times higher if man is unemployed or has part-time employment		Not employed		Least violence in homes of retired men; victim often physically/mentally impaired	
All races; reported most by minorities; blacks more than whites (2:1)		Highest, racial minorities; lowest, blacks		Highest, American Indians, orientals, minorities; blacks = 12%, whites = 88%, also reported as no difference	

Continued

TABLE 19-3   Profile of the violent family   cont'd

Identifying data	Child physical abuse		Child sexual abuse	
	Abuser	Victim	Abuser	Victim
Religion	Highest, one or more parents of minority religion; lowest, Jewish	Mixed religious background	Highest, highly religious family, rigid inflexible belief system; lowest, realistic balance of religion in family belief system	
Education	Most violent, high school diploma for both men and women; least violent, grammar school dropout or some college education	Mostly preschool; if in school, performance may be poor (stress symptom)	Inaccurately presented. Often high school and some college	Grammar and high school student; performance may be poor (stress symptom)
Residence	Large city most often Evenly distributed in United States		Evenly distributed in United States	

be resolved with aggression, and the lowering of inhibitions against violence caused by the use of alcohol and other central nervous system depressants (Hanrahan, Campbell, & Ulrich, 1993). In fact, family violence may result from the interactions of many of these factors.

Table 19-3 outlines the results of many research studies regarding the profiles of violent families. The nurse, on initiating a relationship with a family, considers these factors.

The nurse who suspects abusive behaviors should meet individually with each member of the family. This subject is a difficult one to discuss, yet it must be explored to prevent further abuse and to break the cycle of intergenerational violence. It is especially necessary that the nurse pursue comments by individuals that appear to suggest that they are the victims of abuse or are concerned about becoming violent toward a family member. John Flynn's (1977) research revealed that "almost all" of his sample of abused wives had sought help from a variety of sources, including police, marriage counselors, or clergy. Frequently these pleas for help were not taken seriously. Instead the person from whom help was sought continued to attempt to keep it hidden.

Barbara Limandri, a nurse, suggested the "most critical element in helping abused women is the nurse's response to the women's disclosure" (1987, p. 10). The box on p. 424 lists the facilitative and inhibitive helper responses identified in Limandri's research. The nurse uses the first set of responses to help women discuss the reality that they are victims of abuse.

Psychologic Variables

As the nurse explores the psychologic variables of the family system, cues such as a lack of warmth within the family; avoidance of the expression of feelings; intense levels of anger, hostility, and aggression; depression; expressions of

TABLE 19-3 Profile of the violent family cont'd

Spouse abuse		Sibling abuse		Elder abuse	
Male	Female	Abuser	Victim	Abuser	Victim
Highest, minority religions and Jewish women; lowest, Protestants and Jewish men		Highest minority religions (excluding Jewish, Catholic, or Protestant)		Protestant	
Victim more often without high school diploma and less often with college education		Most violent if father/male highly educated and mother/female high school diploma or some college education		High school diploma or some college	
Most violent husbands, high school diploma; least violent, grammar school dropout or some college	Most violent, wives without high school diploma				
Evenly distributed in United States	Abused by male in large city or rural area; rate decreased by half in suburbs	Higher rates in rural area and large cities Not Southern phenomena		Limited data, evenly distributed with more reports in large cities Not Southern phenomena	

guilt, hopelessness, worthlessness, powerlessness, cynicism, and bitterness; and maladaptive grieving are considered important in identifying a family coping with multiple stressors. Feelings of hopelessness can usually be identified by one or more of the following cues:

- Inability to set goals
- Perception of unachieved outcomes as personal failure
- Emphasis is on failure in light of accomplishments while healthy
- Rigid adherence to the possibility of achieving goals only when healthy
- Making no effort to consider alternatives
- Increasing agitation over accomplishing nothing
- Verbalization of self-doubt, therapy, and life
- Verbalization of giving up as the only solution
- Giving up

During the assessment of psychologic variables the nurse observes how the family perceives itself and its health problems. Some families tend to distort reality, frequently by means of unconscious denial, projection, and/or fantasy formation. The result is rationalization by means of blaming, scapegoating, and wishful thinking as the family tries to solve its problems. The reliance on these coping mechanisms leads to the perpetuation of family myths. Cues that reflect rigid family rules include comments such as, "We are a strong family so none of us cry," or "We'd be okay if everybody like you would leave us alone."

Spiritual Variables

As highlighted in Table 19-1, cues of extremely rigid spiritual beliefs, opposing religious loyalties, and an overdependence on supreme powers frequently are observed among families that are prone to violence. In addition, the families "may not participate in therapy because of their belief that a supreme being will solve the problems, if it is His will" (Shealy, 1988, p. 555).

RESPONSES TO ABUSED WOMEN

Facilitative helper responses

- Helper asking woman if abuse is occurring
- Helper identifying described behavior as abusive
- Helper acknowledging seriousness of abuse
- Helper expressing belief in woman's description of abuse
- Helper acknowledging that woman does not deserve the abuse
- Helper being directive in exploring resources
- Helper telling the man to stop the abuse
- Helper aiding woman to consider full range of available options
- Helper avoiding telling woman what to do
- Helper aiding woman to assess her internal strengths
- Helper suggesting tangible resources (e.g., shelters, financial aid)
- Helper offering support groups with other abused women
- Helper active in listening and empathizing

Inhibitive helper responses

- Helper demonstrating irritation/anger with woman
- Helper blaming woman
- Helper advising woman to accept abuse as better than nothing
- Helper refusing to help until woman leaves abuser
- Helper aligning with abuser
- Helper disbelieving woman
- Helper not responding to abuse disclosure
- Helper advising woman to leave abuser

From "The therapeutic relationship with abused women" by B. Limandri, 1987, *Journal of Psychosocial Nursing, 25*(2), p. 11. Copyright 1987 by Charles B. Slack. Reprinted by permission.

Sociocultural Variables

Sociocultural variables can be the most difficult to assess in a caring and empathetic manner because of the wide differences of cultural orientations among families encountered by community health nurses. When the nurse and the family members have different cultural backgrounds, misunderstandings frequently arise. Toni Tripp-

Reimer and Sonja Lively aptly illustrated this phenomenon with the following case study:

A case of reported child abuse was reported recently to the staff of a county mental health facility. The case involved a Vietnamese refugee family newly arrived in the United States. The referral was made by a school nurse who, while conducting routine physical assessments, identified long bruised areas on the chest and back of a girl in the second grade. However, rather than being caused by incidents of child abuse, the marks were the results of the lay practice or dermabrasion *(cao gio),* a standard home treatment for the symptoms of fever, chills, and headaches that accompany "wind illness." This practice consists of applying oil to the back and chest of the child with cotton swabs. The skin is massaged until warm and then rubbed with the edge of a copper coin until marks (bruises) appear. Thus the parents had not been abusing the child but rather were following a culturally prescribed and sanctioned mode of folk therapy (1988, p. 185).

To avoid misunderstandings such as this, the nurse must be aware of the cultural orientation of the family. (Chapter 3 presents detailed information regarding cultural issues.)

As sociocultural variables are reviewed, the nurse assesses the way members communicate with each other. Depending on the family's cultural orientation, the avoidance of eye contact, excessive agreement or disagreement, and individuals' interrupting each other, changing the topic, silencing some members, and being sarcastic may indicate an altered family. Conversations often are dominated by vague, confusing, unempathetic, negative, critical, and mixed messages.

The family's methods of role allocation and handling of role relationships are considered under the sociocultural dimension. Cues include parent-child role reversals, role deficiencies, disengagement, enmeshment, and rigid role assignments. These behaviors are demonstrated by inappropriate role expectations; that is, they do not correspond to the individual's age, developmental phase, and capabilities.

Enmeshment and disengagement are two extremes of the range of family interaction patterns. **Enmeshment** refers to a pattern in which the sharing among the members of the system is extreme and intense. Individuality and independence are viewed negatively. An example of enmeshment occurred in a family that reacted to the 14-year-old daughter's request to see a movie with two school friends by telling her what a "bad girl" she was for wanting to do something away from the family and then punishing her by giving her extra housework to do. At the other extreme is **disengagement.** In this pattern, rigid, impermeable boundaries separate the members of the system. Thus interactions among the individuals within the family seem to lack response and connection. A sense of abandonment pervades the system because communication among the members is discouraged. An example of disengagement is the case of a 10-year-old who brings home a report card that none of the family members review.

Neither pattern promotes interdependence, which may be defined as "the close relationships of people that involve the willingness and ability to love, respect, and value others, and to accept and respond to love, respect, and value given by others" (Hanson, 1984, p. 306).

Two specific role patterns frequently observed in families coping with multiple stressors are scapegoating and enabling, both of which develop unconsciously within the system.

Scapegoating occurs when one member bears the blame for the problems confronting the family. Frequently, a child or a member with a chronic health problem falls into this role. This person then unconsciously acts out the family's conflict by developing a problem or symptoms of a physical, psychologic, or social nature. The other members of the system unite to focus on the scapegoat's situation. They further express their frustration and anger toward this person for causing the family problems.

Enabling is defined as any behavior that encourages an individual to continue acting in a specific manner primarily by shielding the person from the consequences of the behavior. An example of enabling is the wife who calls her husband's boss to explain that her husband is too ill to work when in reality he has a hangover. In effect, the wife is saving her husband from the consequences of his behavior, rewarding him, and thus encouraging (enabling) him to continue the pattern.

Developmental Variables

In assessing developmental variables, the nurse observes the family for its knowledge of both individual and family developmental tasks (see Chapter 18). Among the variables that cause altered behaviors within a family is insufficient knowledge of the different phases of growth and development. Frequently, this lack of knowledge causes parents to have unrealistic expectations of their children; for example, a mother who believes her 13-month-old daughter should be toilet trained.

In altered families the nurse may observe high levels of **regression,** and behavior and thinking processes that are appropriate for earlier phases of growth and development, in individual members and in the system itself. Frequently, this regressive behavior occurs because those involved are so overwhelmed by a stressor that they believe they cannot resolve the situation.

Stressors

According to Betty Neuman (1983), the family system faces many stressors throughout its life. **Stressors** are forces that produce a reaction from the system, which tends to create instability within it. Stressors can affect an organism either negatively or positively. Neuman emphasizes that the manner in which the family reacts to the stressor depends on its subjective perception of the problem. Furthermore, the family's potential for change as it reacts to stressors is contingent on its previous coping patterns, especially the rigid use of defensive patterns such as the denial or the rejection of help from others. However, the reality is that a family who can cope with a stressor shows adaptive facility; that is, the ability to change.

Neuman (1983) identifies three types of stressors: intrafamily, interfamily, and extrafamily. **Intrafamily** (within the unit itself) **stressors** include the allocation of roles and conflict among the members. An important intrafamily reaction occurs because family stressors tend to require role changes. This reaction may then be experienced as a stressor.

Interfamily stressors occur as the family interacts with other systems in the environment that directly influence the family, such as schools, health care agencies, or the workplace. The nurse, in initiating a relationship with a family, also becomes an interfamily stressor.

Extrafamily stressors occur as the family is influenced indirectly by political, social, and cultural issues. This type of stressor includes limited housing resources, political decisions that restrict the minimum wage and cut back health care funding, and cultural stigmas that perpetuate the myths of hopefulness and helplessness of individuals who experience problems related to alcoholism or mental illness. The nurse needs to be aware that all these forces may be at work and that the effects of these stressors require continual assessment as the nurse cares for the family.

Influence of lines of defense and lines of resistance. All these previously described behaviors and cues result in a weakening of the family's flexible and normal lines of defense and flexible line of resistance.

Neuman (1983) views the flexible line of defense as an accordion-like buffer for the system that aims to prevent stressors from invading the system. It is able to expand and contract rapidly as the system encounters stressors. The normal line of defense represents the usual level of wellness of the system (Neuman, 1983). It represents the standard of wellness for the family as it protects the basic structure of the system by preventing stressor invasion of the core. The lines of resistance are the system's last line of defense from stressor invasion of the basic structure (Neuman, 1983). When a family is overwhelmed by multiple stressors, the flexible line of defense is unable to change as needed to respond to the everyday stressors of life. In effect, it will no longer provide a buffer zone to screen out the pressures from these problems.

When the flexible line of defense is not functioning effectively, the family's normal line of defense is under constant pressure to help it address the immediate pressures of daily existence. The result is that the family's normal level of adaptation, or state of wellness, becomes relatively low.

Finally, the flexible line of resistance is under constant attack as it tries to protect the family's basic energy resources. As demonstrated by the variables already described, this line becomes rigid. Thus the sense of interdependence within the family is limited because members are unable to rely on one another.

The weaknesses of these protective lines result in the family's increased susceptibility to the threat of stressors. The thrust and penetration ability of even weaker stressors becomes relatively strong as the family's resistance level and its ability to change are lowered. At this point death of the family may be close (Reed, 1993) as it attempts to prevent the stressors from destroying its limited energy resources and integrity as a unit.

NURSING DIAGNOSIS

After assessing the family system, the nurse formulates the nursing diagnoses that provide the focus for planning and evaluating care. If a family system is determined to fit the category of altered family processes, the nurse identifies the stressors—intrapersonal, interpersonal, and/or extrapersonal—that are confronting the unit and creating the alteration. Possible nursing diagnoses include the following:

- Ineffective family coping related to substance abuse
- Ineffective family coping related to family violence
- Ineffective family coping related to hopelessness

PLANNING AND INTERVENTION

After formulating the nursing diagnoses, the nurse and family establish the goals for intervention and the plan of intervention. The nurse attempts to capitalize on the strengths of the system that were identified during the assessment.

Engaging the Family in Care

In planning care for families with altered processes within Neuman's theoretical framework, the nurse primarily uses the secondary and tertiary prevention/intervention strategies. Thus the overall goals of nursing intervention will be to "attain/maintain [a] maximum wellness level"

(Neuman, 1983, p. 249). This is accomplished by supporting the internal and external resources of the system to strengthen the family's flexible and normal lines of defense and line of resistance. The result is strengthening the family's abilities to withstand the threats of stressors in the future in an adaptive manner.

The nurse, however, does not employ these terms when meeting with the members to establish the goals. Instead, the nurse uses nontechnical language to emphasize the family's ability to confront its problems so that it may experience a healthier future.

Capitalizing on Strengths of the Family System

The nurse continues to encourage the family to capitalize on its strengths. Frequently the family is so overwhelmed by the stressors it is facing that it is unable to recognize any assets or even the potential for change. It is important that the nurse emphasize the family's ability to attempt to carry on despite difficult circumstances (Fleishman, Home, & Arthur 1983).

The nurse must be sensitive to the deep level of loyalty that tends to exist within families. Consequently, the nurse should move slowly, at the family's pace, and not expect to accomplish major changes quickly. The nurse must especially be sensitive to the fact that "unlike the stable family, the severely disturbed family is heavily invested in its own stabilization, often resorting to old dysfunctional patterns with increased vigor, especially when threatened by imminent breakdown. It can tolerate a challenge to its rules only slowly and with thought-out consequences for the family" (Weitzman, 1985, p. 476).

The nurse must acknowledge that these families are interested primarily in regaining a sense of stability by returning to their previous level of wellness.

Empathizing With the Family's Predicament

The nurse initially empathizes with the family's difficulties, acknowledges past efforts to gain help, and attempts to reduce the level of conflict among family members. The nurse must maintain a balance between accurately recognizing the gravity of the problems that confront the family and maintaining the belief that there is hope and help for the system. The nurse must remember that the family's usual manner of coping with stressors to maintain stability has been developed over a long period of time. Changing this pattern of response will also require a great expenditure of time, energy, and work on the part of each member of the system (Reed, 1993).

To accomplish these objectives the nurse initially can assume an authority position within the unit, taking the role of a warm and concerned, yet controlling, person who can meet the adults' needs for support and direction (Lynch & Tiedje, 1991).

Encouragement of Realistic Goal Setting

In establishing goals, the nurse should discuss with family members how each would like the situation within the family to be different. The nurse should encourage the members to be realistic but also to identify some solutions to their problems.

It is imperative that the nurse focus the discussion on current, here-and-now problems so that the family does not become overwhelmed by past problems and interpersonal conflicts. The nurse also encourages members to express the anger, hostility, and frustration they are feeling while avoiding the ventilation of numerous grievances against each other, such as constant complaints by parents about their children. These accusations lead only to increased tension in the family and may cause the family to reject the nurse's help because of the resultant discomfort. Instead the nurse should listen to the complaints one time, elicit the individual's feelings regarding them, and then focus the family's attention on what can be done to improve the situation, at least minimally.

Encouragement of the Acceptance of Three Primary Rules

In meeting with the family, the nurse should encourage the acceptance of three primary rules. First, everyone present has an opportunity to speak and to participate. Second, only one individual speaks at a time. Thus, while one is speaking, all others should be listening and focusing their attention on what is being said (Fleishman et al., 1983). Third, individuals will not be "permitted to attack one another (verbally or otherwise), be overly critical, disruptive or punitive" (Weitzman, 1985, p. 480).

Relabeling All Members of the System as Victims

Being part of an altered family means that an individual experiences intense anger and a feeling of hurt. Frequently one member is blamed for the family's problems and failures. It is important that the nurse avoid perpetuating this belief. To counteract this phenomenon the nurse attempts to redefine the problem as one that affects the whole family and every person within it. "This is best done by focusing on how each person is, in fact a 'victim' of the problem" (Fleishman et al., 1983, p. 27).

IMPLEMENTATION

After considering the principles already presented, the nurse then works with the family to develop realistic plans of care related to the family's priority nursing diagnoses. Three suggested plans are offered here.

Ineffective Family Coping Related to Substance Abuse

When the nursing diagnosis of ineffective family coping related to substance abuse has been formulated, the nurse and the family members work toward achieving the goals of avoiding substance abuse and developing more adaptive coping mechanisms. The plan of care might include some of the following nurse-centered interventions.

Primary prevention

1. Recognize the reality that substance abuse may be a threat to the stability of the family, and plan how the family may attempt to prevent the invasion of this stressor.
2. Use stress as a positive intervention strategy by encouraging the family to view stress as a challenge it can meet. Empathize with how difficult

this may be in light of the family's other stressors (Feigenbaum, 1986).
3. Educate members regarding the effects of various substances such as alcohol, diazepam (Valium), cocaine, and marijuana. Discuss terms such as *physical* and *psychological dependencies,* and *tolerance* and *cross-tolerance.*
4. Support the efforts of members toward positive coping and functioning.

Secondary prevention

1. Recognize the extent of invasion of the family system by substance abuse, especially the phenomena of psychological and physical dependencies.
2. Mobilize and optimize the family's resources and energy by focusing on the reality that substance abuse is a problem that can be overcome.
3. Encourage the family members to observe within themselves the signs of enabling, denying, and minimizing. Encourage the family to confront the reality of this stressor (substance abuse) directly, and emphasize that avoidance will compound the severity of its impact.
4. Motivate the family to seek treatment for this problem with education regarding the fact that substance abuse affects every member of the family and that the sooner treatment is sought, the weaker these effects will be.
5. Facilitate the seeking of appropriate treatment. If physical dependence is present, the individual should be referred to a detoxification unit. Once withdrawal from the physical effects of the drug and/or alcohol has occurred, participation in a rehabilitation program is helpful. This program should include educational sessions, along with individual, group, and family psychotherapy. During the rehabilitation program the persons who have been abusing the substances should begin attending self-help support groups such as Alcoholics Anonymous, Narcotics Anonymous, or Women for Sobriety. After discharge from the program, active and frequent participation in the therapeutic work of these support groups is necessary to maintain sobriety. Attending meetings daily during the first year of sobriety is recommended. Family members also should attend similar meetings of groups such as Al-Anon, Al-Ateen, and Adult Children of Alcoholics.

6. Support the family's efforts toward health by empathizing with the difficulty of recovery and the need for a day-by-day commitment. Help the members focus on the here-and-now instead of the future.

Tertiary prevention

1. Coordinate the family's efforts to seek and follow through on treatment for substance abuse as already explained.
2. Support the family's efforts to cope with family members' relapses as they try to maintain sobriety.
3. Educate family members regarding adaptive coping mechanisms, such as sublimation, to deal with stressors that attempt to invade the flexible line of defense of both the individual and the family system.
4. Educate regarding the effects of substance abuse.

Ineffective Family Coping Related to Family Violence

When the nursing diagnosis of ineffective family coping related to family violence has been selected, the nurse and family members work toward achieving the goals of avoiding violence as a means of coping with stressors and developing more adaptive coping mechanisms. The plan of care might include some of the following interventions.

Primary prevention

1. Classify violence as a stressor that may threaten a family's stability.
2. Educate the family regarding the dynamics of anger, frustration, aggression, hostility, and violence. Empathize with members' feelings that "it's difficult to cope when you reach your breaking point."
3. Support the members' efforts, especially sublimation, to develop adaptive methods of coping with anger and frustration.
4. Provide information to the parents on how to discipline their children in nonviolent ways, such as the withdrawal of privileges or time-out periods.
5. Educate the parents regarding the stages of child development so that they become aware of the normal characteristics of a maturing individual.

Teach the use of reinforcement of positive behaviors as a parenting technique.

6. Educate the parents regarding the importance of their having time alone together, without the children or older family members, so that their relationship may be sustained.
7. Support each member's attempts to build a positive sense of self-esteem. Emphasize each person's ability to continue trying to cope, despite overwhelming stressors.
8. Encourage the family to build support systems through interactions with other families and significant others.
9. In addition to working with families, the nurse should become politically active to bring about social changes to reduce violence.

Secondary prevention

1. After the invasion of the family by the stressor of violence, protect the system's basic structure by recognizing the existence of family violence as early as possible.
2. Use the theories and skills of crisis intervention to help the family members confront the reality of the abusive situation.
3. Depending on the legal implications of the nature of the violence, if warranted, report the incidence of abuse to the proper authorities. Each state requires that nurses report suspected child abuse or neglect: physical abuse, emotional abuse, some forms of physical neglect, and sexual abuse. Failure to report results in specific penalties (Munro, 1993).

The nurse should include the following information in a report to the authorities (Rhodes, 1987):

- Name and address of child
- Name and address of parent or caretaker
- Age and present location of child
- Nature and extent of injuries
- Any evidence of previous injuries such as scars or healing bruises
- Name, age, and condition of other children in the home
- Parent's or caretaker's description of injury
- Person responsible for injury (if known) or name of person caring for the child at the time of the injury

AGE-SPECIFIC ANTICIPATORY GUIDANCE INTERVENTIONS

Infants, toddlers, preschoolers

Teach parents about developmental stages, child's capabilities, risks for injuries, age-appropriate games and toys, as well as when and how to set limits and discipline without hitting. If guns are in the house, tell parents they should be stored unloaded in a locked area, separate from the ammunition, which should also be locked away.

Elementary-school-aged children

Teach parents about developmental stages, a child's changing interests, peer pressure, as well as limit setting and discipline. Talk with child about how to stay out of trouble; e.g., why an activity might be "wrong," what the consequences could be, and how to suggest a different activity. Ask the child, "Do children pick on each other at your school?" and "What do you think about that?" Help children explore what they could do to avoid an argument with others. By the age of eight the child can be guided in developing ways to avoid confrontations over insults and arguments. Give concrete examples such as, "I don't want to fight with you," or "I don't want to fight about this." Review gun safety with parents.

By 10 to 11 years of age, children should be encouraged to avoid alcohol because of its disinhibiting effects, which increase impulsive behavior and therefore the risk of violence. Give information about high-risk situations to avoid; e.g., peers drinking, lack of adult supervision, presence of gang members or teens upholding "tough" reputations. Teach them to avoid reliance on a "reputation" to keep them safe, and teach specific ways to defuse volatile situations. Role playing to illustrate behavior choices and talking about problems are both techniques a child can use to learn how to offer a confronting person a face-saving "out." These techniques may also help children to internalize new behaviors.

When the child is age 11 or 12, guide her or him in a discussion about depression and the signs of depression. Strongly emphasize that even severe depressions pass. Encourage the child to consider with whom she or he can discuss feelings, and where she or he can go for help if depressed. Review verbal responses to insults and arguments with the child. Review gun safety with parents.

Adolescents, age 13 to 19 years

Review tobacco, alcohol and drug use, safer sex and condom use, seat belt and helmet use. Stress the possible outcome of riding with someone who has been drinking. Review dealing with a depression, maintaining gun safety, and avoiding potentially violent situations. Role play giving an aggressor a face-saving "out," illustrate techniques for effective avoidance of physical violence.

From "Preventing violence through primary care intervention" by C. Roberts & J. Quillian, 1992, *Nurse Practitioner, 17*(8), p. 67.

- Statement summarizing why child abuse is suspected
- Any other information that may be helpful in establishing the cause of the injury or that will provide assistance to the child

Currently nurses are mandated by law to report only incidences of suspected child abuse. Situations that involve the abuse of adults, such as spouse or elder abuse, are not covered under these laws. Wide variations exist concerning how the legal system addresses these episodes of adult violence.

The health care and legal systems view family violence from two widely different philosophies, control versus compassion (Gelles & Cornell, 1990). The compassionate view is that the abusive parents are also victims themselves. Thus intervention involves the support of both abuser and family by providing homemaker services, health and child care, and other supports. The opposite view, that of control, involves aggressive intervention, including the punishment of violent behaviors. The abuser is considered fully responsible, and consequences include removal of the child from the home, separation of the abused wife from her violent spouse, and full criminal prosecution of the offender.

Problems are inherent in each approach. One recommendation combines both: the use of control in assessment and compassion in treatment

STEPS IN THE PREVENTION OF INTIMATE VIOLENCE

The central goal of programs and policies aimed at family violence is to prevent violence. The findings presented in this book clearly point to the fact that some fundamental changes in values and beliefs will have to occur before we see a real decrease in the level of violence in the family. Looking toward the future, there are a number of policy steps that could help prevent intimate violence.

(1) Eliminate the norms that legitimize and glorify violence in the society and the family. The elimination of spanking as a child-rearing technique, the promotion of gun control to get deadly weapons out of the home, the elimination of corporal punishment in school and of the death penalty, and an elimination of media violence that glorifies and legitimizes violence are all necessary steps. In short, we need to cancel the hitting license in society.

(2) Reduce violence-provoking stress created by society. Reducing poverty, inequality, and unemployment and providing for adequate housing, feeding, medical and dental care, and educational opportunities are steps that could reduce stress in families.

(3) Integrate families into a network of kin and community. Reducing social isolation would be a significant step to help reduce stress and increase the abilities of families to manage stress.

(4) Change the sexist character of society. Sexual inequality, perhaps more than economic inequality, makes violence possible in homes. The elimination of "men's work" and "women's work" would be a major step toward equality in and out of the home.

(5) Break the cycle of violence in the family. This step repeats the message of step 1—violence cannot be prevented as long as we are taught that it is appropriate to hit the people we love. Physical punishment of children is perhaps the most effective means of teaching violence, and eliminating it would be an important step in violence prevention.

Such steps require long-term changes in the fabric of society. These proposals call for such fundamental change in families and family life that many people resist them and argue that they could not work or would ruin the family. The alternative, of course, is that not making such changes continues the harmful and deadly tradition of family violence.

From *Intimate violence in families* (p. 139) by R. Gelles & C. Cornell, 1983, Beverly Hills, CA: Sage. Copyright 1983 by Sage Publications. Reprinted by permission.

---

trol in assessment and compassion in treatment (Gelles & Cornell, 1990).

This dilemma confronts the nurse who suspects family violence. It is imperative, however, that the nurse first follow the mandates of the state and then work to coordinate the treatment plan that is established for the family.

4. If the abuse involves adults, support the victim's efforts to deal with the situation.

5. Facilitate appropriate intervention for all family members. The abuser especially will benefit from individual and group psychotherapy to learn adaptive methods of handling frustration and to develop a higher level of self-esteem (Swift, 1986). Refer victims to group-support programs that will help them to realize they did not deserve the abuse and also to increase their levels of self-esteem. Encourage other family members to attend meetings of self-help support groups to help them recognize how they have been affected by the violence within their homes.

6. Refer the family members to Parents Anonymous. One study (Hunka, O'Toole, & O'Toole, 1985) analyzed the functioning of one of these support groups to identify how the group process effected change. The authors concluded that

the group becomes a surrogate family through the process of identification and emotional bonding. Veteran members resocialize a new member . . . to learn new ways of coping with their psychological problems, their feelings toward the child, and means to handle the crisis. At the same time, they learn to identify and relinquish old, maladaptive behavior. . . . Emotional bonding in PA also tends to increase the abusive parent's self-esteem (p. 29).

Tertiary prevention

1. During reconstruction of the family's stability and health, acknowledge the need to break the vicious cycle of intergenerational family violence.
2. Support the members' efforts to deal with stressors in nonviolent manners.
3. Acknowledge the reality that relapses may occur and should be discussed immediately.
4. Encourage the members to continue to participate in the activities of self-help support groups such as Parents Anonymous.
5. If the violence has led to the break-up of the family, support the members' efforts to start a new life.

Ineffective Family Coping Related to Hopelessness

When the nursing diagnosis of ineffective family coping related to hopelessness has been selected, the nurse and family members work toward fulfilling the goals of gaining a sense of hope for the future and developing more adaptive coping mechanisms. The plan of care might include some of the following nurse-centered interventions (Neuman, 1988).

Primary prevention

1. Classify hopelessness as a stressor that may be a threat to the family's stability, and prevent the invasion of this stressor. NANDA defined hopelessness as a "subjective state in which an individual sees limited or no alternatives or personal choices available and is unable to mobilize energy on own behalf" (Bruss, 1988, p. 28).
2. Provide information to the family regarding its existing strengths as a basis for facing problems that seem overwhelming.
3. Emphasize the positive value of stress as a challenge rather than a threat.

Secondary prevention

1. Protect the basic structure of the family by recognizing hopelessness as an invader as soon as possible (Bruss, 1988). Verbal cues of hopelessness are considered to be most significant.
2. Optimize the resources of the family toward stability and energy conservation by encouraging it to find "clues which substantiate hope, [feel it]

has something to anticipate, and [discover] a sustaining supernatural love" (Miller, 1983, p. 297).
3. Educate the family members to develop the coping skill of maximizing experiences; that is, to appreciate to the fullest extent even the smallest positive event (Miller, 1983). The box below lists activities the nurse can suggest to help clients achieve a state of hopefulness.
4. Empathize with the client's frustration and fatigue in feeling that everything appears hopeless and how difficult it is to attempt to change this feeling.

Tertiary prevention

1. Support the family's efforts to sustain a sense of hope while recognizing that relapses will occur.
2. Acknowledge the difficulty of sustaining hope, and educate the family in coping with the difficulties.

EVALUATION

The nurse evaluates the effectiveness of nursing intervention for families with altered processes by analyzing whether changes have occurred within the system. Positive outcomes are re-

---

ACTIVITIES OF DAILY LIVING THAT MAY HELP MAXIMIZE HOPEFUL EXPERIENCES

- Savor the richness of coffee in the morning.
- Note the crystal-clear blue sky.
- Feel the warmth of a sunbeam.
- Watch activities of animals in a tree outside a window.
- Share children's experiences.
- Note loving characteristics of a significant other.
- Appreciate expressions of caring concern.
- Build highlights into each day, such as meals, visits, inspirational reading.
- Study a favorite photograph or painting.
- Listen to a favorite song or symphony on the radio.

From *Coping with chronic illness* (p. 293) by J. Miller, 1983, Philadelphia: Davis. Copyright 1983 by F.A. Davis Co. Modified by permission.

flected in the strengthening of the unit's flexible line of defense, which enables it to respond in a more adaptive manner to the everyday stressors of life. In effect, these families then have a more effective buffer from stressors. In terms of the nursing diagnoses discussed in the previous section, family members might maintain sobriety, react adaptively to feelings of anger and frustration, or maintain a sense of hope even in the face of problems.

Cues of the reactions of the family's normal line of defense are also evaluated. Although realistically this line would be strengthened by the nursing intervention, it probably will be functioning at a relatively low level because of the over-whelming odds facing the altered family compared with a healthy family.

The system's flexible line of resistance will also be strengthened by the intervention, which will allow the family greater interdependence and an increased ability to adapt to change.

In evaluating the effectiveness of the nursing intervention, the nurse should observe for small markers of progress and recognize that they are positive signs of the family's advancement toward health.

The following case study highlights some of the important components of the nursing process applied to a family coping with multiple stressors that develop into altered processes.

■ CASE STUDY

Margaret T. is a married, 32-year-old mother of three. She has been discharged from the hospital against medical advice after a 3-day stay with a medical diagnosis of diabetes mellitus and a compound fracture of the left proximal humerus (upper portion of the arm). She had initially gone to the emergency room of the hospital for treatment of her "broken arm" after a "fall down the basement stairs." During her examination the physician determined that she also was experiencing symptoms of diabetes mellitus. She was admitted to the hospital for further tests that confirmed that diagnosis. Her left arm has been immobilized in a sling, and she has been referred for physical therapy twice a week.

During Margaret's stay in the hospital, the nurse who specialized in diabetes education taught Margaret how to administer insulin injections and modify her diet. The nurse observed that Margaret appeared depressed and sullen, avoided eye contact, and answered all questions with one or two words. The nurse also noted that Margaret had not had any visitors during her stay. The nurse decided that home care follow-up was indicated because Margaret seemed vague and insecure about her condition even though she verbalized a complete understanding of her diet and was able to administer her injections safely. The visit was planned for the day after discharge.

During the first home visit the nurse found that Margaret had given herself the injection but had not eaten because "there was no food in the house." She explained, "My husband didn't have time to shop while I was in the hospital." The nurse also observed that the house appeared cluttered but was relatively clean. A case of empty beer bottles was sitting on the counter.

Margaret appeared very tense and agitated. She told the nurse, "Let's get this over with fast before my husband wakes up. He'll be upset if he sees a stranger here. I wish you'd just leave me alone. I'll be fine. As soon as my eight-year-old daughter gets home from school, she'll go shopping for me."

The nurse empathized with Margaret's feelings and then emphasized the importance of eating scheduled meals and following the prescribed menu. Margaret then began crying and said, "I can't believe this has happened to me. I've never been sick before. How am I going to handle my kids? They're driving me crazy. Besides, I have to get back to work because my husband isn't working now."

The nurse asked Margaret if she could look for something she could make her for breakfast. Margaret hesitantly agreed. While the nurse prepared oatmeal, she encouraged Margaret to talk about her family.

Margaret smiled as she mentioned her eight-year-old daughter and said, "She's my biggest help. She cleans the house when I don't have the time and looks after my other two kids." Her other children are a six-year-old son and a five-year-old daughter. Margaret sounded angry when she mentioned her son, saying, "He never listens to me." She added, "I don't know how much more of him I can take. Even spanking him with the belt doesn't make him behave."

The nurse noted that Margaret never mentioned her husband. So she said, "Tell me about your husband." Margaret averted her eyes and looked fearful. She whispered, "He's asleep now. He had a very bad night."

The nurse followed up by focusing on the husband's use of alcohol and specifically asked if her husband was the cause of her arm injury. Margaret answered that he had thrown her down the stairs when he was drunk. She added, "I know he didn't mean it. He's a wonderful husband and father when he isn't drunk. We just have to act better so he'll love us enough to stop drinking."

The nurse explained that his alcohol abuse was not a result of the behavior of Margaret and her children. She also emphasized that Margaret was going to have to have help if she was going to regain her physical health. She gave Margaret the name of a local priest whose parish supplied groceries to families in need. The nurse also gave Margaret the number of Parents Anonymous, adding, "If you feel like talking to some-one when you feel like exploding at your son, call this number any time, day or night." The nurse encouraged Margaret to consider attending Al-Anon meetings as soon as she felt better. The nurse also arranged for home visits three times a week for 2 weeks to help Margaret adapt to her new diet and medication regimen. Margaret tentatively agreed.

At the completion of the first visit, the nurse completed a family assessment and formulated the following list of priority nursing diagnoses:

- Lack of knowledge and financial resources related to following regimen for diabetes
- Ineffective family coping related to alcohol abuse
- Potential ineffective family coping related to wife and child abuse

When the nurse visited again the next morning, Margaret appeared calmer and more rested. She had given herself an injection and had eaten breakfast made with food donated by the local parish. Margaret explained that her husband had become very angry when the food had been delivered, had left the house, and had not returned. The nurse empathized with the difficulty of Margaret's situation and then emphasized that help was available. The nurse then began to formulate a plan of care for Margaret and her family as shown in Table 19-4.

TABLE 19-4   Nursing care plan for Margaret T. and her family

Assessment	Nursing diagnosis	Plan/intervention	Evaluation
Physical	Lack of knowledge and financial resources related to following diabetic regimen	Identify knowledge of self-care regarding diabetes mellitus; encourage call to welfare for help with food stamps and medical supplies.	Client will verbalize principles of self-care and will secure funds for needed food and supplies.
Behavioral patterns	Ineffective family coping related to alcohol abuse	Implement plan of secondary intervention as discussed above.	Family members will avoid use of alcohol.
Social system	Potential ineffective family coping related to wife and child abuse	Implement plan of secondary intervention as discussed above.	Family members will avoid use of violence to express feelings.

Chapter Highlights

- Families coping with multiple problems tend to experience conflict, disorganization, and severe levels of anxiety, and often perceive a crisis as an overwhelming burden. Other characteristics include a tendency to encourage dependency and learned helplessness and to be suspicious of outsiders.

- Behaviors observed within families coping with multiple stressors may include alcoholism, drug abuse, violence, hostility, overly rigid spiritual beliefs, and unrealistic expectations of other family members.

- The nurse must be aware of his or her own attitudes toward a family coping with multiple stressors and not let these attitudes affect the care given.

- Enmeshment is an interaction pattern in which sharing among family members is extreme and individuality is viewed negatively.

- Disengagement is a pattern in which family interactions seem unresponsive and unconnected.

- Scapegoating occurs when one family member is blamed for the family's problems.

- Enabling is behavior by one family member that encourages another family member to act in a dysfunctional manner.

- Stressors that affect a family may be intrafamily, interfamily, and extrafamily stressors.

- In a family coping with multiple stressors the flexible line of defense is not functioning effectively, which places constant pressure on the family's normal line of defense.

- The NANDA nursing diagnosis that describes families with a minimum level of wellness is altered family processes: addictive behavior.

- In formulating a care plan, the nurse should engage the family in care, capitalize on the strengths of the family system, empathize with the family's predicament, encourage realistic goal setting, allow all members to participate in discussions, and view all members as victims.

- The nurse uses primary, secondary, and tertiary prevention in implementing the plan of care.

 CRITICAL THINKING EXERCISE

A community health nurse receives a referral from a hospital discharge planner to visit an elderly gentleman with prostate cancer the day after he goes home. The referral calls for a dressing change and irrigation of a suprapubic tube. The nurse is let in by a 28-year-old son who has obviously been drinking. He directs the nurse to an upstairs bedroom that is very dirty and cluttered. The room has torn shades on the windows and no wallpaper on the walls. A dog can be heard barking in the next room. The elderly gentleman, who cannot get out of bed by himself, asks the nurse to get him some breakfast and change his wet sheets. The son remains downstairs and only responds when asked for clean bedding. The nurse, after taking care of the man's immediate needs, makes a diagnosis of ineffective family coping.

1. Write a short paragraph describing how you would feel about giving care to this family.
2. Describe and analyze the altered processes observed in this home.

REFERENCES

Blum, K. (1991). *Alcohol and the brain.* New York: Free Press.

Bohn, D., & Parker, B. (1993). Domestic violence and pregnancy—health effects and implications for nursing practice. In J. Campbell, & J. Humphreys (Eds.). *Nursing care of survivors of family violence* (pp. 156-172). St. Louis: Mosby.

Bruss, C. (1988). Nursing diagnosis of hopelessness. *Journal of Psychosocial Nursing, 26*(3), 28-31.

Campbell, D., & Campbell, J. (1993). Nursing care of families using violence. In J. Campbell, & J. Humphreys (Eds.). *Nursing care of survivors of family violence* (pp. 290-317). St. Louis: Mosby.

Campbell, J. (1992). A review of nursing research on battering. In C. Sampselle (Ed.). *Violence against women: Nursing research, education, and practice issues.* (pp. 69-81). New York: Hemisphere Publishing Corporation.

Campbell, J., & Fishwick, N. (1993). Abuse of female partners. In J. Campbell, & J. Humphreys (Eds.). *Nursing care of survivors of family violence* (pp. 68-104). St. Louis: Mosby.

Carson, R., Butcher, J., & Coleman, J. (1988). *Abnormal psychology and modern life.* Boston: Scott, Foresman & Co.

Feigenbaum, J. (1986). Utilizing the nursing process with patients who abuse alcohol and drugs. In M. Mathewson (Ed.). *Pharmacotherapeutics: A nursing process approach* (pp. 119-136). Philadelphia: Davis.

Fleischman, M., Home, A., & Arthur, J. (1983). *Troubled families: A treatment approach.* Champaign, IL: Research Press Co.

Flynn, J. (1977). Recent findings related to wife abuse. *Social Casework, 58,* 13-21.

Foley, T., & Grimes, B. (1987). Nursing intervention in family abuse and violence. In G. Stuart., & S. Sundeen (Eds.). *Principles and practices of psychiatric nursing* (pp. 925-970). St. Louis: Mosby.

Fulmer, T., & Cahill, V. (1984). Assessing elder abuse: A study. *Journal of Gerontological Nursing, 10*(12), 16-20.

Gelles, R., & Cornell, C. (1990). *Intimate violence in families.* Beverly Hills, CA.: Sage.

Hanrahan, P., Campbell, J., & Ulrich, Y. (1993). Theories of violence. In J. Campbell & J. Humphreys (Eds.). *Nursing care of survivors of family violence* (pp. 3-35). St. Louis: Mosby.

Hanson, J. (1984). The family. In C. Roy (Ed.). *Introduction to nursing: An adaptation model* (pp. 519-533). Englewood Cliffs, NJ: Prentice-Hall.

Hunka, C., O'Toole, A., & O'Toole, R. (1985). Self-help therapy in parents anonymous. *Journal of Psychosocial Nursing, 23*(7), 24-31.

Kelley, S. (1985). Interviewing the sexually abused child: principles and techniques. *Journal of Emergency Nursing, 11*(5), 234-241.

Kim, M., McFarland, G., & McLane, A. (1993). *Pocket guide to nursing diagnoses* (5th ed.). St. Louis: Mosby.

Limandri, B. (1987). The therapeutic relationship with abused women. *Journal of Psychosocial Nursing, 25*(2), 8-16.

Lynch, I., & Tiedje, L. (1991). Working with multiproblem families: An intervention model for community health nurses. *Public Health Nursing, 8*(3), 147-153.

McKinney, G. (1976). Adapting family therapy to multideficit families. In F. Turner (Ed.). *Differential diagnosis and therapy in social work* (pp. 109-118). New York: The Free Press.

Meister, S. (1984). Family well-being. In J. Campbell, & J. Humphreys (Eds.). *Nursing care of victims of family violence* (pp. 53-73). Reston, VA.: Reston.

Miller, J. (1983). Inspiring hope. In J. Miller (Ed.). *Coping with chronic illness: Overcoming powerlessness* (pp 287-299). Philadelphia: Davis.

Millor, G. (1981). A theoretical framework for nursing research in child abuse and neglect. *Nursing Research, 30*(2), 78-83.

Munro, J. (1993). The nurse and the legal system: Dealing with abused children. In J. Campbell & J. Humphreys (Eds.). *Nursing care of survivors of family violence* (pp. 343-358). St. Louis: Mosby.

Nelson, J. (1983). *Family therapy: An integrative approach.* Englewood Cliffs, NJ.: Prentice-Hall.

Neuman, B. (1983). Family intervention using the Betty Neuman health-care systems model. In I. Clements, & F. Roberts (Eds.). *Family Health: A theoretical approach to nursing care* (pp. 239-254). New York: Wiley.

Reed, K. (1993). Adapting the Neuman systems model for family nursing. *Nursing Science Quarterly, 6*(2), 93-97.

Rhodes, A. (1987). Identifying and reporting child abuse. *Maternal-Child Nursing Journal, 12*(6), 399.

Roberts, C., & Quillian, J. (1992). Preventing violence through primary care intervention. *Nurse Practitioner, 17*(8), 62-64, 67-70.

Shealy, A. (1988). Family therapy. In C. Beck, R. Rawlins, & S. Williams (Eds.). *Mental health-Psychiatric nursing* (pp. 543-575). St. Louis: Mosby.

Swift, C. (1986). Preventing family violence: Family-focused programs. In M. Lystad (Ed.). *Violence in the home: Interdisciplinary perspectives* (pp. 219-249). New York: Brunner/Mazel.

Tilden, V. (1989). Response of the health care delivery system to battered women. *Issues in Mental Health Nursing, 10,* 309-320.

Tripp-Reimer, T., & Lively, S. (1988). Cultural considerations in therapy. In C. Beck, R. Rawlins, & S. Williams (Eds.). *Mental health-Psychiatric nursing,* (p. 185). St. Louis: Mosby.

Van Hasselt, V., Morrison, R., Bellack, A., & Hersen, M. (1988). *Handbook of family violence.* New York: Plenum Press.

Weitzman, J. (1985). Engaging the severely dysfunctional family in treatment: Basic considerations. *Family Process, 24,* 473-485.

Wilson, H., & Kneisl, C. (1991). *Psychiatric nursing.* Menlo Park, CA.: Addison-Wesley.

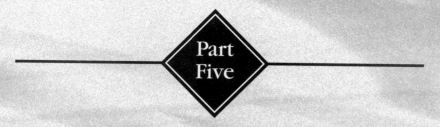

Caring for Clients at Risk

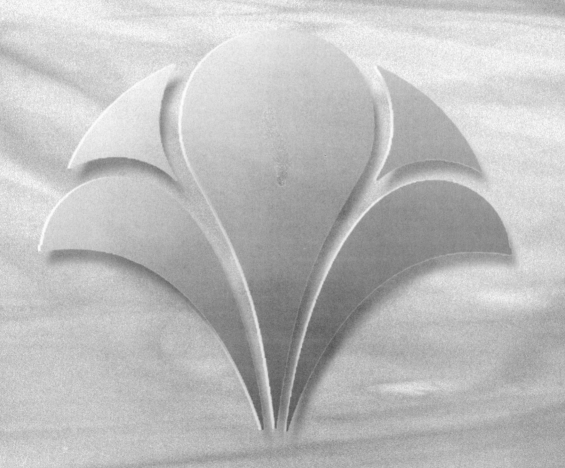

This part focuses on caring for clients at risk. Common communicable diseases are described in Chapter 20. The chain of transmission, clinical interventions, and methods of prevention are included. Viral hepatitis, HIV and AIDS, and drug resistant strains of tuberculosis are discussed. The reasons for the increase in the incidence of tuberculosis are analyzed.

Chapter 21 presents the concerns surrounding the care of a chronically ill person in the home and includes the effect that the illness may have on the family. Several concepts are discussed that may apply to a client or a family with a chronically ill member.

Chapter 22 deals with clients at risk because of developmental disabilities. Nursing concerns relative to this special aggregate are described.

Chapter 23 provides information about clients who are chemically dependent. Selected theories concerning the reasons for chemical dependency are presented.

Finally, Chapter 24 describes the special needs of selected high-risk aggregates. The homeless population, migrant workers, and refugees have been selected for discussion. The expanded role of the nurse as advocate is discussed.

20

CLIENTS WITH
COMMUNICABLE DISEASES

Joan M. Cookfair   ◆   John Flannery

The body's immune system can be thought of as flexible lines of resistance
that help a person to defend against a stressor.

Betty Neuman

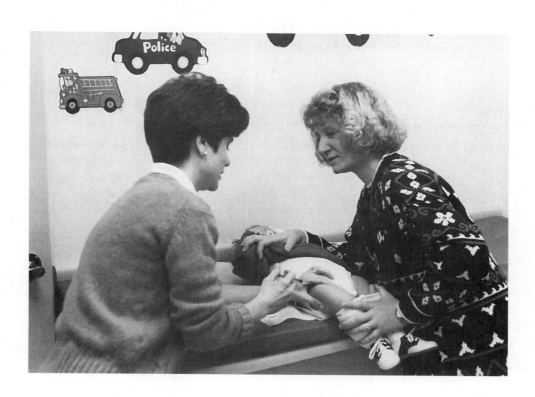

OBJECTIVES

At the conclusion of this chapter the student will be able to:

1. Define the key terms listed.
2. Understand the concept of communicability.
3. Describe relevant immunity in individuals and populations.
4. Discuss the impact of altered immunity on the incidence and prevalence of disease in individuals and populations.
5. Understand how surveillance is facilitated.
6. Identify and describe selected communicable diseases.
7. Understand some of the complex issues surrounding the nursing care of the client with HIV/AIDS.
8. Understand some of the complex issues surrounding the nursing care of the client with HIV/TB.
9. Apply the concepts of primary, secondary, and tertiary prevention to communicable disease.
10. Understand and apply the principles of infection control.

KEY TERMS

Acquired Immunodeficiency
   Syndrome (AIDS)
Anergy
Basic structure
Communicable disease
Contact investigation
Direct transmission
ELISA (enzyme linked
   immunosorbent assay)
Flexible lines of defense

Human immunodeficiency
   virus (HIV)
Immunity
Incubation period
Indirect transmission
Lines of resistance
Means of exit
Neuman systems model
Normal line of defense
Pathogen

Period of communicability
Portal of entry
Reservoir
Surveillance
Susceptible host
T-4 cells
Tuberculosis
Universal precautions
Western blot test

WHAT IS A COMMUNICABLE DISEASE?

A **communicable disease** is any disease that is transmitted from one person to another directly, by contact with excreta or other discharges from the body; or indirectly, via substances or inanimate objects, such as contaminated drinking glasses, toys, or water; or via vectors, such as flies, mosquitoes, ticks, or other insects (Glanz, Anderson, & Anderson, 1990). Most often the causative agent of disease is viral, bacterial, fungal, or protozoal.

MODE OF TRANSMISSION

The manner of transfer of a disease is called the mode of transmission. Transmission occurs from human being to human being or from animal to animal by direct contact through some portal of entry. For example, upper respiratory infections are spread by droplet infection from person to person. An infected person can pass it by such activities as sneezing, coughing, or even laughing. Gonorrhea, which is caused by a bacteria, is spread through contaminated body fluid, most often through the reproductive tract.

Indirect transmission of disease occurs when a disease is transferred via a vehicle (food or water), vector (insect), or through the air. Following are examples of communicable diseases that are transferred in one of these ways.

- Salmonella, is vehicle borne; it is transmitted by contaminated food or water.
- Rocky Mountain spotted fever, which is transmitted by fleas on grass or pets, is vector borne.
- An example of an airborne communicable disease is tuberculosis, which is transmitted by droplet air infection.

Before the advent of water purification, salmonella, the bacteria responsible for a number of gastrointestinal diseases including typhoid fever (*S. typhi*), was responsible for many deaths. The bacillus is excreted in the feces of infected persons and is spread by contaminated food (particularly shellfish) and water. Even before the identification of the causative agent, epidemics were stopped in England by the discovery of the mode of transmission and the subsequent water purification campaign (see Chapter 1). The disease still

surfaces today in areas where water becomes contaminated.

Most communicable diseases can be said to be transmitted by means of a chain of infection (Figure 20-1). There are six links in the chain, which are listed as follows:

1. The pathogen or infectious agent
2. The reservoir
3. The portal of exit from the reservoir
4. The mode of transmission
5. The portal of entry to the person
6. The susceptible host

The chain of infection is often used as a model to illustrate the series of events necessary for transmission. A break in any link in the chain can prevent infection from spreading.

The infectious agent, or **pathogen,** is the first link in the chain and is necessary for any transmission to occur.

A **reservoir,** which is a location where the agent can survive and perhaps multiply, is also necessary. People are the most common reservoirs. A person may be in the **incubation period,** which is the time between exposure to an agent and noticeable clinical symptoms (illness), and still be infectious. A person may also harbor an infectious agent and not become ill. This individual will possibly be a carrier reservoir. Food may be a reservoir for infectious agents. Water, damp or soiled linens, urine, blood, and feces

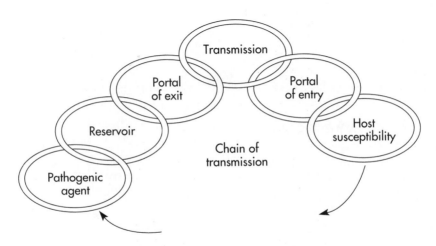

FIGURE 20-1 The chain of infection.

may also be reservoirs. All contaminated material, such as dressings, soiled linen, and so on, from people who are infected may be a possible reservoir.

A **means of exit** from the reservoir is the third link in the chain. Microorganisms leave people and inanimate objects through various routes. The mouth and the respiratory system are important routes for infectious agents to leave the body, as are blood and contaminated body fluids.

The mode of transmission is the fourth link. As discussed earlier, the transmission can occur in various ways; through direct contact; by air; by a vehicle, such as food and water; or by a vector.

Direct transmission occurs when a person touches another person in a way that will transmit an infection. Indirect contact can occur when an individual who is infected touches his mouth to an object, such as a cup, and transfers an infectious agent to the cup. Another person may touch the cup and contract that agent.

Vehicle-borne infection may be spread by a substance such as food, water, or dust. Particles containing infection may be ingested, inhaled, or administered parenterally. The research highlight below illustrates how water can be a vehicle to spread infection.

Vector-borne infection is transmitted by a so-called chain of transmission. Rickettsiae can be transmitted in this way. Figure 20-2 illustrates how the rickettsiae, which causes Rocky Mountain spotted fever, can be spread.

The **portal of entry** into a person is the fifth

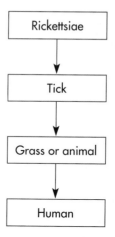

FIGURE 20-2   Chain of transmission of Rocky Mountain spotted fever.

link in the chain of infection. The same routes that allow escape from the body generally allow the entrance of infection.

The **susceptible host** is the last link in the chain. If the host is able to resist the pathogen when it enters the body, the infectious agent will be fought off by the host's immunosystem, and clinical symptoms will not occur. If the host's resistance is compromised, or if the pathogen is extremely virulent, the person is at risk for becoming ill. Nutritional status, hormonal balance, age, sex, and heredity all contribute to an individual's susceptibility. Frequently, susceptibility may be enhanced by the presence of another disease process.

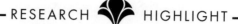

RESEARCH HIGHLIGHT

Water-Related Disease Outbreak, 1985

An outbreak of typhoid fever *(Salmonella typhi)* occurred after cross-contamination between parallel sewer lines during maintenance procedures in 1985. All cases were associated with the drinking of chlorinated but unfiltered water. This outbreak of water-borne typhoid fever was the first to be reported in the United States or its territories since 1974.

From "Water-related disease outbreaks" by the Centers for Disease Control, June 1988, *Morbidity and Mortality Weekly Report, 37,* 55-2, p. 16.

INCUBATION PERIOD

The time between exposure to a pathogenic organism and the onset of the symptoms of disease is called the incubation period (Glanz et al., 1990). The length of time that elapses is often influenced by an individual's immune system.

PERIOD OF COMMUNICABILITY

The **period of communicability** encompasses the time span during which contact with an infected person is most likely to result in the spread of infection (Glanz et al., 1990).

IMMUNITY

Immunity, or resistance to a particular disease or infection, can vary in an individual or in a population on a day-to-day basis, particularly in terms of resistance or lack of resistance to communicable diseases.

Two types of immunity are active and passive. Active immunity to a specific disease or infection may be heightened by the natural acquisition of antibodies as a result of a specific infection or by the acquisition of antibodies through immunization by injection with weakened or killed toxins. Passive immunity may be acquired naturally, passed from the mother to the fetus in utero. It also may be acquired by the injection of gamma globulin or antibodies to a specific disease. Passive immunity generally is long term.

An individual with active or passive immunity thus may respond adequately to prevent illness (clinical symptoms) if immunity is strong when an infection invades the body.

Immunity, however, is relative, and protection that had been adequate can be overcome by excessive strength of an infectious agent. It can also be diminished by (1) some forms of immunosuppressive chemotherapy; (2) infection that has weakened cellular immunity; or (3) the aging process. The client's inherent belief system, values, and culture can affect his or her level of immunity. For example, the Amish, who do not believe in artificial immunization, recently experienced an outbreak of polio in Pennsylvania. Areas close by the Amish community where children (and sometimes adults) had been immunized against the disease were not affected.

Immunity may be diminished in an individual by exposure to extreme heat or cold or a prolonged disease state. Excessive stress, whether psychologic, biologic, or physical, can reduce an individual's immunity (Beneson, 1985). The stressors may be internal or external.

A population's resistance to disease is affected by the level of immunity of the majority of the population, the environment in which the population lives, and in some measure, the socioeconomic level. It also may be affected by accessibility to health services. For example, teams of health professionals have vaccinated a sufficient number of people against smallpox (variola) so that since 1977, *no* cases have been reported anywhere in the world. Thus, the disease has ceased to exist in human reservoirs, and in 1980 the World Health Organization declared global immunity to smallpox (Beneson, 1985). This is not to say that everyone in the world has been vaccinated against smallpox; in fact, immunization is not recommended anymore. At this time, one reported case of smallpox anywhere in the world probably would result in massive immunizations on a global scale.

Application of Betty Neuman's Systems Model to the Concept of Immunity

The **Neuman systems model** can be used to visualize the dynamics of relative immunity. Figure 20-3 depicts the model. The **flexible lines of defense** are represented by the outer broken lines of the model. They form the outer boundary or the external influence on an individual or population group. According to Neuman, each line of defense contains similar elements related to five variables: physiologic, psychologic, developmental, sociocultural, and spiritual. Ideally the flexible lines of defense protect the client from stressor invasions. They are relative and can vary in individuals and populations depending on factors previously mentioned. Climate, developmental stage, socioeconomic group, culture, exposure to infection, accessibility to health care, level of air pollution, and effective public health services are some of the variables.

The **normal line of defense** is depicted by the solid larger circle in the model. It represents the individual's or the population's usual well-

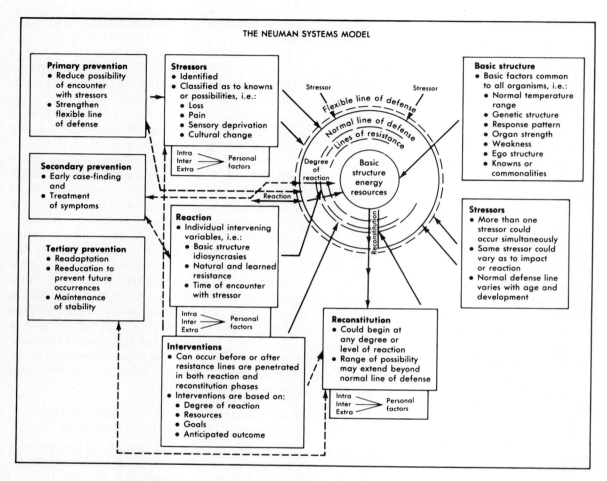

FIGURE 20-3　The Neuman Systems Model. *(Courtesy Betty Neuman, PhD.)*

ness state. If a stressor breaks through the normal state, lines of resistance are activated. The normal line of defense is influenced by coping patterns, lifestyle factors, developmental and spiritual influences, and culture. The normal line of defense, or usual wellness state, can remain the same, become reduced, or expand after treatment of a stressor reaction (Neuman, 1989).

The **lines of resistance,** shown by the inner broken concentric circles around the basic structure are constantly changing. They represent known and unknown factors internal to the individual or group that become activated upon the invasion of a stressor. An example of an individual's line of resistance is the body's mobilization

of white blood cells or immune system mechanisms upon the invasion of a biologic stressor. In a community, on the other hand, local, state, and federal agencies would mobilize to combat a biologic stressor that threatened to turn into an epidemic.

The **basic structure,** represented by the small inner circle, consists of survival factors common to the individual or population that preserve the basic integrity of the system; for example, innate genetic factors, strengths and weaknesses of system parts, and basic energy resources. Stressors that penetrate this inner circle can cause severe illness or death both in an individual and within the community.

SURVEILLANCE

Surveillance, or monitoring, of the incidence and prevalence of communicable diseases through accurate record keeping and data collection can alert health professionals to the possibility of dangerous outbreaks of disease in populations. Local health departments and private physicians report communicable diseases to the State Health Department, which sends information to the Centers for Disease Control in the United States. In Canada, regional health departments and physicians report to the province and then to the Laboratory Center for Disease Control. Ultimately, most countries report the occurrence of infectious disease to the World Health Organization (WHO). This is the method whereby WHO has estimated that there are approximately 2.5 million cases of AIDS worldwide. (See section on HIV/AIDS.)

PRIMARY PREVENTION

Illness caused by a specific infective agent or its toxic products can cause much suffering and sometimes death. Community health nurses need a firm knowledge of the agent, the mode of transmission, the incubation period, and the period of communicability of each disease. They also need to know the clinical symptoms and the appropriate nursing interventions to prevent the disease, if possible, and to plan secondary and tertiary care if it occurs. Many common communicable diseases are listed in Table 20-1. The table includes the name of the disease, the causative agent, the mode of transmission, the incubation period, the period of communicability, the clinical symptoms, the nursing interventions, and the best method of prevention known at this time.

Preventing occurrence of a disease through active immunization is one method of primary prevention. The American Academy of Pediatrics has recommended a schedule of immunizations for infants and children (see Chapter 13). It is recommended that adults receive boosters of the measles vaccine and polio vaccine before international travel. Tetanus and diphtheria toxoids should be given routinely as boosters every 10 years. Table 20-2 depicts dosing schedules for individuals who are traveling to areas where the diseases the immunizations protect against may exist.

SECONDARY PREVENTION

Preventing the manifestation of clinical symptoms by screening for the presence of an agent may enable the nurse to plan interventions before a client becomes ill. For example, frequency of tuberculin testing depends on the client's risk of exposure and on the prevalence of tuberculosis in a population group. A positive purified protein derivative test can indicate the presence of the bacillus. Chemotherapy may be started before the client becomes clinically symptomatic.

TERTIARY PREVENTION

The prevention of disability after illness has become evident can be accomplished by appropriate nursing intervention. A gonorrheal infection can cause pelvic inflammatory disease, which can lead to sterility in a woman. Appropriate administration of antibiotics to stop the spread of the infection can prevent the occurrence of both events.

PROBLEMATIC COMMUNICABLE DISEASES

Modern research, antibiotics, and adequate public sanitation have eliminated, or brought under control, many communicable diseases. This has been especially true in developed countries. A mobile world population and social conditions have caused some infectious diseases to resurface; for example, hepatitis and tuberculosis. In addition, HIV/AIDS another infectious process, has become a threat to mankind worldwide.

Hepatitis

Hepatitis, or inflammation of the liver, is most often caused by viral infection. A vaccine is available to protect children and adults from acquiring hepatitis B. Hepatitis B is discussed later in the chapter. Hepatitis D cannot cause inflammation unless B is present. Hepatitis C is transmitted by blood and body fluids, but is a fairly mild disease. There is no long-term prevention available universally for hepatitis A and E at this time (Smith, 1993). Therefore, these two forms are preventable only by education of the public and intervention to establish adequate public sanita-

Text continued on p. 451.

TABLE 20-1 Common communicable diseases

Disease	Agent	Mode of transmission	Incubation period	Period of communicability	Clinical symptoms	Nursing intervention	Prevention
Escherichia coli 0157 H 7	Bacteria	Fecal, oral	Hours	n/a	Severe diarrhea, destruction of red cells, kidney failure	Symptomatic	Avoid undercooked beef or hamburger and raw, unpasteurized milk; good hand-washing
Diphtheria	Bacteria	Direct contact or articles soiled from lesions	2-5 days	2-4 weeks	Lesions of tonsils, pharynx, and nose; serious in infants. High mortality rate in children under 2 years of age	Symptomatic; possible tracheostomy care; monitor carefully	Immunization
Fifth disease *Erythema infectiosum*	Unknown	Unknown	5-10 days	Unknown	Mild fever, erythema over face, generalized maculopapular rash	Acetaminophen for fever, fluids; treatment of symptoms	None
Influenza	Viral	Droplet infection	1-3 days	Directly before, during	Sore throat, cough, fever, muscle pain, weakness	Symptomatic bed rest, aspirin & fluids	Yearly immunization
Impetigo	Contact with lesions			During infection	Vesicles, lesions	Antibacterial soap, antibiotics	Use of individual linens, hand-washing
Lyme disease	Spirochete	Vector borne	3 days to 3 weeks	n/a	History of tick bite (*erythema chronium migrans* (ECM) followed by arthritic, cardiac, and neurologic symptoms	Symptomatic	Spray infected grassy areas, wear protective clothing, daily inspection of household pets

TABLE 20-1 Common communicable diseases cont'd

Disease	Agent	Mode of transmission	Incubation period	Period of communicability	Clinical symptoms	Nursing intervention	Prevention
Mumps	Viral	Droplet infection	18 days	48 hours before swelling occurs	Mild fever, swelling of one or more salivary glands	Acetaminophen for fever, soft foods, liquids, limited activity, isolation	Immunization
Poliomyelitis	Viral	Direct contact (fecal/oral)	3-35 days	36 hours before symptoms, 72 hours after	Fever, headache, stiffness of neck, paralysis of muscles of neck and swallowing. Sometimes minor, sometimes fatal; may cause paralysis	Treat symptoms as they occur; appropriate isolation techniques	Immunization
Rocky Mountain spotted fever	Rickettsiae	Vector-borne ticks	3-12 days	n/a	High fever, rash, neurologic symptoms	Acetaminophen for fever, antibiotics, symptomatic	Spray infected grassy areas, wear protective clothing, daily inspection of household pets
Rubella (German measles)	Viral	Droplet infection; crosses placental barrier	16-18 days	1 week before & 4 days after onset of rash. Infants who have congenital rubella shed virus for months after birth	Low-grade fever, headache, coryza, conjunctivitis, macular rash in some cases. Teratogenic effects in congenital rubella to the fetus in utero	Limited activity, acetaminophen for fever; fluids. Keep away from pregnant women	Immunization, immunoglobulin (Ig) serum to pregnant women exposed to rubella

Continued

TABLE 20-1   Common communicable diseases   cont'd

Disease	Agent	Mode of transmission	Incubation period	Period of communicability	Clinical symptoms	Nursing intervention	Prevention
Rubeola (red measles)	Viral	Droplet infection	8-13 days	Just before symptoms appear and about 4 days after the rash is gone	High fever, hacking cough, conjunctivitis, irregular red lesions (Koplik's spots) with blue-white centers in mucous membranes of mouth, red maculopapular rash, generalized malaise	Limited activity, acetaminophen for fever, cough syrup if needed. Protect eyes from light; soft foods, push fluids. Monitor carefully; isolation	Immunization
Scabies	Mite	Skin-to-skin, undergarments, soiled bed clothes	2-6 weeks	Until treated	Tiny linear patches on skin that itch	Lindane (Kwell)	None
Scarlet fever	Streptococci	Direct or indirect	1-3 days	10-21 days	Fever, skin rash, strawberry tongue	Acetaminophen for fever, rest, antibiotics, soft foods, fluids	Limit spread of infection
Shigellosis	Bacillus	Fecal, oral transmission; contaminated food	1-3 days	During acute infection and sometime after	Severe diarrhea; often afebrile	Nonirritating diet, Kaopectate, similar medications	Avoid contaminated water/food
Streptococcal sore throat	Streptococci	Direct or indirect through objects or hands	1-3 days	10-21 days	Fever, sore throat, enlarged cervical lymph nodes	Acetaminophen for fever, pain; fluids, limited activity, antibiotics	None
Tetanus	Bacillus	Spores in soil, street dust, lacerations and burns	4-21 days	None	Painful muscular contractions of neck and trunk muscles; may be fatal	Symptomatic	Immunization

TABLE 20-1 Common communicable diseases · cont'd

Disease	Agent	Mode of transmission	Incubation period	Period of communicability	Clinical symptoms	Nursing intervention	Prevention
Tinea capitis (ringworm)	Fungus	Direct or indirect contact	10-14 days	As long as lesions are present	Scaly patches and papules that spread; may itch, may cause baldness	Lindane (Kwell); advise to wash all contaminated clothing	None
Varicella (chicken pox)	Viral	Droplet infection	2-3 weeks	1-2 days before rash, 6 days after appearance of vesicles	Slight fever, vesicular skin eruption	Acetaminophen for fever, limited activity, soft foods, fluids, baking soda baths	None
Venereal: Chlamydia	Trachoma	Sexually transmitted	Unknown	Unknown	Urethritis, pelvic inflammatory disease	Medications as ordered, comfort measures	None
Gonorrhea	Gonococcus	Sexually transmitted	2-7 days	Until treated	Purulent discharge	Antibodies	Education
Hepatitis A	Viral	Fecal, oral	2-6 weeks	While ill	Loss of appetite, fatigue, jaundice	Isolation of towels and dishes; separate toilet and bed; good hand-washing; sterilize dishes; treat patient symptoms	Eliminate possibility of contamination
Hepatitis B	Viral	Blood borne	45-180 days	While ill; leads to carrier state	Loss of appetite, fatigue, jaundice	Use universal precautions; treat patient symptoms	Hepatitis vaccine
Herpes	Viral	Intimate contact	2-12 days	When lesions are weeping	Painful, weepy vesicles in infected area	Burrow's soaks, keep dry and clean	Education
HIV	Viral	Blood borne	Average 4 years to active disease	Lifetime	Fatigue, various opportunistic infections	Monitor medical regime, use universal precautions	Education
Syphilis	Treponema pallidum	Sexually transmitted	3 weeks	Unless treated 2-4 years	Primary lesion, rash, systemic effect	Antibodies	Education

TABLE 20-2 Dosing schedules for travel immunizations

Vaccine	Primary series	Booster interval
Cholera	Two doses 1 week or more apart (0.5 ml SC or IM); (pediatric dose 0.3 ml for 5-10 yrs of age, 0.2 ml for 6 mos-4 yrs of age)	6 mos
Immune globulin (hepatitis A protection)	One dose IM in the gluteus muscle (2 ml dose for 3 mo protection; 5 ml divided dose for 5 mos); pediatric dose 0.02 ml/kg for 3-mo trip; 0.06 ml/kg for 5-mo trip)	Boost at 3- to 5-mo intervals depending on initial dose received
Japanese encephalitis (JEV) (Japanese manufacture, Biken Brand)	Three doses given 1 week apart (1 ml SC ≥ 3 yrs old; 0.5 ml SC < 3 yrs old)	One dose at 12-18 mos, then at 4-yr intervals
Meningococcus (A/C/Y/W-127)†	One dose* SC	None. (Variable immunogenic response in children < 4 yrs; revaccination for this group recommended after 2-3 yrs who continue to be at high risk)
Plague	First dose (1 ml IM); second dose (0.2 ml IM) 4 wks later; dose 3 (0.2 ml IM) 3-6 mos after dose 2	Boost if the risk of exposure persists: give the first 2 booster doses (0.1-0.2 ml) 6 mos apart; then give 1 booster dose at 1-2 yr intervals as needed
Rabies, human diploid cell vaccine (HDCV)	Three doses (0.1 ml ID) on days 0, 7, and 21 or 28	Boost after 2 yrs or test serum for antibody level. Must not use chloroquine prophylaxis until 3 wks after completion of vaccine series
Rabies (HDCV) or rabies vaccine absorbed (RVA)	Three doses (1 ml IM in the deltoid area) on days 0, 7, and 28	Boost after 2 yrs or test serum for antibody level
Tickborne encephalitis	Three doses, given subcutaneously on days 0, 30, and 180	Boost at 3- to 5-yr intervals
Tuberculosis (BCG vaccine)†	One dose percutaneously with multiple-puncture disc; ½ strength for infants < 1 mo old	Revaccination after 2-3 mo in those who remain tuberculin neg to 5 TU skin test
Typhoid, injectable	Two doses (0.5 ml SC or IC) 4 or more wks apart; pediatric dose (< 10 yrs old) 0.25 ml	Boost after 3 yrs for continued risk of exposure
Typhoid, injectable (not acetone-killed and dried vaccine)		Boost with 0.1 ml ID every 3 yrs
Typhoid oral (Ty21A)	One capsule PO every 2 days for four doses (> 6 yrs old)	5 yrs
Yellow fever†	One dose (0.5 ml SC); pediatric dose 0.5 ml SC for > 6 mos old	10 yrs

SC, subcutaneous; IM, intramuscular; ID, intradermal; PO, by mouth

* See manufacturer's package insert for recommendations on dosage.

† Caution, may be contraindicated in patients with any of the following conditions: pregnancy, leukemia, lymphoma, generalized malignancy, immunosuppression caused by HIV infection or treatment with corticosteroids, alkylating drugs, antimetabolites, or radiation therapy.

Information from "Immunizations for international travelers" by E.C. Jong, 1991. In *The Travel Medicine Advisor* by E.C. Jong, J.S. Keystone, R. McMullen (Eds.), Atlanta: American Health Consultants. Adapted by permission.

tion, particularly for sewage disposal plants and public water supply.

Mode of transmission. Hepatitis A and E are commonly spread by the fecal/oral route. Poor handwashing techniques, close contact with an infected person, and consumption of contaminated food or water can all lead to the transmission of infection.

Incubation period. Two to six weeks.

Period of communicability. During the course of the disease.

Clinical symptoms. Children may complain of diarrhea and be asymptomatic. Any child who has jaundice should be screened for hepatitis. Adults will complain of fever, anorexia, nausea, and vomiting, all of which will be followed by dark urine and jaundice.

Nursing intervention. Hepatitis is treated symptomatically. Close contacts, and individuals traveling to countries where poor sanitation exists, should be encouraged to get an injection of serum immunoglobin, which will protect them for a few months. In the United Kingdom, a vaccine has been developed that gives protection against hepatitis A. When it becomes available the general population should be encouraged to seek it out (Jacobs, 1993). A vaccine is available for protection against hepatitis B.

Prevention. Nurses should encourage adequate public sanitation, teach good handwashing techniques, and encourage individuals exposed to hepatitis A, or those traveling to underdeveloped countries, to get human immunoglobin injections before clinical symptoms appear. The individual will acquire temporary passive artificial immunity. Universal precautions should be used to prevent the spread of hepatitis B. Hepatitis vaccine should be encouraged.

HIV/AIDS

Acquired immunodeficiency syndrome (AIDS) was first reported in the literature in 1981. It was at this time that there was an alarming increase in the incidence of *pneumocystis carinii pneumonia*. Further study revealed that many of those who were diagnosed with this virulent form of pneumonia were young homosexual men who were found to have significantly

impaired immune systems. In addition, the increased incidence of Kaposi's sarcoma among these young men was most unusual given that this rare form of cancer was found most frequently in older men. The Kaposi's sarcoma that affected these men was much more aggressive than that which affected older men, and therefore was of particular concern.

It was in 1982 that the Centers for Disease Control and Prevention (CDC) in the United States established the term AIDS. **Human immunodeficiency virus (HIV)** was later found to be the causative agent of HIV disease including AIDS.

Epidemiology. Although most of those who were diagnosed with AIDS in the early 1980s were gay men, this newly identified epidemic was affecting other populations, including injection-drug users, hemophiliacs, and blood transfusion recipients. As the epidemic has spread and is better understood, it is clear that AIDS has affected all segments of society, both in North America and worldwide.

As of March 31, 1993, there were 289,320 persons diagnosed with AIDS in the United States (CDC, 1993). Of this total, 252,363 of the reported cases were male, and 32,477 were female. The remaining 4480 cases were children under 13 years of age. Of the total number of diagnosed AIDS cases in 1993, 182,275 persons have died. It is estimated that there are over one million persons in the United States who are infected with HIV. In Canada, there were 7770 reported cases of AIDS as of April, 1993 (Laboratory Center for Disease Control, 1993a). Of these, 7285 were men, 406 were women, and there were 79 pediatric AIDS cases reported.

Globally, the World Health Organization (WHO) reported a cumulative total of 611,589 AIDS cases as of December, 1992 (WHO, 1993). For a number of reasons, including delays in reporting, WHO believes that the number of reported AIDS cases does not reflect the actual number of cases. WHO has estimated that there are approximately 2.5 million AIDS cases worldwide, and that there are as many as 13 million men, women, and children infected with HIV. Although there are many more men than women who are infected with HIV in North America, the picture worldwide is much different. In sub-Saharan Africa, the infection rate between men and women is proportionately equal, with one in 40 men and one in 40 women estimated to be infected with HIV. Because many women infected with HIV in any country are at childbearing age, transmission of mother to fetus or infant has become an important public health concern because more children are infected with HIV before, during, or after child birth than at any other time or by any other means.

Mode of transmission. HIV is found predominantly in the blood, semen, and vaginal secretions of an infected person (CDC, 1993b). Although HIV has been isolated in tears, saliva, amniotic fluid, and cerebrospinal fluid, these fluids have not been implicated in the transmission of HIV (CDC, 1987). HIV has also been isolated in breast milk, although it is not clear whether HIV-infected mothers can transmit the virus to their children through breast feeding (CDC, 1993b).

Given the poor prognosis for those diagnosed with AIDS, the issue of transmission has been a subject of intense concern, which in some cases borders on hysteria. The fact is, with our present understanding of HIV and AIDS, transmission of HIV is, for the most part, preventable. There are specific behaviors that one must engage in, or conditions that must be present, that put individuals at risk for contracting HIV. These include the following:

- Sexual intercourse (vaginal or anal) with an infected partner. (Exposure to infected semen through artificial insemination can also transmit HIV.)
- Sharing needles contaminated with HIV
- Receiving a transfusion of HIV-infected blood or contacting infected blood through organ transplant
- Perinatal transmission
- Significant exposure to body fluids of an HIV-infected person

Of these, sexual transmission is the predominant means of transmission. In North America, most reported AIDS cases have been found to be men who have sex with men, although the CDC reports that AIDS among heterosexuals has increased by 21% between 1990 and 1991 (CDC, 1993a). Table 20-3 identifies the category, or means, of exposure for all reported AIDS cases in the United States. The practice of sharing contaminated needles when injecting drugs is also an effective means of transmitting HIV. It is important to note, however, that HIV is not gender- or lifestyle-specific. More accurately, HIV is transmitted through various behaviors that might put one at greater risk for contracting the virus. This fact has important implications for nurses in terms of primary prevention with respect to transmission of HIV. Educational programs must focus on reducing or eliminating behaviors that put individuals at risk. Strategies to reduce the

TABLE 20-3 The number of AIDS cases in the United States reported by category to CDC through March 31, 1993

Category	No. male	No. female	No. children	Total
Men who have sex with men	160,345	n/a	n/a	160,345
Injecting-drug use	49,962	15,816	n/a	65,778
Men who have sex with men and inject drugs	18,041	n/a	n/a	18,041
Hemophilia/coagulation disorder	2,460	59	194	2,713
Heterosexual cases	7,540	11,638	n/a	19,178
Receipt of blood transfusion, blood components, or tissue	3,280	2,104	315	5,699
Other/undetermined	10,735	2,860	84	13,679
Mother with or at risk for HIV infection	n/a	n/a	3,887	3,887

possibility of transmission of HIV, including promotion of safer sex techniques and needle exchange programs, have been found to greatly reduce the transmission of HIV.

In addition to specific behaviors that might put one at greater risk of contracting HIV, there are other important means of transmission. The contact with blood and blood products have been found to be an effective means of transmission of HIV. Before the availability of HIV testing in 1985, individuals who received transfusion of blood or blood products were at a greater risk of contracting HIV. In the United States, as of March 31, 1993, persons with hemophilia and recipients of blood transfusions accounted for 8412 of all reported cases of HIV. The incidence of HIV transmission as a result of receiving a transfusion of blood or blood products has been virtually eliminated in Canada and the United States since the routine testing of donated blood for HIV was implemented in 1985.

Perinatal transmission has also been implicated in the transmission of HIV. The World Health Organization estimates that approximately 30% of infants born to mothers who are HIV positive will become HIV positive themselves (WHO, 1992). The detection of HIV infection in infants is complicated because of maternally acquired antibodies to HIV, which may or may not indicate the presence of HIV infection in the newborn. As a result, newborns of HIV-positive mothers must be monitored closely over time to determine their HIV status.

Another important consideration in the transmission of HIV is that of a significant exposure to the body fluids of an HIV-infected person. This is particularly important for nurses and other health care workers who may be at risk for occupational exposure to blood and other body fluids in the course of their work. The CDC reports that 32 health care workers in the United States have seroconverted to an HIV-positive status following occupational exposure to the blood or body fluids of an HIV-infected individual. The most common kind of occupational exposure involved needlestick injuries. Gerberding (1988) reported that the risk of transmission of HIV following a percutaneous exposure is less that 1.0%.

It is believed that the risk of transmission of HIV following skin or mucous membrane exposure to HIV-infected blood is somewhat less than percutaneous exposure. Despite the relatively low risk of transmission of HIV as a result of exposure to blood and body fluids of an HIV-infected individual, it is crucial that nurses and other health care workers take appropriate precautions to reduce the possibility of occupational exposure. Of course, the transmission of HIV is only one important consideration in the prevention of transmission of a communicable illness. Exposure to and transmission of hepatitis B, salmonellosis, and other communicable diseases pose potential occupational risks to nurses.

Universal precautions. Nurses and other health care providers have been forced to reexamine their approach to common infection control practices in efforts to reduce the risk of transmission of HIV to health care workers, or conversely, from health care worker to client. Because most individuals who are infected with HIV are initially asymptomatic and in fact may not know their HIV status, it is imperative that all individuals be approached as though they may potentially be infected with HIV, hepatitis B (HBV), or other potential communicable diseases transmitted through blood or other body fluids. Applying a universal approach to the handling of body substances for all clients eliminates the need to know an individual's HIV status to reduce the risk of HIV transmission. It also prevents the use of inappropriate precautions solely based on a person's lifestyle or sexual orientation. The CDC (1987) recommends the adoption of **universal precautions** (see box on page 454) as a means to prevent the transmission of HIV, HBV, and other blood-borne pathogens. In adopting universal precautions, there are important underlying principles that are useful in clinical practice. First and foremost, precautions are universally applied to all individuals when handling blood and other body fluids. Second, precautions are action driven versus diagnosis driven. This means that precautions are implemented based on the activity that the nurse will be engaged in rather than implementing precautions only when a definitive medical diagnosis is

UNIVERSAL PRECAUTIONS

Because medical history and examination cannot reliably identify all clients infected with HIV, HBV, or other blood-borne pathogens, blood and body-fluid precautions should be used consistently for all clients. This approach previously recommended by CDC, referred to as universal blood and body-fluid precautions or universal precautions, should be used in the care of all clients.

1. All health care workers should routinely use appropriate barrier precautions to prevent skin and mucous membrane exposure when contact with blood or other body fluids of any patient is anticipated. Gloves should be worn for touching blood and body fluids, mucous membranes, or nonintact skin of all patients, for handling items or surfaces soiled with blood or body fluids, and for performing venipuncture and other vascular access procedures. Gloves should be changed after contact with each patient. Masks and protective eyewear or face shields should be worn during procedures that are likely to generate droplets of blood or other body fluids to prevent exposure of mucous membranes of the mouth, nose, and eyes. Gowns or aprons should be worn during procedures that are likely to generate splashes of blood or other body fluids.

2. Hands and other skin surfaces should be washed immediately and thoroughly if contaminated with blood or other body fluids. Hands should be washed immediately after gloves are removed.

3. All health care workers should take precautions to prevent injuries caused by needles, scalpels, and other sharp instruments or devices during procedures; when cleaning used instruments; during disposal of used needles; and when handling sharp instruments after procedures. To prevent needlestick injuries, needles should not be recapped, purposely bent or broken by hand, removed from disposable syringes, or otherwise manipulated by hand. After they are used, disposable syringes and needles, scalpel blades, and other sharp items should be placed in puncture-resistant containers for disposal; the puncture-resistant containers should be located as close as practical to the use area. Large-bore reusable needles should be placed in a puncture-resistant container for transport to the reprocessing area.

4. Although saliva has not been implicated in HIV transmission, to minimize the need for emergency mouth-to-mouth resuscitation, mouthpieces, resuscitation bags, or other ventilation devices should be available for use in areas in which the need for resuscitation is predictable.

5. Health care workers who have exudative lesions or weeping dermatitis should refrain from all direct patient care and from handling patient-care equipment until the condition resolves.

6. Pregnant health care workers are not known to be at greater risk of contracting HIV infection than health care workers who are not pregnant; however, if a health care worker develops HIV infection during pregnancy, the infant is at risk of infection resulting from perinatal transmission. Because of this risk, pregnant health care workers should be especially familiar with and strictly adhere to precautions to minimize the risk of HIV transmission.

Implementation of universal blood and body fluid precautions for all patients eliminates the need for use of the isolation category of "Blood and Body Fluid Precautions" previously recommended by the CDC for patients known or suspected to be infected with blood-borne pathogens. Isolation precautions (e.g., enteric and "acid fast bacillus") should be used as necessary if associated conditions, such as infectious diarrhea or tuberculosis, are diagnosed or suspected.

Modified from "Recommendations for prevention of HIV transmission in health care settings" by the Centers for Disease Control, 1987, *MMWR, Morbidity and Mortality Weekly Report, 36* (Suppl 25[35-185]).

known. The key to implementing universal precautions is based on the nurse using his or her judgement about the likelihood of exposure to blood or other body fluids and then determining which barriers are most appropriate, if any. Another important factor bears repeating. Percutaneous exposure to HIV and HBV poses the most significant risk to nurses and other health care providers in an occupational setting (Gerberding, 1988). Thus, the special handling of needles postinjection is crucial in preventing the transmission of HIV and other blood-borne pathogens.

Pathology. In 1983, teams of researchers in France and the United States identified the causative agent of AIDS. The virus was referred to as the human T-cell lymphotropic virus, type III (HTLV-III) (Gallo, et al., 1983), and lymphadenopathy-associated virus (LAV) (Barre-Sinoussi, et al., 1983). In 1986, an international committee on taxonomy of viruses agreed that the causative agent of AIDS would be called the human immunodeficiency virus, or HIV (Coffin, et al., 1986). In 1986, a subtype of HIV was identified which has been referred to as HIV-2 (Clavel, et al., 1986). This new strain of HIV was found to be prevalent in Western Africa, parts of Europe, and recently in the United States. Subsequently, the routine testing of blood and blood products for the presence of HIV-2 antibodies was initiated.

The devastating effects of HIV come from its affinity for certain types of cells, including T-4 helper lymphocytes, bowel epithelium, and brain cells, among others (Levy, 1988). Of particular importance is the infection of T-4 helper lymphocytes **(T-4 cells)** with HIV. T-4 cells are crucial in coordinating the body's overall immune response. HIV, a retrovirus, infects T-4 cells and integrates with the host cells' DNA by using the enzyme known as reverse transcriptase. HIV may remain dormant for several months or years until it is activated to produce more virus, thus ultimately killing the host cell and infecting others. The factors or mechanisms that trigger activation are not clearly understood. The severe depletion of T-4 cells results in the range of opportunistic infections and other illnesses characteristic of AIDS. The lengthy dormant period between initial infection with HIV and the onset of symptoms associated with T-4 cell depletion holds important implications for nurses in terms of secondary prevention. Interventions geared toward health promotion that include diet, stress management, health monitoring, and other important health strategies may be instrumental in prolonging the latency of the virus and the health of the client.

HIV testing. The routine screening for antibodies to HIV began in 1985. The two tests which are used to screen for antibodies to HIV include the enzyme-linked immunosorbent assay (ELISA) and the Western Blot. **ELISA** is used for the initial screening for HIV antibodies. A positive ELISA is always followed with a confirmatory **Western Blot test.** A negative ELISA may mean one of two things. It may indeed indicate that the person or blood being screened has not been exposed to or infected with HIV. It may also mean that the person has been infected with HIV but has not, at the time of testing, developed antibodies to HIV. The period between infection with HIV and the development of antibodies (seroconversion) is often referred to as the window period. This window period, in which a person is infected with HIV but has a negative HIV test, can last anywhere from 3 to 6 months on average (Chateauvert, Duffie, & Gilmore, 1990). Again, this has important implications for the nurse or health care provider who counsels an individual undergoing testing for HIV antibodies. For clients who believe that they may have been exposed to HIV through risk behaviors or other conditions, it is prudent for the nurse to advise the client to modify risk behaviors to avoid further exposure and to prevent the possibility of transmission to others. It is also recommended that periodic testing be conducted to confirm test results.

Spectrum of HIV disease. Over the natural history of HIV disease, we have come to know a tremendous amount about the course of the illness, and HIV infection, including AIDS, is now viewed as a chronic illness. The CDC developed a classification system for HIV infection in 1986 that was subsequently revised in January, 1993. Table 20-4 provides a summary of the CDC classification system.

The 1993 revision of the HIV classification system was significant because it expanded the criteria necessary for an AIDS diagnosis (see Table 20-5). The criteria were expanded to include the following:

1. A CD4+ T-lymphocyte (T-4 cell) count of less than 200.
2. Pulmonary tuberculosis
3. Recurrent pneumonia
4. Invasive cervical cancer

TABLE 20-4 Centers for disease control classification system for HIV infection

Group I	Acute infection
Group II	Asymptomatic infection
Group III	Persistent generalized lymphadenopathy
Group IV	Other diseases
	Subgroup A: Constitutional disease
	Subgroup B: Neurologic disease
	Subgroup C: Secondary infectious disease
	Category C-1: Diseases as specified in CDC surveillance definition for AIDS.
	Category C-2: Other specified infectious diseases
	Subgroup D: Secondary centers
	Subgroup E: Other conditions

The presence of these four conditions is important because it provides for more accurate diagnostic criteria and opportunities for health care follow-up. The addition of T-4 cell counts is significant because it represents the current trend in medical care and treatment of persons with HIV disease. T-4 counts are used as an important prognostic indicator for persons with HIV infection.

Treatment of HIV. Although HIV/AIDS has been recognized for only a short period, relative to other communicable diseases, tremendous strides in treatment have occurred. In the ab-sence of an effective vaccine against HIV infection, the main thrust of treatment is two-fold: (1) antiviral therapy; and (2) treatment of secondary infections and diseases associated with a compromised immune system.

The use of antiviral therapy including Zidovudine (AZT) has proven successful in prolonging the lives of persons infected with HIV (Williams, Mindel, & Weller, 1989). There are, however, side effects associated with the use of AZT, including nausea and vomiting, anemia, and myelopathy. The initiation of AZT therapy and other antivirals is often based on T-4 cell counts of less than 500/cubic millimeter (Mansell, 1992). In addition to antiviral therapy, there are numerous other chemotherapeutics and treatments for HIV-related conditions.

In conjunction with and complementary to the medical treatment of HIV, nursing interventions and care in the management of HIV-related conditions is crucial to the alleviation of symptoms experienced by many persons living with HIV/AIDS. Table 20-6 provides a summary of common nursing diagnoses (North American Nursing Diagnosis Association, 1988) that are prevalent in the provision of nursing care for these persons.

Many opportunistic infections affect the gastrointestinal tract. Adding to this problem are many of the drugs used to combat the opportunistic infections (see Table 20-7). Care plans for altered nutrition and alteration in elimination follow.

TABLE 20-5 1993 revised classification system for HIV infection and expanded AIDS surveillance case definition for adolescents and adults (Centers for Disease Control and Prevention, 1993)

CD4+ T-cell categories	(A) Asymptomatic acute primary HIV or PGL*	(B) Symptomatic not (A) or (C) conditions	(C) AIDS-indicator conditions
1) less than 500/uL	A1	B1	C1
2) 200-499/uL	A2	B2	C2
3) less than 200/uL AIDS-indicator T-cell count	A3	B3	C3

* PGL: persistent generalized lymphadenopathy

TABLE 20-6 Nursing diagnoses of persons with HIV/AIDS

- Breathing pattern ineffective
- Body temperature altered; elevated
- Nutrition altered; less than body requirements
- Altered bowel elimination; diarrhea
- Mobility impaired
- Fatigue
- Diversional activity deficit
- Skin integrity impaired
- Sensory perceptual alterations
- Self-care deficit
- Comfort altered; pain
- Potential for infection
- Ineffective individual/family coping
- Impaired gas exchange
- Alterations in thought processes
- Alterations in emotional integrity (anxiety, fear, and grieving)

Alteration in nutrition. This diagnosis includes less than body requirements related to decreased intake secondary to nausea, vomiting, dysphagia, fatigue, difficulty swallowing, and changes of taste and smell. Interventions include the following:

1. Assess nutritional state daily. Note weight, caloric/fluid intake and output.

2. Monitor serum/urine electrolytes, protein, albumin, CBC, glucose, and acetone levels as necessary.

3. Provide dietary planning. Encourage small, frequent, high-calorie, high-protein meals.

4. Provide oral care before and after meals to decrease anorexia and stomatitis (side effect of chemotherapeutic medicines).

5. Provide sufficient time for client to eat/assist with meals as necessary because fatigue may prevent patient from eating. Eliminate unpleasant odors/sights from the environment to decrease stimulation of the gag reflex. Restrict fluids before, during, and immediately after meals. Allow client to sip fluids or ice chips between meals. Ensure client remains sitting upright after meals.

6. To decrease dysphagia, difficulty chewing, or painful swallowing, ensure client avoids rough or

TABLE 20-7 Nutrition-related problems from drug therapies for AIDS

Drug therapy	For treatment of	Gastrointestinal impact of drug
Acyclovir	Herpes	Diarrhea, nausea, vomiting
Adriamycin	KS	Nausea, vomiting, diarrhea, stomatitis, esophagitis
Amphotericin B	Meningitis	Anorexia, weight loss, nausea, vomiting, diarrhea
AZT, retrovir	HIV	Nausea, vomiting, anemia
Bactrim	PCP	Nausea, vomiting, thrush
Bleomycin	KS	Nausea, vomiting, diarrhea, anorexia, stomatitis
Clotrimazole	Candida	Nausea, vomiting
DFMO	PCP Cryptosporidium	Diarrhea
DHPG	CMV	Nausea, vomiting
Ethambutol HCL	MAI	Nausea, vomiting, anorexia
Ethionamide	MAI	Anorexia, nausea, vomiting, metallic taste
Ketoconazole	Candida	Nausea, vomiting, diarrhea, constipation
Pentamidine IV	PCP	Hypoglycemia, diarrhea, dysphagia
Pyrimethamine	Toxoplasmosis	Diarrhea, vomiting, anorexia
Vincristine	KS	Weight loss, dysphagia, nausea, vomiting, stomatitis, anorexia, constipation

CMV, Cytomegalovirus; KS, Kaposi's sarcoma; MAI, *Mycobacterium avium-intracellulare;* PCP, *Pneumocystis carinii* pneumonia
From "Nutritional assessment and management" by R.C. Elbein, 1992. In M.L. Galantino (Ed.), *Clinical assessment and treatment of HIV: Rehabilitation of a chronic illness* (p. 50). Thorofare, NJ: SLACK Incorporated.

coarse foods, spicy or acidic foods, extremely hot or cold foods, sticky foods (peanut butter), alcohol, and tobacco. Client should eat foods at room temperature if possible. Popsicles can be used to numb oral pain. For clients who develop a distaste for red meat, try using a meat marinade before cooking or use other protein sources such as eggs, peanut butter, tofu, cheeses, poultry, and fish.

7. Teach client deep-breathing techniques to decrease stimulation of the vomiting center. Administer antiemetic as prescribed.

8. Encourage family to visit during meal times and bring in favorite foods from home (if tolerated). Social isolation leads to depression, which can contribute to a lack of interest in eating.

9. Offer supplements between meals.

10. Administer tube feedings/total parenteral nutrition (TPN) as ordered if patient becomes unable to eat or swallow. Isotonic fluids will help prevent diarrhea.

Alteration in elimination. This diagnosis includes diarrhea related to malabsorption secondary to primary intestinal infection with HIV, secondary opportunistic gastrointestinal infection, malignancy, chemotherapy, radiation, drug reaction, tube feeding intolerance, lactose intolerance. Interventions include the following:

1. Assess consistency of stools for presence of blood, fat, and undigested material. Assess frequency of stools and cause of diarrhea. (Diarrhea as a result of drug reactions is treatable.) Auscultate bowel sounds.

2. Monitor stool cultures to provide information on infectious organisms.

3. Maintain accurate intake and output records. Monitor any change in fluid status. Assess for signs and symptoms of hypovolemia, including cool, clammy skin, increased heart rate, decreased respirations, or a decrease in urinary output.

4. Monitor for potential electrolyte imbalance. Assess for anxiety, confusion, muscle weakness, cramps, weak pulse, and a decrease in blood pressure.

5. Encourage patient to consume 3 liters (12 cups) or more of fluid daily. Suitable fluids include water, gatorade, noncarbonated drinks, caffeine-free drinks, and diluted fruit juices.

6. Provide small, frequent meals. Avoid high fiber, high-fat foods. Also avoid hot, cold, or spicy foods. Peel all fruits and grate raw vegetables. Encourage foods high in potassium, such as bananas, avocados, and potatoes; foods high in sodium, such as cheeses, dried fruits, preserved meats; foods high in protein, such as cottage cheese, cream cheese, boiled low-fat milk, yogurt; and foods high in carbohydrates, such as white bread, toast, crackers, noodles, pasta, white rice.

7. Assess perianal area for excoriation. Provide meticulous skin care. Wash perianal region with soap and water, pat dry, and apply ointment. Vaseline, A & D ointment, and zinc oxide minimize burning of the skin and act as a barrier, thereby decreasing discomfort.

8. Monitor tube feedings. Consider diluting strength or decreasing amount.

(Original care plan from Ms. Cynthia Anslow, 1994, nursing student at D'Youville College. Printed by permission.)

Psychosocial issues. In addition to the physical implications associated with HIV disease, there may be devastating emotional and social reactions for the person diagnosed with HIV infection. Despite the changing nature of HIV disease in North America, many still view HIV as a virus that affects gay men, injection drug users, and prostitutes. The unfortunate discrimination that persons living with HIV/AIDS often experience as a result can lead to withdrawal, social isolation, and rejection at a time when the person may most require support. Persons living with HIV/AIDS may find it difficult to reveal their HIV status for fear of discrimination not only by their family and friends, but also from insensitive care providers. This could result in the person neglecting his or her health needs by not accessing available health and social services.

Learning of an HIV diagnosis can also result in a range of individual responses that, in some ways, are not highly different to the responses that others with a chronic or terminal illness might experience. The person diagnosed with HIV may experience feelings of anger, guilt, anxiety, depression, and fear. In addition, given the many physical, psychologic, and social losses that are associated with HIV disease, it is essential that the nurse have an understanding of the psychologic and emotional impact that these losses have on an individual. The stages of death and dying identified by Kubler-Ross (1969) provide a useful framework in our understanding of these losses and the associated psychologic responses. These responses include denial, anger, bargaining, depression, and acceptance.

Given the poor prognosis of individuals diagnosed with AIDS, treatment must not only focus on an individual's physical needs, but must incorporate the person's whole being, including the emotional and spiritual domains. In doing so, the nurse will assist the person living with HIV/AIDS to mobilize his or her coping strategies in dealing with the effects of HIV infection, thus enhancing his or her quality of life.

Palliative care for persons living with HIV/AIDS. Despite the many advances that have been made in the treatment and care of persons living with HIV/AIDS, there is still no cure. Available treatment options have varied effectiveness, and with the progression of HIV disease, the focus of care and treatment shifts from aggressive treatment to supportive or palliative care.

Palliative care is a philosophy of care in which quality of life for the person with a terminal illness becomes the major focus. Both the person with HIV/AIDS and his or her family are viewed as the unit of care. The client's autonomy is respected, and he or she plays a central and integral role in care planning and treatment. The hospice team promotes a dignified, comfortable life until death.

There are numerous hospices or palliative care programs throughout the United States and Canada. Within the last 6 years, Casey House Hospice in Toronto, Canada, has admitted over 450 persons living with AIDS to the 13-bed residential facility and home hospice program. The Casey House program is modeled on traditional hospice philosophy, which emphasizes symptom management within a holistic approach to care. Since opening in March of 1988, Casey House staff have identified numerous factors which are unique to AIDS palliative care. One of the most significant factors is the notion of active versus palliative treatment for persons living with HIV/AIDS. The dilemma arises in determining which treatments are active and which are palliative. For example, the use of ganciclovir administered through a central venous line is a commonly used medical treatment in preventing or delaying the progression of CMV retinitis and subsequent blindness in these clients. In addition, there are numerous antibiotic and other medical treatments used in controlling symptoms associated with a variety of opportunistic infections related to HIV. The question that then faces AIDS hospice staff is: What constitutes palliative versus active treatment in an AIDS hospice setting? This dilemma is perhaps best illustrated in the following case study.

■ CASE STUDY

Mark is 29 years old. He first learned of his HIV status 5 years ago. In appearance, Mark was physically healthy until 6 months ago, when he developed severe, intractable diarrhea. Despite several interventions, Mark lost over 50 pounds in the ensuing months. Last month, Mark was admitted to a hospital. His physical decline was rapid, with numerous concurrent infections and insidious dementia related to HIV. He depends on others to meet his basic physical needs. Although Mark has a supportive network of friends and family, they have had significant difficulty in dealing with his diagnosis and deteriorating health. Following discussion with the health care team, his family, and his friends, Mark has opted for nutritional supplement through a nasogastric tube. This intervention has slowed his progressive weight loss.

Mark hopes for a cure for AIDS. He very much wants to live and continues to take a range of antiviral, antifungal, and other related medical treatments to control his symptoms. Mark has goals he still wants to accomplish in his life. Mark was referred to Casey House for palliation.

Both persons living with AIDS and the disease itself have challenged the traditional concept of palliative care as we have known it. Words such as *active treatment* and *acute care* hold limited value within an AIDS hospice setting. Concepts such as "symptom management with comfort" and "quality of life" perhaps hold more value in determining the appropriateness of admission to a hospice or palliative care program. As treat-

ments for HIV- and AIDS-related conditions continue to advance, it will become increasingly difficult to differentiate between chronic and palliative care.

Hepatitis B

Hepatitis B (HBV) is a viral infection that primarily affects the liver of infected persons. HBV is one of three distinct liver infections, which also

--- RESEARCH HIGHLIGHT ---

Occupational Exposure to Bloodborne Diseases and Universal Precautions

In response to the need for a valid and reliable tool to assess the attitudes of health care workers toward universal precautions and exposure to bloodborne diseases, an instrument was developed to measure how these attitudes affect behaviors. The Health Belief Model (HBM) served as the theoretical framework for the design of this instrument. The first part of the instrument contained five questions that elicited the subjects' exposure to blood-borne diseases and formal training in universal precautions, and the second part consisted of 37 items accompanied by a five-point likert scale to measure each subject's responses to the items reflecting the five (perceived susceptibility and seriousness, benefits and barriers-action, and health motivation) HBM constructs. The higher numbers (5 and 4) represented high self-perceptions of seriousness or susceptibility to blood-borne diseases, high agreement with use of universal precautions UP, or high health-related motivation, and the lower numbers (1 and 2) represented the opposite extreme. An uncertain response (3) was considered neither high nor low.

One hundred nurses in a large metropolitan region in the Midwestern United States volunteered to anonymously respond to the questionnaire, and 24 of the 100 nurses volunteered for retesting by placing their identity (name and address) on a cover sheet that accompanied the questionnaire. These subjects were retested 2 weeks later, and a coded questionnaire was returned in a self-addressed envelope. While the region in which the

questionnaire was administered had a low prevalence of blood-borne diseases, especially HIV/AIDS, 85% of the respondents had cared for clients with blood-borne diseases, 55% had cared for clients with HIV/AIDS, and 30% had cared for clients who died of AIDS. Homogeneity of the sample (nurses attending a professional organization meeting [$n = 60$] or enrolled in graduate level nursing courses [$n = 40$]), its size, and the voluntary nature of participation were limitations identified in this study.

Eighty-seven percent of 98 subjects had received training in universal precautions, and 63% of 98 subjects reported experiencing a needlestick injury. The internal reliability estimates for the total scale, for which there was a 100% return, were .74 and .77 after deletion of the six-item health motivation subscale. The test-retest reliability was significant for each subscale, and for the total score. Construct validity was evident by independent factoring of the four subscales (health motivation deleted) of the HBM. Data supported that the four constructs, with the exception of health motivation, from the HBM are appropriate and theoretically supported when measuring health care workers attitudes toward universal precautions and blood-borne diseases. It was recommended that further studies be conducted with a variety of health care workers throughout the country, and continued testing with refinement of the instrument be achieved before attempts at generalization and initiation of strategies to attain adherence to universal precautions.

From "Occupational exposure to bloodborne diseases and universal precautions" by M.M. Grady, L.A. Shortridge, L.S. Davis, & C.S. Klinger. 1993. *American Association of Occupational Health Nurses Journal, 41*(11), 533-540.

include hepatitis A and hepatitis C. The onset of hepatitis B is usually insidious, although in a small number of cases, fulminating hepatitis with acute hepatic necrosis can occur. Symptoms include anorexia, abdominal discomfort, nausea and vomiting, and jaundice. Fever may or may not be present, and individuals infected with HBV may sometimes have a rash (Beneson, 1985). Incubation of HBV ranges anywhere from 45 to 180 days. Individuals infected with HBV can remain infective from before the onset of symptoms to many years as a chronic carrier. HBV is detected by serum testing for hepatitis B surface antigen (HBsAG).

Mode of transmission. HBV is primarily a blood-borne pathogen, although it has been isolated in virtually all body fluids. The body fluids that have been implicated in the transmission of HBV include blood, semen, vaginal fluids, and saliva (Beneson, 1985). HBV is transmitted through the exposure to blood of an infected person and through sexual contact with an infected person. Infants can contract HBV during birth through exposure to blood of an infected mother. Because of the potential of exposure to blood in an occupational setting, health care workers should strictly adhere to universal precautions to prevent exposure to HBV.

Treatment. Primary prevention of HBV is crucial to reduce the prevalence and incidence of HBV. For nurses and other health care workers, routinely practicing universal precautions is an important and effective means of preventing occupational exposure to HBV. In addition, there are synthetic vaccines available that have proven highly effective in preventing the transmission of HBV. Active artificial immunization with the use of vaccines provides protection in 80 to 95% of persons who receive immunization (CDC, 1993). Vaccines are administered in three intramuscular doses. The first injection is followed at subsequent intervals of 1 to 6 months. The CDC recommends that infants be immunized against HBV by administering HBV vaccines at birth, followed by injections at 2 months and 6 to 18 months.

Individuals exposed to HBV should be given hepatitis B immune globulin within 24 hours of the exposure or HBV vaccine within 7 days of ex-

posure. A combination of both could be employed by the treating physician. Medical interventions for individuals who develop symptoms of hepatitis B are limited in their effectiveness. Nursing interventions must be geared toward promoting rest and maintaining adequate hydration and nutrition.

Tuberculosis

Epidemiology. Forty years ago, **tuberculosis** (TB) was a major health threat to adults and children in the United States and Canada. A combination of research and aggressive public health case findings decreased the incidence by an average of 5% annually. It became, virtually, a disease of the past.

In 1985, the disease began to resurface. It has continued to increase annually. This phenomenon is the result of several factors:

1. An estimated 1.0 million persons in the United States are infected with HIV, and therefore will contract a wide range of illnesses, including tuberculosis, as a result of a weakened immune system.

2. An estimated 10 to 15 million persons in the United States are infected with *Mycobacterium tuberculosis,* the organism that causes TB.

3. In 1990, approximately 5% of all AIDS patients also had TB. In some areas, as many as 58% of persons with TB are HIV seropositive.

4. Individuals infected in their 30s and 40s who never progress to active tuberculosis may do so as the aging process depletes their immune system.

Globally, 20% of the population is infected with the tubercule bacillus (bacterium), according to WHO. Refugees, coming from underdeveloped countries, may have become infected with TB in their country. They may show no signs of active disease when they enter the United States and Canada, but progress to active disease after they are here. They then become a danger to others in terms of being able to pass on the infection.

Individuals infected in their 30s and 40s, but never treated because of the absence of active disease, may experience an altered immune state as they age. If this occurs, they could progress to an active disease state without becoming reinfected.

Tuberculosis disease does not develop in everyone who is infected with tuberculosis bacillus. In the United States, about 90% of infected persons remain infected for life and never develop symptoms of TB. But in about 5% of infected persons, disease develops in the first or second year after infection, and in another 5% it develops later in life. (This varies with age and immunologic status.) The risk that active TB will develop in a person infected with both TB and HIV is about 8% per year. In contrast, the risk that it will develop in a person infected only with TB is 5% to 10% during a lifetime.

Tubercule bacillus infection in a person who does not have the active disease is not considered a case of TB. Persons with TB infection who do not have the active disease cannot infect others, usually have a positive reaction to the tuberculin skin test, usually have a negative chest radiograph and no clinical symptoms of TB, and have tubercle bacilli in their bodies. Although contained, these bacilli remain viable and capable of producing active disease at any time.

The development of HIV-related TB disease can follow either of two courses. First, if a person who has latent TB infection also becomes infected with HIV, active TB may develop as HIV weakens the person's immune system. Second, if a person who has preexisting HIV infection becomes infected with TB, TB infection may progress rapidly to disease.

Mode of transmission. TB is a communicable disease caused by the bacterium *Mycobacterium tuberculosis,* often called the tubercle bacillus. It is spread from person to person through the inhalation of airborne particles containing *M. tuberculosis.* These particles, also called droplet nuclei, are produced when a person with infectious TB of the lung or larynx (pulmonary TB) forcefully exhales, such as when coughing, sneezing, speaking, or singing. These infectious particles can remain suspended in the air and inhaled by someone sharing the same air. Tuberculosis is transmitted in closed areas where

ventilation is poor. The risk of transmission increases when susceptible persons share air for prolonged periods with a person who has untreated pulmonary TB. Persons who have TB in extrapulmonary sites (not including laryngeal TB) are usually not considered infectious to other people.

Incubation period. During the first few weeks after infection, tubercle bacilli can spread from their initial location in the lungs (usually in the lower portions), to the lymph nodes in the center of the chest, and then to other parts of the body by way of the bloodstream. Tubercle bacilli can reach all areas of the body, but they often travel to the areas that are most susceptible to TB disease, such as the upper portions of the lungs, the kidneys, the brain, and the bones. Within 2 to 10 weeks, the body's immunologic response to the tubercle bacilli usually prevents the bacteria from multiplying and spreading more. In persons with depressed immunity, the disease may manifest clinical symptoms within 4 to 6 weeks.

Pathology. TB infection may occur when droplet nuclei are inhaled through the nose and mouth and then move down the trachea into the lungs and along the branches of the airways (the bronchi) until they reach the small air sacs of the lungs (the alveoli). Tuberculosis infection usually begins in the alveoli, where tubercle bacilli are initially able to multiply.

Most cases of TB (approximately 85%) are pulmonary TB because they occur in the lungs. But disease may occur at any site in the body, such as the larynx, the lymph nodes, the brain, the kidneys, or the bones (extrapulmonary TB). Extrapulmonary TB and unusual presentations of pulmonary TB are more common among HIV-infected persons than among persons not infected with HIV.

The signs and symptoms of TB vary according to the location of the disease. General signs and symptoms may include fatigue, feeling ill, loss of appetite, weight loss, fever, and night sweats. In addition to the general signs and symptoms, pulmonary TB usually causes a cough, chest pain, coughing up sputum, and sometimes coughing up blood (hemoptysis); TB of the spine may cause pain in the back; and TB of the kidney may

TABLE 20-8 Selected clinical characteristics of persons with tuberculosis infection, active pulmonary tuberculosis, or extrapulmonary tuberculosis

	TB infection	Active pulmonary TB	Extrapulmonary TB
Skin test result	Usually positive	Usually positive	Usually positive
Signs and symptoms	None	Cough, hemoptysis, fever, night sweats, weight loss, fatigue, chest pain, and anorexia	Depends on affected site in body General signs and symptoms: fever, night sweats, weight loss, fatigue, feeling ill, and loss of appetite
Infected	Yes	Yes	Yes
Infectious	No	Usually (before effective treatment)	Usually not

cause blood in the urine. Table 20-8 summarizes selected clinical characteristics of persons with TB infection, active pulmonary TB, or extrapulmonary TB.

Prevention. Screening with a tuberculin skin test to determine the presence of infection remains the best way to target persons at risk of developing the disease (and possibly spreading it) (Dowling, 1991).

The Mantoux tuberculin skin test is the recommended method of skin testing to determine whether a person is infected with *M. tuberculosis.* Multiple-puncture tests should not be used because the results are less reliable. The Mantoux skin test is performed by injecting 0.1 ml of 5 tuberculin units of purified protein derivative intradermally, usually on the forearm. The patient's arm is examined 48 to 72 hours later for induration (palpable swelling) around the site of injection. The diameter of the indurated area across the forearm is measured. The area of erythema (redness) around the indurated area does not indicate infection with *M. tuberculosis* and should not be measured. A positive reaction to the tuberculin test usually means the patient has been infected with *M. tuberculosis.* A tuberculin skin test reaction of 5 or more millimeters of induration is considered positive.

All persons known to have or suspected of having HIV infection should be given a purified protein derivative tuberculin skin test. Persons infected with both TB and HIV may have a false-negative skin test reaction because of anergy. **Anergy** is the inability to mount a delayed-type hypersensitivity response to skin test antigens because of immunosuppression that may be caused by certain medical conditions, such as HIV infection, or drugs. According to recent studies, HIV infection can depress tuberculin reactions even before the signs and symptoms of HIV infection develop.

Testing for anergy. Because persons with HIV infection are more likely to have an anergic response to a tuberculin skin test, these persons should be evaluated for DTH anergy at the time of tuberculin testing.

For anergy testing, Mantoux tuberculin testing should be accompanied by Mantoux testing with two DTH antigens; for example, Candida, mumps, or tetanus toxoid. The reactions should be measured 48 to 72 hours after the test is administered. Induration of 3 or more millimeters to any of the antigens is considered evidence of DTH responsiveness; failure to respond to all of the antigens is considered anergy. In general, persons who respond to DTH antigens but who have a negative reaction to tuberculin are not considered infected with *M. tuberculosis.* HIV-infected persons who are anergic (and thus have a negative reaction to tuberculin skin test) and who are at increased risk for TB should be considered for preventive therapy.

Tuberculin skin test reaction in persons vaccinated with BCG. Outside the United

States, many countries use Bacille Calmette-Guérin (BCG) vaccination as part of their TB control activities, especially for infants. The size of tuberculin skin test reactions caused by BCG vaccination varies by the strain and the dose of the vaccine, the age and the nutritional status of the person at vaccination, the number of years since vaccination, and the frequency of tuberculin testing. After BCG vaccination, it is usually impossible to distinguish between a tuberculin skin test reaction caused by mycobacterial infection or by vaccination. However, BCG-induced tuberculin skin test reactivity wanes over time. Also, because BCG is used more often in countries where the prevalence of TB is high, BCG-vaccinated persons are more likely to have been exposed to TB. Therefore, these persons should be considered infected with *M. tuberculosis* if they have a positive reaction to 5 tuberculin units of purified protein derivative tuberculin. They also should be evaluated for TB disease and managed accordingly.

Preventive therapy for TB infection. Preventive therapy can reduce the risk of TB by more than 90% if taken correctly by infected persons. The recommended preventive therapy regimen is isoniazid, at a dosage of 5 mg/kg daily for adults and 10 mg/kg daily for children to a maximum of 300 mg, for at least 6 continuous months for adults and 9 continuous months for children. For HIV-infected persons, preventive therapy is recommended for at least 12 months. Patients given preventive therapy should be monitored monthly for adherence to therapy and for drug side effects, especially the signs and symptoms of hepatitis.

Anergic persons who are at increased risk for TB but who choose not to take preventive therapy should be informed about the signs and symptoms of TB and instructed to report promptly for medical evaluation if any of these develop.

Persons who have a positive skin test result and persons with TB symptoms (regardless of the skin test result) should be evaluated with a chest radiograph to rule out pulmonary TB. Almost any abnormality on a chest radiograph may indicate TB. The radiograph may even appear entirely normal while sputum or lung fluid specimens are culture-positive for *M. tuberculosis.*

Patients who have abnormal chest radiographs should have sputum specimens collected for acid-fast bacilli examination. For this examination, the specimen is smeared onto a glass slide and stained with a fluorochrome stain or a conventional stain, such as Ziehl-Neelsen or Kinyoun. Laboratory personnel use the microscope to look for acid-fast bacilli on the smear. These bacilli are bacteria that remain stained even after they have been washed in an acid solution. Tubercule bacilli are one kind of acid-fast bacilli. Fluorochrome stains offer two advantages over conventional stains: they make the acid-fast bacilli easier to see, and they allow slides to be examined much more quickly.

Because acid-fast bacilli are not always tubercle bacilli, patients who have positive smears do not necessarily have TB. Furthermore, patients who have negative smears may have TB because negative smears do not rule out the possibility of TB. A culture result that is positive for *M. tuberculosis* is the only definitive proof of TB disease. Nevertheless, TB treatment should be started if the smear is found to be positive before the culture results are known. Drug susceptibility testing is recommended for the first *M. tuberculosis* isolate for all patients, and it should be performed on additional isolates if culture results remain positive after the patient has received 3 months of therapy or if the patient does not seem to respond to therapy. Drug susceptibility results should be promptly reported to the health care provider and the health department.

Contact investigation. Contact investigation, one of the best ways to find other persons who require treatment or preventive therapy for TB disease or infection, should begin as soon as a person is suspected of having TB. All new TB cases and suspected cases should be promptly reported to the health department by the health care provider. Early reporting is essential for the prompt evaluation of contacts of persons who have infectious TB. If a person's medical history and clinical findings suggest TB, health care workers should not wait for culture results before starting a contact investigation. Contact investigations are usually performed by the staff of health department TB control programs, although hospital infection control officers and the staff of correctional and long-term care facilities may also conduct them.

Evaluations should be convenient for the contact. This may require that tuberculin testing and sputum collection be done in the field and that transportation to facilities be provided for radiographic and other examinations. The evaluation should proceed in an orderly manner, starting with persons who are most likely to have been infected, such as members of the client's immediate family or others who have recently shared the same indoor environment with the infected client for prolonged periods. The highest priority should be given to rapid examination of close contacts who are children and persons who are HIV infected because they are at high risk for active disease if infected with TB. For example, life-threatening TB meningitis or miliary TB can develop in newly infected children within weeks of infection unless preventive therapy is administered.

Close contacts of highly infectious persons, especially high-risk contacts, such as children and immunosuppressed persons, should be considered for preventive therapy even if their initial tuberculin skin test result is negative (less than 5 mm). A second skin test should be given 12 weeks after contact with the infectious person ended; if this result is also negative, preventive therapy may be stopped.

The HIV-infection status of contacts alters the approach to both the investigation and the use of preventive therapy. Appropriate counseling and HIV testing for contacts whose HIV status is unknown is advisable. HIV-infected contacts should be considered for preventive therapy, regardless of their tuberculin skin test results.

Multidrug-resistant TB. An extremely serious aspect of the TB problem in the United States is the recent increase in multidrug-resistant TB (MDR TB). From 1990 through late 1992, CDC investigated eight outbreaks of MDR TB in hospitals and correctional facilities in New York, Florida, and New Jersey. These outbreaks have included almost 300 cases. Some cases were caused by organisms resistant to at least seven antituberculosis drugs. Most of the patients in these outbreaks were infected with HIV. Mortality among patients with MDR TB in these outbreaks ranged from 72% to 89%, and the median intervals between TB diagnosis and death ranged from 4 to 16 weeks.

Following are descriptions of persons who are at high risk for drug-resistant TB: persons who have been recently exposed to drug-resistant TB, especially if they are immunocompromised; TB patients who failed to take medications as prescribed; TB patients who were prescribed an ineffective treatment regimen; and persons previously treated for TB. Clinicians who are not familiar with the management of patients who have MDR TB or patients who have been exposed to MDR TB should seek expert consultation.

Tuberculosis and HIV/AIDS are the community health nurses' challenges for the coming decade. An understanding of tuberculosis and how to prevent its spread makes it possible to eliminate it. HIV/AIDS remains a threat and a mystery. Multidrug-resistant TB requires careful supervision and ongoing evaluation to determine the effectiveness of treatment.

Nursing interventions for persons with active tuberculosis. Nurses should explain the importance of compliance with the medical regime prescribed (see Table 20-9). Failure to comply may make it more difficult to rid the client of active disease. It may also allow the immune system time to develop some immunity to the medication. Persons with infected sputum should be taught to use tissues when they cough or sneeze and to properly dispose of them. While the sputum is positive, the client should keep linens, dishes, and bedding separate. Ventilation of rooms is important. Institutional settings are being advised to place active tuberculosis clients in negative-pressure rooms, with the air from the room vented directly to the outside.

Nurses and other health care workers must implement work practices and use personal protective equipment to protect themselves and other clients from the spread of the disease. Nurses need to be aware of the necessity to prac-

TABLE 20-9   Dosage recommendations for the treatment of TB in children* and adults

	Dosage					
	Daily dose		Twice-weekly dose		Thrice-weekly dose	
Drugs	Children	Adults	Children	Adults	Children	Adults
Isoniazid	10-20 mg/kg Max. 300 mg	5 mg/kg Max. 300 mg	20-40 mg/kg Max. 900 mg	15 mg/kg Max. 900 mg	20-40 mg/kg Max. 900 mg	15 mg/kg Max. 900 mg
Rifampin	10-20 mg/kg Max. 600 mg	10 mg/kg Max. 600 mg	10-20 mg/kg Max. 600 mg	10 mg/kg Max. 600 mg	10-20 mg/kg Max. 600 mg	10 mg/kg Max. 600 mg
Pyrazinamide	15-30 mg/kg Max. 2 gm	15-30 mg/kg Max. 2 gm	50-70 mg/kg	50-70 mg/kg	50-70 mg/kg	50-70 mg/kg
Ethambutol**	15-25 mg/kg Max. 2.5 gm	15-25 mg/kg Max. 2.5 gm	50 mg/kg	50 mg/kg	25-30 mg/kg	25-30 mg/kg
Streptomycin	20-40 mg/kg Max. 1 gm	15 mg/kg Max. 1 gm	25-30 mg/kg	25-30 mg/kg	25-30 mg/kg	25-30 mg/kg

*Children = 12 years of age and younger.
**Ethambutol is generally not recommended for children whose visual acuity cannot be monitored (children less than 6 years of age). However, ethambutol should be considered for all children with organisms resistant to other drugs, if susceptibility to ethambutol has been demonstrated or susceptibility is likely.

tice with an awareness of prudent infection control.

Tuberculosis is usually curable if it is diagnosed early and if effective treatment is instituted without delay. Tuberculosis must be treated for a long time compared with most other infectious diseases. If treatment does not continue for a sufficient length of time (at least 6 months), enough tubercle bacilli may survive to make the client ill and infectious again; also, ineffective treatment may foster the development of drug-resistant mycobacteria.

INFECTION CONTROL

Nurses in the community and in the hospital setting must assume the responsibility to adhere to scientifically accepted principles of infection control, and monitor the performance of those for whom the profession is responsible. In home nursing this would include home health aides and registered nurse assistants.

A knowledge of the modes and mechanisms of the transmission of pathogenic organisms must be supplemented with an understanding of engineering and work practice controls that re-

duce the opportunity for exposure of the client and health care worker to potentially infectious material.

Engineering Controls

Engineering controls seek to eliminate or isolate the hazard. For example, providing continuous protection from needle stick injury can be accomplished by providing a mechanism to safely cover the sharps immediately after use. This would mean using self-sheathing needles (Figure 20-4), disposal containers, and trays to store and transport syringes. It is also important to provide puncture-resistant containers for the disposal and transport of needles and other sharps, and splatter shields on medical equipment.

The provision of negative-pressure units for persons who are institutionalized and have active tuberculosis is mandatory in some states. This provides a process whereby all air is exhausted out of the room and into an area separate from the main ventilation system. Also recommended are Hepa filters (high efficiency particulate air filters) whenever possible. In the home, commercial air filters placed in the client's room would

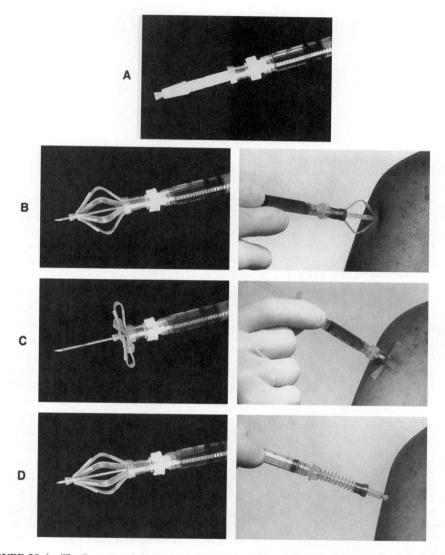

FIGURE 20-4 The Protector Self-Covering Hypodermic Needle by InjectiMed, Inc. **A,** Ready. Needle with protector covering ready for use. **B,** Plunge. Needle tip is exposed only when spring cover is compressed during use. **C,** Inject. **D,** Withdraw from injection site. Protector passively covers the needle. (From *AIDS and HIV infection* (p.202) by D.E. Grimes & R.M.Grimes, 1994, St. Louis: Mosby.)

assist in cutting down the number of tuberculosis nucleii in the immediate area.

Work Practice Controls

Work practice controls include treating all blood and body fluids as if they are known to be infectious with HIV or HBV, and treating all needles as if they were contaminated. Also recommended as work practice controls are avoidance of unnecessary use of needles and other sharps, not recap-

---

TUBERCULOSIS PROGRAM REQUIRED BY OSHA

1. Protocol for early identification of individuals with active TB.
2. Medical surveillance.
3. Evaluation and management of employees who test positive.
4. AFB isolation rooms.
5. Training and information.
6. Respiratory fit testing.
7. Accident prevention signs.
8. Access to employee exposure and medical records.

PRECAUTIONS REQUIRED BY OSHA

OSHA blood-borne pathogen

In December 1991, the Occupational Safety and Health Administration (OSHA) Blood-borne Pathogen Standard 1910:1030 took effect. This standard imposes a requirement on employers to implement an exposure control plan for the protection of employees from HIV and HBV. Training of all employees concerning the risk of blood-borne disease exposure and the principles of universal precautions, including the use of personal protective equipment, preventive practices, the nature and location of the exposure control plan, and procedures for exposure follow-up, is required annually.

Universal precautions

Universal precautions is OSHA's required method of control to protect employees from exposure to all human blood and other potentially infectious material. The term *universal precautions* refers to a concept of blood-borne disease control that requires that all human blood and certain human body fluids are treated as if known to be infectious for HIV, HBV, and other blood-borne pathogens.

Body substance isolation (BSI)

Body substance isolation is a control method that defines **all** body fluids and substances as infectious. BSI incorporates not only fluids and materials covered in the standard, but expands coverage to include all body substances. BSI is an acceptable alternative to universal precautions, provided facilities that use BSI adhere to all other provisions of the OSHA standards.

---

ping needles or, when necessary, using an appropriate one-handed technique. Sharp instruments should be passed from one worker to another by use of designated safe zones. Sharps should be dissembled by use of forceps or other equipment. Sharps should not be left on a field, tissue should not be held with fingers, and forceps suture holders or other instruments should be used when suturing. Hand washing is the single most important work practice control that can be used. The use of gloves does not omit the need for hand washing. Rings and watches should be removed; the hands should be rubbed briskly together to create a lather with an appropriate soap. The hands should be rinsed by holding them downward, and dried with a paper towel. The faucet should be turned off with a dry paper towel. In the home, there may not be a clean sink to wash hands in. In this case the nurse must provide antiseptic towelettes to cleanse the hands and then must dispose of them appropriately. Good personal hygiene in a general way is important to protect the client and oneself. Adequate rest, clean hair, clean uniforms, and clean shoes when entering a client's home will be helpful. Some nurses keep a washable pair of slippers in their bag to eliminate wearing street shoes or boots into a client's home. Good patient hygiene is important. The nurse should make sure that the aide or whoever is responsible for the client's personal care in the home changes clothing often, keeps bed linens clean, and includes oral and perineal care when it is appropriate. Disposal of wastes in a prudent manner is imperative. For example, the nurse or aide should use nonsterile gloves to remove a dressing and sterile gloves to apply the new dressing. Not reporting to work if a respiratory or enteric infection is present will protect the client and the nurse. The protection of the client is especially important if the client has a compromised immune system.

Personal Protective Equipment

Personal protective equipment should be made available to all nurses, especially those working in the community. Typical protective wear are latex or vinyl gloves, ventilation devices for performing mouth-to-mouth resuscitation, protective eye wear and disposable gowns or aprons if splashing should occur, and face masks made with Hepa filter material. For those nurses giving care to persons who have active tuberculosis, Hepa filter masks are essential.

Blood-borne pathogen standards and the protocol recommended by OSHA to prevent the spread of tuberculosis are presented in the boxes on page 468. Nurses need to be aware of these standards and protocol and implement them in their practice.

Chapter Highlights

- Communicable diseases are most often caused by the following agents: viral, bacterial, fungal, or protozoal.

- The mode of transmission of an agent can be direct; for example, droplet infection, or indirect; for example, water borne or vector borne.

- Some diseases, for example Rocky Mountain Spotted Fever, have a chain of transmission: Rickettsiae to Tick to Grass or Animal to Human.

- There is an incubation period of the time between exposure to a pathogenic agent and symptoms of disease.

- Period of communicability is the time span during which contact with an infected person is likely to result in the spread of infection.

- Immunity can be active or passive; it may be acquired naturally or artificially. The level of immunity in an individual or a population can vary, particularly with respect to communicable diseases.

- Betty Neuman's client systems model can be used to illustrate the concept of relative immunity.

- Primary prevention of communicable diseases is accomplished through immunizations, education, and adequate public sanitation.

- Screening for communicable diseases allows the nurse to practice secondary prevention by planning interventions before a client exhibits symptoms of a disease.

- Tertiary prevention is used to limit disability after an individual has symptoms of a disease.

- Because of a mobile world society and changing social conditions, hepatitis and tuberculosis are increasingly problematic.

- HIV is spread through direct contact of body fluids, which can occur by means of sexual activity, intravenous administration of drugs with contaminated needles, transfusions of contaminated blood or blood products, or transfer from mothers to infants in utero through the placenta or through breastfeeding.

- Because of compromised immunity, the client with AIDS is susceptible to many infections that normally would be resisted by the body's immune system.

CRITICAL THINKING EXERCISE

Local health department officials issued an alert about a town's water supply. Persons with weakened immune systems were advised to boil their tap water before drinking it because of high levels of turbidity. Several days of strong winds had stirred up a nearby lake that is the source of the town's water. The health department warned of a risk of contamination from organisms such as bacteria and protozoans.

1. What high-risk aggregates in this town would most likely be affected by the water?
2. Describe and give examples of persons who may have impaired immunity.

REFERENCES

Anslow, C. (1994). Original care plan submitted for course work at D'Youville College.

Barre-Sinoussi, F., Chermann, J.E., Rey, F., et al. (1983). Isolation of a T-lymphotropic retrovirus for a patient at risk for acquired immunodeficiency syndrome. *Science, 220*(868).

Beneson, A.S. (1985). *Control of communicable diseases in man* (14th ed.). Washington, DC: American Public Health Association.

Bennet, C., & Searl, S. (1982). *Communicable diseases handbook.* New York: Wiley & Sons.

Braunwald, E., Thorn, G., Adams, R., Isselbacker, K., & Petersdorf, R., (Eds.). (1987). *Harrison's principles of internal medicine* (11th ed.). New York: McGraw-Hill.

Centers for Disease Control and Prevention. (1986). Classification system for human T-lymphotropic virus type III/lymphadenopathy-associated virus infection. *Morbidity and Mortality Weekly Report, 35*(344).

Centers for Disease Control and Prevention. (1987). Recommendations for prevention of HIV transmission in health care settings. *Morbidity and Mortality Weekly Report, 36*(1S).

Centers for Disease Control and Prevention. (1988, June). Water-related disease outbreaks, *Morbidity and Mortality Weekly Report, 37*(55).

Centers for Disease Control and Prevention. (1992, December). 1993 revised classification system for HIV infection and expanded surveillance case identification for AIDS among adolescents and adults. *Morbidity and Mortality Weekly Report, 41,* RR-17.

Centers for Disease Control and Prevention. (1993a, March). *CDC quarterly HIV/AIDS report: Exposure categories* (Document No. 320201). Atlanta, GA: Author.

Centers for Disease Control and Prevention. (1993b, March). *CDC quarterly HIV/AIDS report: Management of exposures to HIV and HBV* (Document No. 23117). Atlanta, GA: Author.

Centers for Disease Control and Prevention. (1993c, March). *CDC quarterly HIV/AIDS report: Statistical projections/ trends* (Document No. 320210). Atlanta, GA: Author.

Centers for Disease Control and Prevention. (1993d, March). *CDC: Viral hepatitis—general information* (Document No. 361300). Atlanta, GA: Author.

Chateauvert, M., Duffie, A., & Gilmore, N. (1990). *Human immunodeficiency virus antibody testing.* Ottawa, Ontario: Canadian Medical Association.

Clavel, F., Guetard, D., Brun-Vezinet, F., et al. (1986). Isolation of a new human retrovirus from West African patients with AIDS. *Science, 233*(343).

Coffin, J., Haase, A., Levy, J.A., et al. (1986). Human immunodeficiency viruses. *Science, 232*(697).

Department of Health, New York State: Official administrative information, July 1, 1993, Series 93-73, Press release.

Dowling, P. (1991). Return of tuberculosis: Screening and preventive therapy. *American Family Physician, 43*(2), 448-465.

Elbein, R. (1992). Nutritional assessment and management and treatment of HIV: Rehabilitation of a chronic illness. In M.L. Galantine (Ed.), *Clinical assessment* (p. 50). Thorofare, NJ: Slack.

Gallo, R.C., Sarin, P.S., Gelman, E.P., et al. (1983). Isolation of human T-cell leukemia virus in acquired immune deficiency syndrome (AIDS). *Science, 220*(865).

Gerberding, J.L. (1988). Occupational health issues for providers of care to patients with HIV infection. *Infectious Disease Clinics of North America, 2*(2), 321-328.

Glanz, W., Anderson, K., & Anderson, L. (1990). *Mosby's medical, nursing, and allied health dictionary.* St. Louis: Mosby.

Glettenberg, J.V. (1990). International affairs: Problems of global control of tuberculosis. *Journal of Professional Nursing, 6*(2), 73, 129.

Grimes, D.E., & Grimes, R.M. (1994). *AIDS and HIV infection.* St. Louis: Mosby.

Jacobs, R. (1993, February 28). Pediatric hepatitis: Where do we stand? *Emergency Medicine,* pp. 83-87.

Jong E. (1992). Immunizations for international travelers. In M. Wolfe, (Ed.), *The medical clinics of North America,* 76(6), 1280. Philadelphia: W.B. Saunders.

Kubler-Ross, E. (1969). *On death and dying.* New York: MacMillan.

Laboratory Center for Disease Control. (1993). *AIDS in Canada: Quarterly surveillance update* (Document No. 110 and 111). Health and Welfare Canada.

Levy, J.A. (1988). The human immunodeficiency virus and its pathogenesis. *Infectious Disease Clinics of North America, 2(2).*

Mansell, P.W.A. (1992). An introduction to the medical management of HIV infection. In M. Galantino, (Ed.), *Clinical assessment and treatment of HIV: Rehabilitation of a chronic illness* (pp. 1-8). New York: McGraw-Hill.

Neuman, B. (1989). *Application of nursing education and practice: The Neuman systems model* (2nd ed.). East Norwalk, CT: Appleton & Lange.

North American Nursing Diagnosis Association. (1988).

Smith, J.P. (1993). Hepatitis C: A major health problem. *Journal of Advanced Nursing, 18,* 503-506.

Trainex Corporation. (1982). *Infection control, the chain of infection.* Garden Grove, CA: Author.

Williams, I., Mindel, A., & Weller, I.V.D. (1989). *AIDS.* New York: J.B. Lippincott.

World Health Organization. (1992). *Current and future dimensions of the HIV/AIDS pandemic: A capsule summary.* Switzerland: Author.

21 CLIENTS WITH CHRONIC ILLNESSES

P. Susan Wagner

The solid meaning of life is always the same eternal thing — the marriage, namely, of some unhabitual ideal, however special, with some fidelity, courage and endurance, with some man or woman's pains.

William James

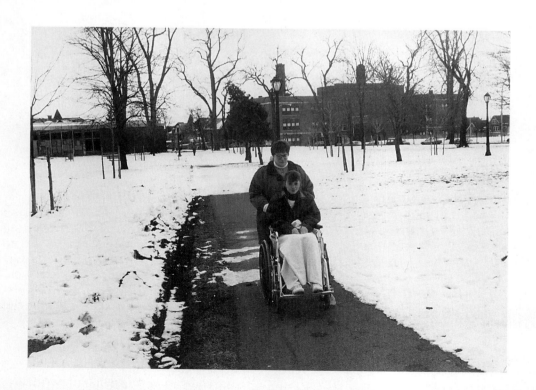

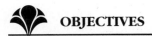

OBJECTIVES

At the conclusion of this chapter the student will be able to:

1. Define the key terms listed.
2. Describe the incidence and prevalence of chronic illness in various populations.
3. Discuss the concept of trajectory and the nature of work imposed by adjustment to a chronic illness from the perspective of the client and of the family.
4. Describe differing response patterns of families to a chronically ill member.
5. Discuss the relationship of a family's available internal and external resources to caregiver burden when there is a chronically ill family member.
6. Explain why accepting help from others is so complex an issue for individuals and families.
7. Describe the importance of timing for the setting of nursing goals.
8. Differentiate between vicious and virtuous communication cycles for the nurse working with a chronically ill client and family.
9. Identify different client and family responses to health care professionals.
10. Describe the difference between the nurse "facilitator" role and the nurse "expert" role.

KEY TERMS

Caregiver burden
Chronic illness
Circular communication diagram
Denial
Disability
Disassociation

Disease
Disenchantment
Guarded alliance
Handicap
Illness

Illness trajectory
Impairment
Normalization
Overcompensation
Sickness

This chapter will attempt to give meaning to the perceptions and responses of the chronically ill or disabled client and family as a foundation for the provision of effective nursing care. Because of their long experience with chronic illness or disability, these clients are experts on their own bodies, their responses to the medical regimens, and the health care system. Their opinions and behavior patterns, and those of their families, often prove frustrating for nurses who have different expectations and goals for interventions. Self-understanding by the nurse is a requirement for respectfully accepting the decisions and actions of clients and families. Unless nurses have some knowledge of their own prejudices, fears, and limitations, and some confidence in their own perceptions, decisions, and competencies, they are ineffective in working with clients. Theoretical frameworks presented as tools for understanding clients will be personally applied through self-assessment study questions.

CONTEXT
Labels, Terms, and Definitions

Evaluations of health and illness depend on the perceptions, value orientations, and knowledge of the people involved (Hamera et al., 1994; Shaw & Halliday, 1992). Disease, illness, and sickness are all terms used to describe states of health, but they have different connotations despite their being used interchangeably. **Disease** refers to objective evidence of "nonhealth, or a state in which the body is suffering from a malfunction of one or more parts" (Dimond & Jones, 1983, p. 3). This evidence includes signs that are visible to others and symptoms that are reported by the affected individual. It is possible for a disease to be diagnosed in an individual without the individual's feeling ill because symptoms are under control. Individuals with epilepsy and diabetes are examples. The term **illness** refers to phenomena that are perceived only by the ill person. These are feelings and perceptions that are usually reported as symptoms. Although it is assumed that disease is the reason for illness, illness can exist without disease. Illness can arise from psychological or social distress. If the symptoms are severe or continue for a period, illness may cause disease. The relationship of stress to gastric ulcers is widely accepted. **Sickness** is the perception of a nonhealthy state by others. It may occur when disease becomes visible or when a person communicates illness to others. Both circumstances result in the alteration of relationships with others. The person involved may behave differently toward others, adopting new roles, and also may be exempted from certain responsibilities by family and friends. It is possible for a person to have disease, feel ill, and not be perceived as sick, such as someone with chronic fatigue syndrome. It is also possible for someone to be treated as sick, but not feel ill or have disease, such as someone exposed to AIDS. When the behavior of the affected individual and others is based on differing evaluations of disease, illness, and sickness, relationships may become very tangled. For the chronically ill, these evaluations may also shift from day to day with changes in the trajectory of the disease. Flexibility is very important for families and for professional staff as they respond to the needs of the ill person. The title of this chapter reflects the centrality of the perceptions of the client for effective nursing interventions.

Chronic illness, according to the National Commission on Chronic Illness, refers to a condition that has one or more of the following criteria: it is permanent, it leaves residual disability, it is caused by a nonpathologic alteration, it requires special training for rehabilitation, and it is expected to require a long period of supervision, observation, or care (Lubkin, 1990). Chronic illness has aspects that correspond to the states of nonhealth described above. It can be described in terms of disease, illness, or sickness according to whether people have a clinical, personal, or social orientation. Other terms that confuse the discussion are impairment, disability, and handicap. **Impairment** is defined as "any loss or abnormality of psychological or anatomical structure or function" (WHO, 1980, p. 46). It is more inclusive than disease. Amputations and the alteration of cultural-, age-, and gender-related attributes would classify as impairments. A **disability** is the consequence of an impairment. It is "any restriction or lack resulting from an impairment of ability to perform an activity in the manner or within the range considered normal for a human being" (WHO, 1980, p. 143). Disabilities are both disease-related and social because they reflect limitations on patterns of behavior. **Handicap** is defined as "a disadvantage for a given individual resulting from an impairment or disability, that limits or prevents the fulfillment of a role that is normal (depending on age, sex, and social and cultural factors) for that individual" (WHO, 1980, p. 183). A handicap does not necessarily mean that there is a functional limitation in all aspects of living. Someone with visual impairment has a handicap that prevents driving a car but that need not interfere with earning a livelihood. The terms used today attempt to be considerate of the feelings of the chronically ill and reduce societal stigma. Labels such as "crippled" and "retarded" are no longer widely used, for example, and terms such as "wheelchair bound" and "mentally challenged" are used instead.

Prevalence of Chronic Illness

In the United States, estimates of the prevalence of chronic conditions range from 50% to 80% of the population, depending on the definitions used (Hymovich & Hagopian, 1992). The statistics are very similar for Canada. The magnitude of the effect on individual capabilities, on family lives, on the health of communities, and on health care costs is enormous. Looking at one subset of the chronically ill population, Balram (1989) stated that 13% of the population has one or more long-term functional disabilities that were not eliminated with the use of an aid and that lasted more than 6 months. Each of those disabled individuals required a family caregiver and altered the life and priorities of a family. The Canadian Health and Activity Limitation Survey (HALS) discovered that over one third of people with disabilities reported out-of-pocket expenses for prescription and over-the-counter drugs not reimbursed by insurance programs, and close to 60% of the adults reported annual incomes of less than $10,000 (1990). The morbidity caused by chronic illness is reflected by the mortality statistics. Eight of the top 12 causes of death in the United States are chronic diseases: heart disease, cancer, cerebrovascular disease, chronic lung disease, diabetes, chronic liver disease, atherosclerosis, and renal disease (Hymovich & Hagopian, 1992). The others are accidents, pneumonia, suicides, and homicides. In Canada, the pattern is similar except that falls are among the top 11 causes of death for women, and homicides for men or women are not (Hum & Semenciw, 1991). The accompanying medical, hospital, and other health care costs cause personal and public concern across North America.

Pless and Perrin (1985) reported that the incidence of chronic conditions in children younger than 18 years of age may be as high as 22%. The majority of conditions are rare, with a few common ones. Mental and sensory impairments and speech, learning, and behavioral disorders were included. Other conditions that have long-term impact on children include chronic respiratory problems, allergies, congenital anomalies, psychiatric problems, nutritional deficiencies, and diseases such as cancer and motor disorders. These conditions may also have repercussions on the child's personal and social well-being, which in itself is a chronic problem. Situations that may create long-term developmental and interpersonal problems, such as abuse, poverty, or homelessness, were not included in these numbers. The Canadian survey (HALS, 1990) completed af-

ter the 1986 census showed that children aged 14 years and under constituted almost 10% of the 3.3 million people with disabilities. Nine percent of those children were classified as severely disabled, 26% required the use of a technical aid, and 26% reported a learning disability (HALS, 1990).

Chronic illnesses in adults are largely caused by a small number of diseases highly prevalent in the population. The list includes heart disease, arthritis, cancer, and diabetes, plus a few conditions that are less common. Adults with chronic conditions often experience limitations in productivity at work or in mobility. About 80% of people over 65 years of age suffer from at least one chronic condition (National Advisory Council on Aging, 1993). Many of those people are restricted in mobility as a result of that condition and therefore have difficulty maintaining activities of daily living independently. Balram (1989) states that 39% of the Canadian population over 65 years of age has a long-term functional disability. Of those, 27% are classified as severely disabled (HALS, 1990). In spite of these figures, 41% of people over 65 years perceive their health status to be better than that of their peers, and 43% perceive it as the same (Health and Welfare Canada, 1993). The chronic disease mortality rate for the elderly is greater than that of younger people, ranging from twice the death rate for hypertension to 17 times the death rate for broken neck of the femur (Hill, 1993).

Trajectory Work

The course of an illness is often called the trajectory, but that phrase does not encompass the complexities experienced by those with chronic illness. Strauss and his colleagues (1984) coined the term **illness trajectory.** The concept encompasses the differences in perception over time of those involved in the situation, the impact on these people, and the identification, organization, and performance of tasks that are associated with management over the course of the illness (Lubkin, 1990). Strauss et al. (1984, p. 64) speak of shaping the trajectory by adapting to events that occur using the coping skills and resources available because control is impossible. Each person involved has a different perspective on the illness trajectory, and each person's efforts are variously directed. The adult client may be more optimistic than the doctor, a spouse more fearful than an elderly parent. The client's efforts may be focused on exercising to regain strength, the physician's on managing the prescriptions to minimize pain during exercise. The spouse's efforts may be in addressing anxieties about his or her skill and knowledge level, the parent's efforts may be directed at providing emotional encouragement to the client. Although some diseases have a fairly predictable course, the projection of trajectory efforts for everyone is difficult. Making plans for the future must include predicting the energy and symptoms of the chronically ill person; the energy and cooperation of family and friends; the priorities compared with other stressors that will exist at that time for all parties involved; the availability of resources such as money, equipment, and facilities; and the flexibility possible if sudden changes occur in any one of the variables. The social impact of the uncertain future of chronic illness is readily apparent.

Stigma: A Response to the Deviance of Disability

Functional disability, brain injury, sensory impairment, and disfigurement can all be reasons for stigma in society. People with these attributes are sometimes excluded from interaction and intimacy and are denied job opportunities or housing (refer to Chapter 22 for more detail). The degree of stigma against those with disabilities varies according to how well the disabled fit the societal norm. People are easier to accept if their illness or disability does not alter their integrity as individuals, their behavior, or their ability to maintain independence in their activities of daily living. Sensory impairment is the easiest disability to overlook because it is so common. Functional disability is the next most readily accepted. A disfigurement is more difficult, particularly if it is on the face or hands. Brain injury is the hardest type of disability for others to accept. The unpredictability of behavior by people with cognitive impairment or head injuries makes life difficult for others.

Everyone has had experience in stigmatizing another person because of prejudices or unpleasant past experiences. Any barrier that interferes with the connection between two people interferes with the potential for an effective relationship. When a relationship is beginning in the presence of a stigma, conversation is initially a challenge because the disability may be a subconscious focus for the "normal" person. When focus is moved to the person instead of the disability, the relationship can be created and maintained because the stigma is gone. The nurse's internal barriers make it impossible for a therapeutic relationship to occur.

Stigmas can include opinions about people with disabilities, racial or gender prejudice, or a rumor or premature judgment of another that is believed without validation. Other internal barriers can include fear of the implications of relating to this person, fear of incompetence, personal anxiety about saying the right thing, or a preoccupation with other personal matters (Dass & Gorman, 1987). For a relationship to be successful, the focus must be on the other person, not on one's self; on his or her needs, not personal needs. Accurate assessments require the ability to be patient, to listen, and avoid or compensate for stigmas that may influence the nurse about a family.

ASSESSMENT OF FAMILIES
Challenges Faced by Families with an Ill or Disabled Member

Families coping with an ill member are challenged by developmental or adjustment tasks that must be addressed if equilibrium is to be maintained. These tasks are in addition to the usual functions and responsibilities of family units described in Chapter 18. Moos and Tsu (1977) identified seven tasks for families with an ill member, and other authors have described similar ones (Butcher, 1994; Canam, 1993; Hanson, 1987; Strauss et al., 1984). The tasks can be applied to client and families in both institutional and community settings and circumstances. See box on page 477.

Preserving emotional balance. Preserving a reasonable emotional balance is very difficult when the chronically ill member's health can change hourly, taking family members' emotions

---

ADJUSTMENT TASKS FOR FAMILIES WITH AN ILL MEMBER

1. Preserving a reasonable emotional balance
2. Preserving a satisfactory self-image
3. Preserving relationships with family and friends
4. Preparing for an uncertain future
5. Dealing with pain and incapacitation
6. Dealing with the treatment environment and special treatment procedures
7. Developing adequate relationships with professional staff

Adapted from "The crisis of physical illness: An overview" (p. 9) by R.H. Moos & V.D. Tsu, 1977, In R.H. Moos, (Ed.), *Coping with physical illness*. New York: Plenum. Copyright 1977 by Plenum Medical Book Co. Adapted by permission.

---

on a roller coaster ride of despair and hope. Members of the family may react very differently to events and are often at different stages in their adjustment to changed priorities and lifestyle. Difficulties with the health care system can create extra frustration.

Preserving a satisfactory self-image. The family identity is threatened when a member has an illness or disability, because all members of the family acquire a social stigma. They are associated with someone who is not normal, not healthy, and thus considered deviant in our society. Not only do others regard them differently, but the family members have similar stigmas against their own relative and must incorporate both into the family identity. The family's history of competence in coping with difficult situations and personal expectations of the unit's future ability to adjust will affect the sense of group self-esteem. The extent of knowledge about the situation, the existing skills of family members, and the degree of commitment to adjust to the situation can threaten or reinforce family confidence.

Preserving relationships with family and friends. People tend to grieve by themselves — some openly tearful, some stoic, some focused on action. The sharing of loss expressed in so many different forms is difficult. If the sharing does not

occur, distances will develop within the family, and it will be more difficult for members to comfort one another. Positive adjustment to the changing capacities of family members requires sensitivity and flexibility in the reallocation of roles and responsibilities within the family. In some families these changes can be negotiated openly. In others, one member decides how the functions are reassigned. The families that retain rigid role expectations in spite of the changing situation will experience much frustration. Disagreements over changing responsibilities may occur frequently, increasing the distance between family members. Illness is difficult for friends to accept as well. Uncertainty about what to say or what to do may prevent friends from visiting or cause the family to isolate itself. Unexpected events may prevent the family from returning visits or sharing activities, so the frequency of contacts with friends or supportive groups in the community may decrease.

Preparing for an uncertain future. One of the hardest tasks required of families with an ill or disabled member is preparing for an uncertain future. If a chronic disability or condition is stable, there is often confidence that life will return to the family's adjusted "normal," so the stress is lessened and made manageable. When the affected person has an unstable condition such as cancer or Alzheimer's disease, uncertainty about the future may be so intense or constant that the situation requires hourly adjustment. It is difficult to plan holidays, plan an evening out, or even plan the dinner meal when symptoms are unpredictable. Even if the future of the affected person is predictable, events that occur to other family members are always a source of uncertainty, such as job loss, children acting out, or illness of a second family member. Outside assistance may be required to cope.

Dealing with pain and incapacitation. Pain and deteriorating abilities are associated with many chronic illnesses. Much symptom management tries to address these problems. Sometimes the pain and incapacitation are a direct result of the treatment received for the chronic condition. People who are admitted to a hospital may become worse while there. They become more malnourished or more ill from side effects of medicines or interventions such as chemotherapy or surgery. Clients and families must be convinced that the suffering will mean better health in the future to consent to and adjust to these negative effects of therapy.

Dealing with the treatment environment and special treatment procedures. Someone who has had experience with a health institution before may be more relaxed or may have increased fear. People who are used to a quiet life without too many interpersonal contacts may consider a hospital to be like Grand Central Station. In addition to the symptoms they have to endure, they may be exhausted just by the environment. Knowing the unwritten rules for behavior, how to obtain satisfaction from the bureaucracy, and how to interpret all of the forms is essential for a satisfactory adjustment to any type of health care. Very few community or institutional organizations provide coaching on these topics for clients or family members.

Developing adequate relationships with professional staff. Clients and families learn very quickly that if they follow the unwritten rules, they will be treated well. If they thank professionals for their trouble, even if it hurts, if they are never irritable, if they are always understanding of late responses to call lights or phone calls, then all will be well. The needs of health personnel to feel useful and appreciated will be met, but client and family needs for information or for appropriate care may not be met. When fear of negative reprisals from health care staff prevents a client or family from expressing their needs or their responses to care, effective therapeutic interactions can not occur. It is unfortunate that professionals sometimes impose these expectations on people who are already coping with significant stresses.

Families that have internal resources or access to external resources are able to cope with these seven challenges in ways that are supportive of family members and the unit as a whole. Families that have many sources of stress and are unable to access the external resources they require will be ineffective in meeting these tasks. These families will have difficulty establishing their own priorities and will also have difficulty in relationships with health personnel. See Family

Responses to Health Professionals later in this chapter.

Family Responses to Chronic Illness or Disability

People adjust to illness or disability by developing behavior patterns. Those patterns are selected, consciously or subconsciously, to meet basic needs (Lantican, Birdwell, & Harrell, 1994). For effective nursing interventions to occur, client and family choices and behavior must be accepted and understood, and the nursing actions must be directed at meeting the underlying needs of that client or family.

Some of the determining characteristics that influence health behaviors include age, sex, socioeconomic status, cultural background, past experience with the health care system, and the perceived meaning of the condition. There are remarkable similarities among authors in the listing of these influencing factors (Azjen & Fishbein, 1980; Moos & Tsu, 1977; Orem, 1991).

An individual's initial adjustment period is around 6 weeks when a chronic illness or disability is diagnosed. During this time a dynamic testing of responses and coping mechanisms occurs by the individual and the family, according to the knowledge, capabilities, and preferences of each. Within 6 weeks, the situation has usually stabilized, and family life has settled into a fairly permanent pattern of behavior. Knafl and Deatrick (1986) have explored the concept of normalization in their attempt to understand these permanent behavioral patterns of families. They articulated three different response types: normalization, disassociation, and denial. This author has added a fourth category, that of overcompensation. Conflict occurs when members of the same family have different responses, or when the client or family selects a response with which health professionals disagree. All four response types have the defining criteria articulated by Knafl and Deatrick (1986); acknowledgment of the impairment, definition of family life, social significance of the impairment, and behavioral strategies (see Table 21-1).

Normalization. **Normalization** is the response most health professionals consider the

TABLE 21-1 Family responses to chronic illness or disability

Type of response	Defining criteria			
	Impairment acknowledged	Definition of family life	Social significance of impairment	Behavioral strategies
Normalization	Yes	Normal	Minimal	Show normalcy
Disassociation	Yes	Abnormal	Very significant	Show abnormality
Denial	No	Normal	None	Show normalcy
Overcompensation	Yes	Normal	Very significant	Show abnormality

Adapted from K.A. Knafl & J.A. Deatrick, 1986, "How families manage chronic conditions: An analysis of the concept of normalization" by *Research in Nursing and Health, 9,* p. 220.

ideal. Recognition of the impairment is shown when the client or family seeks professional help for symptoms that cannot be handled independently. Family life, priorities, and activities remain normal, as they were before the impairment, with adjustments made for the differing skills and abilities of the affected person. Explanation of the impairment to others occurs matter-of-factly because the social significance is minimal (Baker & Stern, 1993; Knafl & Deatrick, 1986). See Case Study on page 482.

Disassociation. This response frustrates health professionals. In **disassociation,** the client or family acknowledges the impairment and gives it great social significance. Family life is considered very different because of this impairment, and behavioral strategies selected demonstrate the abnormality. They disassociate from "normal" families by choice and may even disassociate from similarly affected families. The impairment has changed their world, and life rotates around the affected member and the special activities required (Knafl & Deatrick, 1986).

These clients and families can show their disassociative response in two different ways. The impairment may be considered so unique that it has made them very special, so they believe special consideration is deserved in all contacts with the health care system and society. Failure of others to consider their unique needs will be interpreted as a lack of understanding of the significance of their concerns. The client's or family's sense of identity and self-esteem is centered in the dependent or the caregiving role, and any questioning of their choices may be interpreted as personal threat or rejection. These clients and families may be very fussy about the care received, may complain frequently, and may seek health care assistance on the slightest provocation. The second kind of disassociative response is not as visible. These clients and families consider the impairment to be very terrible and very socially significant. It may be concealed from as many people as possible. They will avoid talking about it but will readily admit that family life is not "normal" and that their activities rotate around the need to preserve equilibrium in the presence of the impairment. People with this type of disassociative response may have an alcoholic family member or one who is mentally ill. A person with situational depression related to an impairment would also fit into this category. Others who try to minimize the significance just do not understand what life is like trying to live with it. Identity has been consumed by the impairment, accomplishments are trivialized, and compliments are rejected.

Denial. The third response category identified by Knafl and Deatrick (1986) is **denial.** These clients and families do not acknowledge the impairment, so family life is normal, it has no social significance, and all behaviors are as they were before the event with the family showing normalcy. There are reasons for the conscious or unconscious selection of denial as a long-term response. If the implications of the diagnosis are too great and there are other pressures in addi-

— RESEARCH ❦ HIGHLIGHT —

Stress in Children With Asthma

Eighty-four children (48 boys and 36 girls) with asthma (documented allergies to environmental agents) between the ages of 8 and 13 ($\overline{X} = 10.5$), assented to respond to the Feel Bad Scale (FBS), an instrument that measures children's perspectives of the frequency and severity of stressors they experience other than their asthma. Criteria from the National Heart, Lung, and Blood Institute served as a guide for the distribution of subjects in relation to age, grade, gender, ethnicity, and asthma severity. It was determined that the children did not differ from nonparticipants with respect to demographic variables, and although the sample was nonrandom, it was viewed as fairly representative of children with asthma. Duncan's Socioeconomic Index was used to determine that parental employment represented all levels of socioeconomic status.

The children completed the instrument in groups at their own pace, but the items were read to the 8- and 9-year-old children. Group scores were compared on age, gender, ethnicity, and severity of illness, item mean scores for frequency and severity of stressors were ranked, and the frequency and severity of specific items related to gender were compared. While mean frequency scale scores did not differ, the one exception to no significant differences in the severity scale scores was gender in that girls recorded significantly higher mean scores than boys. Feeling left out of the group and not being good enough at sports were serious stressors for both genders, but an item analysis disclosed that the stressor feeling left out of the group occurred significantly more often for girls than for boys.

Because the mean scores for frequency and severity did not significantly differ from the scores of the original sample, these results suggested that children with asthma experience similar levels of stress as their peers and perceive the stressors in much the same way. Children with and without asthma reported "feeling sick" as the most frequently reported stressor, and pressure to try something new and having parents separate as most severe although not experienced very frequently.

Possible reasons for these results were explored from a developmental standpoint because children experience stressors related to self-concept and school, family, and peer relationships, and in this instance, they have the added stressor of illness. It is within this context that children with asthma should be considered by parents, teachers, and health professionals. Nurses, in providing guidance for care, could possibly reduce or minimize potential conflicts by exploring parents' and children's concerns associated with the resumption of activities. In addition, plans for intervention could extend to the school system to educate teachers-coaches not only about the health problem and measures for intervention (*i.e.*, exercise-induced asthma), but also in regard to coping strategies to modify school-peer related stressors. Peers should also be included because of the significance of peer contingency and shared stressors. Further research is required, perhaps on a longitudinal level, to explore the reasons for childrens' choices and to use other instruments to ascertain perceptions in similar situations.

From "Sources of stress in children with asthma" by M. Walsh & N.M. Ryan-Wenger, 1992, *Journal of School Health, 62*(10), 459-463.

tion to this health problem, the diagnosis may be denied to maintain equilibrium (Whyte, 1992). People tend to postpone bad news for as long as possible. Admitting to the diagnosis may also mean admitting several other needs: for lifestyle change, for dietary change, for altered roles, for a different future, for change of occupation, for financial insecurity, or more. Individuals and families have resources to adjust to only a few events

at the same time. It may be too stressful to adjust to all implications at once. When circumstances change that increase the energy available within the family, or when symptoms become so severe that the diagnosis cannot be denied any longer, then the behavior pattern will change. Professional intervention will have very little effect until the client or family is ready to listen.

Denial is not a common response. Avoidance

behaviors may be part of a disassociative or over-compensatory behavior pattern. Sometimes avoidance of the issue reflects a focus on normalization through attempts to plan for the future. Health professionals are very quick to label people as being in denial when they appear to be coping "too well" and do not want to talk about the condition. The difficulty is sometimes within the health professional. Identifying with the client, the professional cannot imagine making a personal adjustment of that magnitude and so cannot accept the apparently calm approach of the client or family as being normalization. The difference is that people denying the impairment do not seek any assistance from the health care system for difficulties, and the normalizing client or family will seek assistance when necessary.

Overcompensation. A fourth category of response to chronic illness or disability, added by this author, is that of **overcompensation.** These clients and families acknowledge the impairment, consider it to have great social significance, and try to maintain as normal a family life as possible. The distinguishing feature is that the behavior emphasizes the "abnormality." Because of the perceived deficiency in one aspect of life, the client or family strives for excellence in another aspect. Someone with a handicapping condition may decide to undertake a task to emphasize how well they are coping, for example, a one-legged person participating in a cross country run, a blind person enrolling in accounting courses, or a child with asthma excelling at athletics. The demonstration of this excellence becomes the driving force and center of the individual or family's existence.

These four response types are presented to assist nurses in understanding the behavior patterns of chronically ill clients and their families, not as a rigid categorization of people. If nurses can identify the client and family patterns, then goals for intervention will be more reasonable, and the nurse will be less frustrated when there is no behavior change. See the following Case Study of family responses to childhood asthma.

Family Resources

In studies of physiologic conditions, more studies have focused on pathology than on normal conditions, and the situation is similar for family research, which has focused on dysfunctional families. The psychology, sociology, health, and family therapy descriptions of healthy family functioning, however, are remarkably similar, even in the absence of definitive research. All families must have access to internal and external resources to perform the tasks required of them and adjust to the unpredictable events that occur within and to families. See Chapter 18 for more details.

Basic resources required for all families are a source of income, adequate housing, and food. Internal resources include the attitudes, skills, and knowledge of the individual members. Previous experience with similar events, previously successful coping strategies, and a belief that the family will be able to adjust are all internal strengths (Linsey & Hills, 1992). Health professionals must respect these resources to gain entry to the family system. When the family recognizes that internal resources are insufficient to meet the demands placed on the unit, then they may seek external assistance. If a family assumes all responsibility for the care of the ill member, refusing offers of help from anyone, stress and frustration may increase for all. Being able to request help is a strength.

The balance maintained between informal and formal sources of help is also an indication of healthy functioning. Informal external resources available to families include extended family members, friends, neighbors, and community groups. If informal resources are relied on very heavily for a long period, caregiver exhaustion may occur. The family may also turn to formal sources of external help such as the health care system. If the family relies entirely on formal sources for help, however, their sense of competence will not grow, and dependence will be the result. A balance between formal and informal sources of help can relieve the family of some tasks but will also support decision-making and competence.

Caregiver Burden

Caregiver burden is a perception that the caregiving responsibilities have negative effects on the emotional or physical health of the caregiver. That perception is most important when held by

■ CASE STUDY

A group of school-aged children had spent much time together in asthma self-management classes sponsored by the Lung Association. The families had been encouraged to enroll their children by the physicians from the Pediatric Asthma Clinic. The wind-up for the classes was a family picnic, to which all of the parents and siblings were invited. It was to be held in a local park where flowers were in bloom. Birch tree pollen and cottonwood fluff would also be a difficulty, but the setting had a playground with a baseball diamond, and many physical activities were planned. Four of the families responded very differently.

Johnny's family was pleased to have the invitation. His parents had been encouraging Johnny to take more responsibility for his health for some time, and they saw this as an opportunity for him to try his new skills in self-assessment and decision-making. He would have to take his inhaler with him, but his parents, as usual, expected him to participate in as many physical activities as he could for as long as he thought he could. They would make sure that the car was parked close to the picnic site in case he had some problems and needed to go to the hospital, but they did not anticipate trouble. He had been on picnics before and really enjoyed playing softball.

Mario's family was very upset with the invitation to the picnic. They had avoided outdoor family activities since his diagnosis with asthma, particularly at this time of year, and thought it an unfair request. Mario had received permission from his teachers not to join in physical activities at school because he was likely to have an attack of asthma, and so the planned picnic activities also worried them. They had enrolled Mario in the self-management classes because he still needed to have his mother beside him to help him handle attacks, and they thought he might feel more secure if he knew more. His mother still intended to make all of the assessment and treatment decisions.

Janine's mother looked at the invitation and knew that it would be impossible to get there. She had enrolled Janine in the classes because the doctor insisted, but she was convinced that they were not relevant. Janine had not gained anything from the classes. She had not made any new friends and saw no reason to change anything she was doing. They both considered the breathing troubles just severe colds with a sudden onset, impossible to prevent anyway. Janine's mother had to work on the day of the picnic, and with the two younger children in day care, it would be unfair to ask the sitter to take all three to the picnic. Re-

the primary family caregiver but is also valid when held by other relatives or professionals who know the family. Situational, behavioral characteristics, and caregiver perceptions indicating vulnerability to caregiver burden and breakdown are listed in box on page 484. Predicting whether the primary caregiver in a family will feel burdened is difficult. The presence of several of these characteristics does not necessarily mean that caregiver burden exists. There may be no burden felt if the caregiver's whole identity rests in the "martyrdom" of giving service to another. However, these characteristics do serve as a red flag for professionals who are attempting to prevent family breakdown. If the client and the family have different responses to the chronic illness or disability, there will be conflict. The client who wants to normalize his or her life may become increasingly frustrated with the enforced

helplessness imposed by a caregiver who is very protective and believes that helping means doing everything for the other person. The stress of the helping relationship for the caregiver may lead to a sense of burden, of not being appreciated, or of being confined to the caregiving role (Reinhard, 1994; Whyte, 1992). If there is agreement of the response, such as the whole family disassociating, caregiver burden may still exist because of the losses incurred to maintain intense focus on the ill person. Losses could include minimal social activities, private time, or personal rewards, in addition to the physical or emotional exhaustion of caregiving duties.

It must be remembered that the use of negative terminology such as burden, strain, and guilt tends to camouflage the positive impact of caregiving relationships. The process of giving care to a loved one can be fulfilling, satisfying, and an

cently separated, she did not want to ask Janine's father because it wasn't that important.

Sara and her family were eager to go to the picnic. She was anxious to show her new friends how well she could play softball. She had managed her own symptoms for 2 years, so the classes were a refresher for her. Sara's parents insisted that she maintain normal activities, believing that if she put her lungs under stress they would improve. The logical outcome was her commitment to school and community sports. She had placed in the city-wide track and field competition for sprints, and her softball team was doing well in its division. Sara insisted on being treated like everyone else and excused herself to go to the bathroom when she needed her inhaler.

Mr. Brant, the nurse who had conducted the asthma self-management classes, intervened with these families according to their response to the chronicity of the asthma. Johnny and his parents were praised for their realistic attitude, which normalized life for their family. They were aware of possible risks and took precautions, but they did not let the asthma interfere with "normal" activities. The disassociative response of Mario's family was harder to address. Mr. Brant informed Mario's mother of her son's increased knowl-

edge level, shown by his behavior at the classes. He supported her concern for her son and listened to her objections to the picnic. The nurse also clearly stated his own opinion that Mario could attend the picnic because he was capable of deciding when he needed help. Janine's mother was difficult to reach for confirmation of attendance at the picnic. When Mr. Brant finally contacted her, it was the day before the picnic, and too late to make alternative child care and transportation arrangements. The denial response of this family was not confronted. Information about asthma, the value of the classes for Janine, and the availability of the nurse was repeated as the conversation was closed. Sara and her family were excited to receive the nurse's call. Mr. Brant listened patiently to their descriptions of how well she would play ball at the picnic. He attempted to minimize the overcompensation response by emphasizing Sara's high scores on the asthma class quiz and praising her positive relationships with the other children. Mr. Brant reminded himself that the role of the nurse is to facilitate healthy choices when the family is open to change and to support families when they are not ready for change by accepting their behavior and informing them of options.

---

opportunity for building personal and family relationships (Findeis et al., 1994). No assumptions should be made about the negative impact of a situation until perceptions are validated with family members.

Assessment Questions as Intervention

Intervention begins as soon as the nurse has contact with the family. The process of needs assessment is an intervention because the family has requested and accepted assistance from a resource external to the family. A home visit is validation of their self-assessment that formal help is required. Whether the admission form is filled in by the client or by the nurse, the process of answering the questions indicates to the family the facts that are considered to be important for their care. If they feel that some of the data are not relevant, they may refuse to provide the in-

formation. It is the nurse's responsibility to explain how the information will be helpful in designing the care plan. The family members will immediately sense whether their opinions are respected and will decide whether to continue contact with this agency.

The assessment of family functioning is difficult. Nurses with chronically ill clients require much more information about family structure, dynamics, and goals than nurses caring for clients with an acute, time-limited illness. Chronically ill clients are or will become experts on their disease, its effect on the family, and the usefulness of the health care system in helping them adjust to living with that disease. Nurses who provide effective care base interventions on the family's perceptions, the family's reality, and the family's hopes for the future. This information is not usually obtained from traditional admission forms.

VULNERABILITY FOR CAREGIVER BURDEN AND BREAKDOWN

Situational factors:

Sharing a household with the dependent

Financial loss for the family

Dangerous behavior of the dependent to self or others

Mental impairment of the dependent

Incontinence of bowel or bladder of the dependent

Unacceptable changes in roles and responsibilities

Isolation of the family by relatives, community, or by choice

Disturbance of caregiver's sleep

Embarrassment of the caregiver

Angry, uncooperative behavior of the dependent

Continuous questions from the dependent

Day wandering by the dependent

Physical assistance required for dependent's walking and transfers

Caregiver or family behaviors:

Lack of knowledge about illness, causes, prognosis, or behavioral implications

Inability to make decisions

Unequal balance of formal and informal supports to assist family

Denial of need for personal time or rewards

Rigidity of role expectations

Members not supportive of one another

History of faulty interpersonal relationships

Caregiver or family perceptions:

Chronically unexpressed feelings of anger, anxiety, guilt, or despair

Being afraid to leave the dependent alone

Sense of being tied down by caregiving responsibilities

Perception that caregiving responsibilities interfere with social life

No good things perceived in caregiver role

Perception that caregiving can only continue for short time longer

Perception that help is needed but unavailable

Conviction that dependent would be better off living elsewhere

Identity defined primarily as caregiver role or as sick role

Low self-esteem and self-confidence

Low motivation and pessimism

Sense of having lost control of one's life

Belief in self or family as basically unhealthy, unsatisfied, or unfulfilled

---

Indirect questions can give the nurse a sense of family priorities and whether relationships are positive, negative, or neutral. Watson and her colleagues at the Family Nursing Unit at the University of Calgary in Alberta, Canada, use assessment questions that are, intentionally, also nursing interventions (1987). These approaches provide the nurse with important information but also require family members to regard their situation from different perspectives, to identify implications of their responses to events, and to articulate their hopes. In this way, the nurse encourages the client and family to grow in self-understanding and be open to alternative methods of coping with their situation. See examples in box on page 485.

Differences. Questions that explore differences give information about which aspects of the current situation are most important to the family. These questions also enable families to

identify their sources of frustration in dealing with a chronically ill member. The differences can be in time, in relationships, or in perceptions.

Triadic. These questions obtain information about relationships among family members by asking one person what he or she thinks about other members of the family. The answer requires some reflection about the priorities of others, which may be different from the priorities of the person being interviewed.

Hypothetical. People are asked to imagine other realities with this type of question. It gives them a chance to articulate their expectations of the future and gives the nurse an insight into their perspective on the present. Sometimes learning needs are shown.

Catastrophic expectation. When people are frustrated or discouraged, sometimes it helps to remind them of their strengths. One way to force

ASSESSMENT QUESTIONS AS INTERVENTION

Difference questions:

How is your husband different now compared with last month?

> Since he had the stroke, I have to help him get dressed and go to the bathroom, walk beside him, and bathe him.

Five years ago, what did you think your life would be like now?

> We thought that after he retired we would travel in the motorhome, visit the children, and see new places.

Triadic questions:

What does your mother like most about caring for your father since his stroke?

> She knows what he needs and is glad to be there whenever he wants help.

What does your father like most about being cared for by your mother?

> She is there whenever he needs her, and he isn't embarrassed when she gives him care.

Do you think your mother will go away for a holiday, as you've been telling her to do?

> No, I guess not. She is giving him better care than anyone else can, and she feels good about doing it.

Hypothetical question:

What do you think will be happening a year from now?

> I expect Dad will be in a long-term care facility because Mom will have worn herself out.

Catastrophic expectation questions:

You are very worried about your mother becoming exhausted. What is the worst thing that could happen?

> If she needs to go to the hospital because her angina came back, it would be bad.

What would you do then?

> I guess I would call my sister, and we would figure out a way of taking care of Dad until Mom was able to do it again. I think we could work something out, maybe using the home care agency.

That sounds reasonable. What can you do to prevent your Mom's angina from coming back?

> I should ask her if she's been to the doctor lately. She does know when to take those pills. Maybe I don't need to worry. She knows how to take care of herself.

---

a client to think positively is to ask what the very worst outcome of the present situation would be and then ask what the client would do. When the reply is made, it is easy to reinforce assessment and problem-solving skills and to praise the identified coping mechanisms. The client may then feel more self-confidence in facing an uncertain future.

PLANNING

Community nurses are often reluctant to draw conclusions about a family on receiving a referral or even after the first contact. It is indeed respectful of the family to validate all information and particularly to validate impressions of others about the family. A comprehensive assessment of any family will occur over a period and will most likely use several contacts with different members and both objective and subjective data. Nevertheless, it is important to use nursing time effectively for the client's benefit as well as that of the employing agency. Planning a working relationship with a family must consider the legitimacy of the professional contact, the point of entry into the family, the attitudes of the family toward outside help, the timing of the professional contact, and the approach to be used.

Legitimacy of Helper

Before entering the family constellation in an ongoing relationship, it is essential to consider the legitimacy of the professional involvement. Orem (1991) has described the legitimacy of the nursing role. There are differences between categories in the degree of nursing involvement in family activities, the commitment held by the family to the interaction, and the likelihood of attaining goals. In the *wholly compensatory* nursing system, the nurse provides complete care to a client or family temporarily or permanently incapable of independently managing activities of daily living. The client or family gives legitimacy to the nurse role by abdicating all responsibility for assessing needs, making decisions, or doing any of the care themselves. An unconscious client or chaotic family without relatives or friends nearby would be in this situation. When activities to maintain health are shared by the client or family and the nurse, a *partially compensatory* nursing system is in effect. Legitimacy arises from the mutual consent to share responsibilities. Most nurse-client and nurse-family relationships fall into this category. When the nurse is in a *supportive-educative* role, the client or family is independent in activities of daily living. The nurse's role is outside, not within, the family structure and occurs in two sets of circumstances. Legitimacy could come from the family's request for information or guidance regarding a particular aspect of their life. Goals may be mutually set and evaluated if there is joint commitment to their attainment. The nurse also functions in a supportive-educative role when responding to potential or actual health needs that the client or family is not yet ready to address. Legitimacy then comes from the professional responsibility of nursing to promote health. Information to increase awareness of risk factors and the assurance of availability of the nurse is all that can be provided legitimately. Any other actions done for that family are nurse-centered, fulfilling the nurse's need to "do something." The client and family have a right to refuse intervention. Actions not respectful of the client's and family's wishes may alienate them. If the family has not admitted a need for help, or if they have not selected the nurse as the professional to deliver that help, then chances of their behavior changing are very low. Nursing goals should be restricted to promoting awareness and trust. When the family recognizes a need and invites the nurse to assist, an active role within the family is legitimized (Luker & Chalmers, 1990).

Point of Entry

The point of entry into the family may be the client with the chronic illness or another family member. The nurse must discover enough about the family to determine the roles each family member assumes. If the person who is the point of entry has no power or influence on decisions that are made regarding the topic in question, then continuing with that person as the primary contact may not be beneficial. For example, if a child is found to have diabetes, the first point of entry into the family may be the child. It is obvious, however, that much of the teaching will be done with the parents. Teaching about medications may use one parent or family member as the point of entry, but coverage of expenses might be a topic that requires the other parent's or another family member's involvement.

Attitudes Toward Being Helped

Independence is precious. Most people are reluctant to admit a need for help, reluctant to request help, and sometimes reluctant to accept help. The helping relationship is complex, because it has implications for self-image, coping styles, and relationships with others. When a nurse identifies a client or family in need, the attitudes toward help must be assessed to plan effective nursing interventions. The goal of the nurse is to assist in a manner that leaves the client or family more competent, more knowledgeable, or more self-confident than they were before the intervention. It is therefore imperative that planning respect the client's and family's attitudes, goals, priorities, and behaviors. A client or family that has requested help has already made many decisions that must be respected by the nurse (see box on page 487).

Recognizing a need for help. Some people may not be able to compare their situation to that of others and may honestly not recognize a need for help. It could be that their life is in so much disarray that they don't know where to start first or that they despair of anything making a difference. They may have no idea what type of assistance would fit their situation. Perhaps so much help is needed or it is so urgent that it is useless to ask. They may feel that if they start to receive help, they would then need it forever, so they may want to postpone admitting the need as long as they possibly can.

Requesting help. People may be reluctant to request help for several different reasons. They may be convinced that the type of help they

HELP QUESTIONS

Recognizing a need for help

1. Do I need help?
2. Will help make any difference?
3. What kind of help do I need?
4. How much help do I need?
5. When do I need the help?
6. For how long will I need this help?

Requesting help

7. Is the type of help I need available?
8. Where can I get this help?
9. How much will this help cost?
10. Do I have to ask for the help?

Accepting help

11. How will I explain receiving this help to others?
12. How will this help make me stronger?
13. Can I accept the help?

---

need is not available or that they cannot choose from so many sources of help. A major factor for many people is the potential cost of requesting help. Even in Canada, health insurance coverage varies from one province to another, and the indirect costs of care like travel, supplies, and lost wages are seldom covered. If the help is expected to be more than the family can afford, often the request is not made. Another impediment is simply having to ask. When someone offers help, it is easier to accept it. Many people consider requesting assistance to be admitting defeat or incompetence.

Accepting help. Even when people have admitted a need and requested the help, sometimes they still refuse the help when it comes. It may be because it carries a stigma, and they are afraid of what neighbors or family will think. A socially acceptable explanation for the help is needed before they are willing to accept it. In an effective helping relationship, the family needs to feel good about receiving the help and be able to justify it to themselves. If they feel worse because they are receiving the help, the relationship between the family and the nurse will be difficult. It is important to emphasize the strengths of individuals and the family system in each nursing in-

teraction with family members. Careful planning that respects the decisions already made by the client and family before they come for help will contribute to effective nursing interventions (Price, 1993; Robinson, 1994).

Timing of Nursing Actions

A sense of timing is best learned from experience, so it is difficult for the beginning practitioner to develop. Timing must be considered in relation to the events that are happening to that family, and the timing of a particular approach must be considered in relation to the family's level of functioning during interaction with the nurse.

Timing in relation to significant events for families. All families and individuals develop behavior patterns that serve them more or less effectively. Human beings are creatures of habit and move out of their traditional response patterns reluctantly. Whenever a significant event occurs in the family, those stable patterns are interrupted. Major points in the developmental stages of individual and family life, such as marriage, first child starting or leaving school, retirement, or death of a spouse all require adjustments. Unexpected events such as loss of job, sudden changes in income, change of residence, or trouble raising children also require adjustment. Changes require reevaluation of personal and family philosophy, priorities, communications, roles, and responsibilities. The search for effective ways of handling the situation may include seeking more knowledge about the event, its implications for behavior and roles, and the predictability of the future. The individual and family members search for coping mechanisms that will best suit their situation and priorities, such as the balance between resources internal and external to the family. There is a 6-week period when the family unit and individual members are uncertain about their behavior, trying one approach, then another. Some people may go into crisis if their perception of the situation, social supports, and coping mechanisms cannot sustain their adjustment to the new circumstances (Aguilera & Messick, 1986). Most people manage to adjust since during this 6-week period they are more open to suggestion, more eager to learn, and more willing to try new approaches. Maximum benefit can be gained from information and alternatives presented at this point, because the clients are ready to act.

In addition to responding to the above life-cycle or situational events, the person with chronic illness also has equilibrium disturbed whenever a significant event occurs in relation to the illness. Important events on the illness trajectory include diagnosis, hospital admissions, hospital discharges, remissions or exacerabations in the disease, and significant changes in medical treatment or health care services required (Strauss et al., 1984). There is a 6-week window of opportunity during the adjustment period when the family and its members are more open to learning about the illness, about their responses to the event, and about new coping mechanisms. At times other than these, families with a chronically ill or disabled member will have a fairly stable pattern of behavior in response to their situation. See the section on responses to chronic illness above. The supportive-educative intervention of health professionals will not be effective at changing the primary response pattern during these stable periods but may increase awareness of need for change. When the family is at a transition point because of a developmental, situational, or illness-related event, the actions of health professionals are more influential because clients and family members are searching for new responses and understandings to guide them in the future. Goals can be more ambitious, because the clients are ready to change.

Timing in relation to family level of functioning. Wright and Leahey (1984) developed a simple framework to assist nurses in planning specific approaches to use with families at particular times. It is based on an assessment of the level of functioning of the individual or family unit according to the predominance of the affective, behavioral, or cognitive domain. A person or family functioning in one domain is entirely preoccupied with concerns in that domain. Attempts to intervene in any other domain will be ineffective because the person's attention and energy just isn't there (Baker & Stern, 1993). Nurses must respect the family's priorities and match the approach used to the current domain

of functioning to be recognized as a helper and trusted by the family. After the family or the individual has connected with the nurse and a trusting relationship has been earned, a shift to another level of functioning may be possible.

People functioning at the *affective* level are completely absorbed in their emotional reaction to the situation. They may be displaying behaviors of anxiety, fear, excitement, joy, or anger. It will be impossible to establish a relationship with them until the nurse has validated those feelings as legitimate and provided the family or person an opportunity to talk about them. Affective behaviors are easily validated by reflective comments that describe behavior or appearance, such as "You look sad today" or "You are very angry." When the individual recognizes that someone has heard them and considers their concerns legitimate, it may be possible to concentrate on learning new information or planning future actions.

The *behavioral* level of functioning is often used by people who cope with stress by doing things rather than by talking about feelings. These people may be absorbed in making arrangements to maintain family activities as much as possible, in keeping to a daily routine in the institution, or in making appointments to obtain more information about the event. Action is comforting for these people, and any nursing intervention that does not relate to action will be interpreted as irrelevant to their concerns. Nurses must validate the preoccupation with action by supporting client decisions regarding priority actions, suggesting alternative people to see or things to do, or, if the family wishes, assuming some responsibility for tasks that need to be done. Only when the nurse accepts the focus of the individual or family on action and responds in kind will the timing of the intervention be appropriate.

The *cognitive* level of functioning is the level at which learning occurs. Many nursing interventions that teach people about the illness or disability are ineffective because the timing is incorrect. If the family is focused on affective or behavioral concerns, their attention will not be on the content of the nurse's teaching. It will be on the mismatch of the nurse's approach to their current concerns. It will be impossible to establish a trusting relationship, and the teaching will be ineffective. When the individual or family have their perceptions and focus validated as appropriate, relaxation and trust are more likely. They will be more open to learning and more able to identify the type of information that will be most useful to them. Their learning needs may be understanding the normalcy of their own behavior and the responses of others in their network or knowledge about the illness event or the treatment required.

The timing of nursing contact with the family determines the priority nursing diagnosis, the goals for nursing interaction, and the nursing approach most likely to be effective in assisting the family.

Priority Nursing Diagnoses

It is important to make nursing diagnoses even before first contact with a family to provide a focus for the first visit. Nursing diagnoses are not final conclusions about the health status of a family; they are tentative guesses about the reasons for strengths and limitations of family functioning. Nursing diagnoses are fluid, dynamic, and continually changing as more information about the family becomes available and as circumstances and priorities change for that family. For a detailed discussion of nursing diagnoses see Chapter 5.

The traditional approach to the selection of priority nursing diagnoses has been for nurses, as the health experts, to define them and evaluate them. It is increasingly recognized that this approach does not work. Consumerism and self-care movements have acquired credibility. A client will refuse care perceived as irrelevant. The most effective nursing diagnoses are identified by the client, who may also have opinions on alternative actions available and the type of help required. The nurse who ignores client opinions shows lack of respect for client self-assessment and goals and cannot develop an effective therapeutic relationship. Therefore, the client or family's priority should be the first nursing diagnosis (Baker & Stern, 1993; Bond, Phillips, & Rollins, 1994). Community nurses may identify additional diagnoses that are not yet recognized as valid by

the client, based on research or past experience with similar families. These additional diagnoses should be noted in the client's record. They give other health professionals valuable insights into the functioning of the family and provide direction for future actions that may promote family competence. These nurse-framed diagnoses are only one professional's opinion, however, and require validation by the family before definitive action is taken. When working with the chronically ill client and family, patience is one of the most difficult lessons to learn. The nurse cannot move any faster than the client and family are prepared to move. See Chapter 18 for a discussion of families and nursing diagnoses.

IMPLEMENTATION
Purpose of Help

Nursing care for families with a chronically ill member can be described according to the purpose of the help, the strategies used, and the philosophical approach. *Affective assistance* means the primary purpose of help is emotional or social support. Relatives and friends in the informal network are the best source of support that reinforces the self-esteem and emotional well-being of the client or family. Help with the tasks of daily living, such as help with errands, shopping, or personal care, is called *instrumental assistance*. Agencies in the formal network such as community nursing and home support organizations offer instrumental assistance, because the client is a stranger, at least initially. Nevertheless, it is common for family and friends to provide both affective and instrumental support to a chronically ill person, and many close personal relationships develop between official helpers and their clients.

Helping Strategies

Another way of classifying nursing activities is by the strategies used to strengthen the family system. Improving family functioning encourages clients and families to recognize internal strengths and have confidence in their abilities to begin coping with the situation. This strategy could include educating family members about the variety of responses to chronic illness or disability; providing information about the course of action, treatment, and possible implications for family life; encouraging reliance on family support and love; and validating perceptions and responses as understandable and normal. Enlarging the structure of the family increases the internal and external resources available to that family. Examples include encouraging the family to accept offers of help, providing information about or referral to community agencies, or redistributing work among others in the family to reduce the burden on the family caregiver and decrease the sense of helplessness felt by the other members. Decreasing disruption of family life can occur by altering the family's social, economic, professional, or physical environment. Actions may include arranging for changes in hospital visiting hours to make life easier for the family, obtaining reimbursement coverage for a service, advocating for the family with other health professionals or organizations, altering the physical environment with a raised toilet seat, or accessing renovation grant monies for a main floor bathroom or a ramp to the front door. See Chapter 18 for more details.

Approaches to Nursing Care

The provision of care to a chronically ill individual and family can be either nurse-centered or client-centered. Nurse-centered care is initiated by the nurse, done by the nurse, and evaluated by the nurse. The client and family may be consulted regarding the care goals, but they are not considered the experts on what is needed, and decisions about priorities and approaches are made by the nurse. Nurse-centered care is appropriate only when the client or family are unable to perform self-care activities independently and are wholly reliant on the nurse to maintain the client's health and well-being (Orem, 1991).

Client-centered care is much more difficult to provide because the control of what happens is shared. The client and family must be full participants and may even be the initiators of the nurse-client interaction. The family retains control, even if the nurse is providing direct assistance with self-care activities. The family and client make the decisions, do as much as they can, and evaluate whether the care met their needs in a satisfactory manner (Ahmann, 1994;

Robinson, 1994; Trnobranski, 1994). The client and family are the experts on the disease or disability as it affects them, on their responses to the medical regimen, and on the response of the health care system to their needs. The nurse retains expertise on specifics of the illness or disability and its treatment, on the possible future course of the condition, on the adaptations other families have made to similar situations, and on the health services available to meet their needs.

Circular Communication Cycle

The key to any effective nursing approach is communication — how it occurs, the nonverbal messages that reinforce or conflict with the words, and the respect for the participants that is or is not evident. Tomm's **circular communication diagram** is one way of showing the complexities of the client-nurse interaction, and it can also be applied to interaction among family members. As Wright and Leahey (1984) describe Tomm's theory, the process of interaction is the focus, not the content. Interactions tend to become repetitive, stable, and self-regulatory patterns, regardless of which topic is discussed. Each member of a dyad contributes to the effectiveness or the ineffectiveness of that interaction. Nurses participate in the interaction and are either part of the problem or part of the solution. Each person has thoughts and feelings that influence behavior in an interaction. That person's behavior will engender a thought and a feeling in the other person, resulting in a behavior by them. In this way, causality of any problems or successes in the interaction is mutually borne by both participants (see Figure 21-1).

Vicious communication cycle. Whenever nurses place a barrier between themselves and the client, a vicious communication cycle occurs. The many sources of barriers include a stigma, a rumor, a psychiatric label, a preoccupation with personal concerns, fatigue, or boredom. All interfere with the nurse's being fully present, alert, and sensitive to the cues and behavior demonstrated by the client. All interfere with effective interactions. Nurses are often preoccupied with the content of an interaction, teaching plan, or details of a client history and may not pay enough attention to the process. When the nurse

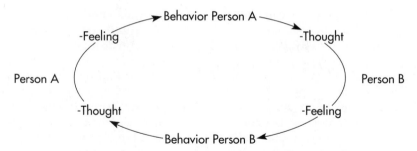

FIGURE 21-1 Circular communication diagram. *(Adapted from* Nurses and families: A guide to family assessment and intervention *(p. 57) by L.M. Wright & M. Leahey, 1984, Philadelphia: F.A. Davis. Copyright 1984 by F.A. Davis Company. Adapted by permission.)*

falls into the trap of responding personally to the client's behavioral symptoms, the nurse is meeting personal needs, not those of the client. A vicious communication cycle is very quickly established. Focusing on changing the behavior of the client will just make both people frustrated and will perpetuate the vicious cycle. The nurse is part of the problem in an interaction that does not work.

Virtuous communication cycle. To change an interaction to a virtuous communication cycle that is effective for both people, the nurse must step back and examine the situation. All human behavior has a reason. The only behavior that the nurse can control is that of the nurse. The key to changing the vicious communication cycle to a virtuous one is for the nurse to stop meeting personal needs and focus on the needs of the client. It requires constant attention to how others may perceive personal behavior. The nurse has a professional responsibility to be part of the solution.

Ineffective communication is often a problem for families with a chronically ill member. People get trapped into a vicious cycle of interaction and do not know how to get out. They focus more and more on their own needs and justifying their own behavior and forget they have some responsibility for things going wrong or not getting better. The role of the nurse is to assist these families to step back and look at what is happening and to assess whether it is possible to alter behavior to enhance family functioning.

EVALUATION OF CARE

People with chronic illness or disability and their families have frequent contacts with the health care system, sometimes for a duration of decades. They become expert at manipulating the bureaucracy to achieve their own needs, and health professionals are often distrustful of them. The traditional role of "expert" has the professional retain control over all aspects of the treatment process. The differing perspectives on who has control and on appropriateness of treatment interfere with effective client-professional interactions. Nursing care should always be evaluated from the initial goals established for the interaction. If the goal is nurse-centered, then it is possible for the goal to be met only by nursing action being taken, regardless of the outcome for the client or the wishes of the family. Nurse-centered goals perpetuate the traditional, expert, nurse-as-doer role, which excludes the client and family from involvement in their own care.

However, there are always two or more perspectives to a situation, so the evaluation of a nurse's interaction with a family must include all points of view. The client, the family caregiver, and the nurse may all have different opinions about the effectiveness of the interactions that have occurred. Each person will match what has happened against the expectations of what should have happened or of what was hoped for. If the goals of all parties were not clarified in the beginning, the nurse may discover that a personal sense of satisfaction with the care delivered has no relevance for clients and family members who feel that their priority needs were not addressed. To maintain a client-centered approach to care, the goals must be client centered: "He will perform this action within one week." The outcome of care should be a family that is more knowledgeable and more competent at handling their own affairs. To ensure that result, the nurse must ensure that the family is intimately involved in the establishment of nursing diagnoses, priorities, intervention strategies, and the evaluation of that care. A self-reliant family will reject efforts that deny them control and involvement but will welcome guidance and facilitation by the nurse who respects their perspectives and decisions.

Family Responses to Health Professionals

People with chronic illness and their families show different attitudes and behaviors when relating to health professionals. Thorne and Robinson (1988) have articulated a framework that helps to explain these differing responses. They interviewed families of chronically ill children and identified three stages in the client or family's relationships with health professionals: naive trust, disenchantment, and guarded alliance.

Naive trust. On first contact with the health care system, the client and family expect to have their opinions regarding diagnosis and treatment listened to and respected. They expect health professionals to be interested in the mechanisms they have developed to deal with symptoms and concerned about the impact of the medical regimen on the daily life of their family. They expect to be part of any decisions made about their care, and they expect health professionals to place importance on how the illness fits into their daily lives. Unfortunately, clients and families usually discover that their trust is ill-founded. Health professionals have their own agenda and their own priorities for treatment, and they are usually not interested in or respectful of the learnings of the client and family regarding the illness and its management at home.

Disenchantment. The client and family slip into the second phase of their relationship with the health care system, **disenchantment,** when they discover that health professionals do not listen to or respect them. They become angry, demanding of information, insistent on participating in decisions regarding treatment, and they may openly disregard professional instructions. The client and family may be unsure of their own expertise but also believe that the health professional cannot be trusted.

Guarded alliance. Some people never move beyond the stage of disenchantment. Most people develop a way of dealing with health professionals that guards their own interests and needs but, of necessity, also forms an alliance with professionals to obtain health system services required. Thorne and Robinson (1989) identify four different approaches to **guarded alliance;** hero worship, resignation, consumerism, and team playing. The approaches can be displayed on a graph with confidence in personal competence on the horizontal axis and trust in the health professional on the vertical axis (see Figure 21-2).

People who adopt a *hero worship* pattern of behavior are convinced that successful handling of the illness is entirely dependent on a single health professional, often a particular physician. They trust completely in that doctor's opinions and actions, and they have low confidence in their own judgment. If that health professional ceases to be available to them, anxiety is very high. They may then have major difficulties in both accessing and accepting services.

People in the *resignation* quadrant have no confidence in health professionals or in themselves. They feel that no one can influence the course of their disease and are resigned to enduring whatever life brings. They lack a sense of control over their world, and if they seek medical help, it is only because it is required to manage symptoms. They have little or no hope and will resist all attempts to build their self-esteem or skills.

Some people with chronic illness or disability adopt behaviors of *consumerism.* They mistrust everyone else and rely on their own investigative and experiential knowledge to guide the manage-

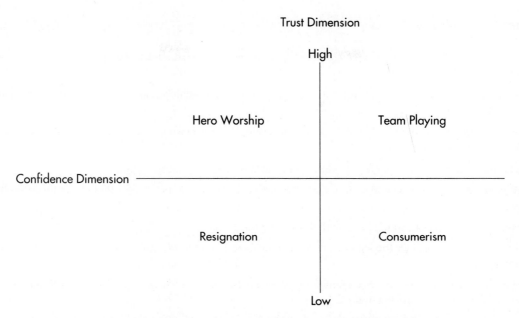

FIGURE 21-2 Dimensions of guarded alliance. *(From "Guarded alliance: Health care relationships in chronic illness" by S.E. Thorne & C.A. Robinson, 1989,* Image: Journal of Nursing Scholarship, Fall 1989, 21*(3), p. 156. Copyright 1989 by Sigma Theta Tau. Reprinted by permission.)*

ment of the condition. Their only contact with health professionals may be to obtain prescriptions they consider necessary and any advice received is not considered reliable. They assume complete responsibility for their own health. They claim personal credit for any successes, but they also accept complete blame if the condition deteriorates. The guilt felt in those circumstances cannot be assuaged.

The most effective response to health care professionals is one of *team playing.* People adopting this response recognize that they have some skills and knowledge and have confidence in their own judgment related to those issues. However, they also recognize that health professionals have areas of expertise and are quite prepared to accept information and consider advice. The key to the concept of mutual trust is the reciprocity of the relationship. The health professional must acknowledge and respect that the person with the illness or disability has expertise in the symptoms, the response to treatment modalities, and the integration of that treatment

regimen into the lifestyle of the family. The client recognizes that the professional has expertise regarding the pathology of the condition, its prognosis, alternative means of treatment, and the side effects and implications of those alternatives. Together, they are able to learn from each other, and more effective, appropriate, and acceptable care should be the result.

The health professional has major responsibility for creating this team playing response that shows mutual trust. People with chronic illness have usually had so many negative experiences with the health care system that they are distrustful. Nurses who use a facilitative, client-centered approach to care have an opportunity to demonstrate respect for client experience, opinions, and knowledge of the condition, thereby earning trust (Robinson, 1994). Clients who respect and trust nurses are more relaxed, more open to learning about their condition, and more open to personal growth. Effective care of the chronically ill client and family requires patience, respect, and self-understanding by the nurse.

Chapter Highlights

- Evaluations of health and illness depend on the perceptions, value orientations, and knowledge of the people involved.

- Over one half of the population of North America has a chronic condition, and about 15% of the population has functional limitations.

- An illness trajectory is unique to the beliefs, characteristics, and experience of the individual client, caregiver, or professional.

- Clients and families develop stable behavioral patterns in response to chronic illness.

- When family resources are insufficient to meet the tasks of adjusting to the chronic illness, caregiver burden may result.

- Assessment questions can stimulate growth in the client or family.

- Planning care must consider the legitimacy of the helper, the point of entry, the attitudes to help, and the timing of care.

- Helping strategies are most effective in building competence when the client or family directs or actively participates in all steps of the nursing process.

- Nurse beliefs, attitudes, or fears may be part of the problem or the solution when interacting with clients and families.

- A professional approach based on respect and client competence will encourage a relationship of mutual trust with clients and families.

 CRITICAL THINKING EXERCISE

Select a family member, friend, or previous client who was a family caregiver for a chronically ill or disabled family member.

1. Identify whether this person perceived or was showing signs of caregiver burden. Justify your example using characteristics of vulnerability for caregiver burden.

2. Was the caregiver aware of the personal risks of caregiving? Were any actions taken to minimize the risks of caregiver breakdown?

3. Were others aware of the existence of or vulnerability to caregiver burden? Were any actions being taken to minimize the stress for the caregiver?

4. Were the actions taken by others perceived by the caregiver as reducing or increasing the stress levels? Why?

5. As a health professional, what approaches would you use with a caregiver who resists help? Why?

REFERENCES

Aguilera, D.C., & Messick, J.M. (1986). *Crisis intervention theory and methodology* (5th ed.). St. Louis: Mosby.

Ahmann, E. (1994). Family-centered care: shifting orientation. *Pediatric Nursing, 20*(2), 113-117.

Azjen, I., & Fishbein, M. (1980). *Understanding attitudes and predicting social behavior.* Englewood Cliffs, New Jersey: Prentice-Hall.

Baker, C., & Stern, P.N. (1993). Finding meaning in chronic illness as the key to self-care. *Canadian Journal of Nursing Research, 25*(2), 23-36.

Balram, C. (1989). Impact of chronic diseases on the health of Canadians: A case for prevention. *Chronic Diseases in Canada, 10*(3), 42-43.

Bond, N., Phillips, P., & Rollins, J.A. (1994). Family-centered care at home for families with children who are technology dependent. *Pediatric Nursing, 20*(2), 123-130.

Butcher, L.A. (1994). A family-focused perspective on chronic illness. *Rehabilitation Nursing, 19*(2), 70-74.

Canam, C. (1993). Common adaptive tasks facing parents of children with chronic conditions. *Journal of Advanced Nursing, 18,* 46-53.

Dass, R., & Gorman, P. (1987). *How can I help? Stories and reflections on service.* New York: Alfred A. Knopf.

Dimond, M., & Jones, S.L. (1983). *Chronic illness across the lifespan.* Norwalk, CT: Appleton-Century-Crofts.

Findeis, A., Larson, J.L., Gallo, A., & Shekleton, M. (1994). Caring for individuals using home ventilators: An appraisal by family caregivers. *Rehabilitation Nursing, 19*(1), 6-11.

Hamera, E.K., Pallikkathayil, L., Bauer, S., & Burton, M.R. (1994). Descriptions of wellness by individuals with schizophrenia. *Western Journal of Nursing Research, 16*(3), 288-300.

Hanson, S.M.H. (1987). Family nursing and chronic illness. In L.M. Wright & M. Leahey (Eds.), *Families and chronic illness* (pp. 2-32). Springhouse, PA: Springhouse Corporation.

Health and Activity Limitation Survey. (1990). *Highlights: Disabled persons in Canada.* Ottawa, Ontario: Statistics Canada.

Health and Welfare Canada. (1993). *Ageing and independence: Overview of a national survey.* Ottawa, Ontario: Supply and Services Canada.

Hill, G.B. (1993). Monograph series on aging-related diseases in Canada: Introduction. *Chronic Diseases in Canada, 14*(1), 1-3.

Hum, L.C., & Semenciw, R. (1991). Mortality patterns in Canada, 1988. *Chronic Diseases in Canada, 12*(2), 16-19.

Hymovich, D.P., & Hagopian, G.A. (1992). *Chronic illness in children and adults: A psychosocial approach.* Philadelphia: W.B. Saunders.

James, W. (1981). *The principles of psychology* (Vol. 1). Cambridge: Harvard University Press.

Knafl, K.A., & Deatrick, J.A. (1986). How families manage chronic conditions: An analysis of the concept of normalization. *Research in Nursing and Health, 9,* 215-222.

Lantican, L.S.M., Birdwell, C.N., & Harrell, R.T. (1994). Physically handicapped individuals in psychotherapy: Some empirical data. *Issues in Mental Health Nursing, 15*(1), 73-84.

Linsey, E., & Hills, M. (1992). An analysis of the concept of hardiness. *Canadian Journal of Nursing Research, 24*(1), 39-49.

Lubkin, I.M. (Ed.). (1990). *Chronic illness: Impact and interventions* (2nd ed.). Boston: Jones and Bartlett.

Luker, K.A., & Chalmers, K.I. (1990). Gaining access to clients: The case of health visiting. *Journal of Advanced Nursing, 15,* 74-82.

Moos, R.H., & Tsu, V.D. (1977). The crisis of physical illness: An overview. In R.H. Moos (Ed.), *Coping with physical illness* (pp. 3-21). New York: Plenum.

National Advisory Council on Aging. (1993). *Aging vignettes.* Ottawa, Ontario: Author.

Orem, D.E. (1991). *Nursing: Concepts of practice* (4th ed.). St. Louis: Mosby.

Pless, I.B., & Perrin, J.M. (1985). Issues common to a variety of illnesses. In N. Hobbs & J.M. Perrin (Eds.), *Issues in the care of children with chronic illness* (pp. 41-60). San Francisco: Jossey-Bass.

Price, P.J. (1993). Parent's perceptions of the meaning of quality nursing care. *Advances in Nursing Science, 16*(1), 33-41.

Reinhard, S.C. (1994). Living with mental illness: Effects of professional support and personal control on caregiver burden. *Research in Nursing and Health, 17*(2), 79-88.

Robinson, C.A. (1994). Nursing interventions with families: A demand or an invitation to change? *Journal of Advanced Nursing, 19,* 897-904.

Shaw, M.C., & Halliday, P.H. (1992). The family, crisis, and chronic illness: An evolutionary model. *Journal of Advanced Nursing, 17,* 537-543.

Strauss, A.L., Corbin, J., Fagerhaugh, S., Glaser, B.G., Maines, D., Suczek, B., & Wiener, C.L. (1984). *Chronic illness and the quality of life* (2nd ed.). St. Louis: Mosby.

Thorne, S.E., & Robinson, C.A. (1988). Health care relationships: The chronic illness perspective. *Research in Nursing and Health, 1988, 11,* 293-300.

Thorne, S.E., & Robinson, C.A. (1989). Guarded alliance: Health care relationships in chronic illness. *Image: Journal of Nursing Scholarship, 21*(3), 153-157.

Trnobranski, P.H. (1994). Nurse-patient negotiation: Assumption or reality? *Journal of Advanced Nursing, 19*(4), 733-737.

Watson, W.L. (1987). Intervening with aging families and Alzheimer's disease. In L.M. Wright & M. Leahey (Eds.), *Families and chronic illness* (pp. 381-401). Springhouse, PA: Springhouse Corporation.

Whyte, D.A. (1992). A family nursing approach to the care of a child with a chronic illness. *Journal of Advanced Nursing, 17,* 317-327.

World Health Organization. (1980). *International classification of impairments, disabilities, and handicaps.* Geneva, Switzerland: Author.

Wright, L.M., & Leahey, M. (1984). *Nurses and families: A guide to family assessment and intervention.* Philadelphia, PA: F.A. Davis.

22

CLIENTS WITH DEVELOPMENTAL DISABILITIES

Karen Cassidy King

Monday's child is fair of face,
Tuesday's child is full of grace,
Wednesday's child is full of woe,
Thursday's child has far to go. . . .

Unknown

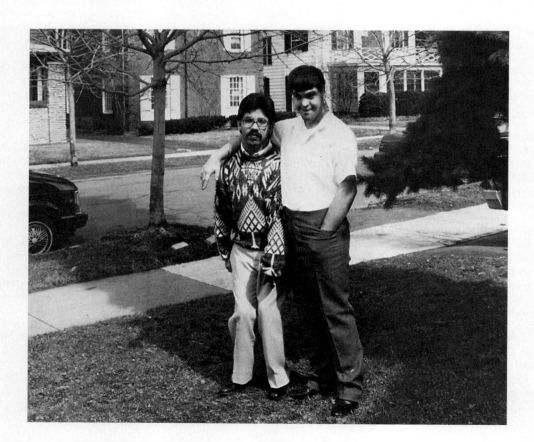

◆ OBJECTIVES

At the conclusion of this chapter the student will be able to:

1. Define the key terms listed.
2. Discuss the reasons individuals with developmental disabilities have become more visible in the community.
3. Describe the impact of developmental disabilities across the lifespan.
4. Describe the role of the community health nurse in the care of individuals with developmental disabilities.
5. Identify selected developmental disabilities.
6. Use the nursing process to address the needs of individuals with developmental disabilities.
7. Use appropriate communication skills in nursing care of individuals with disabilities.

KEY TERMS

Autism
Cerebral palsy
Developmental disability

Disability
Down syndrome

Learning disability
Mental retardation

During their lifetimes, individuals with disabilities have frequent contacts with nurses in the community. Individuals with disabilities encounter community-based nurses in such places as physicians' offices, primary care centers, health departments, clinics, schools, and their homes. Contact with community nurses most often focuses on preventive health, since preventive health efforts are important for individuals with disabilities and chronic illness.

Technology has decreased the gap between people without disabilities and people with them; an individual with a motorized wheelchair is no more "handicapped" than an individual traveling through an automatic door or down the aisles of the shopping mall (Johnson, 1992). Today, disabled people say the biggest problem facing them is discrimination and not their physical limitations (Johnson, 1992).

A disability that affects one member of the family also influences the other members of the family. It is important for the nurse to work with all family members to help identify their strengths and manage the problems related to the individual's disability (Drapo & Patrick, 1989). Nurses are strategically positioned to undertake a vital role in assisting the person with a developmental disability and the family with advocacy, problem solving, and decision making.

WHAT IS DISABILITY?

Traditionally, disabilities have been defined medically, but recently, definitions of disability have become broader. The World Health Organization (WHO) (1981, p. 8) defined a disability as "any restriction or lack of ability to perform an activity in the manner, or within the range, considered to be typical for a human being."

Disability is a general term used for a functional limitation that interferes with a person's ability, for example, to see, walk, lift, hear, or learn. It may refer to a physical, sensory, mental, or emotional condition.

A **developmental disability** is any mental and/or physical disability that has an onset before age 22 years and is likely to continue indefinitely. It can limit major life activities. This term includes individuals with mental retardation, cerebral palsy, autism, epilepsy (and other seizure disorders), sensory impairments, congenital anomalies, traumatic accidents, or conditions caused by disease (polio, muscular dystrophy) (Research & Training Center on Independent Living, 1990).

The Americans with Disabilities Act (ADA) of 1990 defines a "disabled" person as one that fits one of the following descriptions:

1. The person has a physical or mental impairment that substantially limits one or more major life activities (such as performing manual tasks, being able to care for oneself, walking, seeing, hearing, speaking, learning, or working).

2. The person has a record of such an impairment.

3. The person is regarded as having such an impairment.

If a person fits any one of these categories, the law protects them.

The ADA definition is a functional rather than a disease-oriented definition. Physical impairment, in the ADA definition, means any physiologic disorder or condition, cosmetic disfigurement, or anatomic loss affecting one or more of the following body systems: neurologic, musculoskeletal, special sense organs, respiratory (including speech organs), cardiovascular, reproductive, digestive, genitourinary, hemic and lymphatic, skin and endocrine. Mental impairment, according to the ADA definition, means any mental or psychological disorder, such as mental retardation, organic brain syndrome, emotional or mental illness, and specific learning disabilities.

BRIEF HISTORY OF THE DISABILITY MOVEMENT

People with various kinds of disabilities began uniting in the 1930s to find ways to improve their lives. Typically, these groups were composed of parents of disabled individuals looking for a cure. Many groups focused on a particular kind of disability. Groups like the National Federation of the Blind and the National Association for the Deaf are examples of such groups.

In the 1960s, these groups recognized that persons with disabilities were systematically being kept out of the mainstream of society. While efforts had been made to provide "special" transportation and "special" schools, individuals with disabilities were still restricted from restaurants and employment. These restrictions, while not intentional, had the same effect as discrimination had on other groups. As a result, individuals with disabilities were kept out of society and were often poor and unemployed.

In the 1970s and 1980s, laws were passed on the state and federal levels that helped people with disabilities enter the mainstream of society (see Table 22-1). Many of these laws were targeted at eliminating architectural barriers in public buildings and increasing access to restrooms. In 1973, a federal law called the Rehabilitation Act was passed. For the first time a nondiscrimination requirement was included in a federal law: federal programs and those programs receiving federal funds could not discriminate against individuals with disabilities.

In 1990, Congress passed the Americans with Disabilities Act (ADA). The ADA is landmark civil rights legislation that extends to people with disabilities the framework of federal civil rights laws that formerly applied to women and minorities. The purpose of the ADA is to provide a clear and comprehensive federal mandate on the elimination of discrimination against individuals with disabilities.

DEVELOPMENTAL DISABILITY ACROSS THE LIFESPAN
Infancy and Childhood

A child who is born with an identifiable disability is usually hospitalized immediately for diagnosis and treatment. This can cause delayed bonding because of the separation of infant and parents. The role of the nurse is to encourage the bonding process. A reciprocally satisfying relationship between children and parents is necessary for children to achieve the task of developing trust. Without a sense of trust, children may have difficulty expressing themselves to others. They may

TABLE 22-1   An overview of legislation for the disabled in the United States

Year	Legislation
1968	**Architectural Barriers Act (Public Law 90-480)** The act mandated that almost any public building constructed or leased by federal funds must be accessible to physically disabled people and that all construction after 1968 using federal dollars must ensure accessibility. The mandates of this law were mostly ignored, and in 1978 Congress created a compliance board to enforce the law.
1971	**Developmental Disabilities Act (Public Law 91-517)** The act stated that each state would receive federal funds to establish and maintain services that are required by developmentally disabled children and adults.
1973	**Rehabilitation Act of 1973 (Public Law 91-453)** This was landmark legislation that authorized vocational rehabilitation services, emphasized services to the severely disabled, and expanded the federal role in service and training programs.
1975	**Developmental Disabilities Assistance and Bill of Rights Act (Public Law 94-103)** This act created a system of advocacy on the state level to pursue legal actions necessary to eliminate problems for those individuals with mental retardation, epilepsy, autism, and cerebral palsy.
1984	**Rehabilitation Amendment (Public Law 98–221)** This amendment modified the definition of "severely disabled" and placed the age limit for disability benefits at 16 years of age.
1990	**The American with Disabilities Act (Public Law 101-336)** This landmark legislation was designed to provide a clear and comprehensive mandate to end discrimination against individuals with disabilities. It addresses issues of housing, employment, public transportation, and communication services.

not believe that they are lovable or that people would want to interact with them. Developmentally disabled individuals needs others to help them meet their needs to some degree, sometimes to a great degree. Children with disabilities needs to develop a sense of trust to reach out for help when needed (Pillitteri, 1992).

Infants with disabilities may not achieve the normal milestones that other infants reach (social smile, laughing out loud, sitting, talking), or they may be delayed in doing so. The nurse should encourage the relationship between parents and child by highlighting the positive things the infant can do.

All children experience the same growth and health problems regardless of whether a disability is present, and all children should receive immunizations according to the recommended schedule. The one exception is that the pertussis (whooping cough) vaccine should not be given to children with uncontrolled seizures or who have neurologic conditions that predispose them to seizures (Batshaw, 1991). Some children with

severe disabilities, especially those who are bedridden or who are susceptible to pneumonia, may benefit from the influenza and pneumococcal pneumonia vaccines.

Toddlers are entering the stage of autonomy and need to master locomotor and language skills. When teaching a toddler with a disability such skills as using a spoon or toileting, tasks should be broken down into small parts. Allowing parents to observe the nurse teaching the child helps them learn the teaching techniques and helps them gain the patience needed to teach their child other tasks. It is important for parents to understand how to break one task down into many smaller tasks (Pillitteri, 1992).

School-Age Children

School-age children with certain, severe disabilities must deal with the problem of losing valuable time in the classroom. This affects the child's academic achievement as well as the child's relationships with peers. The community

TABLE 22-2 Nursing actions that encourage a sense of industry in the school-age child with a developmental disability

Category	Actions
Nutrition	• Allow choices of food and respect preferences. • Provide small servings that can be easily finished, encouraging accomplishment.
Medication	• Teach child the name of each medication. • Teach child the action of each medication. • Allow child to choose the sight of IM or IV injections when possible.
Rest	• Establish clear limits for periods of rest (i.e., reading and watching television is all right, playing games is not).
Hygiene	• Respect the modesty of the school-age child as being at an adult level. • Allow as many choices as possible in bathing, personal hygiene schedule, and clothing choices.
Stimulation	• Encourage school work. Encourage activity that ends in a product (putting together a puzzle instead of playing a video game). • Do not suggest competition games for children younger than 10 years of age.

Adapted from *Maternal and child health nursing* by Pillitteri, A., 1992, Philadelphia: J.B. Lippincott Co.

health nurse should encourage the child to keep in contact with friends during times at home or during hospitalizations. It is important for the child to keep up with homework so as to continue to progress, which facilitates positive self-esteem (Pillitteri, 1992).

It is especially important for the child with a disability to develop a sense of independence. A child with a disability may not develop a sense of industry if he or she is unable to participate in activities that can be accomplished. The nurse can assist the school-age child with a disability by choosing activities that can be completed satisfactorily by the child to provide him or her with a sense of accomplishment (see Table 22-2). It is better for the nurse to choose a task that is too simple but that the child can perform well than one that is more complicated and that the child cannot master (Pillitteri, 1992).

The advocacy role of the nurse is important for the child in the classroom. The nurse should work collaboratively with the classroom teacher in developing effective learning strategies for the child.

The community health nurse should be familiar with the condition of the child with a disability and the complications that can occur. Some parents become "experts" on the care of their

child and the particular disability. The nurse should listen very attentively to the parents. At times, parents can become impatient with nurses who appear to be inattentive or unaware of the knowledge base they have. The nurse should be familiar with community resources that may be of assistance to the family.

Children with a long-term disability may need adapted educational programs or individualized instruction. They may miss school more often than their classmates and may fall behind unless special plans are made to keep them with their school group. By federal law (Public Law 99-457, Education of the Handicapped Amendment), a school system must provide educational opportunities in the least restrictive setting possible (beginning with preschool). Federal law mandates an Individual Education Plan (IEP) for each child with a disability that includes a statement of the child's current level of education performance, a statement of long-term goals and short-term instructional objectives, the specific special education and related services to be provided, the amount of time the student will spend in regular educational programs, the projected dates for the services, and the appropriate procedures and criteria for evaluating success in meeting the goals and objectives (Batshaw, 1991). Every parent is entitled to a copy of the child's IEP. The community health nurse should be a strong advocate so that the best educational program available is provided for the child (Downey, 1990).

Adolescence

The effect of disability can be most detrimental during adolescence. The major task of adolescence is to establish a personal identity. An adolescent with a disability may have difficulty with a positive sense of identity. Some of the greatest difficulties experienced by the adolescent with a disability include exerting independence, achieving success in school, and establishing close relationships. The loss of many hours of school because of illness or frequent hospitalizations may result in the inability to pursue a desired career.

A disability can cause depression in adolescents. This places them at a high risk for drug abuse and suicide. The nurse can help these individuals realize that they are not so different from other individuals who must learn to compromise in making decisions about their life for other reasons (lack of money, lack of ability or qualifications, extra personal responsibilities) (see Table 22-3).

It is a myth that sexual development in individuals with a disability differs from individuals without disabilities. An adolescent with a disability has the same sexual development, confusion, and drives as the rest of the adolescent population. And as with their nondisabled peers, the nurse should be aware that the adolescent with a disability may lack knowledge and education about sexuality. The nurse can be an important resource for the adolescent with a disability.

Adulthood

During adulthood, persons with disabilities have a wide range of capabilities and needs. Very few mandated programs exist for adults in terms of education, medical care, housing, or recreation. Legal guardianship, marriage, child bearing, and institutionalization are tough issues that arise for the adult with disabilities and their family members.

Some adults with disabilities are eligible to collect Supplemental Security Income (SSI), which includes cash benefits and Medicaid coverage, as well as Social Security Disability (which is not SSI). This income can be supplemented with work earnings without jeopardizing the SSI or Medicaid benefits.

Advances in medical technology and changing societal attitudes have led to a longer life for the individual with disabilities. Some adults with Down Syndrome will develop Alzheimer's disease. About 10% of individuals with severely profound mental retardation develop recurrent aspiration pneumonia. Adults with cerebral palsy may develop spinal cord injuries as they age (Batshaw, 1991).

TABLE 22-3   Nursing actions that encourage a sense of identity in the adolescent with a developmental disability

Category	Actions
Nutrition	• If adolescent is on special diet, discuss role of individual diet preferences with a dietitian. Respect food preferences.
Dressing changes	• Ask for suggestions to make appearance of dressing acceptable. • If soaks are needed, have the adolescent time the treatment when feasible.
Medications	• Teach name, action, and possible side effects of medicines. • Allow the adolescent to select the site of IM or IV injections when possible.
Rest	• Contract with adolescent for time and length of rest periods.
Stimulation	• Encourage school work. It may be necessary to divide school work into manageable work units to avoid fatigue and frustration. • Encourage adolescents to keep in contact with school friends during hospitalizations and illnesses through telephone and letters.

SELECTED DEVELOPMENTAL DISABILITIES
Cognitive Impairments/Mental Retardation

The term cognitive impairment encompasses any type of mental deficiency. The term **mental retardation** (MR) is often used synonymously with cognitive impairment. MR is the most common developmental disability in the United States and affects 3% of the population. The definition of mental retardation has three components: (1) The IQ score of a mentally retarded child is below 70, (2) mental retardation is a nonprogressive disorder evident during childhood, and (3) a mentally retarded individual has an impaired ability to adapt to his or her environment (Batshaw, 1991).

Categories of mental retardation include mild MR (IQ 55-69), moderate MR (IQ 40-54), severe MR (IQ 25-39), and profound MR (IQ less than 25). The causes of severe MR are related primarily to genetic, neonatal and perinatal, infancy and childhood, and social-cultural-familial factors (Drapo & Patrick, 1989).

Nurses play a major role in identifying children with MR. Delayed developmental milestones are the major clues. Parental concerns related to developmental delays when compared with other siblings should be taken seriously. Mental retardation is recognized most frequently at birth, age 3 years, and age 6 years (Drapo, 1989).

The goal of caring for children with MR is to promote optimum development. Specific strategies of nursing care for the child with MR are to educate the child and the family, to teach the child self-care skills, and to help the family plan future care (Wong, 1993).

Children with MR should be "mainstreamed" into regular classrooms to allow them opportunities to engage in social activities and other experiences with peers. This process of normalization makes available the experiences and opportunities of everyday life.

Down Syndrome (Trisomy 21) and Other Chromosomal Abnormalities

Down syndrome is the most common chromosomal abnormality of a generalized syndrome, occurring in 1 in 800 live births. It gets the once-common but now unacceptable name mongolism from the particular facial characteristics that resemble those of the Mongol race (Wong, 1993). It occurs more often in children of women over the age of 35 years. As maternal age increases, the incidence of Down syndrome increases. Down syndrome affects both sexes equally and is found in every race and culture (Drapo & Patrick, 1989).

The cause of Down syndrome is an extra number 21 chromosome. There are a number of medical complications of Down syndrome. Approximately 40% are born with a congenital heart defect. Hypothyroidism occurs in 10%. The spinal column in the upper neck may be unstable and a sudden jolt can lead to spinal cord damage. Most individuals with Down syndrome fall in the range of moderate mental retardation (Batshaw, 1991).

The nurse can be reassuring to the parents by providing information to show that help is available. It is often helpful for the family to have peer support from another family with a child with Down syndrome.

The nurse should assist the adolescent with Down syndrome and his or her family in learning appropriate behavior with behavior modification techniques. By the end of schooling at age 21 years, individuals with Down syndrome may have some "survival" reading and math skills that will allow them to be self sufficient in many areas. The level of independence depends on the level of intelligence. To the greatest extent possible, the adult with disabilities should be encouraged to take care of himself or herself, make meals, do housework, and travel by bus (Batshaw, 1991). Because an individual with disabilities may outlive his or her parents, long-term planning regarding future living arrangements is important.

Cerebral Palsy

Cerebral palsy (CP) is the term used to describe disorders of movement and posture resulting from brain damage at birth or during childhood. It is not preventable, and damage commonly occurs during the first few months of pregnancy. With CP there is nonprogressive damage to the brain with the primary effect on the muscles. There are three types of CP: (1) spastic cerebral palsy (damage occurs in the pyramidal tract of the brain that initiates voluntary movement), (2) extrapyramidal cerebral palsy (damage occurs in the extrapyramidal tract), and (3) mixed-type cerebral palsy (damage occurs in both areas; brain damage may be extensive). About 60% of children with CP are mentally retarded.

Symptoms of early CP in infants include absence of normal reflexes, irritability, feeding problems, poor motor development, and poor muscle tone (Drapo & Patrick, 1989). The nurse should be an active member of the interdisciplinary team that may also include a speech and hearing therapist, social worker, occupational therapist, physical therapist, nutritionist, neurologist, and pediatrician.

Common problems in infants with CP are irritability and feeding disorders. In older children, drooling, constipation, contractures, dislocations, and decubital ulcers are common concerns (Batshaw, 1991).

One of the most important nursing interventions is emotional support for the child and the family. The nurse should be knowledgeable of community resources for the child with CP and the family. In the home, modifications to promote the child's independence should be encouraged.

Autism

Autism is a syndrome, the major symptoms of which include delayed and abnormal language, inability to relate to people, and stereotyped, repetitive behaviors (Batshaw, 1991). Other common symptoms include need for social isolation, resistance to change in routine, abnormal responses to sensory stimuli, insensitivity to pain, and specific limited intellectual problems (Pillitteri, 1992). Autism appears to result from abnormal brain development in the areas of the limbic and cerebellum areas.

There is no specific treatment for autism. One of the most important nursing measures is support to the family, especially the parents. Many emotional demands are placed on a family with a child with autism. It is important that the parents do not reject the child even though it seems that the child is rejecting the parents. Teaching the child how to behave in a social situation is challenging but very important. This usually begins with teaching the child to maintain eye contact then by role-playing various situations. Behavior modification is vital for autistic children. Parents should be encouraged to find regularly scheduled respite care. Autistic characteristics generally improve in adolescence. Level of functioning depends largely on intelligence and speech skills.

Learning Disabilities

A **learning disability** describes a permanent condition that affects the way an individual with average or above-average intelligence takes in, retains, and expresses information (Research & Training Center on Independent Living, 1990). Learning disabilities have been distinguished from mental retardation, neurologic impairment, and emotional impairments. The Education for All Handicapped Children Act of 1975 (Public Law 94-142) defines learning disability as a "disorder in one or more of the basic psychological processes involved in understanding or in using language, spoken or written, which may manifest as imperfect ability to listen, speak, read, write, spell or do mathematical calculations." This definition of learning disability does not include those children with mental retardation, emotional disturbance, or visual, hearing, or motor handicaps.

There are more than 100 types of learning disabilities. Symptoms of a learning disability can be recognized by an astute nurse. Problems in language, motor skills, and behavior develop long before school problems do. If the child exhibits problems following instructions, is easily distracted, has a short attention span, and needs to be told the same thing repeatedly, the nurse should suspect a learning disability. Because children with learning disabilities do not learn readily from past experiences, parents often have difficulty with disciplining these children.

Families need special support in dealing with a child with learning disabilities. Siblings should not be compared with each other but should be told honestly that the child has a learning disability.

RESEARCH ❧ HIGHLIGHT

Play and Children With Autism

Eight boys and one girl with autism between the ages of three and six years were matched for gender, age, and parental socioeconomic status with developmentally normal children for the following purposes: (1) to compare the play of children with autism with the play of children without dysfunction in their homes, and (2) to examine the relationships between children's play performance and their communication, social, and motor abilities.

A modified version of the Preschool Play Scale (PPS) was used to evaluate videotaped free play activities of children in a room chosen by their parents in their home consisting of 15 minutes of unstructured play immediately followed by 15 minutes of structured play. The Vineland Adaptive Behavior Scales (VABS), a standardized, norm-referenced evaluative instrument, was used to elicit information from parents during interviews about their children's adaptive behavior in four domains: (1) communication, (2) daily living skills, (3) socialization, and (4) motor skills.

The children with autism differed significantly (had lower scores) from their developmentally normal peers on the total PPS score and in the participation dimension, which was one of the four domains listed above included in the total. In addition, the children with autism had significantly lower VABS total scores than their normally developing counterparts. PPS total scores were significantly correlated with VABS total scores for both (autistic and peers) groups, while PPS total scores were not significantly correlated with the mental or chronological age variable for either group. The adaptive ability of communication (VABS score) correlated significantly with the play (PPS total score) performance of children with autism. The domain of socialization (VABS score) correlated significantly with the normally developing group's total PPS score.

The results of this study suggest that deficits in social development are a central feature of autism. The findings support the continued use of play to assess skills, particularly in socialization, and to therapeutically intervene in the development of interpersonal interactions of preschool children with autism. Future research endeavors could focus on the learning styles of children to facilitate and maintain interest in a variety of play activities and to initiate strategies to enhance children's interaction with their environment.

From "Play and preschool children with autism" by G. Restall & J. Magill-Evans, 1994, *American Journal of Occupational Therapy, 48*(2), 113-120.

HEALTH PROMOTION AND PREVENTION OF DEVELOPMENTAL DISABILITIES

The nurse can play a vital role in the primary prevention of developmental disabilities through health education. Health education includes sex education, family planning, prevention of gynecologic infections, and emphasis on adequate prenatal care. There are complex relationships between prevention of developmental disabilities and development in utero and during infancy. It is important for the nurse to educate the client regarding nutrition, environmental modification, and especially immunization, which prevents disabling conditions that can result from childhood infections.

Nurses involved in well-child care settings are in a prime position to evaluate developmental delays. Systematic assessment of development and planned screening programs are important to detect delays. Through early identification, treatment programs can be instituted to maximize the developmental potential of the child. Children may risk developmental delays because of an environment that is not conducive to growth and development. The role of the nurse is one of case finding and referral.

NURSING PROCESS

The nurse's main goal is to help the family remain intact and functioning at the maximum level possible. The nurse should form a partnership with the family that encourages input, ac-

DISABILITY ETIQUETTE

Basic guidelines

- Make reference to the person first, then the disability. Say "a person with a disability" rather than "a disabled person." (The latter is acceptable in the interest of conserving space when documenting patient care.)
- The term "handicapped" is derived from the image of a person standing on the corner with a cap in hand, begging for money. People with disabilities do not want to be recipients of charity. They want to participate equally with the rest of the community. A disability is a functional limitation that interferes with a person's ability to walk, hear, talk, learn, and so on. Use "handicap" to describe a situation or barrier imposed by society, the environment, or oneself.
- Remember, a person with a disability is not chronically sick or unhealthy. He or she is often just disabled.
- A person is not a condition, so avoid describing a person in such a manner. Do not present someone as an "epileptic" or "a post polio." Say instead, "a person with epilepsy" or "a person with polio."
- Leaning on a person's wheelchair is similar to leaning or hanging on a person and is usually considered annoying and rude. The chair is part of one's body space.
- When offering assistance to a person with a visual impairment, allow that person to take your arm. This will enable you to guide, rather than propel the person. Use specific directions, such as "left 100 feet" or "right 2 yards," when directing a person with a visual impairment.
- When planning events such as health education or screening programs that involve persons with disabilities, consider their needs before choosing a location. Even if people with disabilities will not attend the event, select an accessible spot. You would not think of holding an event where other minorities could not attend, so do not exclude people with disabilities.
- To get the attention of a person who has a hearing impairment, tap him or her on the shoulder or wave. Look directly at the person and speak clearly, slowly, and expressively to establish if the person can read lips. Not all people with hearing impairments can read lips. Those who do rely on facial expressions and body language for understanding. Stay in the light and keep food, hands, and other objects away from your mouth. Shouting will not help. Written notes will.
- When talking to a person in a wheelchair for more than a few minutes, place yourself at eye level with that person. This will spare both of you a sore neck.
- When greeting a person with severe loss of vision, always identify yourself and others. Remember to identify persons to whom you are speaking. Speak in a normal tone of voice and indicate when the conversation is over. Let the person know when you move from one place to another.

From PARAQUAD, 5100 Oakland Ave, Suite 100, St. Louis, MO 63110-1426. Used by permission.

countability, and responsibility for the care of the disabled member (Wong, 1993). The effectiveness of the nurse rests on a personal awareness of her attitude toward individuals with disabilities. The nurse must make an honest appraisal of her own attitudes and prejudices. This process usually requires direct involvement and personal experiences with persons with disabilities (Burgess, 1990).

Assessment

The nursing assessment may involve a broad general assessment, such as the general development of the individual, or a specific functional pattern, such as mobility. The ability to identify developmental lags and deviations is based on the nurse's working knowledge and understanding of usual growth and development.

The nurse should assess the family system in the following areas: knowledge of the family's available support systems, including family members, colleagues, and friends; and the family's perception of the disability. Other important areas to assess are knowledge of the condition before the diagnosis was made, the influence of religion and culture, perceived causes of the condition, and the effects of the disabled individual on the family system.

Nursing Diagnoses

Many nursing diagnoses should be considered in the care of the individual with disabilities and their families. It is important to remember the emotional impact a diagnosis of disability may have on the family. The philosophical approach to imparting the diagnostic information will, in part, determine the family's ability to cope with a potentially difficult situation (Burgess, 1990). Labels, once applied, are likely to stick for many years. It is important to be very careful when "labeling" an individual with a disability.

One cannot generalize about the affect an individual with disabilities will have on the family unit. Families seek truthful, accurate information presented in a empathetic manner. A sensitive and caring atmosphere will provide support for families in coping with their feelings.

Planning

The nursing plan depends to a large extent on the disability. The following are basic goals for all families with an individual with disabilities.

1. Provide support at the time of diagnosis.
2. Accept the family's emotional reactions.
3. Help the family cope.
4. Foster reality adjustment. (Wong, 1993, p. 521)

Planning for the future should be a gradual process. The family should cultivate realistic expectations for the disabled member.

Interventions may include assessing the meaning of crisis for the family, counseling regarding the diagnosis, providing parents with ongoing teaching about the child's growth, addressing development and health care needs, giving help in the planning of activities of daily care, relieving stress of the caretakers, and identifying program choices for the child (Burgess, 1990).

TABLE 22-4 Preferred terminology when referring to disabilities

Words/phrases to avoid	Preferred words/phrases
cripple/handicapped/handicap/invalid (Literally, invalid means "not valid." Don't use it.)	person with a disability/disabled/disability
victim/afflicted with (e.g. victim of cerebral palsy)	person who has/person who experienced/person with (e.g. person who has cerebral palsy)
restricted, confined to a wheelchair/wheelchair bound (The chair enables mobility. Without the chair, the person is confined to bed.)	uses a wheelchair
normal (Referring to non-disabled persons as "normal" insinuates that people with disabilities are abnormal.)	nondisabled
deaf mute/deaf and dumb	deaf/does not voice for themselves/nonvocal
birth defect	disabled since birth/born with
crazy/insane	emotional disorder/mental illness
fits	seizures
slow	developmental delay
abnormal, burden, condition, deformed, differently abled, disfigured, incapacitated, imbecile, maimed, moron, palsied, pathetic, physically challenged, pitiful, poor, spastic, stricken with, suffer, tragedy, unfortunate	blind (no visual capability)
	deaf/profoundly deaf (no hearing capability)
	hearing impaired (some hearing capability)
	visually impaired (some visual capability)
	hemiplegia (paralysis of one side of the body)
	paraplegia (loss of function in lower body only)
	quadraplegic (paralysis of both arms and legs)

From PARAQUAD, 5100 Oakland Avenue, Suite 100, St. Louis, MO, 63110-1426. Used with permission.

Evaluation

The needs of the entire family should be considered in the evaluation of nursing care.

The effectiveness of nursing interventions is determined by continual reassessment and evaluation of care based on the following observational guidelines and expected outcomes:

1. Observe the response of the family members to the diagnosis and the types of questions or concerns that they have.

2. Interview the family regarding their knowledge and understanding of the condition; observe if they have incorporated suggestions from the health care providers.

3. Observe the response of professionals to reactions such as denial, guilt, and anger, and note whether supportive interventions are used with the family.

4. Observe the communication patterns in the family and the ability to discuss feelings about issues such as the impact of the family member with a disability on the marriage or additional care responsibilities; investigate the family's use of services, such as self-help groups or other community resources (Wong, 1993, p. 538).

COMMUNICATION SKILLS IN NURSING CARE OF INDIVIDUALS WITH A DISABILITY

The nurse should keep in mind clear communication techniques in caring for individuals with disabilities. By using words that convey dignity, the nurse encourages equality for everyone. The use of words that express dignity for the individual will give them dignity and encourage the therapeutic relationship between nurse, individual, and family (see Table 22-4). The box on page 505 provides an introduction to the basic guidelines of disability etiquette.

Chapter Highlights

- Disability is a general term used for a functional limitation that interferes with an individual's functional ability.

- A developmental disability is any mental and/or physical disability that has an onset before age 22 years and is likely to continue indefinitely.

- Many individuals with disabilities began forming groups and were proactive in the past. Federal legislation has evolved that prohibits discrimination against people with disabilities.

- Infants with disabilities need a supportive, positive relationship with their parents to establish trusting relationships throughout their lifetimes.

- Toddlers need to master skills in becoming autonomous. School-age children need to be encouraged to keep up with school work and social activities and friendships. Adolescents with a disability need to establish a sound personal identity, incorporate the disability, and gain self-esteem.

- Planning for the adult with disabilities includes confusing issues such as legal guardianship, marriage, employment, and independent living. Long-range planning is vital for adults with disabilities.

- Mental retardation or cognitive impairment is the most common developmental disability in the United States. Nurses play a major role in the identification of delayed developmental milestones.

- Down syndrome is the most common chromosomal abnormality of a generalized syndrome and involves many medical complications.

- Cerebral palsy is the term used to describe unpreventable disorders of movement and posture resulting from brain damage at birth.

- Autism is a syndrome resulting from abnormal brain development that results in delayed and abnormal language, inability to relate to others, and repetitive behaviors.

- A learning disability is a permanent condition that affects the way an individual with average intelligence or above-average intelligence takes in, retains, or expresses information.

- The main goal of the nurse in caring for the individual with disabilities is to help the family remain intact and functioning at the maximum level possible. This involves an understanding of the disability, family coping, and community resources.

- Communication skills are critical in developing therapeutic relationships with the individual and family.

 CRITICAL THINKING EXERCISE

A special education teacher has children in his class he considers at high risk because of their varied disabilities. The teacher's goal is to educate them, but he is unclear how to proceed. The children that he feels are at high risk include a child with cerebral palsy who is nonverbal, a blind child, a deaf child, and a child who is moderately retarded and experiences violent episodes of acting out.

1. Using the communication skills and basic guidelines for disability etiquette described in the chapter, write a list of guidelines for the teacher to use when attempting to teach these children.
2. What would be your concerns as a nurse?

REFERENCES

Batshaw, M.L. (1991). *Your child has a disability.* Boston: Little, Brown.

Burgess, A.W. (1990). *Psychiatric nursing.* Norwalk, CT: Appleton & Lange.

Drapo, P., & Patrick, C. (1989). Nursing strategies: Alterations in development. In R.L. Foster, M.M. Hunsberger, & J.J. Anderson (Eds.), *Family-centered nursing care of children* (pp. 1038-1076). Philadelphia: W.B. Saunders.

Downey, W.S. (1990). Public law 99-457 and the clinical pediatrician. *Clinical Pediatrics, 29,* 158.

Johnson, M. (1992). *People with disabilities explain it all for you.* Louisville, KY: The Advocado Press.

Pillitteri, A. (1992). *Maternal and child health nursing.* Philadelphia: J.B. Lippincott.

Research & Training Center on Independent Living. (!990). *Guidelines for Reporting and Writing About People With Disabilities,* (3rd. ed.), Lawrence, KS: University of Kansas.

Wong, D.L. (1993). *Whaley & Wong's Essentials of Pediatric Nursing,* (4th ed.), St. Louis: Mosby.

World Health Organization Expert Committee on Disability Prevention and Rehabilitation. (1981). *Disability prevention and rehabilitation.* Technical Report Series 668, Geneva: Author.

Acknowledgements

The author wishes to express sincere thanks to Cass Irvin, Access to the Arts, for her candid consulting regarding disabilities. Thanks to Mrs. Rita DeToma for her help and advice on the sections relating to parenting, and to Dr. Marianne Hutti, Associate Professor of Nursing, Louisville, Kentucky, for her editorial assistance.

23

CLIENTS WITH CHEMICAL DEPENDENCIES

Elizabeth Schenk

Overall, 70.4 million Americans older than 12 years of age have tried some kind of illicit drug at least once in their lifetime.

(National Institute on Drug Abuse, 1986)

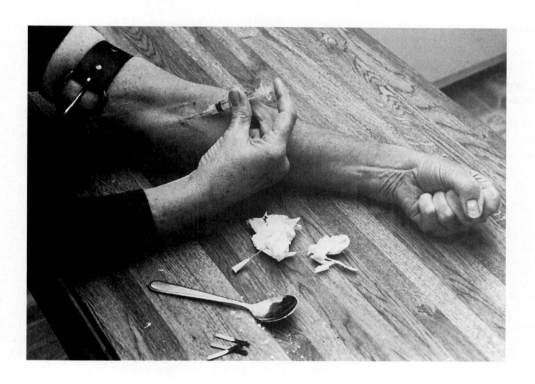

OBJECTIVES

At the conclusion of this chapter the student will be able to:

1. Define the key terms listed.
2. Describe the terms *dependence* and *tolerance* as they relate to drug and alcohol use.
3. Describe what is meant by *enabling behavior.*
4. State two theories that have been proposed to explain the development of chemical dependency.
5. Describe four disorders associated with substance abuse and chemical dependency.
6. Describe what is meant by the term *drug addiction.*
7. Cite at least four populations that are at risk for chemical dependency.
8. Discuss the relationship of acquired immunodeficiency syndrome (AIDS) to substance abuse.
9. Name at least 10 common substances of abuse.
10. Describe aspects of primary, secondary, and tertiary prevention in relation to substance abuse.
11. Explain one way the nursing process may be applied to substance abuse.

KEY TERMS

Alcoholics Anonymous
Alcoholism
Amphetamines
Barbiturates
Cannabis
Chemical dependency
Deliriants
Designer drugs

Detoxification
Drug abuse
Drug addiction
Drug habituation
Fetal Alcohol Syndrome
Hallucinogens
Intervention
Narcotics

Physical dependence
Psychological dependence
Stimulants
Substance abuse
Tolerance
Tranquilizers
Withdrawal syndrome

It is important for the community health nurse to understand substance abuse because of the number of persons it affects. The nurse who works in the community is in a unique position to assist in many different ways in the detection, treatment, and rehabilitation of substance abusers.

ISSUES AND TRENDS IN SUBSTANCE ABUSE

The use of alcohol predates recorded history. Cultures from many parts of the world have used alcoholic beverages to celebrate important events. Alcohol has been consumed as medicine, as a form of magic, and as a part of worship services. In America there have been various legal views on the use of alcohol. In 1642 drunkenness was punishable by a fine. In 1790 a law was passed that gave every soldier a portion of daily liquor. Prohibition, which forbade the production or sale of alcoholic beverages, was enacted in 1919 and repealed in 1933. Even today the use of alcohol is sanctioned by society.

The history of nonmedical drug use goes back thousands of years. As early as 5000 BC the Sumerians referred to a "joy plant" (believed to be the opium poppy plant). Since then, drugs have played a significant role in almost every culture. In the United States the first national awareness of a drug problem occurred in the mid-1860s during the Civil War, when injured and wounded soldiers became addicted to the morphine that was used to relieve pain. In recent years the incidence of drug abuse has risen.

Between 1940 and 1960, drug abuse in the United States was considered to be a ghetto-related phenomenon. As drug use increased, this view was proved untrue. As patients sought drugs from physicians to make them feel better, more and more psychoactive drugs were prescribed. Today Americans classify drug abuse as the number one problem in the United States.

One current trend in substance abuse is the high incidence of acquired immunodeficiency syndrome (AIDS) that occurs with intravenous (IV) drug abuse. The number of persons with AIDS has increased each year, and the reason for the shift in infection source from homosexual white men to a broader group is attributed mainly to IV drug use. Nearly 75% of women with AIDS were infected when either they or their sexual partners used drugs. Because blood-to-blood contact is the most efficient mode of transmission of the human immunodeficiency virus (HIV), sharing a needle is a more certain way of spreading the disease than is sexual contact. In addition, drug abusers do not take the responsibility to protect themselves and others from the spread of the disease as have homosexual men and women (Long, Phipps, & Cassmeyer, 1993).

SCOPE OF THE PROBLEM

Alcoholism is defined as the extreme dependence on excessive amounts of alcohol (Mosby's Medical, Nursing, and Allied Health Dictionary, 3rd ed., 1990, p. 40), is a common health problem that may exacerbate other health disorders. Excessive alcohol consumption can lead to coma or death from acute alcohol poisoning or to numerous other health problems if the drinking continues over a long period of time. (Associated disorders are discussed later in this chapter.)

Estimates are that about 90 million persons use alcohol, and at least 18 million are alcohol abusers or "problem drinkers." In addition, alcoholism affects the functioning of another 30 million friends and relatives of alcohol abusers (Fitzgerald, 1988). Industries lose billions of dollars annually because of effects of alcoholism. This figure includes medical expenses, lost wages, decreased production, motor vehicle accidents, and crime.

The costs of alcohol-related problems in the United States have been estimated to exceed $70 billion per year with an additional $44 billion attributed to problems related to drug use (Rice et al., 1990). It has been found that approximately half of all traffic fatalities are alcohol related. In addition, the incidence of burn victims who are intoxicated at the time of injury ranges from 37% to 64%, and the number of drowning victims who were under the influence of or had been exposed to alcohol is 38%. There has been found a high correlation of alcohol abuse in victims of suicide. Studies of emergency room visits have shown that between 20% and 37% of trauma victims use alcohol (United States Department of Health and Human Services, 1990).

It is difficult to estimate the number of persons addicted to drugs. Overall, 70.4 million Americans older than 12 years of age have tried some kind of illicit drug at least once in their lifetime (USDHHS, 1990), a figure that constitutes about 37% of the population in this age range. The greatest number (33%) have tried marijuana, whereas 11% have experimented with cocaine. The highest rate of use of hallucinogens and inhalants is among young persons. Despite the fact that its prevalence rate is low, heroin is of great concern because it is taken intravenously and can contribute to the spread of AIDS.

During the past century there has been a large increase in chemical dependence among adolescents, women, and elderly persons. Chemical dependency can be defined as the total psychologic and physical state of a person who is addicted to drugs or alcohol. In most parts of the world the rate of chemical dependency increases as income increases. The media also influences drug use.

THEORIES OF CAUSATION

Numerous theories have been suggested to explain the causes of chemical dependency. These theories have been divided into the following three main categories:

1. Physiologic
   a. Genetotrophic — related to genetically determined biochemical defect
   b. Endocrinal — caused by dysfunction of the endocrine system
   c. Genetic — 30% to 50% risk of alcoholism developing in sons or daughters of alcoholic parents; in 60% of cases, alcoholism will develop in identical twins of an alcoholic parent
2. Psychologic
   a. Oral fixation — resulting from lack of a warm, loving relationship with a mother figure during childhood
   b. Behavioral learning theory — association of alcohol ingestion with a positive experience leads to substance abuse
3. Sociocultural or cultural
   a. Cultural — relationship between various groups in society and incidence of alcoholism
   b. Moral — substance abuse as moral fault or sin of the alcohol abuser (Kirk & Bradford, 1987)

Ongoing research continues to determine the causes of **substance abuse,** the overindulgence in and dependence on a stimulant, depressant, or other chemical substance. No one theory has been found to be all-inclusive. It is apparent, however, that alcohol-addicted persons share common personality characteristics, which include dependency, denial, and delusion. Substance abuse has been found to occur at higher rates in some families. It is likely that the origin of substance abuse is multicausal.

FACTORS THAT PLACE POPULATIONS AT RISK
Poverty

Although the incidence of substance abuse has not been found to be positively correlated with poverty, it is not uncommon to find a greater number of persons addicted to drugs and alcohol among those who live in poverty, inasmuch as drug use may result in lost jobs, income, and family. The irresponsibility that usually accompanies chemical dependency makes it difficult for these persons to hold a job and follow through on financial obligations. Thus they become poor.

The impoverished substance abuser poses a special challenge to the community health nurse because of the inadequate resources available to treat those who are without financial resources. The person may want help but may be unable to obtain it. In addition, the impoverished substance abuser may turn to drug dealing or trafficking as a way to escape poverty. It is not uncommon for young persons to earn thousands of dollars a day through drug dealing, which may seem like an easy escape from poverty.

The homeless. It may be difficult to intervene in treatment of the homeless. Generally the prognosis for this population is poor because of the difficulty in changing patterns of behavior. Detoxification centers, shelters, and other short-term programs that offer medical care, food, and shelter are located in most metropolitan areas. These resources often are inadequate, and long-term provisions for care are not readily available (Wagner & Menke, 1991). (Problems of the homeless are discussed in Chapter 24.)

Culture

A relationship has been found between various groups in society and the use of substances. Jews, Mormons, and Moslems, for instance, have a low rate of alcoholism, whereas the rate among the French is high, and the Soviet Union recently reported a serious problem with alcoholism. Although the reason for this incidence may be in part cultural, experts believe that further study is needed to reach definitive conclusions.

Alcohol abuse among Native Americans and native Alaskans is well documented and presents a challenge for the nurse who works with these populations. A major cause of death among Native Americans is directly related to alcohol abuse, including accidents, cirrhosis, suicide, and homicide (Andre, 1979).

More than 70% of Hispanic men drink, and the prevalence of alcohol-related problems is higher among Hispanics now than among black or white men.

As a whole, Asian Americans have the lowest level of alcoholism and alcohol-related problems of all racial and ethnic groups in the United States (USDHHS, 1990).

In some cultural groups, drinking is viewed as socially acceptable and may be the focus of get-togethers. There are few sanctions against drunken behavior, and the goal of drinking usually is to get drunk. This outlook almost always leads to problems with alcohol. In addition, drinking is believed to be a way to escape feelings of anger and helplessness, which are often caused by forced assimilation into modern mainstream society. Even today, native Americans who leave the reservation for urban settings often experience long periods of unemployment, which may lead to the use of drugs and alcohol.

To help decrease substance abuse, the community health nurse who deals with persons from a different culture needs to be aware of these cultural influences. Involving this population in the planning of effective prevention and treatment programs is essential to positive change.

Youth

A high-risk group for the development of substance abuse is the youth population. **Drug abuse,** the use of a drug for a nontherapeutic effect, has increased drastically among this group in the United States and other countries. Explanations that have been offered for this increase include the affluence of society and increased leisure time and financial resources as compared with youth of the past.

Drug and alcohol use among adolescents also can serve as a rite of passage from childhood into adulthood. It is associated with the risk-taking and rebellious behavior that is often characteristic of adolescents attempting to determine their own identities. Further, the influence of the peer group usually is stronger than that of the family or church. It has been found that adolescents drink more frequently and more heavily as the extent of drinking among their peers increases.

Certain groups of adolescents have been found to be at increased risk for drug or alcohol abuse. These include the following:

- School dropouts
- Girls who have had a pregnancy
- Youths from economically disadvantaged homes
- Children of drug- or alcohol-abusing parents
- Victims of child abuse
- Youths who have had trouble with the law
- Youths with history of mental health problems
- Youths who have attempted suicide in the past
- Youths with long-term physical pain (Schwartz & Wirtz, 1990).

It also has been found that youth tend to use a variety of mood-altering substances; two substances that are prevalently abused are alcohol and marijuana. Initial experimentation with drinking often takes place within the home and with parental approval. As the adolescent becomes older, the drinking takes place outside the home. Although many youths may identify daily drinking as dangerous, they see no harm in getting drunk at a party.

Adolescents who are substance abusers also may exhibit other problem behaviors, including delinquent behavior, precocious sexual behavior, poor school performance, and a high dropout rate from school. Alcohol-related accidents among this group are common, as are other forms of violence and suicide.

The community health nurse who assists in the treatment of adolescent substance abusers must consider the stability of the family (see the next section in this chapter concerning the family, as well as Chapter 19). Also, identification and treatment of the adolescent can be extremely difficult and expensive. This group generally is treated most effectively in treatment centers equipped with special adolescent services. In addition, it is important to keep in mind normal adolescent developmental tasks and how they affect the problem of substance abuse. Substance abuse can prevent the adolescent from successfully moving through developmental phases.

Family Patterns

Alcoholism and drug abuse have been found to occur more frequently in some families; 50% of all alcohol abusers have an alcohol-addicted parent, grandparent, brother, or sister. Children of alcoholic parents are twice as likely to experience alcohol-related problems as are children of nonalcoholic parents (Fitzgerald, 1988). It also has been found that the children of alcoholic relatives tend to feel a personal immunity to alcoholism because they are certain that they are familiar with the consequences and would never allow themselves to develop such a problem. Family members are affected either directly because of physical, sexual, or emotional abuse or indirectly because of the unpredictability of the alcohol abuser's behavior.

In addition, children and spouses of chemically dependent persons tend to feel a sense of shame and guilt and often exist in isolation from their peer group. They may feel that they have a unique and devastating problem that others are incapable of understanding. Children brought up in a home with alcoholic parents will carry the scars for a lifetime if they do not receive appropriate therapy and help (Rivinus, 1991).

Chemical dependency has a disruptive effect on the entire family. Family members often become involved with the alcohol abuser's behavior to the extent that their behaviors become compulsive patterns of dysfunctional reactions that include enabling behavior. Psychiatric treatment of family members, or school and behavioral problems of children should alert the nurse to explore the presence of a substance-abuse problem in the family. Chemical dependency must be seen as a family disease, and chemically dependent persons must be treated as part of the family unit if they are to have the best chance to remain abstinent (Captain, 1989).

Jackson (1954) identifies the following seven stages through which the family passes in adjusting to alcoholism or substance abuse:

- Stage 1 — Attempts to deny the problem (episodes of excessive drinking are rationalized and not discussed)
- Stage 2 — Attempts to eliminate the problem (as the use becomes more of a problem, the spouse may try to control the drinking by throwing out the alcohol or by buying it, and the family becomes more isolated)
- Stage 3 — Disorganization of the family (the family equilibrium breaks down, hostility is expressed, children are caught in the middle, and financial and legal problems are common)
- Stage 4 — Efforts to reorganize despite the problem (spouse or child assumes a great deal of the alcohol abuser's responsibility and treats the alcoholic as a child)
- Stage 5 — Attempts to escape the problem (marital separation or divorce may occur, or if the family unit remains intact, the family arranges its lifestyle around the alcohol abuser)
- Stage 6 — Reorganization of part of the family (the spouse and children make a new home without the alcohol abuser, who may threaten or beg to get back into the home)
- Stage 7 — Recovery and reorganization of the whole family (if the alcohol abuser maintains sobriety, the family may reunite, but the adjustment may not be easy)

Through ongoing work with individuals and families in the community, the nurse can observe for signs and symptoms of drug or alcohol use. Much of this information can be gained through work in the home setting. The assessment of the family should include a three-generation health history that asks about substance abuse, the presence of significant physical illnesses, social behaviors such as difficulty with the law, and any history of violence or child abuse. There should also be a current nuclear family history obtained.

Babies of Addicted Mothers

Women who are addicted to substances during their pregnancies can cause damage to their babies. The number of such infants is increasing; one estimate is that about 10% of newborns suffer from the effects of substance abuse, including the following:

1. The infant is born with an actual addiction and experiences withdrawal symptoms of varying degrees.
2. The infant becomes ill because of the drug's toxic effects.

3. The infant has brain damage or other congenital problems because of the teratogenic characteristics of the drug (Zuckerman, 1989; Jacques & Snyder, 1991).

Fetal alcohol syndrome is a set of congenital abnormalities. The problems associated with it have been documented over a long period of time. Women who drink excessively during pregnancy have a higher incidence of infants with birth defects such as mental retardation, growth disorders, and malformed body parts. These women also have a high incidence of spontaneous abortions, stillbirths, and infant deaths. Even moderate drinking can cause birth defects in infants.

The problem of babies of addicted mothers is an area well-suited for intervention from the community health nurse. Education and monitoring during pregnancy can prove helpful; the family with an infant suffering from problems caused by addiction will need a great deal of assistance in providing the required care.

One area of need that has been identified to aid this population is the treatment center that can treat the pregnant substance abuser, as well as the mother and baby together after the birth.

Many children, including newborns and infants, are being abandoned by their parents. This seems to be more common with crack cocaine use. Crack addiction has led to the creation of the "boarder-baby" (babies boarded in maternity, pediatric, and other settings). One example of a home that boards babies of addicted mothers is Hale House in New York City. This has also led to an increase in "kinship" foster care placement, a situation in which blood relatives are licensed and paid to be foster parents. In other cases, grandparents, especially grandmothers, often of advanced age, are being forced to care for their children's children (Dumas, 1992).

Women

The incidence of chemical dependency in women has increased dramatically in the twentieth century. The ratio between alcoholic men and alcoholic women is steadily decreasing. One interesting but alarming statistic is the increase in the percentage of young women drinking in the past 20 years (USDHHS, 1990). Women are also more likely to be dually addicted or polydrug abusers.

It has been common for society to view chemically dependent women as immoral, whereas the man who is an alcohol abuser is seen as "macho" or "just having fun." The stigma of being a woman substance abuser may increase the denial by all concerned and further handicaps her from obtaining treatment. Studies have found that the family tends to deny the woman's drinking problem longer than does the family of a male, inasmuch as it is difficult for family members to accept that their wife, mother, or daughter has a drinking problem. Because they have been able to conceal their drinking for a longer period of time, women have often been known as "closet" drinkers. They have also been protected from facing the consequences of their substance abuse; for example, women are less likely to receive citations for driving while intoxicated (DWI) than are men (Hennessey, 1992).

Women are also more likely to go to a family physician for vague complaints and receive a prescription for a mood-altering drug such as diazepam (Valium) or chlordiazepoxide (Librium). These drugs are often combined with alcohol consumption, which leads to polyaddictions and cross-tolerance.

The Elderly

The problem of substance abuse among elderly persons is receiving more attention as the true nature of the problem is coming to light. Estimates are that perhaps 5% to 10% of persons older than 60 years of age are alcohol or drug abusers. These problems often develop as a result of stress, loss, depression, and other negative aspects of aging. Alcohol is the substance most abused by the elderly, followed by prescribed mood-altering drugs (Chenitz, 1990). It has been stated in at least one source that between 50% and 60% of older adult men use alcohol on a routine basis well into old age (USDHHS, 1990).

Older persons who began to have drinking problems early in life may exhibit signs of late stages of alcoholism, including liver cirrhosis, polyneuropathy, malnutrition, alcohol-related dementia, Wernicke-Korsakoff syndrome, and cerebellar degeneration. The progression seen in long-term chronic alcohol abusers covers a period of 20 to 40 years, whereas deterioration in persons who begin drinking heavily in later years is relatively rapid.

Chemical dependency in the elderly often goes undetected and untreated (Curtis, 1989). The effects of the abuse may be explained as a sign of senility or chronic brain syndrome or as a natural consequence of growing older. Also, society may view substance abuse in the elderly as untreatable or may believe that the elderly deserve this "pleasure" in life (Parette, 1990). The community health nurse can be invaluable in detecting chemical dependency in an elderly person with a history of malnutrition, falls, depression, or other alcohol-related physical disabilities (Krach, 1990).

Nurses

Nurses have been found to be at high risk for the development of substance abuse and chemical dependency. Although it is difficult to estimate precisely the incidence in nurses, the American Nurses' Association (ANA) estimates that between 6% to 8% of nurses have a substance abuse problem (Green, 1989). Identification of these nurses may be extremely difficult because they often resist treatment because of the stigma. Traditionally, nurses have been believed to be immune from such problems or to know better, and society may view nurses who abuse alcohol with disdain. In addition, affected nurses may fear legal or licensing reprisals, which may prevent them from seeking help.

Nurses are at risk for chemical dependency for a number of reasons. The work is viewed as stressful and demanding with few positive rewards (Green, 1989). Nurses may feel they have little control over their own working situations. They also have ready access to many mood-altering drugs, especially narcotics, which are the drugs most abused by nurses. Often, however, substance abuse in a nurse begins with legal prescriptions for drugs. The nurse continues to obtain a supply of drugs from legal sources for as long as possible and begins to divert drugs only when the addiction worsens. Some nurses have been found to come from dysfunctional families

and may enter nursing to feel good about who they are. Because of this co-dependent behavior, they are at increased risk of developing substance abuse themselves (Zerwekh & Michaels, 1989).

The community health nurse should be aware of the possibility of chemical dependency in colleagues. Some signs of substance abuse in nurses include excessive absenteeism and tardiness, excessive medication errors, illogical charting, keeping isolated at work, poor judgment and mistakes, appearing at work early and staying late, and signs of drug withdrawal. As the chemical dependency worsens, so will the job performance. Behavior that interferes with job performance should be documented.

Just as is the case with the general public, nurses tend to turn their backs on chemically dependent colleagues. They may enable them by covering up for them, ignore them for fear of getting involved, or refuse to admit the possibility of an alcohol or drug problem. However, the worst thing that a nurse can do regarding a chemically dependent colleague is to do nothing (Green, 1989).

Most states have now established peer-assistance programs that offer assistance to the impaired nurse. These programs usually are linked with a state board of nursing or a professional organization, or both. Specific information about these programs can be obtained from the American Nurses' Association.

COMMON SUBSTANCES OF ABUSE
Alcohol

Alcohol is a central nervous system depressant. The so-called stimulating effect of alcohol occurs because the first areas affected are the higher centers of the brain that control judgment and self-control. As alcohol intake increases, other areas of the brain are also affected. Unconsciousness may occur, respirations may slow, and death may result.

Alcohol does not require digestion and is absorbed in both the stomach and the intestine. An empty stomach increases absorption. After ingestion, small amounts of alcohol are lost through breathing and in the urine, but 90% of alcohol is broken down by the liver. The active ingredient

TABLE 23-1 Effects of varying blood alcohol levels

Level (mg)	Effect
50-75 (0.05-0.075%)	Pleasant, relaxed state, mild sedation, loosening of inhibitions
100-200 (0.1-0.2%)	Overt signs of intoxication: loosening of the tongue, clumsiness, beginning emotional changes
200-400 (0.2-0.4%)	Severe intoxication: difficulty speaking, stumbling, emotional lability
400-500 (0.4-0.5%)	Stupor, coma
>500 (0.5%)	Usually fatal

in alcoholic beverages is ethyl alcohol, or ethanol. A 12-ounce bottle of beer, a four-ounce glass of wine, and 1½ ounces of "hard liquor" contain similar amounts of alcohol.

Alcohol has a diuretic effect. Increased amounts of electrolytes, including potassium, magnesium, and zinc, may be excreted in the urine of a heavy drinker. Prolonged use of alcohol has a toxic effect on the mucosa of the intestine, which results in decreased absorption of thiamine, folic acid, and vitamin B_{12}.

Alcohol is not converted to glycogen, and it provides the body with calories but no minerals or vitamins. One ounce of alcohol provides 200 kcal, but these are "empty calories." This accounts for malnourishment in many alcohol abusers who maintain near-normal body weight.

Blood alcohol levels depend on the amount of alcohol ingested and the size of the individual. Most states designate blood alcohol serum levels of 100 mg/100 ml (0.10%) as the legal limit for driving a motor vehicle. Higher blood alcohol levels have increasingly more side effects (Table 23-1).

In 1987 the average annual consumption of alcohol in adults in the United States was equivalent to 1.34 gallons of beer, .39 gallons of wine, and .83 gallons of distilled spirits. Males are more likely to drink and be heavy drinkers than women (USDHHS, 1990).

Stimulants

Stimulants are natural and synthetic drugs that have a strong stimulating effect on the central nervous system (CNS) and are accompanied by a feeling of alertness and self-confidence. When stimulants reach the brain, they cause the neuron transmitters to fire off messages too quickly. Other results include dilation of the pupils, increases in pulse and blood pressures, reduction of fatigue, reduction of appetite, and an increase in concentration. When the feeling of alertness wears off, however, the person experiences fatigue and depression, as well as a feeling of lethargy and anxiety. Drugs included in this category are amphetamines, cocaine, caffeine, and nicotine (Fitzgerald, 1988). These drugs will be discussed separately.

Stimulants have the potential to produce **tolerance,** the ability to endure drugs without apparent injury, but usually they do not cause symptoms of physical withdrawal. Psychologic dependence is common. Side effects of stimulant use include restlessness, dizziness, insomnia, headaches, diarrhea, constipation, and lack of appetite. Persons who ingest a large amount of stimulants over a period of time may experience extreme agitation and anxiety. Death may occur as a result of a cerebral hemorrhage or heart attack. Collapse from exhaustion during the use of stimulants can occur. Withdrawal can lead to profound depression and suicide.

Amphetamines

Amphetamines are synthetic psychoactive drugs that are available in capsule or tablet form. Current belief is that amphetamines increase the release of norepinephrine. The resulting stimulation increases alertness, concentration, learning ability, and attention span. Medical uses of amphetamines include the treatment of narcolepsy, obesity, fatigue, and depression. Methylphenidate

(Ritalin), an amphetamine-like drug, often is used to treat children who are hyperactive. Commonly used amphetamines and their brand names are dextroamphetamine (Dexedrine), metamphetamine (Methidrine), and amphetamine (Benzedrine). Street names include pep pills, dexies, bennies, ups, speed, crystal, meth, and whites.

Cocaine

Cocaine (gold dust or champagne of drugs) has been called the recreational drug of the 1980s. The statistics for cocaine use are alarming. Twenty one million persons have tried cocaine, and nearly three million use the drug on a regular basis (House, 1990). Cocaine is a psychoactive drug that comes from the leaves of the South American coca bush. It was first used by the members of early South American tribes, and its use was encouraged by the Spaniards, who found that the natives worked longer and harder and needed less food when they used cocaine.

At one time cocaine was used as an ingredient in many products, including syrups, nasal sprays, cigarettes, liquors, and cola beverages. It also was recommended, at one time, as a treatment for alcoholism. In 1914, the nonmedical use of cocaine was prohibited. It is used medically as an anesthetic of choice for some procedures of the nose and throat and as a part of Brompton's mixture, which is administered for pain control in patients with cancer.

Cocaine is similar to the neurotransmitter norepinephrine. It mimics norepinephrine's action in carrying neuron impulses between cells. With the use of cocaine the brain cuts back on its own production of norepinephrine; when the cocaine "high" wears off, the supply of norepinephrine is depleted, which leads to the cocaine "crash." Continuous use of cocaine can result in a more permanent depletion of the neurotransmitter, which produces a parkinsonian-like syndrome (House, 1990).

Cocaine is ingested by sniffing, smoking, or injection. Cocaine may also be "free-based," a process of heating the drug to separate it from impurities. When free-based cocaine is injected, it produces a high that is more intense and short-lived than when cocaine is smoked.

A newer form of cocaine that is now readily available in most locations is called "crack," a mixture of cocaine and common baking soda and water. It gets its name from the sound it makes as it is used. Crack is heat resistant and reaches the brain faster and in higher concentrations, producing a more intense euphoria within about six seconds. The high is also more intense because crack contains as much as 90% pure cocaine, whereas cocaine hydrochloride may contain only 15% to 25% of pure cocaine. The feeling of exhilaration lasts a much shorter time, however: generally five to seven minutes in contrast with 30 minutes after using powdered cocaine. It is less expensive than other forms of cocaine and is considered highly addicting (Fitzgerald, 1988). Other street names for cocaine include blow, coke, dust, flake, nose candy, rock, snow, super-blow, toot, and white (Povenmire, 1990).

Chronic sniffing of cocaine can destroy the nasal tissues. Smoking it can cause lesions in the lungs. Tolerance and psychologic dependence can develop, and an overdose can cause convulsions, respiratory paralysis, and death. A cocaine psychosis has been reported that is characterized by a loss of pleasure and orientation, by hallucinations, and by insomnia. Abrupt withdrawal from cocaine does not lead to physical withdrawal (Dubiel, 1990).

Caffeine

Caffeine is the most accepted and most used psychoactive substance in the United States. Many beverages, medications, and other products contain caffeine. It has been used as an additive in carbonated beverages since the early 1900s. Because of its availability and widespread use, most persons do not view caffeine as a drug.

In its pure state, caffeine is a white powder or consists of white, needle-shaped crystals. It stimulates the CNS, the digestive system, and the kidneys. Body metabolism is increased, and blood pressure is raised. Large doses of caffeine cause tachycardia, headaches, nervousness, insomnia, and stomach distress. Physical dependence occurs with a regular intake of 350 mg for an adult (a cup of brewed coffee contains 75 to 155 mg).

Withdrawal symptoms are severe headache, irritability, and fatigue (Abadinsky, 1993).

Nicotine

Nicotine is one of the most widely abused drugs today. It is far easier to become addicted to cigarettes than to alcohol or other drugs. Although the prevalence of nicotine use has shown a downward trend across race, gender, and educational levels, there are still approximately 50 million smokers in the United States. The rate of decline has been slower in women and in those of a lower educational level. There has been a significant decline among adolescents.

Smoking also is physically damaging. It has been linked to heart and blood vessel disease, chronic bronchitis, emphysema, and cancer.

Cigarette smoking is the leading cause of preventable death, with 350,000 deaths per year directly related to cigarette smoking. More than 1000 people die from the effects of smoking each day in the United States (Koop, 1988).

The tobacco plant belongs to the genus *Nicotiana,* a member of the nightshade family. Evidence has been found that tobacco use occurred as early as 200 AD. Tobacco is ingested by chewing or inhaling. The nicotine in tobacco acts as a stimulant to the CNS and also acts as an appetite depressant.

Nicotine is present in the brain within a few seconds of the beginning of smoking. Smokers claim that smoking produces relaxation; however, smoking releases epinephrine, which may cause psychologic stress. Withdrawal symptoms include a decrease in heart rate, weight gain, impairment of psychomotor performance, nervousness and anxiety, headaches, fatigue, and insomnia.

Barbiturates

Barbiturates are synthetic drugs that are classified as sedative-hypnotic agents. They are derived from barbituric acid and are used medically to treat high blood pressure, epilepsy, and insomnia and to sedate patients before and during surgery.

Barbiturates are swallowed (capsule or elixir form), used as a suppository, or injected. Drugs of this class were first synthesized in the early 1900s. Street names of barbiturates include yellow jacket (pentobarbital), red devil (secobarbital) phennie (phenobarbital), blue heaven or blue devil (amobarbital), barbs, downs or downers, rainbows, blues, and goof balls.

Barbiturates cause depression of the CNS, including slowing of physical and mental reflexes. Continued use of these drugs can cause physical and psychologic dependence and tolerance. Barbiturates produce feelings of well-being, euphoria, and relief from anxiety. Side effects include difficulty in breathing, lethargy, nausea, and dizziness. Alcohol and other CNS depressants potentiate the effects of barbiturates. Withdrawal symptoms include irritability, restlessness, anxiety, and sleep disturbances. In severe form, withdrawals may cause convulsions and delirium (Abadinsky, 1993).

Tranquilizers

Drugs classified as **tranquilizers** generally are referred to as major and minor tranquilizers. The major tranquilizers include drugs used to treat psychiatric illnesses and generally are not abused.

Minor tranquilizers are psychoactive drugs that are taken to reduce anxiety. First developed in 1950, they are commonly prescribed and are available in capsule, tablet, and liquid forms. Common types of tranquilizers are those found in the benzodiazepine family and include chlordiazepoxide (Librium), diazepam (Valium), oxazepam (Serax), lorazepam (Ativan), and clorazepate (Tranxene). It is estimated that more than 65 million prescriptions are written yearly for Valium, 75% by physicians who are not psychiatrists (Fitzgerald, 1988).

Hallucinogens

Hallucinogens are drugs — both natural and synthetic — that affect the mind and produce changes in perception and thinking. Included in this category are phencyclidine (PCP), lysergic acid diethylamide (LSD), mescaline, psilocybin, and 3,4-methylenedioxyamphetamine (MDA). Hallucinogens are found on the streets in a wide range of forms, including powder, peyote buttons, mushrooms, capsules, and tablets. LSD may

TABLE 23-2   Common street names of hallucinogens

Drug	Street name
LSD	Acid, barrels, blotter, domes, microdots, purple haze, windowpane
Mescaline	Buttons, cactus, mesc, mescal buttons
MDA	Love drug, mellow drug of America
Psilocybin	Magic mushroom, shroom
PCP	Angel dust, animal tranquilizer, crystal, dust, hog, embalming fluid, KJ killer, peace pill, synthetic marijuana

be found on blotter paper, chips, and sheets of paper, including tattoos or stamplike pictures of cartoon figures. Hallucinogens usually are taken orally, although MDA may be sniffed or injected. These drugs sometimes are placed on sugar cubes or mixed in other food. PCP may be sprinkled on marijuana and smoked. When it is combined with marijuana, it is called *sheba.* PCP may be injected or snorted. Some common street names for hallucinogens are listed in Table 23-2.

Most of the effects of hallucinogens are psychologic, although nausea and vomiting are common reactions. These drugs act as stimulants at first and produce depressed appetite, dilated pupils, and increases in body temperature and heart and respiration rates. Hallucinogens have a profound psychologic effect that is often described as a process of amplication, with the drug acting as a catalyst. These processes are called "trips." A person's attempts to resist the effects of the drug seem to increase the chances of a negative experience, or a "bad trip." These negative experiences are characterized by tremendous confusion, unpleasant sensory images, and extreme panic. With large doses of PCP there may be respiratory or cardiac arrest. Flashbacks may occur with the use of hallucinogens; that is, the user reexperiences the effects of the drug without having taken it again (Abadinsky, 1993).

Narcotics

Narcotics are drugs that are derived from the opium poppy or are produced synthetically. In the nineteenth century tincture of opium was called God's own medicine (GOM). In general,

narcotics lower the perception of pain. Narcotics include heroin, morphine, opium, codeine, meperidine, and methadone. Narcotics are injected, sniffed, smoked, or taken by mouth. Street names for heroin include H, horse, junk, hard stuff, smack, and scag.

Effects of narcotics include shallow breathing; reduced hunger, thirst, and sexual drive; and drowsiness. The user may experience euphoria, lethargy, heaviness of the limbs, and apathy. Overdose of narcotics can cause coma, convulsions, respiratory arrest, and death. If narcotics are injected, there is a risk of hepatitis or AIDS and other infections such as septicemia. With narcotics, tolerance and physical and psychologic addiction develop. Withdrawal may be painful and requires medical supervision.

Cannabis

Cannabis, or marijuana, comes from the Indian hemp plant, *Cannabis sativa.* It can grow wild; it is also fairly easily cultivated. It grows throughout the world, and its use has been recorded as long ago as 2700 BC. It usually is smoked as a cigarette (joint or reefer) or in a pipe or "bong." Slang terms for marijuana include dope, grass, herb, joint, pot, reefer, roach, smoke, snuff, and weed. Marijuana has been used for medical and nonmedical uses for more than 3000 years. Its popularity as a street drug began in the nineteenth century, and it is commonly abused today. Hashish or hash is more concentrated than marijuana and produces more intense symptoms. The primary psychoactive agent of marijuana is tetrahydrocannabinol (THC) (Fitzgerald, 1988). In low doses it acts as a mild sedative. In higher doses it has properties similar to the hallucinogens.

Marijuana's role in reducing eye pressure in glaucoma and in controlling side effects of chemotherapy is being evaluated. Physical effects of marijuana include drying of the eyes and mouth, increase in appetite, reddening of the eyes, and impairment of short-term memory. It raises the heart rate and blood pressure while lowering the body temperature and producing loss of coordination and possible confusion. Research shows that marijuana may affect chromosome division and cause birth defects (Zuckerman et al., 1989). Persons who smoke marijuana have been found to have a lowered resistance to infection. Also, the tar content of marijuana cigarettes is 7% to 20% that of regular cigarettes, and thus may lead to respiratory problems (Fitzgerald, 1988). Marijuana is fat-soluble and may be stored in the body for as long as several months.

Psychologic effects of marijuana include an altering of perception by the senses. The user has a sense of well-being and intoxication, although depression and panic may occur. Marijuana is psychologically addictive, and anxiety reactions may occur.

Deliriants

Deliriants are any chemicals that give off fumes or vapors that, when inhaled, produce symptoms similar to intoxication. They may be called inhalants. The fumes or vapors from inhalants are sniffed through the nose, or the vapors are put into a bag or captured in a balloon to increase the concentration of the inhaled fumes.

The history of the use of inhalants is traced back to ancient Greece. Sniffing of commercial products and solvents was first documented in the 1950s. Deliriants or inhalants have a psychoactive or mood-altering effect when the vapors are inhaled and sniffed. Most inhalants fall into one of three categories: solvents, aerosol sprays, or anesthetics. Solvents include commercial products such as glue, gasoline, kerosene, lighter fluid, "white out," and nail polish remover. Aerosol products include hair sprays, deodorant, insecticides, and cookware sprays. Anesthetics that are used recreationally include ether, chloroform, and nitrous oxide. Amyl nitrate and butyl

nitrate, drugs used for treatment of cardiac disease, also are abused; these fall into a category called whippets.

Almost all inhalants are CNS depressants that slow the user's heart rate, brain activity, and breathing. Other effects include slurred speech, blurred vision, inflamed mucous membranes, light-headedness, ringing in the ears, watering eyes, loss of coordination, and excessive nasal secretions. With high doses, the user may lose consciousness or have seizures. The effects are immediate and usually last 20 to 45 minutes.

The prolonged use of inhalants may lead to liver, kidney, blood, and bone marrow damage. The sniffing of toluene, found in gasoline and commercial cleaners, has been linked to irreversible brain damage, which can manifest as forgetfulness, inability to think clearly, depression, irritability, hostility, and paranoia. Use of large amounts of aerosols or solvents can cause death as a result of cardiac arrest after arrhythmias. Death from inhalants usually is caused by suffocation because of the displacement of oxygen in the lungs. Sniffing of inhalants from a bag or balloon increases the risk of suffocation (Abadinsky, 1993).

Designer Drugs

Designer drugs are synthetic, organic chemical variations of drugs that are commonly abused. They are also known as analogs. These designer drugs are created by underground chemists and designed to act like controlled substances (Seymour, 1989). The molecular structure of the drug is altered, thus making the drug legally unrestricted. One of the dangers of designer drugs is that a change in chemical structure may also change the length of action, the effects, or the possible side effects of the drug. An example of an analog is the drug methylenedioxymethamephetamine (MDMA). This drug has been nicknamed "Ecstasy." It was first patented in 1914 but did not receive a great deal of attention until it was rediscovered in the late 1970s. This analog of methamphetamine was reported to cause acute euphoria and to produce long-lasting positive changes in attitude and self-confidence. Some symptoms of use mimicked those of LSD, but MDMA was not felt to produce the severe side ef-

TABLE 23-3   Chemical use history

Classification	Drug name	Date of last use	Amount	Frequency	Length of use	Usual amount	Method of use
Barbiturates							
Tranquilizers							
Alcohol							
Marijuana							
Opium							
Heroin							
Narcotics							
Cocaine							
Stimulants							
Hallucinogens							
Inhalants							
PCP (dust)							
Amphetamines							
Caffeine							
Hash/hash oil							
Analgesics							
Others							

fects commonly found with amphetamines. Unfortunately, the use of this analog has been found to cause damage to nerve cells that results in parkinsonian-like symptoms (Abadinsky, 1993).

CHEMICAL DEPENDENCY

Alcoholism and drug addiction are commonly referred to as **chemical dependency**. Most modern definitions of dependence concerning drug addiction and alcoholism consist of two parts—physical and psychologic dependence. **Physical**

dependence refers to a physiologic state in which the continuous and prolonged consumption of a drug or alcohol leads to the user's adaption to its presence. **Tolerance** then develops. If the use of alcohol or drug use stops, withdrawal symptoms occur. **Psychologic dependence** refers to the craving for a drug or alcohol.

The terms *habituation* and *addiction* also have been used to define the nature and extent of drug use. **Drug habituation** includes repeated use of a drug to a point to which psychologic dependence occurs. **Drug addiction** includes craving, psychologic dependence, and physical dependence (Long, 1993).

Dual Diagnosis

Chemical dependency is a primary illness; however, chemically dependent persons often have other psychologic problems, such as depression or anxiety. Many problems disappear when drinking and drug use cease. It is important to diagnose and treat chemical dependency before other psychologic problems are investigated.

Psychiatric and psychologic symptoms may, however, make recognition of an addiction more difficult. Determining the correct diagnosis is a task for an expert in chemical dependency and psychiatry or psychology. Persons with a dual diagnosis may be more difficult to treat and may require treatment with medication such as antidepressants.

USE OF THE NURSING PROCESS
Assessment

It is important to collect both subjective and objective data about the client suffering from alcoholism. Subjective data include the person's normal using or drinking pattern, as well as the date and time of the last drink or use of drugs. The specific drink or drug used and the quantity used is important. Table 23-3 shows a chemical use history form that may be helpful in determining a drinking or drug-using pattern.

Any past history of tremors, hallucinations, delusions, or delirium tremens (DTs) should be assessed. Past periods of abstinence, normal diet patterns, the presence of problems (e.g., legal, occupational, or family), and any family history of chemical dependency are evaluated. The occurrence of blackouts is considered diagnostic. It is important for the community health nurse to remember that the defense mechanism of denial will be present in both the substance abuser and the family in untreated chemical dependency. The information gained from the affected person may not always be accurate, and it is helpful to validate it with family members or significant others (Tweed, 1989).

Objective data that can be important include an abnormal response to preoperative medica-

tion, anesthesia, or sedatives. The existence of tremor, morning nausea, or skin conditions should be assessed, as well as mental functioning, general behavior, and the relationship of weight to height. The occurrence of tachycardia, hypertension, neuropathies, and petechiae is significant. The presence of ascites and a positive result of a blood alcohol, urine alcohol, or drug screen should alert the community health nurse to take an in-depth history. Another objective sign in the IV drug abuser is track marks. If the person has been injecting into the veins, needle marks or small scabs may be present on the hands, forearms, or instep. The abuser may attempt to hide sites of injection and use the veins of the penis or the conjunctival vessel of the eyelid.

Diagnosis

A diagnosis of psychoactive substance dependence, including alcoholism, is based on the specific criteria presented here (Kirk & Bradford, 1987).

1. At least three of the following signs indicate psychoactive substance dependence:
   a. Substance often taken in larger amounts or over a longer period than intended
   b. Persistent desire for the substance or one or more unsuccessful efforts to cut down or control substance use
   c. A great deal of time spent in activities necessary to get the substance, taking the substance, or recovering from its effects
   d. Frequent intoxication or withdrawal symptoms when the individual is expected to fulfill a major role obligation at work, school, or home
   e. Important social, occupational, or recreational activities given up or reduced because of substance use
   f. Continued substance use despite knowledge of having a persistent or recurrent social, psychologic, or physical problem caused by or exacerbated by the use of the substance
   g. Marked tolerance: need for markedly increased amounts of the substance to achieve intoxication or the desired effect
   h. Characteristic withdrawal symptoms

i. Substance often taken to relieve or avoid withdrawal symptoms

j. Persistence of some symptoms of the disturbance for at least one month or repeated occurrences over a longer period of time

Diagnostic tests. Routine blood tests often reveal abnormalities that are directly related to alcoholism. These include elevated liver enzymes, hypoglycemia, and abnormal blood protein levels. Magnesium levels may be decreased. It is not uncommon to find anemia and other evidence of poor nutrition in alcoholic clients.

One diagnostic test used to detect drug abuse is the urine or blood drug screen. The amount of time after use that drugs can be detected in the urine varies from a very short time for alcohol and cocaine to a long time for benzodiazepines and cannabis. It is possible to have a minimally positive drug test result for cannabis because of a long period of "passive inhalation" from close contact with someone smoking and exhaling marijuana fumes. Urine testing usually is not used to detect alcohol because it is metabolized very rapidly. Alcohol blood levels are much more accurate. The breathalyzer test is used by law enforcement agencies to determine alcohol levels in the blood.

Nursing diagnoses. Nursing diagnoses by the community health nurse for the person with substance abuse depend on the condition and nursing assessment of the person. The diagnoses may include the following:

1. Activity intolerance
2. Anxiety
3. Coping, ineffective individual and family
4. Denial, ineffective
5. Fear
6. Fluid volume, excess or deficit
7. Health maintenance, altered
8. Home maintenance management impaired
9. Incontinence, bowel or bladder
10. Infection, potential for
11. Injury, potential for
12. Knowledge deficit
13. Mobility, impaired physical
14. Noncompliance
15. Nutrition, altered: less than body requirements

16. Self-care deficit
17. Self-esteem, disturbance in
18. Sensory-perceptual alteration
19. Social interaction, impaired
20. Spiritual distress
21. Thought processes, altered
22. Violence, potential for

Implementation

Primary prevention. Prevention of chemical dependency is a complex issue, partly because of the almost unlimited financial resources of the illicit drug industry, and its power. Primary prevention attempts to prevent alcohol and drug problems before they begin. Legal efforts have been made to restrict the sale of alcohol to minors and to institute heavier penalties for driving while intoxicated and for drug trafficking. The federal government also has scheduled drugs according to their addictiveness. Unfortunately, many of these efforts have not been highly successful. Other efforts have been aimed at monitoring the influence of mass media on attitudes and behaviors.

Education is, in part, the key to prevention. This includes teaching fairly young children about the dangers of alcohol use and abuse. Many elementary schools now start these programs as early as the first or second grade. In addition, working with children can help to increase their self-esteem so that they may be better able to avoid peer pressure to drink or use drugs as they become older. This is similar to strategies that promote prevention by improving an individual's ability to deal with the environment without drug use. These strategies include problem solving, assertiveness, stress management, parenting, and values clarification. The goal is to help individuals improve interpersonal relationships, communication, and self-esteem.

The Drug Free School Act of 1986 requires elementary, middle, and high schools to have programs to encourage a drug-free school environment.

One such program is Project Dare. This program works in school to prevent chemical abuse and dependency during school years by providing accurate information about alcohol and drug use, teaching students decision-making skills, showing students how to resist peer pressure, and giving ideas for alternatives to drug use (Ohio Department of Education, 1989).

Another attempt to educate persons involves families and employers of alcohol and drug abusers. They are taught that alcoholism is a disease that needs treatment. Alcohol abusers usually are surrounded by persons who enable their substance use and abuse; for example, the spouse who calls the employer to say that the drunk or hung-over mate is sick with the flu. Without this enabling behavior, which includes making many excuses for the affected person, the substance abuser might seek help sooner.

Community health nurses are in an excellent position to implement substance-specific primary prevention for clients and families. All the settings in which community health nurses work offer opportunities to introduce the subject of substance abuse in day-to-day health care and teaching. These settings include schools and occupational and clinic sites.

Secondary prevention. Prompt diagnosis and treatment can be important in assisting alcoholic abusers to once again become productive members of society. More and more programs are being developed to detect substance abusers; some are occupational programs or employee-assistance programs. These programs generally accept the assumptions that the most clear-cut mechanism for defining problems related to drug use is the immediate supervisor's awareness of impaired performance on the job and that chemical dependency is accepted as a medical problem. Generally, disciplinary procedures are suspended while the person receives treatment.

Planned confrontation (intervention). Some people still believe that it is only when the alcohol abuser desires and seeks help that treatment can be effective. Unfortunately, often by the time an alcohol-dependent person realizes the need for help, much has been lost. Recently, a process called **intervention** has been used to assist the alcohol abuser in asking for help. Interventions are planned confrontations by individuals who care about the addicted person. These individuals present facts or data about specific and descriptive events. The tone of the intervention should be nonjudgmental. The goal of the intervention is to have the alcohol abuser see and accept reality so that the need for help is realized. It is best to have immediate help available (Johnson, 1987).

Tertiary prevention. The goal of tertiary prevention is to end the compulsive use of alcohol or other drugs, or to minimize the negative effects of the use of thorough treatment and rehabilitation. The prevention of complications such as infections, neuropathy, and myopathies is a goal of treatment.

Nursing care. Care for the alcohol- or drug-addicted client in the acute phase involves detoxification efforts to prevent acute **withdrawal syndrome.** Withdrawal syndromes are physical reactions that occur after cessation or after a severe reduction in intake of drugs or alcohol. **Detoxification,** the removal of the toxic effects of alcohol or drugs from a patient, is undertaken in a controlled setting or under supervision of the physician or nurse. The person is closely watched and treated for complications as needed.

The initial goals for nursing care focus on maintaining the safety of the client. Prevention of injury, often from seizure activity, is important, as well as the maintenance of an intact airway. As the client begins to feel better, the nurse works to help facilitate a decrease in anxiety and the beginning of acceptance of the need for help. Later, the client is assisted in making positive changes in lifestyle to maintain sobriety.

Medications. Medications used in the initial period of detoxification include chlordiazepoxide (Librium) or a similar drug. The drug is used in decreasing doses for its sedating and anticonvulsant effects during detoxification. The dosage can be as great as 50 mg every 3 hours in the first 24 hours. Anticonvulsant therapy may include phenytoin (Dilantin) and magnesium sulfate. The anticonvulsant agent may be continued longer if the person has a history of seizures.

Specific medications may differ from setting to setting. In some, alcohol or paraldehyde is used in the detoxification process. Whatever medication is used, it is important to realize that alcohol and drug abusers may initially require large doses of medication to safely withdraw from the substance.

Another medication, which may be used in the treatment of alcohol abuse, is disulfiram (Antabuse), which blocks the enzymatic action needed to metabolize alcohol. If the person drinks, the drug will cause symptoms of nausea, vomiting, palpitations, and general sick feelings. Antabuse is used voluntarily by the person as a help in maintaining sobriety. It is important for the community health nurse who deals with the person on an Antabuse regimen to realize what effects will occur if the person drinks while taking this drug.

Methadone maintenance. One approach to the treatment of narcotics addiction is the methadone maintenance program. Methadone is a synthetic drug, and the average daily dose is much less expensive than is heroin or morphine. The drug is given legally as a part of a rehabilitation program. Methadone itself is addictive. Because methadone is easily available through legal channels, some experts believe that it is essentially the same as taking maintenance doses of other drugs such as insulin. Other persons disagree, however, because they believe that the use of methadone encourages addiction and replaces one drug with another.

Nutrition therapy. Many alcohol-addicted persons enter treatment with a history of poor nutrition. They may have received most of their calories from alcohol or have no appetite for food. As the condition of the alcohol abuser improves, the appetite usually improves also. The emphasis is on three well-balanced meals a day, with free access to snacks. Many clients find that they crave sugar in this period. If the alcohol-dependent person has problems with cirrhosis of the liver, dietary modifications may be needed. In cases of delerium tremens (DTs), intravenous or nasogastric feedings may be necessary. In the acute withdrawal period, vitamin supplements including thiamine are almost always used.

Associated disorders of alcohol withdrawal. When alcohol is not available to a person in whom a physiologic dependence has developed, withdrawal symptoms occur. These symptoms range from mild tremors to severe agitation and hallucinations. The type and seriousness of the symptoms depend on several factors.

Alcohol abusers at high risk for serious symptoms include older persons, persons with a previous history of delirium tremens, persons with nutritional problems, and persons with other illnesses. Symptoms of alcohol withdrawal include diaphoresis, tachycardia, elevated blood pressure, tremors, nausea and/or vomiting, anorexia, restlessness, hallucinations, and convulsions.

The tremors associated with alcohol withdrawal usually are seen six to 48 hours after the last drink. They may persist from three to five days. The hands are involved first, but the tremors may become generalized, with involvement of the feet, tongue, and trunk. Seizures may occur from 12 to 24 hours after the last drink. Usually these are grand mal seizures and are not preceded by an aura.

Delirium tremens (DTs) is an acute complication of alcohol withdrawal that interferes with brain metabolism. The rate of death of persons who experience DTs can be as high as 15%, even with treatment. Signs that indicate DTs may occur include tremors, increased activity, confusion and disorientation, fear, and an elevated temperature. DTs often occur suddenly, three to four days after the last drink. The condition lasts from two days to a week but at times can last as long as four weeks.

Other disorders that occur with substance abuse include those found in Table 23-4.

Addicted persons who inject drugs are at risk for diseases such as hepatitis and AIDS. Often, they share needles and equipment or reuse them without sterilization between periods of use. They also demonstrate resistance to more responsible use because of blackouts or the character traits that accompany drug addiction.

The possibility of contracting AIDS is one of the high risks for persons who use drugs intravenously. AIDS has become an epidemic in the United States. By May of 1991, 132,510 cases of AIDS had been reported in America, and it was estimated that another one to 1.5 million people are infected but asymptomatic. Populations at high risk for HIV exposure include intravenous drug users, who often share needles.

The problem of AIDS in drug-addicted women is steadily increasing. Currently, almost 20,000

TABLE 23-4 Disorders associated with alcohol abuse

Body system	Disorder
Hepatic	Hepatitis, cirrhosis, fatty liver
Gastrointestinal	Cancer of the mouth and esophagus, irritation of the stomach or pancreas, difficulty in absorbing food
Neurologic	Organic brain disease with confusion, Wernicke-Korsakoff syndrome, disorders of peripheral nerves (neuropathies)
Cardiovascular	Enlarged heart, high blood pressure, increased cholesterol levels, low blood sugar, anemia, coronary artery disease, congestive heart failure, arrhythmias
Musculoskeletal	Disorders of muscles (myopathies), trauma, gout
Immunologic	Increased susceptibility to infection
Skin	Abscesses, rashes
Psychologic	Depression, anxiety, passive-aggressive personality, antisocial personalities, food addictions (bulimia or anorexia nervosa)

women have AIDS. This figure makes up 12% of the AIDS population. Fifty percent of this group abuse drugs intravenously. An increasing number of HIV-positive clients are manifesting AIDS and AIDS-related complex. HIV infection effects black and Hispanic women unequally. Women of color represent only 19% of all women nationwide, but they comprise 72% of all women with AIDS (Dumas, 1992).

Education. Educating the alcohol-addicted person about the disease of alcoholism is very important. Education includes teaching about the disease concept, medical aspects of the disease and accompanying complications, the need for continued abstinence, and signs and symptoms of relapse. The importance of aftercare, including Alcoholics Anonymous (AA), of being honest with physicians and dentists, and of learning how to express feelings in a more positive way is stressed. This area is one in which the community health nurse can be extremely helpful and effective in assisting the person and family in recovery issues. It also is important to educate the person about what drugs to avoid, as well as about products that contain alcohol, such as mouthwash, cough syrup, and aftershave lotion.

Rehabilitation. The treatment objective for substance abuse is to assist persons to completely stop using the substance and to under-

stand that they can never take one drink or mood-altering drug without the danger of relapse. Alcohol- and drug-addicted persons who are not currently using their substance of choice are not considered cured, only recovering. Treatment may take place in an inpatient setting or in an outpatient clinic. There is more and more emphasis on treatment in the outpatient setting. This emphasis has occurred partly because of financial concerns of insurance companies but also because few studies have demonstrated a significant difference between inpatient and outpatient treatment. Further, outpatient treatment allows the person to remain in a familiar setting.

Group therapy is often used. Its goal is to enable the person to see the relationship between the abused substance and the negative consequences that have resulted. Positive reinforcement, caring, emotional support, and encouragement are also very important. The group can point out negative behaviors and defense mechanisms and offer possible solutions to its members' problems. Many recovering alcoholics attend AA meetings or similar 12-step groups.

Alcoholics Anonymous is an international nonprofit organization, founded in 1935, that consists of abstinent alcoholics, whose purpose is to help other alcoholics stop drinking and maintain sobriety through group support, shared experiences, and faith in a power greater than themselves. These groups serve self-acknowledged substance abusers whose goal is to stay sober and help other substance abusers gain sobriety. AA groups meet regularly in most communities. Some groups are listed in the local telephone book or in a local directory of meetings. A telephone call to AA will bring help in the form of a returned call or a visit from an AA member to the alcohol-addicted person who desires help.

AA and other similar programs are founded on 12 steps (see box at right) that assist the alcohol abuser to admit his or her powerlessness over alcohol and other drugs. Other groups that have been formed as a result of the success of AA include Al-Anon, Families Anonymous, and Overeaters Anonymous.

Peer assistance programs for nurses. Over the last decade many states have developed programs to assist nurses who are impaired by either alcohol or drug use. Before the start of peer assistance programs the nurse often would be fired, or be free to move to another facility where the abuse could continue.

Peer assistance programs have several goals: (1) to assist the impaired nurse to receive treatment; (2) to protect the public from the untreated nurse; (3) to help the recovering nurse reenter nursing in a systematic, planned, and safe way; and (4) to assist in monitoring the continued recovery of the nurse for a period of time. The reentry of the nurse may include a restriction on passing narcotics or other drugs for a designated period (Green, 1989).

These programs are based on one nurse helping another nurse. Most volunteers in these programs are recovering nurses or nurses who work in the area of chemical dependency or psychiatric nursing.

Evaluation

Evaluation of clients with chemical dependency involves input from the clients themselves, as well as from family members or significant others, employers, or teachers. Questions to consider include whether the affected persons are staying sober and abstinent and whether they are

THE 12 STEPS OF ALCOHOLICS ANONYMOUS

1. We admitted we were powerless over alcohol—that our lives had become unmanageable.
2. Came to believe that a power greater than ourselves could restore us to sanity.
3. Made a decision to turn our will and our lives over to the care of God as we understood Him.
4. Made a searching and fearless moral inventory of ourselves.
5. Admitted to God, to ourselves, and to another human being the exact nature of our wrongs.
6. Were entirely ready to have God remove all these defects of character.
7. Humbly asked Him to remove our shortcomings.
8. Made a list of all persons we had harmed, and became willing to make amends to them all.
9. Made direct amends to such people whenever possible, except when to do so would injure them or others.
10. Continued to take personal inventory and when we were wrong promptly admitted it.
11. Sought through prayer and meditation to improve our conscious contact with God as we understood Him, praying only for knowledge of His will for us and the power to carry it out.
12. Having had a spiritual awakening as a result of these steps, we tried to carry this message to alcoholics, and to practice these principles in all our affairs.

The Twelve Steps are reprinted with permission of Alcoholics Anonymous World Services Inc. Permission to reprint the Twelve Steps does not mean that AA has reviewed or approved the content of this publication, not that AA agrees with the views expressed herein. AA is a program of recovery from alcoholism. Use of the Twelve Steps in connection with programs and activities which are not patterned after AA but which address other problems does not imply otherwise.

able to function in society with minimal anxiety. Their medical condition should be under fairly good control, and they should demonstrate positive coping mechanisms. Sleeping patterns, nutritional status, and self-concept all should show improvement. Last, the community health nurse needs to assess the entire family system, to ensure that all members are moving toward recovery.

Chapter Highlights

- The community health nurse frequently sees the problem of substance abuse in the community.

- Alcoholism and drug addiction are commonly referred to as chemical dependency.

- Dependency may be psychologic and physical and is defined as the need to continue the use of drugs and/or alcohol to prevent withdrawal.

- Efforts to prevent chemical dependency have included legal and educational efforts.

- Persons with chemical dependency also may suffer from a psychiatric diagnosis (called dual diagnosis).

- At least 18 million persons are considered "problem drinkers" in the United States today.

- There is a genetic component to the development of chemical dependency.

- Alcohol provides the body with "empty calories," and heavy drinking can cause damage to many body systems, especially the liver.

- Denial and delusion commonly are seen in persons with untreated chemical dependency.

- Substance abusers may require large doses of medications to prevent withdrawal symptoms during detoxification.

- Many of the problems found in alcoholism may be a result of nutritional problems.

- The so-called stimulating effects of alcohol occur because the first areas of the brain affected are the higher centers that regulate self-control and judgment.

- Alcoholics Anonymous, or a related 12-step group, has been found to be highly effective in treatment of the alcoholic and his or her family because it helps the person accept his or her powerlessness over drugs or alcohol.

- The basic types of drugs that are commonly abused are stimulants, depressants, hallucinogens, narcotics, cannabis, and deliriants.

- Caffeine is the most accepted and most widely used psychoactive drug in the United States.

- Drug addiction includes craving, psychologic dependence, and physical dependence.

- Drug-addicted persons who inject drugs are at increased risk for the development of AIDS and hepatitis.

- Nurses are at increased risk for the development of alcoholism and chemical dependency.

CRITICAL THINKING EXERCISE

A group of nursing students is assigned to a rehabilitation unit for persons who have been diagnosed as being chemically dependent. The students ask their instructor what causes the illness. She replies that several theories have been suggested to explain it.

1. Describe the three theories in detail that are outlined in this chapter. Apply each to a client from a different developmental stage. Write an appropriate nursing care plan for each of these clients.

2. Analyze the reasons why there are a greater number of chemically dependent persons from lower socioeconomic groups than there are from higher socioeconomic groups.

REFERENCES

Abadinsky, H. (1993). *Drug abuse: An introduction.* Chicago: Nelson-Hall Publishers.

Adams, F. (1988). Drug dependency in hospital patients. *American Journal of Nursing, 88,* 477-481.

Alcoholics Anonymous. (1976). New York: Alcoholics World Services.

Andre, J. (1979). *The epidemiology of alcoholism among American Indians and Alaskan natives.* Albuquerque: Indian Health Service.

Captain, C. (1989). Family recovery from alcoholism: Mediating family factors. *Nursing Clinics of North America, 24,* 55-68.

Chenitz, W. et. al. (1990). Drug misuse and abuse in the elderly. *Issues in Mental Health Nursing, 11,* 1-16.

Curtis, J.R., Geller, G., Stokes, E.J., Levine, D.M., & Moore, R.D. (1989). Characteristics, diagnosis, and treatment of alcoholism in elderly patients. *Journal of the American Geriatrics Society, 37*(4), 310-16.

Dubiel, D. (1990). Action stat! Cocaine overdose. *Nursing 90, 20*(3), 33.

Dumas, L. (1992). Addicted women: profiles from the inner city. *Nursing Clinics of North America, 27*(4), 901-915.

Fitzgerald, K. (1988). *Alcoholism: The genetic inheritance.* New York: Doubleday.

Frances, R. (1991). Substance abuse. *Journal of the American Medical Association, 265*(23), 3171-3172.

Frances, R. & Miller, S. (Eds.). (1991). *Clinical textbook of addictive disorders.* New York: The Guilford Press.

Green, P. (1989). The chemically dependent nurse. *Nursing Clinics of North America, 24,* 81-94.

Hennessey, M. (1992). Identifying the woman with alcohol problems: The nurse's role as gatekeeper. *Nursing Clinics of North America, 27*(4), 917-924.

House, M. (1990). Cocaine. *American Journal of Nursing, 90,* 40-45.

Hughes, T. (1989). Models and perspectives of addiction: Implications for treatment. *Nursing Clinics of North America, 24,* 1-12.

Jack, L. (1989). Use of milieu as a problem strategy in addiction treatment. *Nursing Clinics of North America, 24,* 69-80.

Jackson, J. (1954). The adjustment of the family to the crises of alcoholism. *Quarterly Journal of Studies of Alcoholism, 1,* 526-586.

Jacques, J., & Snyder, N. (1991). Newborn victims of addiction. *RN, 54*(4), 47-51.

Jesse, R. (1989). *Children in recovery.* New York: W. W. Norton and Co.

Johnson, V. (1987). *Intervention.* Minneapolis: Johnson Institute.

Kirk, E., & Bradford, L. (1987). Effects of alcohol on the CNS: Implications for the neuroscience nurse. *Journal of Neuroscience Nursing, 19,* 316-335.

Koop, J. (1988). The health consequences of smoking-nicotine addiction: A report of the Surgeon General. Washington DC: United States Department of Health and Human Services.

Krach, P. (1990). Discovering the secret: Nursing assessment of elderly alcoholics in the home. *Journal of Gerontological Nursing, 16*(1), 32-38.

Leccese, Arthur, P. (1991). *Drugs and society: Behavioral medicines and abusable drugs.* Englewood Cliffs, New Jersey: Prentice Hall.

Levy, G., & Hickey, J. (1991). Fighting the battle against drugs. *RN, 54*(4), 44-47.

Levy, S., & Rutter, E. (1992). *Children of drug abusers.* New York: Lexington Books.

Lindenberg, K. et al. (1991). A review of the literature on cocaine abuse and pregnancy. *Nursing Research, 40,* 69-75.

Long, B., Phipps, W., & Cassmeyer, V. (1993). *Medical-surgical nursing: A nursing process approach.* St. Louis: Mosby.

Mosby's Medical, Nursing, and Allied Health Dictionary (3rd ed.) (1990). St. Louis: Mosby.

Nuckols, C., & Greeson, J. (1989). Cocaine addiction: Assessment and intervention. *Nursing Clinics of North America, 24,* 33-44.

Ohio Department of Education. (1989). Drug Abuse Resistance Education: D.A.R.E. information brochure. Columbus, Ohio. Ohio Department of Education and Ohio Association of Chiefs of Police and Attorney General's Office.

Parette, H. (1990). Nursing attitudes toward the geriatric alcoholic. *Journal of Gerontological Nursing, 16*(1), 26-31.

Povenmire, K. (1990). Recognizing the cocaine addict. *Nursing 90, 20*(5), 46-48.

Rice, D. et al. (1990). *The economic costs of alcohol and drug abuse and mental illness.* San Francisco: Institute for health and aging.

Rivinus, T. (1991). *Children of chemically dependent parents.* New York: Brunner/Mazel, Inc.

Schuckit, M. (1989). *Drug and alcohol abuse: A clinician's guide to detoxification and treatment.* New York: Plenum Medical Book Co.

Schwartz, R., & Wirtz, P. (1990). Potential substance abuse: Detection among adolescent patients. *Clinical pediatrics, 29,* 38-43.

Seymour, R. et al. (1989). *The new drugs: Look alikes, drugs of deception, and designer drugs.* Center City, Minn: Hazeldon Foundation.

Tweed, S. (1989). Identifying the alcoholic client. *Nursing Clinics of North America, 24*(1), 13-32.

U.S. Department of Health and Human Services. (1990). *Seventh Special Report to the U.S. Congress on Alcohol and Health: From the Secretary of Health and Human Services.* (DHHS Publication No. ADM 90-1656). Rockville, MD: USDHHS, National Institute on Alcohol Abuse and Alcoholism.

Vandegaer, F. (1989). Cocaine: The deadliest addiction. *Nursing 89, 19,* 72-74.

Wagner, J., & Menke, E. (1991). Stressors and coping behaviors of homeless, poor, and low-income mothers. *Journal of Community Health Nursing, 8*(2), 75-84.

Williams, E. (1989). Strategies for intervention. *Nursing Clinics of North America, 24,* 95-108.

Zerwekh, J., & Michaels, B. (1989). Co-dependency: Assessment and recovery. *Nursing Clinics of North America, 24,* 109-120.

Zuckerman, B., Frank, D.A., Hingson, R., Amaro, H., Levenson, S.M., Kayme, H. (1989). Effects of maternal marijuana and cocaine use on fetal growth. *New England Journal of Medicine, 320,* 762-768.

HIGH-RISK AGGREGATES IN THE COMMUNITY

Joan M. Cookfair

Identifying aggregates within the population which are at high risk to illness, disability, and premature death, and directing resources toward them is one of the most effective approaches for accomplishing the role of Public Health Nursing.

American Public Health Association

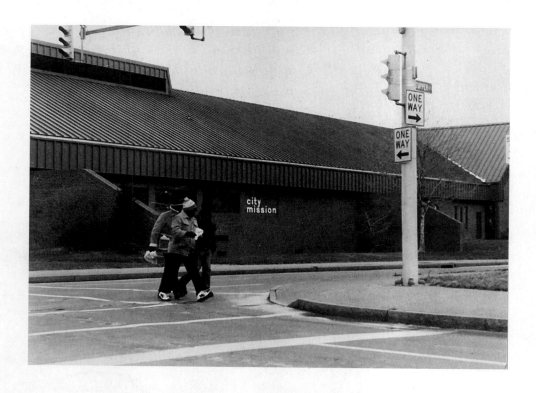

OBJECTIVES

At the conclusion of this chapter the student will be able to:

1. Define the key terms listed.
2. Understand the concept of aggregate-focused nursing.
3. Describe the lifestyles and/or circumstances of selected high-risk aggregates.
4. Discuss possible nursing interventions that would raise the level of wellness of each of these aggregates at primary, secondary, and tertiary levels.
5. Describe and discuss the nurse's role in aggregate-focused practice.

KEY TERMS

Aggregate

High-risk aggregate

Homeless

Migrant laborers/agricultural workers

Refugees

Nurses working in the community have traditionally focused on individuals and families when planning nursing interventions. The American Nurses' Association (ANA) and the American Public Health Association (APHA) have challenged community health nurses to broaden their practice. The ANA definition of community health nursing includes the responsibility to provide holistic care to groups in the community while the APHA includes a directive to improve the health of the entire community (see Chapter 1). Interventions with individuals and families are important parts of providing health to the entire community; however, to improve the health of the entire community, nurses need to move toward providing health care to persons at an aggregate level.

An **aggregate** is a collection of individuals who share similar characteristics. Health care can be provided to aggregates in many settings. For example, school nurses can establish programs to assist children with nutritional deficits. Occupational health nurses can set up programs to promote safety awareness in persons who are working in high-risk occupations. Community health nurses can set up programs for the homeless, mi-

grant workers, abused women and children, infants under one year, persons with AIDS, the frail elderly, refugees, and other groups within the community. Nurses may also teach newly diagnosed diabetic patients to adapt to an altered lifestyle. Aggregates may not be in the same geographic community, depending on their defining attributes; they are defined as aggregates because of their shared characteristics.

Lillian Wald, as early as the 1800s, saw that political and environmental factors such as poverty and pollution can create groups of people with special needs. Her nurses improved the health of the poor and of newly arrived immigrants through nursing interventions and political activity. Their actions raised the level of health of the entire community. In today's world, these groups of individuals with special needs might be called high-risk aggregates. A **high-risk aggregate** is described as a collection of individuals who, because of lifestyle or other circumstances, are at high risk for illness, disability, or premature death.

The nurse who identifies a high-risk aggregate can plan helpful interventions for the total group, instead of planning for each separate indi-

■ CASE STUDY

A nurse who worked in a special school for pregnant adolescents assessed their unique health problems in the following manner.

Assessment and Diagnosis

To determine their specific needs and knowledge deficits, the nurse met with each student as she entered the school and asked questions about her past and present health history and her source of prenatal care. If the student was not receiving prenatal care, she was referred to a provider. Students were made aware that the school nurse would be available for counseling while they were at school and that a public health nurse would visit them after the baby's birth. The initial physical examination included determination of blood pressure and weight and a urinalysis.

The nursing diagnosis for the students as a group included potential for high-risk pregnancy related to young age (teenager) and lack of prenatal care.

Planning and Intervention

The goals of the program were to maintain the students' health during pregnancy and to ensure their de-

livery of healthy babies with normal birth weights. (Low birth weight is considered five pounds, eight ounces or less.)

In an effort to do as much preventive counseling and intervention as possible, students were encouraged to weigh in frequently so that the nurse could talk with them. Also, visual aids with important information about nutrition, infant development, exercise, and pregnancy were placed on bulletin boards in strategic locations throughout the building.

A student group was formed for group counseling sessions. Some of the topics covered were physical and psychologic changes of pregnancy; the processes of labor and delivery; and birth control. In addition, much time was spent on nutrition.

Evaluation

Students who completed this program showed a lower incidence of low–birth-weight babies than did population groups with similar demographic statistics served by the city health department's maternity clinics (Higgs & Gustafson, 1985, pp. 130, 131).

---

vidual within the group. This is because the characteristics that place them at risk are similar. For example, family caregivers of Alzheimer's patients need respite from 24-hour supervision. Day care for the affected person, personal care aides, or other family members can all help to provide that respite and should be frequently accessed for the caregiver. All persons with chronic illness need appropriate education and counseling to encourage them to be compliant with prescribed treatments that will help them to remain at the highest possible level of wellness. The frail elderly need services that will enable them to continue their activities of daily living and maintain some control of their lives. The case study above describes an identified high-risk aggregate, pregnant adolescents.

THE HOMELESS

Homeless persons represent an aggregate that is particularly at risk for disability, injury, or prema-

ture death. They suffer from a lack of food, clothing, medical services, and social support. Without safe refuge, they are vulnerable to criminal acts such as robbery, assault, and rape. For homeless persons, recovery from an illness can be hampered by inadequate wound care, poor nutrition, and exposure. They are at high risk for episodic and chronic health problems. Homeless children may not be adequately immunized, and they experience many upper respiratory infections and ear infections (Miller & Lin, 1988).

Chronic physical problems of older homeless adults include disorders of the legs and feet, which occur disproportionately compared with persons in the general population. Many homeless have no place to lie down at night; thus, edema and loss of valve competence in legs and feet often result (Lamb, 1984). Lack of compliance with prescribed medical treatments may occur because of inability to access needed supplies. An outcome may be frequent exacerbations of existing chronic illnesses. Infestation may

TABLE 24-1 Presenting medical diagnoses in 434 homeless patients seen in a free clinic in New York City

Diagnosis		Number
Acute or chronic alcoholism		160
Drug use, intravenous or subcutaneous		102
Trauma		80
Assault	32	
Accidental	38	
Burns	10	
Respiratory infection		76
Active pulmonary tuberculosis		54
Leg ulcer, cellulitis		41
Acute gastrointestinal disease		22
Seizure disorder		16
Jaundice or ascites		15
Venereal disease		7
Gonorrhea	5	
Primary syphilis	2	
Osteomyelitis		2

From *Providing services for the homeless: The New York City program* (p. 82) by A. Leaf & M. Cohen, 1982, City of New York: Human Resources Administration. Reprinted by permission.

occur because of shared clothing and lack of sanitary conditions. Sexually transmitted diseases are a problem (see Table 24-1). According to recent studies, the homeless are increasingly at risk for drug-resistant tuberculosis. Screening the aggregate for possible infection is difficult because of their constant movement. Follow-up is hampered by the lack of an address or phone. There sometimes is simply no way to get in touch with homeless persons.

The Causes of Homelessness

The causes of homelessness are varied. They are frequently economic, occasionally the result of personal crisis, and sometimes the result of illness. Depression and alienation from society can also be a factor.

Economic causes. Loss of employment can result in homelessness for an entire family. Once a family on the edge of poverty loses its home, finding a new job or even applying for government funding becomes a major problem. Persons with low incomes may lose their homes because of cutbacks in government assistance, or in some cases, urban renewal may destroy housing that was affordable to persons on very limited budgets.

Personal crisis. Women who run from abusive situations sometimes have nowhere to go. Adolescents who rebel from parental authority or abusive parents may also find that there is no available housing or they may have no way to access social services that might be available to them.

Mental illness. The trend toward releasing the mentally ill to community-based housing began in the 1960s. A comparison of two principle groups in Philadelphia, persons who are homeless episodically and persons who are homeless chronically, described the typical chronic homeless person as white, older than 40 years of age, and schizophrenic. The chronically homeless person may also be a substance abuser and have other health problems (Arce, Tadlock, Vergare, & Shapiro, 1983). Although well intended, the idea of placing the mentally ill in the least restrictive environment, or "deinstitutionalization," was not totally successful. Community-based housing is not the total answer. Some halfway houses and supervised group homes meet the needs of mentally ill persons well. However, there must be more consideration given as to the best possible solution for assisting the seriously mentally ill to remain as healthy as possible. Most certainly it cannot be life on the streets.

By far most of the newly identified homeless are young adult males. They are usually from minority groups, and may also come from low income, sometimes dysfunctional families. Lack of support systems, lack of job skills, and lack of available employment leaves these young men with nowhere to go but the streets.

In the United States, Vietnam veterans comprise 37% of the homeless population (Blakely, 1992).

It is difficult to collect statistics on the actual number of homeless persons in the United States and in Canada because of their transitory life style, but it is estimated that on any given night there are 600,000 homeless persons in the United States alone (Lindsay & Gottesman, 1992).

TABLE 24-2   Demographic characteristics of homeless subjects

Characteristic	Percentage of subjects
Gender	
Male	91.4
Female	8.6
Race/ethnicity	
Black	47.0
Caucasian	26.9
Hispanic	24.1
Other	2.0
Age (in years)	
Under 18	4.7
18-20	3.8
21-30	30.9
31-40	30.6
41-50	15.7
51-60	10.9
Over 60	3.3

From "The homeless population" by D.L. Vredevoe, P. Shuler, & M. Woo, 1982, *The Western Journal of Nursing Research, 14*(6), p. 732. Copyright 1992 by Safe Periodicals Press. Reprinted by permission.

Table 24-2 describes some of the demographic characteristics of this aggregate. Large cities, such as Los Angeles, New York, and Toronto, have large numbers of homeless. However, they can be found in most major cities, affluent suburbs, and rural areas; and the number of homeless is growing each year.

The Homeless Assistance Act

The Homeless Assistance Act of July, 1987 (PL100-77), defined a homeless person as an individual who lacks a fixed, regular, and adequate night-time residence or an individual who has as a primary residence a shelter, a welfare hotel, a transitional residence, or a public or private place not designated as a regular sleeping accommodation for human beings (Mayo, 1992).

Proposed Solutions

There is no one cause of homelessness; there is also no one solution. Some communities have come up with their own plans to assist this unfortunate group of people.

Wichita Sedgewick county task force for the homeless (Jeffers & Okeson, 1992) indicated three solutions that could assist homeless persons:

1. Coordinate services within the community.
2. Develop more low-cost housing and job-training opportunities.
3. Address the health care needs of the homeless and other low income persons (Figure 24-1).

In one year alone (1991), the Charleston Interfaith Crisis Ministry provided 66,911 shelter nights to the homeless. During this time, homeless persons made 2490 visits to nurses and physicians on site. Each day, 242 lunches were served, and social workers saw 372 persons per month. This service group strives to assist people to attain employment and housing (Mayo, 1992).

On a national level, in the United States, Congress passed the Homeless Persons' Survival Act in 1986. It included the following provisions:

- Homeless persons living in shelters are now eligible for food stamps. In addition, food stamps may be used by homeless people to buy prepared meals served in nonprofit agencies.
- Federal agencies may not bar anyone without a fixed address from receiving benefits from Supplemental Security Income, Medicaid, social security, Medicare, aid to dependent children, or the veterans administration.

We know what some of the causes for homelessness are and what some of the predictable needs are. Planning to help reduce the incidence and risk can be done at primary, secondary, and tertiary levels.

Primary prevention can be done by advocating for more low-income housing and job and education programs for unskilled people. Chapter 31 of this text recommends writing letters to government officials at national and local levels to lobby for clients. In addition, nurses can seek ways to immunize this population despite the transient lifestyle and the difficulty in follow-up. Teaching adaptive health practices when possible would be helpful. Lobbying for a humane solution to the problem of housing persons with mental illness is of paramount importance.

Secondary prevention can be done by screen-

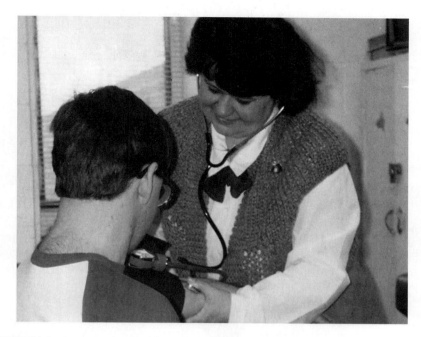

FIGURE 24-1   A community health nurse performs a health assessment for a homeless client.

ing persons in temporary shelters for beginning disease states that have not yet manifested themselves in clinical symptoms. Hypertension and diabetes are examples of treatable chronic illnesses that can be controlled if diagnosed in the early stages.

Tertiary prevention can come about by teaching the importance of compliance with prescribed medical regimes, referring for rehabilitative services, assisting with palliative care when necessary, and counseling individuals and families who have experienced loss of employment and loss of their homes.

Nurses who care for the homeless have to be aware of the need to advocate for them. They must also be able to give needed information and to refer appropriately. It is also imperative for the nurse to refrain from judgmental or punitive behavior. An acceptance of the homeless person's transient state and a sincere effort to plan short-term and long-term nursing interventions will benefit them. For example, providing lists of available shelters, soup kitchens, and sources of medical care will assist homeless persons in obtaining short term needs. Referral to available so-

cial services and counseling centers may assist homeless persons for the long term. Lobbying for affordable housing, job training programs, and expanded mental health care could actually help eliminate the problem of homelessness.

Although the homeless can be found anywhere, they seem to be predominantly an urban phenomenon. High-risk aggregates in rural areas may differ; for example, migrant workers may be the aggregate assessed by the nurse as the most in need of health care services.

MIGRANT AGRICULTURAL WORKERS

Migrant laborers, or **migrant agricultural workers,** move regularly to find work. They are usually poor and may have language barriers that make communication difficult. Their mobile lifestyle prohibits consistent long-term health care. For the most part, the patterns of migratory travel follow crop harvesting needs. The east coast migratory stream begins in Florida, and the mid-continent stream starts in south Texas, as does the West coast stream (Figure 24-2). Some migrant workers travel a few hundred miles while others travel thousands of miles. According

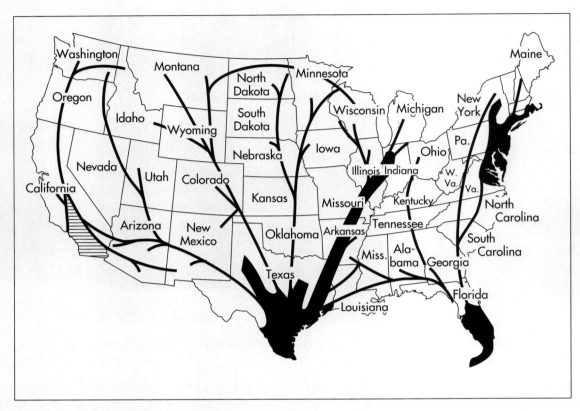

FIGURE 24-2 Major patterns of migratory travel. From *Health for the nation's harvesters* (p. 24) by A. Johnston, 1985, Farmington Hills, MI: National Migrant Worker Council Inc.

to the government Migrant Health Services, a migrant agricultural worker is "an individual whose principal employment is in agriculture on a seasonal basis, who has been so employed in the last 24 months, and who establishes, for the purposes of such employment, a temporary abode."

Using this definition, it was estimated that the total migratory population in the United States numbered 3.5 million. Many migrant workers are from minority groups such as African Americans, Native Americans, and Hispanics. Some are Mexican nationals who enter the United States illegally. Recently there have been increasing numbers of workers from Central America, Nicaragua, Guatemala, and El Salvador, who leave their countries to find work. What all of them have in common is that they are very poor, and they are desperate. Therefore, they will put up with working conditions that are substandard for

fear of being sent back to their country of origin (Johnston, 1985).

The most heavily traversed section of the United States–Mexico border is a strip that runs 15 miles east along the Pacific Coast. Here, the border is marked by a chain-link fence. In many places this fence is trampled or torn. The town of San Ysidro, California, which is across from Tijuana, is a border town. Nobody knows how many illegal immigrants slip through its legal port of entry. One estimate is 5000 per day. These illegal immigrants carry their most precious belongings in knapsacks or plastic supermarket bags and they will do anything for poor wages to earn their keep (Barach, 1990).

The Story of the Mistecs

The Mistecs and the Zapotec Indians come from a place in Mexico named Oaxaca. It is 1600 miles south of the border, and its residents are very poor. There are 570 villages in Oaxaca. None of them are prosperous, and outmoded farming methods have rendered much of the land impossible to grow crops. On one of the farms near San Diego, California, that employs some of the Mistecs, the conditions are unconscionable. The Indians live in camps because they cannot afford apartments in the town. Most do not speak English, and they stay close to the camps because of fear of being misunderstood. One camp in the town, which was built on a dry creek bed, consists of shacks made of scavenged lumber and cardboard. The shacks were constructed by the workers themselves. There are no toilets and there is no electricity or running water. Trash and excrement lie about. Groceries are purchased from a truck that drives through the camp. In the winter, the Mistecs suffer from the cold. They use kerosene and candles to light the shacks, and there are frequent fires. Pages from magazines and newspapers are stuffed into the walls for insulation. In other camps, the workers live in "spider holes;" they dig a pit and cover themselves with branches. They are frequently paid in cash so that taxes do not have to be deducted and the pay can be far below union scale. All are saving money to go home (Barach, 1990).

Beginning in 1986, the Immigration Reform and Control Act (IRCA) allowed workers to enter the country legally for a period of 11 months if farmers could document their inability to obtain United States citizens as workers (Barach, 1990). Many of these individuals bring their dependents with them, as do migrant workers who are citizens of the United States. Thus, women and children make up a large part of the migrant work force (Johnston, 1985).

Occupational hazards associated with this particular aggregate are exposure to sun and heat, muscular strains from heavy lifting, dermatitis from exposure to plant substances such as peach fuzz, respiratory conditions caused by weather and pollution, and accidents and bruises caused by incorrect operation of farm machinery. There is also a lack of available running water and toilets on many farm sites. Poor sanitation is common.

In 1984, Occupational Safety and Hazards Administration (OSHA) released proposed requirements that agricultural employers provide toilets, potable water, and handwashing facilities for their workers (Johnston, 1985). In spite of OSHA's efforts, migrant agricultural workers continue to have health problems in excess of the national norm because many employers disregard OSHA's standards. They also do not access health care as often as they should because of lack of insurance, lack of education, and lack of accessibility.

Common health problems among the children of this aggregate are upper respiratory problems, severe ear infections, dermatitis, and severe diarrhea. In addition to the occupational hazards mentioned earlier, both children and adults may suffer toxic reactions to pesticides applied to the crops.

The Migrant Health Act (see Table 24-3) set aside special funding for health programs targeted at this group of people by the federal government. It has been extended in one form or another since that time.

In December of 1979, the General Assembly of the United Nations stressed the tragic conditions of migrant workers worldwide. These conditions were in part a result of international conflict. The assembly composed a document aimed at assisting those who were working outside of their countries of origin. Following years of negotiations, a multinational human rights instrument was adopted by the assembly. The document gave workers the right to leave any state without restrictions and return to their country of origin. The document also gave the workers the right to life under the law, and guarded them against inhuman, degrading treatment or punishment. The document forbade slavery, servitude, and forced or compulsory labor (United Nations, 1991).

Persons do not remain migrant workers by choice. If given the opportunity, they move on to other occupations. Those who move on are replaced by the poorest, least educated, and most vulnerable groups among the general population. Their health and environmental surroundings remain substandard, in spite of government-sponsored migrant health programs. The question of how to raise the quality of life of migrant work-

TABLE 24-3   Migrant Health Act, 1962-1985

Legislative authority & effective date	Annual appropriation ceiling*	Eligible grant applicants	Services eligible for grant assistance	Persons eligible to receive grant-assisted service	Significant changes not otherwise noted
Public Law 87-692; added sec. 310 to Public Health Service Act: effective Sept. 1962	Not more than $3 million for each of 3 fiscal years ending 6-30-65	Public or private nonprofit organizations	Services of family health service clinics and other projects to improve migrants' health services or conditions	Migratory farm workers and their families	
Public Law 89-109; renewed Sec. 310 for 3 years; effective Aug. 1965	Increased ceiling to $7, $8, and $9 million, respectively, for 3 years ending 6-30-68	Same	Added "necessary hospital care"	Same	None
Public Law 90-574; renewed Sec. 310 for 2 years; effective Oct. 1968	Increased ceiling to $9 million for fiscal year ending 6-30-69 and $15 million for fiscal year ending 6-30-70	Same	Same	Same	Joint Conference Senate and House: "This program should be considered as a permanent and separately identifiable program, subject to periodic-Congressional review"
Public Law 91-209; renewed Sec. 310 for 3 years; effective March 1970	Increased ceiling to $20, $25, and $30 million, respectively, for 3 years ending 6-30-73	Same	Added "continuity in health services"	Added "Other seasonal farmworkers and their families"	Made DHEW Secretary rather than PHS; Surgeon General responsible for awarding grants; mandated a National Advisory Council

TABLE 24-3 Migrant Health Act, 1962-1985 cont'd

Legislative authority & effective date	Annual appropriation ceiling*	Eligible grant applicants	Services eligible for grant assistance	Persons eligible to receive grant-assisted service	Significant changes not otherwise noted
Public Law 93-45; renewed Sec. 310 for 1 year; effective June 1973	Increased ceiling to $26,750,000 for fiscal year ending 6-30-74	Same	Same	Same	None
Public Law 94-63; substituted new section 319 for Sec. 310; effective July 1975**	Set ceiling at $26,750,000, $39 million, and $44 million for 3 fiscal years ending 6-30-77	Wording changed to "public and nonprofit private entities"	Defined eligible services and arrangements in detail; added "project planning and development" and "acquisition and modernization of buildings"	Defined eligible population in detail	Provided priority for high impact areas and consumer-sponsored projects; mandated consumer governing board for each project; specified character of National Advisory Council's membership
Public Law 95-626; extended Sec. 319 as Sec. 329 for 2 years; effective Nov. 1978	Set ceiling at $40.8 million and $52 million for 2 years ending 9-30-81 (fiscal year-end date was changed)	Same	Added health education and social service; prepaid care under specific conditions; etc.	Same	Defined duties of project governing board; etc.
Public Law 97-35; extended Sec. 329 for 3 years; effective 1981	Set ceiling at $43, $47.5, and $51 million, respectively, for 3 years ending 9-30-84	Same	Same	Same	None
Public Law 99-280 (S.1282): 1986, for 2 years, effective 1987	$45,400,000	Same	Migrant workers	Same	Focused on health centers

Continued

TABLE 24-3   Migrant Health Act, 1962-1985   cont'd

Legislative authority & effective date	Annual appropriation ceiling*	Eligible grant applicants	Services eligible for grant assistance	Persons eligible to receive grant-assisted service	Significant changes not otherwise noted
Public Law 100-386; 100th Congress, 1988; for 3 years 1989, 1990, 1991	$48,500,000	Same	Migrant workers	Same	Extended to focus specific health centers for the health management of infants and pregnant women
Public Law 101-527; 101st Congress 1990			Migrant workers		Established an office of minority health to establish long-range and short-range goals that relate to disease prevention, health promotion, service delivery, and research for minority health in the United States
Public Law 102-531; 102nd Congress 1992; 1994-1997	$205 million	Activities for making progress toward health objectives for the year 2000	Migrant workers	Vulnerable populations	More state involvement

From *Health for the nation's harvestors* (p. 142) by A. Johnston, 1985, Farmington Hills, MI: National Migrant Worker Council Inc. (First eight entries only.) Remaining entries from specific United States Public Law documents.

* The actual appropriation for a particular fiscal year is usually lower than the ceiling set by Congress. Thus in the Program's first year, the appropriation was $750,000 rather than the authorized $3 million.

** The law was completely rewritten in 1975 adding a great deal of detail regarding eligible projects, eligible recipients of grant-assisted services, arrangements for service, etc. The original purpose was not changed.

ers, to increase their level of wellness, is complex and not easily answered. Many workers are so poor and desperate that they will work for low wages without complaint. Their nomad-like existence discourages any continuity in education and many groups remain semi-literate for generations. Language barriers are also a problem, as are cultural differences. The workers are not able to understand things like OSHA standards. In addition, those who complain probably would be fired. They have no valued skills and there are always other workers to take the place of those who move on or are fired. Interventions to assist migrant workers would need to be aggressive and planned at primary, secondary, and tertiary levels.

Primary prevention would be best if started at a federal level. Advocating for enforcement of OSHA standards would be a good beginning. Education for children and adults, perhaps onsite, would decrease functional illiteracy and increase language skills. Outreach programs to teach health-related topics would be appropriate. Nutritional supplements and a safe water supply would have to be made available to the workers.

Secondary prevention might include screening of infants, children, and adults in the health centers and house-to-house for beginning disease states.

Tertiary prevention might include treatment of existing health problems with an emphasis on possible toxic reactions to pesticides.

Migrant workers comprise what is probably one of the most disenfranchised aggregates in North America. Targeting them as a vulnerable group in need of special services should be made a nursing priority.

REFUGEES

Refugees comprise a high-risk aggregate about which there is little written. The United States has been called the "melting pot" for a diverse group of settlers. Canada has experienced, through the years, an influx of people who are from the dominant population group. In both the United States and Canada these individuals have come as immigrants. Immigrant status does not occur unless someone petitions on that person's behalf. The process is similar in both the United States and Canada. The person who petitions may be a family member or an individual willing to take responsibility for that person. Thus, the immigrant does not become a public charge or a drain on the community resources (United States Department of Immigration Information Services, 1993).

A refugee comes to the new country as a global homeless person with no city or country of origin. He or she is completely dependent on the state to which he or she applies for resettlement. Starting in 1975, refugees began arriving from countries vastly different from those of the caregivers available to them. The cultural differences, therefore, were also vast. In some instances, the refugees spoke languages unrelated to English. Recently, there has been an increase in persons arriving from Africa, South Asia, and the former Soviet Union (Muecke, 1992).

The nursing research on refugees, which was begun a decade ago, focuses on Indochinese refugees. From 1979 to 1980 the influx of persons in both the United States and Canada was from Cuba and Haiti. All of these new persons have strained and challenged the health care systems of the receiving countries. Public health nurses in particular have had to be vigilant and aware of the stressors the refugees may be experiencing and the cultural disparity between themselves and this high-risk aggregate. Many refugees who come to the new country may have histories of deep trauma and loss. Some may come from very rural areas. They settle in low socioeconomic locations with no idea of how to use support systems available to them. They grieve for lost relatives and cope in ways known to them in their country of origin (Muecke, 1992).

■ CASE STUDY

A community health nurse received a referral to visit an infant seen at a hospital emergency room for recurrent pneumonia and failure to thrive. Information on the referral included the fact that the family was non-English speaking. The spoken language was Imaric. The family members also spoke some Arabic. Taking an interpreter with her, the nurse gathered the following information. The family consisted of a 60-year-old widow, a 19-year-old son, a 15-year-old daughter, a 10-year-old son, a four-year-old grandson whose mother was still attempting to get out of Africa, and a three-month-old boy whose mother was the 15-year-old. The health state of the three-month-old was the reason for the referral. An assessment of the infant revealed a temperature of 104° F, rales in both lungs, and an inability to suck on his bottle. The family was giving him his medicine but was not giving Tylenol or attempting to push fluids. They did have cold cloths on his head. A phone call to the physician who had written the referral resulted in admission of the child to the hospital to get him past his present crisis. Following discharge, the infant was referred for follow-up care. The order for follow-up was broad and focused on teaching and counseling for the caretakers of the infant.

On the first visit following the child's discharge, the nurse did a family assessment to determine what kinds of intervention might be necessary (Figure 24-3).

The goal of the nurse was to create a safer environment for the child. It seemed evident that the whole family would need to become involved to create this environment. The head of the family was a widow, A. Mohammed, who had lost her husband and six of her children as a result of civil war in her country. She brought her remaining children and her grandchildren to America so they would be safe. However, she did not feel safe in her present environment, an apartment in an urban area that had a high crime rate. Sirens were heard all the time. "Bad men were on the street," and her apartment had been broken into. Food had been taken. The nurse realized that no teaching could take place until the woman felt safe, so the nurse referred her to social services. Efforts were begun to move the family to government housing where security was assured. Within two months this was accomplished. The 15-year-old mother was also referred to a supplemental feeding program for her baby.

The next visit went well. A. Mohammed had developed a nice rapport with the interpreter. That rapport extended to the nurse.

Contact was made with the school nurse to try to obtain free dental care for the children and the parent. After some delay, this was accomplished through a local university.

In an effort to do as much health prevention counseling as possible, the nurse scheduled biweekly visits and focused on the baby, weighing him weekly and praising the mother when he began to gain weight.

A local church was contacted and asked for donations of baby furniture and appliances that the family did not have. Members of the church became interested in the family and brought clothes and other needed items. Church members began to provide needed transportation to clinic appointments and other places. The general health of the family began to improve.

Evaluation: 6 months after the nurse began the visits, the baby had gained enough weight that he was no longer considered failing to thrive. There were no more episodes of pneumonia. When he began to show signs of an upper respiratory infection, the mother was able to call the clinic doctor and arrange treatment for him. All of the family members, with the exception of Mrs. Mohammed, were progressing well with their English. The nutrition of the family vastly improved, and the four-year-old had a normal hemoglobin level. The family seemed to be adjusting well. They began reaching out to others in their neighborhood and joined a mosque nearby. The people from the church continued to be involved, and even helped the two teenagers to obtain jobs. The social worker called the family regularly and visited at intervals as needed to help fill out forms and so on. The family was discharged from nursing care, although the nurse called weekly for some time to assess their health status.

Client name: A. Mohammed	Case no.: 2340
Client address: 33 Maple Lane	Phone no.: 872-5555

Reason for admission: Follow-up care; teaching & counseling, infant post pneumonia, failure to thrive.

Family constellation:

Name	Relationship	Age
A. Mohammed	mother	60
S. Mohammed	son	19
F. Mohammed	daughter	15
T. Serahan	grandson	4
F. Mohammed	son	10
F. Terahan	grandson	3 mos

Social history:

Name	Ethnicity	Occupation	Income
A. Mohammed	Black/Ethiopian	housewife	welfare
S. Mohammed	" "	attends school	"
F. Mohammed	" "	" "	"
T. Serahan	" "	" "	"
F. Mohammed	" "	" "	"
F. Terahan	" "	infant	"

Neighborhood data: Affluent _____ Moderate _____ Poverty __X__

Adequate utilities: Yes __X__ No _____

Neighbors: Friendly _____ Noncommittal __X__ Hostile _____

Transportation: Convenient _____ Accessible _____ Not available __X__

Health care facilities accessible: Yes _____ No __X__

Family health care data:

Present family illnesses (list) __Infant pneumonia, failure to thrive. T.Serahan__ appears anemic, F. Mohammed abscessed teeth. All of family are very thin.

Past action taken when family member ill _____
folk remedies _____

Family dynamics:

Role of each member A. Mohammed, head of household; others dependent children

Leadership: Patriarchal _____ Matriarchal __X__ Egalitarian _____ Democratic _____

Communication style: Open _____ Closed _____ Direct _____ Indirect __X__

Values system: Family _____ Religion __X__ Materialism _____ Ethnic beliefs __X__ Health _____

Health beliefs: Myths __X__ Old wives' tales _____ Cultural beliefs __X__ Fact _____

Family priorities: __safety__

FIGURE 24-3 Comprehensive family assessment tool and care plan.

continued

Family coping skills:

	Adequate skills	Needs assistance
Communication patterns: Express thoughts and feelings with one another		X
Emotional support: Encourage and care about one another		X
Community interaction: Involved in community activities, maintain friendships		X
Accepting help: Able to tap resources when needed		X
Flexibility of roles: Able to adjust responsibilities in change or crisis		X
Crisis management: Draws family together, viewed as a growth experience		X

Family wellness behaviors:

	Acceptable habits	Needs improvement
Nutritional status		X
Exercise program	X	
Alcohol consumption	X	
Drug habits	X	
Smoking	X	
Sleep patterns	X	
Stress management		X
Practices preventive health care		X

Risk factors identified: _Knowledge deficit regarding care of sick infant. Altered nutrition, less than body requirements due to lack of food and poor dental health. Ineffective family coping related to stress, high anxiety._

Notes: _Need an interpreter when visiting the family. Language is Arabic._

Signature _____

Home Care Nurse

FIGURE 24-3 Cont'd.

Chapter Highlights

- An aggregate is a group of individuals who share similar characteristics.

- A high-risk aggregate is a group of individuals who share similar characteristics or experience common factors that place them at risk for disease, disability, or death.

- The homeless are at risk. They are defined by the Homeless Assistance Act of 1987 as individuals who lack a fixed, regular, and adequate night-time residence or as persons who have as a primary residence a shelter, a welfare hotel, or a public or private place not designated as a regular sleeping accommodation for human beings.

- Primary, secondary, and tertiary care for the homeless include coordinating services within the community, screening for beginning health problems, and addressing the health care needs of the homeless population.

- Migrant workers are a high-risk aggregate because of their transient life-style, their low socio-economic status, and their lack of education and frequent problems with communication.

- Primary, secondary, and tertiary care for migrant workers include advocating for enforcement of OSHA standards and outreach programs to assist them, screening infants, children, and adults for beginning disease states, and treating existing health problems.

- Refugees are high-risk aggregates because they come to a new country stateless and completely dependent on the state to which they apply for resettlement. Often they do not know the customs or the language of the country in which they settle.

- To be effective, case management for refugee families would need to include a knowledge of the cultural disparity between the nurse and the client or family.

- The nurse who identifies with a high-risk aggregate can plan interventions for the total group instead of for only one individual within the group because the characteristics that place them at risk are similar.

 CRITICAL THINKING EXERCISE

A facility that provides temporary shelter to homeless persons is awarded a grant to expand services to include health care. The nurse practitioner they hire is expected to implement the grant.

1. Describe some of the health problems homeless persons are at high risk for.

2. Analyze the reasons you think they are at high risk for these particular problems.
3. Apply the answers you have given to questions one and two to develop a plan to provide health care at a walk-in clinic that will be established.

REFERENCES

American Public Health Association, Division of Nursing. (1981). *The definition and role of public health nursing in the delivery of health care.* Washington, DC: Author.

Arce, A., Tadlock, M.J., Vergare, M.J., & Shapiro, S. (1983). A psychiatric profile of street people admitted to an emergency shelter. *Hospital and Community Psychiatry, 34,* 812-817.

Barach, B. (1990, December 17). A reporter at large, LaFrontera. *The New Yorker Magazine,* 72-93.

Blakely, B. (1992). Nursing the homeless: Problems and solutions. *National Student Nurses' Association Imprint, 39*(5), 67-69.

Goldman, H.H., Gattozzi, A., & Taube, A. (1981). Defining and counting the chronically mentally ill. *Hospital and Community Psychiatry, 32*(1), 17-27.

Higgs, Z., & Gustafson, D. (1985). *Community as client: Assessment and diagnosis.* Philadelphia: Davis.

Jeffers, J., & Okeson, D. (1992). Homelessness in the Midwest. *National Student Nurses' Association Imprint, 39*(5), 70-72.

Johnston, H. (1985). *Health for the nation's harvestors: A history of the migrant health program and its economic and social setting.* Farmington Hills, MI: National Migrant Worker Council Inc.

Lamb, R. (1984). *The homeless mentally ill: A task force report of the American Psychiatric Association.* Washington, DC: American Psychiatric Association.

Leaf, A., & Cohen, M. (1982, December). Providing services for the homeless: The New York City program. *City of New York Human Resources Administration,* p. 82.

Lindsay, A.I., & Gottesman, M. (1992). Overview: Homelessness in America. *National Student Nurses' Association Imprint, 39*(5), 60-62.

Mayo, K. (1992). Homelessness in the south: Excerpts from student journals. *National Student Nurses' Association Imprint, 39*(5), 64-66.

McEwen, M., & Kemp, C. (1994). Teaching strategies for operationalizing nursing's agenda for healthcare reform. *Nurse Educator, 14*(1), 10-13.

Miller, D.S., & Lin, E.H.B. (1988). Children in shelters and homeless families: Reported health status and use of health services. *Pediatric, 81,* 668-673.

Muecke, M. (1992). Nursing research with refugees: A review and guide. *The Western Journal of Nursing Research, 14*(6), 706-715.

United Nations, Department of Public Information. (1991). Convention on migrant workers adopted. *U. N. Chronicle, 28,* 80-81.

United States Immigration. (1994) Washington, DC: Information Services (interview).

United States Public Law. Public Law 99-280, S.1282 (April 24, 1986); Public Law 100-77 (July, 1987); Public Law 100-386 (Aug. 10, 1988); Public Law 100-436 (Sept. 20, 1988); Public Law 101-527 (Nov. 6, 1990); Public Law 102-531 (Oct. 27, 1992).

Vredevoe, D.L., Shuler, P., & Woo, M. (1992). The homeless population. *The Western Journal of Nursing Research, 14*(6), 732.

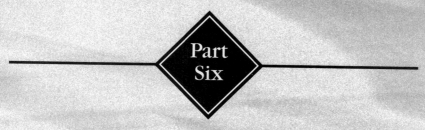

Part
Six

Home Health Care

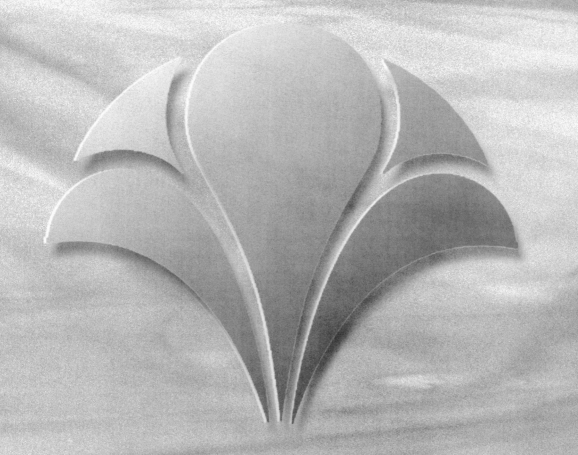

Home health care has become incredibly challenging. Clients being discharged from the hospital to go home may require highly technical services or planning for extensive long-term care. The nurse may be part of a discharge planning team, a client family advocate, or the provider of highly skilled technical care.

Chapter 25 describes the role of the nurse as a discharge planner. Material is presented that will enable the student to understand the difficulties of the task and the necessity for an interdisciplinary focus.

Chapter 26 focuses on the role of the nurse when providing care in the home. A broad overview of the complex problems encountered in planning care of clients in the home is provided. Concepts about approaches to case management are included.

DISCHARGE PLANNING AND CONTINUING CARE

Patricia A. O'Hare

Discharge planning aims to ensure continuity of care and helps sick and well persons and their families to find the best solutions to their health problems, at the right time, from the appropriate source, at the best price, and on a continuous basis for the required period of time.

National League for Nursing

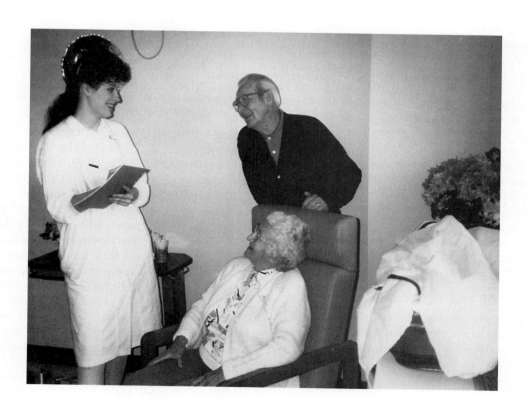

OBJECTIVES

At the conclusion of this chapter the student will be able to:

1. Define the key terms listed.
2. Discuss the role of discharge planning in the overall delivery of health care today.
3. Discuss the discharge planning process.
4. Discuss the components for providing continuity of care.
5. Analyze the nurse's role in discharge planning for continuity of care.
6. Describe the role of the community health nurse as home care coordinator.

KEY TERMS

Activities of daily living
Acute care case management
Continuing care
Continuity of care
Continuum of care

Cost-effective care
Discharge planning
Instrumental activities of daily
   living

Level of care
Referral
Uniform Needs Assessment
   Instrument (UNAI)

Discharge is a time of transition, as the client moves from hospital to home or to other care settings. Discharge planning for the provision of continuing care is one of the major elements in the overall delivery of health care today. It is the link from the hospital to the community for continuity of care. Discharge planning must be carried out in all settings involved in the continuum of care, such as hospitals, home health agencies, nursing homes, physicians' offices, ambulatory care settings, health maintenance organizations (HMOs), and adult day-care centers.

HISTORICAL PERSPECTIVE

The concept of assessing needs and planning for ongoing care is not new. *Charities and the Commons,* a publication of Bellevue Hospital in New York City in 1906-1907, refers to

"a nurse whose entire time and care is given to befriending those about to be discharged. She inquires into their circumstances, finds out whether they have home or friends to return to; if necessary, secures ad-

mission for them into some other curative or consolatory refuge" (Bellevue Hospital, 1906, p. 125).

Some referral systems for continuity of nursing care began as early as 1910 (Smith, 1962). One study (Carn & Mole, 1949), conducted by a joint committee of the National Organization for Public Health Nursing and the National League of Nursing Education, reported that 30 public health nursing agencies throughout the United States had liaison referral systems in conjunction with 43 hospitals. Another report (Smith, 1962) noted the increased interest in follow-up nursing services for clients after their discharge from the hospital in the period between 1946 and 1961. This report also identified the need for nursing involvement in discharge planning. Knowing which clients to assess for ongoing needs was considered the critical first step.

A follow-up publication, *Nursing Service Without Walls* (Wensley, 1963, p. 38), presented criteria that would be useful in alerting hospital staff members to patient needs for referrals to community services. These criteria were as follows:

- The complexity of a procedure, such as administration of a medicine or a treatment, that requires professional assistance in the home
- An indication that a client and/or family are unable to give care or do not understand directions for follow-up care
- Signs that the client and/or family are unable to accept or are disturbed by some aspect of the condition or care
- Evidence of need for reinforcement and clarification of instruction that was started in the hospital
- The expressed needs of clients for follow-up nursing service when professional personnel have corroborated the appropriateness of public health nursing to meet those needs
- Some aspect of the physical or social environment at home and outside the hospital that may interfere with a client's satisfactory self-care; for instance, an elderly client living alone or with an elderly spouse, or at a distance from the clinic that makes frequent trips difficult.

These criteria are as relevant today as they were in 1963. Indeed, the need has always existed for nurses to be involved in the planning for continuing care of patients. That need is even greater today, given the dynamics of the health care delivery system and societal and demographic changes. This chapter explores the concept of discharge planning, why it is important today, and the nurse's role in the process. Although discharge planning must be carried out in all settings, the examples in this chapter focus on the hospital. However, the principles apply whether the nurse is practicing in an outpatient clinic, physician's office, or nursing center. The process is client-centered and concerned not only with planning and arranging for ongoing care, but also with measuring the outcomes of that plan of care. Continuity of care communicates an ongoing, uninterrupted process (**continuing care**) with forward and backward movement occurring based on patient needs.

CURRENT PERSPECTIVES
Definitions of Discharge Planning

The American Nurses' Association (ANA) in 1975 stated that

Discharge planning is the part of the continuity of care process which is designed to prepare the patient or client for the next phase of care and to assist in making any necessary arrangements for that phase of care, whether it be self-care, care by family members, or care by an organized health care provider (ANA, 1975, p. 3). The purpose of discharge planning is twofold: (1) **continuity of care:** coordinated delivery of ongoing services as needed; and (2) **cost-effective care:** that is, to move the person to the appropriate level of care as quickly as possible. **Level of care** is determined by client needs and may be designated as acute, subacute, skilled, intermediate, custodial/domiciliary, or chronic. Discharge planning takes place within a **continuum of care,** which is an integrated system of health and social services representing all levels of care from wellness care to hospice care.

In 1985 the National League for Nursing (NLN) defined discharge planning as that "which aims to ensure continuity of care, helps sick and well persons and their families find the best solutions to their health problems, at the right time, from the appropriate source, at the best price, and on a continuous basis for the required period of time" (Hartigan & Brown, 1985, p. 9). Discharge planning is not an end point; it is a process, a linking mechanism that requires collaboration, communication, and coordination between the client and family and all other members of the health care team. By nature, discharge planning is interdisciplinary because no one discipline can provide all services to the client.

Legislation Affecting Discharge Planning

The 1985 definition of discharge planning differs from the 1975 definition in that the economics of care are addressed for the first time. The "price" of care has become a major concern worldwide. In the United States the Social Security Act amendments of 1983 provided sweeping changes in the area of hospital reimbursement for persons on Medicare. Public Law (PL) 98-21, Title VI, ushered in prospective payment for hospitals for services to persons on Medicare on the basis of diagnosis-related groups (PL 98-21, 1983). This legislation provided a major impetus for hospitals to review their admissions and to reduce the length of hospitalization, both of which have major implications for the public at large and for health care delivery in general.

Recent Changes Affecting Health Care Delivery

The present importance of discharge planning in providing continuity of care is a result of the following changes in health care delivery:

1. The prospective payment system, with its 473 diagnosis-related groups for Medicare reimbursement to hospitals, resulted in a decrease in the average length of stay. Medicare predicts, and agrees to pay, a set amount for certain diagnoses, regardless of the amount of time the client spends in the hospital. Early discharge increases the hospital's revenues. Because of early discharge, the client's follow-up needs are more complex.

2. Fiscal austerity in all sectors of the health care environment has resulted in decreased resources, not only in acute care but also in home care and long-term care.

3. Changing demographic patterns have resulted in an expanding aging population, the fastest-growing segment of which is the group aged 85 years and older. This segment of the population has increased in number by 65% in the last decade (United States Department of Health and Human Services [USDHHS], 1987). Those persons older than 85 years are often frail and have chronic health problems that require ongoing care. Although persons aged 65 years and older represented only 12% of the United States' population in 1984, it is projected that this group will account for 31% of total personal health care expenditures (American Association of Retired Persons [AARP], 1988).

4. Managed care organizations, such as Health Maintenance Organizations (HMOs), Preferred Provider Organizations (PPOs), and networks of providers called point-of-service plans, have increased. These financing and delivery systems continue to increase in number over solo practitioners, fee-for-service, and indemnity plans. From a health services perspective, the effects of managed care on service planning and delivery is widespread, affecting choice of providers and caps on services. The nursing literature refers to *managed care* within the framework of coordinated care or case management, with the goals being to standardize appropriate resource utilization, foster collaborative team practice, facilitate

continuity of care, promote job satisfaction, and decrease length of stay (DelTogno, Olivas, & Harter, 1989). Within this framework of managed or coordinated care, the case management plan for long- and short-term outcomes is developed (McGinty, Andreoni, & Quigley, 1993).

THE PROCESS OF DISCHARGE PLANNING

It is becoming increasingly important for nurses in all settings to be involved in planning for ongoing care. The hospital is part of the community, as are such settings as the home, the nursing home, and the adult day-care center. Regardless of where the nurse practices, it is necessary to view the client from a holistic perspective as a member of a family and of a community. Clients cannot be separated from their environments, and the nurse cannot be concerned with meeting only immediate needs. It is essential to know from where the client came, the place to which he or she is going, available help, other responsibilities of that caregiver, available resources in the community, eligibility requirements for those services/resources, and the process whereby the client can gain access to them. The discharge planning process for ensuring continuity of care parallels the nursing process. The components of the discharge planning process are as follows:

- Assessment of needs
- Analysis and diagnosis of needs
- Outcome identification
- A plan for how to meet those needs
- Implementation of the plan
- Evaluation of the outcome(s) of the plan

Assessment and Diagnosis

Assessment is the initial step. It involves data collection to identify and validate needs to diagnose current and continuing care needs. Assessment is an ongoing, cyclical process, with plans changing as necessary. In addition, the effect of the illness or health problem on the client and family requires attention (Figure 25-1). Data that are collected regarding client needs are validated with the client and family/significant other and with the physician.

Clients with high-risk factors, such as living alone, lacking insurance, being elderly (65 years of age or older), having specific diagnoses (e.g.,

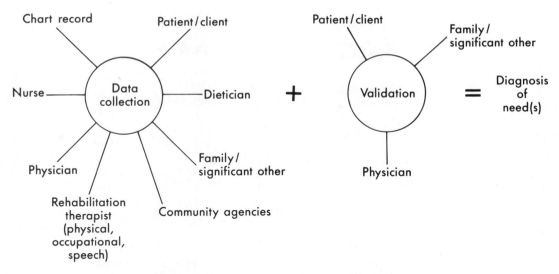

FIGURE 25-1   Assessment process components of discharge planning.

cancer, stroke, confusion, or amputation), and having frequent hospital readmissions, usually are screened in the hospital for continuing care needs. What may be overlooked, however, is the level of the client's functioning before hospitalization and the projected level of functioning as services are provided and care is received. Level of functioning must be defined to include not only the **activities of daily living,** such as bathing, dressing, toileting, transfer, continence, and feeding, but also the **instrumental activities of daily living,** which include shopping, light housekeeping, taking medications, handling finances, and using the telephone and transportation. The Manitoba Longitudinal Study on Aging (Shapiro, 1986) found that one of the best predictors of need for home care, after age, is the client's level of difficulty in coping with instrumental activities of daily living.

Assessment includes considering whether the client is dealing with a short-term or a long-term illness and the possible changes in lifestyle or role that may occur as a result of the illness or health problem. The box on p. 556 provides a framework that is useful for all nurses in hospital discharge planning.

A nursing history obtained as part of the admission database is also used. This nursing history provides the initial data for interacting with the client and family in planning care. The nurse

on the unit shares this information and the current treatment needs of the client with the other members of the interdisciplinary team. This team may include the physician, social worker, discharge planner or continuing care coordinator, dietitian, rehabilitation therapists, and others. Sharing of this information might take place at weekly discharge planning rounds or client care rounds. These rounds provide a mechanism for case finding and assessment for the discharge planner, with input from the staff nurse as an essential part of appropriate planning. The data are analyzed, diagnoses of current and continuing care needs are determined, and plans are made with the client, the family, and relevant health care providers to meet those needs.

Outcome Identification

Outcome identification is the establishment with the client of measurable goals to resolve health problems, maintain health status, or foster health promotion. These outcomes provide a way of knowing whether care needs have been met.

Planning and Implementation: Teaching and Referral

Teaching and referral are part of the discharge plan. As noted in the box on p. 556, health teaching, or client (patient) and family teaching, is an integral part of discharge planning. In the current

GUIDELINES FOR HOSPITAL DISCHARGE PLANNING TO BE USED BY HOSPITAL NURSE

Section I: overview

Refer to basic information already on the admission fact sheet of the chart, which includes: name, address, phone number, age, sex, marital status, occupation, place of employment, admitting diagnosis, insurance, and person to contact in emergency. The nurse would question whether this person would be available to help if assistance was needed after discharge. The nurse is trying to determine the patient's personal support system; that is, who the patient can and does depend on.

Section II: interaction/impact

Looking at the client, family, and diagnoses, consider the following:

What *concerns* does the client and family have about the hospitalization, diagnosis, or treatment?

Lifestyle — How do the diagnoses, treatments, and their implications, if any, affect the client and family lifestyle?

Will the condition interfere with the client's present occupation or profession now or in the future? Is the situation short-term or long-term?

Assistance

Can the client care for him/herself?

If the client cannot care for self, who can assist him?

What other responsibilities does this person have?

Is professional assistance needed?

Is assistance needed continuously or periodically?

What about insurance coverage for financial considerations?

Section III: home needs

Consider the *home environment* in terms of space, stairs, location of toilet, etc.

Supplies or equipment needed in the home:

What supplies will the client be taking home from the hospital with him; e.g., irrigating equipment, dressings, walker, etc.?

What equipment will the family need to have in the home when the client comes home; e.g., hospital bed, commode chair, wheelchair, etc.?

Referral for follow-up nursing in the home. Was the client known to a Community Nursing/Home Health Agency before admission? Does the community health nurse know that the client is in the hospital?

Is the form on the chart for referral to the Community Nursing/Home Health Agency?

Transfer or discharge to another facility

If the client was in a nursing home before admission, is the nursing home holding the bed for him, or must he reapply for admission?

If the client is to be discharged to a nursing home or a community residential facility, is the "Patient Transfer Form" on the chart? This form needs to be completed and sent with the client to the facility.

Section IV: health teaching re: diagnoses and implications

Specific teaching as indicated looking at the physiological and psychological changes in terms of resulting needs

Physical care required — mobility, continence, etc.

Dressings

Catheters

Special diets

Therapies — physical, occupational, speech

With the information elicited by means of these guidelines, the nurse has a database for anticipating needs and planning with the client/family/significant other and other disciplines for continuity of care during hospitalization and after discharge.

hospital environment of shortened lengths of stay, it is not possible for all teaching to be completed by the time of discharge from the acute care hospital. It is critical that all teaching be documented and recorded in terms of client/ family ability to perform procedures, to state names and purposes of drugs, and so forth. It is also essential that plans be made for continued teaching in the community through referral to the community health nurse. Referrals to home health agencies must include an account of teaching to date and those objectives still to be achieved. Whether the discharge planner or the staff nurse makes the referral to the home health agency, the staff nurse is responsible for documenting on the referral form the care provided to the client during hospitalization. This care includes the teaching content and an assessment of that teaching in terms of client/family learning and their ability to perform the care activities. For example, if a family has been taught decubitus care, the nurse would document the following:

- Description of the stage and condition of the decubitus ulcer
- Description of the ulcer care procedure
- State how many times, if any, the family or caregiver has observed the procedure
- State how many times, if any, the family or caregiver has demonstrated the procedure
- State the family's understanding of what to do and why
- State the overall ability and willingness of the family/caregiver to do the procedure at home
- State the supplies or equipment needed in the home and whether they have been obtained or ordered.

It is important that the community nurse receive this information so that continuing care can be maintained. The case studies at the end of the chapter illustrate the discharge planning process and the nurse's role.

Evaluation

Although the discharge plan for the posthospitalization period can be evaluated by the discharge planner and can occur at a place other than the hospital unit, the staff nurse on the unit needs to be informed of outcomes of referrals to home health agencies. This feedback from the nurse in the community includes the effect of teaching that was begun in the hospital, and the ability of the client or family, or both, to provide the care. This information allows the unit nurse to plan and adjust with regard to future nursing interventions with other clients and families. This feedback from the agency can be communicated either in writing or through a follow-up telephone call, depending on the protocol established by the hospital and the agency.

COMPONENTS FOR PROVIDING CONTINUITY OF CARE

The major components for providing continuity of care are the care plan, education of the client and family, and the referral.

The Care Plan

The discharge plan should be identified specifically as part of the care plan. Not every client requires referral to another agency or facility, but every client should be assessed for continuing care needs. All nursing diagnoses must be reviewed from the perspective of ongoing needs. For example, at the time of discharge, it is critical for the nurse to determine the meaning of any unresolved nursing diagnoses in terms of continuing care needs and ongoing planning. A revision has been proposed of NANDA'S taxonomy of conditions that necessitate nursing care (Fitzpatrick, et al. 1989). The revision provides several possible examples. Under the category *Human Response Pattern: Moving* is the nursing diagnosis "physical mobility, impaired." If this alteration or impairment in physical mobility is an unresolved problem at the time of discharge, the nurse should incorporate this problem into the discharge plan. It may mean that a referral for physical therapy after hospitalization is indicated, or it may mean that equipment such as a wheelchair is needed, or both. Basically, all nursing diagnoses require review from the standpoint of possible implications for interventions for meeting continuing care needs.

Education of the Client and Family

Education involves the assessment of learning needs, readiness for learning, and level of understanding, as well as the use of principles of teaching and learning. The nurse must be cognizant of the effects of stress on learning and the importance of repetition and return demonstration throughout the educational process. Also involved in the process are assessment of continuing care needs and evaluation of client learning.

The Referral

A **referral** is a written or verbal communication for services. Referrals are made as needed for home care or services such as those provided by a social worker, a dietitian, or rehabilitation therapists. Referrals need to be thought of as mechanisms for communication, coordination, and collaboration between and among care settings and disciplines.

REVIEW OF CRITICAL PROCESS INFORMATION

The information needed in carrying out the discharge planning process in any setting includes the following:

- Knowledge of the client's prior health status
- Current level of care needed
- Projected level of care needed
- Projected time frame for moving the client to the next level of care
- Therapy(ies) and teaching that should be accomplished before moving the client to the next level of care
- Ability and willingness of family or caregiver to provide care
- Financial resources of the client
- Available community resources and eligibility requirements

In all settings the client and family need to be involved in decision making regarding ongoing care. Yet, the assurance of consistent assessment in all settings remains a problem.

Uniform Needs Assessment Instrument

There is a need in health care today for an assessment tool or tools that can be used across care settings. The Omnibus Budget Reconciliation Act (OBRA) of 1986 attempts to address this identified need. OBRA '86 mandated that the Secretary of the Department of Health and Human Services develop a "uniform needs assessment instrument" that does the following (U.S. Congress, 1986):

(A) Evaluates:
    (i) the functional capacity of an individual
    (ii) the nursing and other care requirements of the individual to meet health care needs and to assist with functional incapacities
    (iii) the social and familial resources available to the individual to meet those requirements

(B) Can be used by discharge planners, hospitals, nursing facilities, other health care providers, and fiscal intermediaries in evaluating an individual's need for posthospital extended care services, home health services, and long-term care services of a health related or supportive nature.

Progress has been made on this task. A draft entitled "Assessment of Needs for Continuing Care" was reviewed by a stratified sample of providers that included hospitals, nursing homes, home health agencies, and other organizations and individuals with expertise in needs assessment. The final meeting of the advisory panel on the development of the uniform needs assessment instrument was held in July, 1989. The panel revised the draft instrument on the basis of a summary and analysis of comments from the stratified sample of providers and other experts in health care. The panel also developed recommendations regarding the use of the needs assessment instrument as follows:

1. The primary purpose should be to determine a client's need for continuing care, and it is not intended to represent a comprehensive geriatric or functional assessment or a care plan.

2. The instrument was developed to evaluate needs for continuing care across various health care settings and is intended as a means of establishing consistency and communicating care needs in the post-acute care community (McBroom, 1989, pp. 1, 3).

After the assessment form was fully developed, a plan evolved for field testing of the instrument.

In June, 1993, a Request for Proposal entitled "Field Testing of Uniform Needs Assessment Instrument" went out from the Health Care Financing Administration (HCFA) Division of Contracts and Grants. This field testing of the **Uniform**

Needs Assessment Instrument (UNAI) is necessary so that HCFA can make an informed decision regarding mandating its use. Among the objectives to be studied are testing the reliability and validity of the UNAI; developing and evaluating a uniform high-risk screen to identify hospitalized Medicare clients who need extensive discharge planning evaluations; demonstrating the administrative feasibility and resources needed for use of the UNAI in hospitals, nursing homes, and home care agencies; and evaluating the effects of the UNAI on the discharge planning process and the outcomes of its use for the client and family (HCFA, 1993).

DISCHARGE PLANNING ROLES
The Home Care Coordinator

A hospital may have a home care coordinator either from its own hospital-based home health agency or from a community-based home health agency. The primary role of the home care coordinator is to facilitate coordination of home care referrals. Medicare will not reimburse home health agencies for discharge planning activities in the hospital. However, once the client's physician has decided that home health services are required and the specific home health agency has been chosen, then reimbursable "coordination" includes the following postreferral activities by the home care coordinator (Lasater, 1983):

1. Explaining agency policies and procedures to the client and family
2. Establishing a home care plan before discharge
3. Ensuring that the agency can meet the client's needs.

The home care coordinator attends hospital discharge planning meetings and suggests follow-up care services. In addition, the home care coordinator is a primary resource person in the education of physicians and hospital staff members with regard to what is involved in home care and the kinds of services that can be provided in the home setting. The home care coordinator's knowledge of the community and community resources is invaluable, especially when the diversity of backgrounds involved and the experience of the discharge planner are recognized.

The Discharge Planner and the Primary Nurse

The discharge planner may be a nurse, a social worker, or in some facilities, a clerical person. It is critical for the nurse to know the discharge planning process that is followed in the facility. OBRA '86 included a mandate to hospitals to provide the discharge planning process as a condition of participation for Medicare. Hospitals, however, may or may not have discharge planning programs in place to implement the process. Each professional nurse has the responsibility for continuity of care planning as an integral part of professional nursing practice. The degree of nursing involvement depends on the structure in place in the facility inasmuch as a knowledge of the policies and procedures for discharge planning is required for continuity of care.

The hospital discharge planner may have one of many titles: discharge planner, continuing care coordinator, disposition coordinator, admission/discharge coordinator, RN discharge coordinator, coordinator of assessments, discharge coordinator, public health coordinator, community health nurse coordinator, or director of client and family services. It is also possible that the designated person is responsible for both utilization review and discharge planning, or quality assurance and discharge planning, or utilization review, quality assurance, and discharge planning.

The role of the staff nurse may include various duties, depending on whether the continuing care needs of the client and family are simple or complex. The simple discharge plan includes client and family teaching and referral; the primary nurse can be expected to coordinate this discharge plan. Complex continuing care needs involve multiple disciplines and resources because of complex physical and perhaps financial and social problems. The staff nurse provides input and is involved in the planning, but is not responsible for the coordination of the complex discharge plan. Two case studies are presented on pp. 561 and 562 to depict the role of the primary nurse in the discharge planning process.

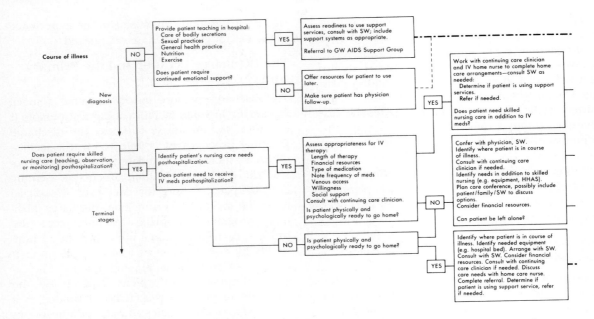

FIGURE 25-2 Discharge planning decisions made by the primary nurse caring for a patient with AIDS. *(Copyright (1989) by Irene Paige, RN, MSN, Continuing Care Clinician. Reprinted by permission.)*

Figure 25-2 provides an additional example, which shows the nurse using the decision-making process to care for a client with acquired immunodeficiency syndrome (AIDS).

In 1995, as concern about the implications of President Clinton's Health Care Reform package heightens, many hospitals are restructuring their care delivery processes. **Acute care case management** with its focus on client outcomes and nurse accountability has strengthened the staff nurse's role in the discharge planning process. The most well known of the acute care models is Zander's model at the New England Medical Center in Boston (Zander, 1991). Critical paths and/or CareMaps™ are essential elements in this model and are at the core of the caregiving process of all disciplines. CareMaps™ plot client problems and nursing diagnoses against a time frame of anticipated client outcomes; CareMaps™ sequence problems, goals, and outcomes to provide a database for continuous quality improvement where variances can be identified as they occur and corrective actions can be taken. Acute care case management can provide a framework within which the nurse on the unit, in collaboration with the client, family, and other disciplines, plots out the activities and the time frame required for inpatient care and the successful achievement of the transition from the hospital to the next level of care. Acute care case management is a client-centered, systematic, multilevel process that includes assessment, education, planning, coordination, and some follow-up postdischarge to achieve predetermined outcomes within an allotted length of stay. How case management and discharge planning interact depends on the model of case management in place in the organization. In-depth discussion of case management and managed care can be found in the literature; for example, in Bower, 1992; Ethridge & Lamb, 1989; Hampton, 1993; Hicks, Stallmeyer, & Coleman, 1993; Lyons, 1993; and Zander, 1991. These case management models are evolving. They involve collaboration among all disciplines involved in care of the client. These evolving delivery systems serve to strengthen the unit nurse's role in discharge planning for continuity of care.

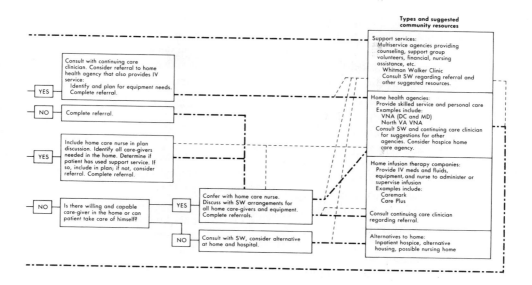

Types and suggested community resources

CASE STUDY

Case study A: a simple discharge plan*
Assessment and analysis

Mr. J is an 81-year-old man admitted to the hospital with a diagnosis of laryngeal cancer. He lives alone in a one-level house in a large senior citizens' housing complex in the suburb of a metropolitan area. He has two adult children, a son and daughter, who live in the metropolitan area. A laryngectomy was performed 10 days previously, and Mr. J is medically ready for discharge. His son and daughter have visited fairly frequently during this hospitalization and have expressed to the primary nurse a willingness to assist their father with his posthospital care. Mr. J is a small, frail-looking man, but he is able to perform his activities of daily living independently and has been in good health most of his life. He is hard of hearing, which he describes as "worse since this surgery." He does not use a hearing aid. He wears glasses for near-vision activities. He has a postlaryngectomy stoma that requires care. Mr. J is able to

clear his secretions but requires infrequent suctioning. His appetite is poor, but he is able to eat. He is unable to speak and communicates by writing. He shakes his head "no" vigorously when questioned about his son and daughter assisting him after he is discharged.

Planning and implementation

The primary nurse institutes the following activities:

1. Assesses Mr. J's feelings about his discharge and the need for follow-up care.
2. Teaches Mr. J how to care for the stoma, how to perform self-suctioning, and details of skin care.
   Teaches Mr. J about the role of adequate nutrition in the healing process. Explores with him how he will go grocery shopping and prepare meals at home. Talks with the dietitian about Mr. J's poor appetite. The dietitian discusses with Mr. J his food likes and dislikes and helps him plan his diet.
3. Organizes a case conference with Mr. J, the social

* The author thanks Irene Paige, R.N., M.S.N., Continuing Care Clinician, for her assistance in developing these case studies.

worker, and Mr. J's physician to discuss concerns about Mr. J's continuing care needs. Mr. J's son and daughter join the group later in the discussion. The primary nurse is especially concerned about Mr. J's safety in going home alone because of his inability to speak, his hearing deficit, and his inability to perform self-suctioning independently at this time. Mr. J agrees to go to his daughter's house immediately after discharge. He also agrees to allow her to assist with his care until he becomes more independent and is able to go to his own home. In addition, it is agreed that a hearing evaluation will be arranged.

4. Begins to teach the daughter stoma care, skin care, and suctioning. The primary emphasis is on the suctioning.
5. Discusses with the physician Mr. J's equipment needs; that is, suction machine, suction catheters, supplies for cleaning the stoma, and stoma covers.
6. Arranges with the equipment company for delivery of the equipment and supplies to the daughter's home.
7. Refers Mr. J to a certified home health agency for follow-up nursing services in the home and requests a visit on the day of hospital discharge to assess that needed equipment and supplies are in the home, and that Mr. J and his daughter know how to

operate the suction machine. In addition, the home health nurse/visiting nurse/community health nurse will evaluate Mr. J's and his daughter's ability to do the suctioning and will continue the teaching in the home.

Evaluation and discussion

Mr. J's case is considered a simple discharge planning situation. However, the expectation is that the primary nurse would be supported by the hospital's continuing care clinician in carrying out this discharge planning process. The continuing care clinician in this situation assisted the primary nurse not only in counseling Mr. J but also including his son and daughter in the assessment and care planning. The continuing care clinician also was the catalyst for the organized care conference, at which time definitive, workable plans were made. It also was critical that the primary nurse make telephone contact with the nurse in the community, in addition to sending a written referral. It is expected that if care questions arise, the community nurse, who has the name and telephone number of the primary nurse in the hospital, will call for additional information and also provide feedback. This is the system that needs to be fostered so that continuing care is provided.

■ CASE STUDY

Case study B: a complex discharge plan
Assessment and analysis

Ms. M is a 38-year-old woman admitted to the hospital with a diagnosis of *Pneumocystis carinii* pneumonia (PCP). Human immunodeficiency virus (HIV) positivity had been diagnosed 2 months previously. Ms. M is divorced, works as a waitress, and has one child, a 20-year-old daughter who lives out-of-town. Ms. M's marriage ended 18 months previously. It was a difficult-marriage that included violent sexual abuse. Ms. M is an intelligent, physically fit woman who lives alone in a city apartment, but has many friends for support. She was treated initially with sulfamethoxazole (Bactrim) intravenously, with poor response. Pentamidine, 180

mg per day, was then begun intravenously for 14 days, which Ms. M tolerated without difficulty. After 2 days on this regimen, the physician indicated that she was ready for discharge and was to continue the course of treatment at home. After the initial respiratory difficulty, Ms. M spent her days in the hospital in a darkened room, occasionally watching television. She refused to talk with a social worker or to have a psychiatric consultation. Ms. M was physically but not psychologically ready for discharge.

Planning and implementation

The primary nurse focused on providing support for Ms. M and making her aware of where she could obtain additional support when she was ready. The primary nurse also instituted the following actions:

1. Assessing Ms. M's response to the anticipated discharge and her willingness and ability to perform self-care regarding the medication schedule and needed monitoring.

2. Teaching Ms. M about her disease process and about the medication, diet, the need to increase her fluid intake, and initiating some limited discussion of sexual practices. The importance of using universal precautions was also discussed (see Chapter 20).

3. Working with other members of the team, such as the continuing care clinician, social worker, physician, and nurse from the infusion company to make

arrangements for Ms. M to receive pentamidine intravenously at home.

4. Discussing Ms. M's situation with the nurse from the home infusion company, who was to administer and monitor the medication after the client's discharge from the hospital.

Evaluation and discussion

The continuing care clinician again was a resource and support person for the primary nurse during this care process. Feedback from the nurse employed by the home infusion company after Ms. M's hospitalization indicated that the client was responding positively to the medication and ongoing care. Although Ms. M at this time has not sought additional support from the AIDS support group, she is aware of its availability.

Chapter Highlights

- Discharge planning is the process of assessing needs and arranging or coordinating services for clients as they move through the health care system.

- Discharge planning should be carried out in all health care settings, including hospitals, home health agencies, nursing homes, physicians' offices, and ambulatory care centers.

- Criteria that indicate the need for further services include complexity of the procedures to be performed, inability of the client and/or caregiver to provide care, and environmental factors that interfere with a client's care.

- The implementation of the prospective payment system in 1983 led to a decreased average length of stay in hospitals and an increased need for follow-up care.

- The discharge planning process begins with an assessment of the client's needs, including an assessment of the client's level of functioning before hospitalization.

- Health teaching, which is an integral component of discharge planning, should be documented in detail to ensure continuity after discharge.

- Referrals are mechanisms for communication, coordination, and collaboration between and among care settings and disciplines. The information communicated should include the client's prior health status, the level of care needed, therapies and teaching to be accomplished, availability of caregivers, financial resources, and available community resources.

- The uniform needs assessment instrument, which is currently in development, will allow for determination of a client's need for continuing care across various health care settings.

- Continuing care needs may be either simple or complex. A simple discharge plan can be coordinated by the primary nurse, whereas a complex plan involves health care providers from multiple disciplines.

- Each professional nurse is responsible for continuity of care planning as an integral part of professional nursing practice.

- Acute care case management strengthens the nurse's role in hospital discharge planning for continuity of care.

CRITICAL THINKING EXERCISE

A community health nurse receives a call from a man who is concerned about his neighbor, an elderly gentleman living alone in an apartment in an urban setting. The elderly man was brought home by wheelchair van after one week in the hospital. He is unable to cook and is homebound. The neighbor has been taking him sandwiches and coffee, but can do no more, and asks what can be done.

On arrival at the elderly gentleman's apartment, the nurse finds him sitting in a chair. His legs are badly swollen and ischemic as a result of peripheral vascular disease. There is a decubitus on his coccyx, his hygiene is poor, and he is profoundly depressed.

The apartment is littered and dirty and there are no groceries.

He states that his only help comes from his friend and neighbor. His only relative lives some distance away. He maintains that his physician had promised him home care, but it never came. He doesn't know what to do.

1. What kinds of assistance will this man need? Write a care plan for him based on the information given.
2. How could a hospital discharge planner have helped this man?
3. What questions will you have for the physician?

REFERENCES

A field nurse for old Bellevue. (1906-07). *Charities and the Commons, 17,* 125.

American Association of Retired Persons. (1988). *A profile of older Americans.* Washington, DC: Author.

American Nurses' Association. (1975). *Statement on continuity of care and discharge planning programs in institutions and community agencies.* Kansas City, MO: Author.

Bower, K.A. (1992). *Case management by nurses.* Washington, D.C.: American Nurses Publishing.

Carn, I., & Mole, E.W. (1949). Continuity of nursing care: An analysis of referral systems with recommended practice. *American Journal of Nursing, 49,* 388-390.

DelTogno-Armanasco, V., Olivas, G.S., & Harter, S. (1989). Developing an integrated nursing case management model. *Nursing Management, 20*(10), 26-29.

Ethridge, P. & Lamb, G. (1989). Professional nursing case management improves quality, access and costs. *Nursing Management, 20*(3), 30-35.

Fitzpatrick, J., Kerr, M., Saba, V.K., Hoskins, L.M., Hurley, M.E., Mills, W.E., Rottcamp, B.E., Warren, J., & Capinito, L.J. (1989). Translating nursing diagnosis into ICD code. *American Journal of Nursing, 89,* 493-495.

Hampton, D.C. (1993). Implementing a managed care framework through care maps. *Journal of Nursing Administration, 23*(5), 21-27.

Hartigan, E.G., & Brown, D.J. (Eds.). (1985). *Discharge planning for continuity of care.* New York: National League for Nursing.

Health Care Financing Administration. (1993). *Field testing of uniform needs assessment instrument* (RFP-HCFA-93-052/PK). Baltimore, MD: Author.

Hicks, L.L., Stallmeyer, J.M., & Coleman, J.R. (1993). *Role of the nurse in managed care.* Washington, DC: American Nurses Publishing.

Lasater, N. (1983). Nurse coordinator reimbursement. *Caring, 89,* 14-16.

Lyons, J.C. (1993). Models of nursing care delivery and case management: clarification of terms. *Nursing Economics, 11*(3), 163-169.

McBroom, A. (1989). Advisory panel on uniform needs assessment instrument completes recommendations. *Access, 7*(3), 1, 3.

McGinty, M.H., Andreoni, V.M., & Quigley, M.A. (1993). Building a managed care approach. *Nursing Management, 24*(8), 34-35.

Public Law 98-21, Title VI. (1983). *Prospective payment for Medicare in-patient hospital services.* Washington, DC: U.S. Government Printing Office.

Shapiro, E. (1986). Patterns and predictors of home care use by the elderly when need is the sole basis for admission. *Home Health Care Services Quarterly, 7*(1): 29-44.

Smith, L.C. (1962). *Factors influencing continuity of nursing service.* New York: National League for Nursing.

Wensley, E. (1963). *Nursing service without walls* (p. 38). New York: National League for Nursing.

U.S. Congress. (1986, October 17). *Omnibus Budget Reconciliation Act: Report to Accompany H.R. 5300.* 99th Cong., sect. 9305.

U.S. Department of Health and Human Services. (1987). *Aging America: Trends and projections* (1987-1989 ed.). Washington, DC: U.S. Government Printing Office.

Zander, K. (1991). Case management in acute care: Making the connections. *The Case Manager, 1,* 39-43.

26

CARE OF CLIENTS IN THE HOME

Joan M. Cookfair ◆ Susan K. Markel

Much that now strikes us as incomprehensible would be far less so if we took a look at the racing rate of change that makes reality seem, sometimes, like a kaleidoscope run wild.

Alvin Toffler

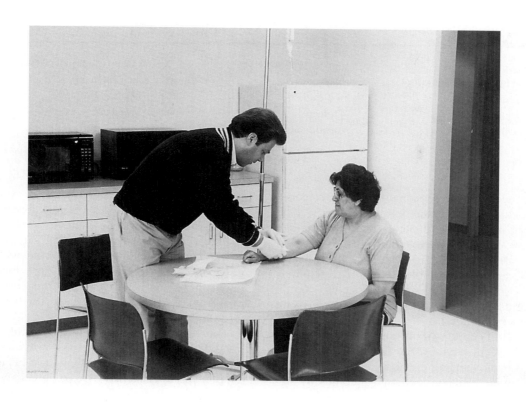

OBJECTIVES

At the conclusion of this chapter the student will be able to:

1. Define the key terms listed.
2. Define home health nursing practice.
3. Define home health care.
4. Describe the Standards of Home Health Care Nursing.
5. Identify the various disciplines involved in home care.
6. Describe the concept of collaborative care.
7. Discuss the difficulties in caseload management.
8. Describe the nurse's actions in an initial home visit.
9. Discuss trends in home health care.
10. Understand the role of the nurse in home health care.

KEY TERMS

Caseload management
Certified home health agency
Home health aide
Home health care
Home health care nursing

High-tech therapy
Hospice
Medicaid
Medicare
Nutritionists

Occupational therapists
Palliative care
Physical therapists
Social worker

The idea that professional nursing care could be provided in the home began early in the 19th century in the United States and Canada (see Chapter 1). Costs were relatively low, and in many cases care was given voluntarily. As health care became more complex and other disciplines became involved, there evolved a need to coordinate and regulate services and to control rising costs (see Chapter 25).

The 20th century has brought about demands for expanded services. Altered family patterns, caused by a changing economy and the fact that most young families need two incomes to survive, have increased the need for paid caretakers in the home. Because the adult or adults that are head of a household often work full-time, more often than not, there is no one to as-

sist with the care of a fragile elderly person who cannot manage the activities of daily living alone, or to care for a chronically ill child.

Both the rising cost of hospital care and the new policy of sending people home who may need complex, technical care, have increased public need for health care professionals who can provide interdisciplinary care in the home (see Chapter 25).

The need to provide palliative care in the home has also increased. Hospice programs have been very successful when they have been coordinated and approached by using a collaborative team approach. It is obvious that home health nursing in contemporary society will have to include collaborative case management. Interaction with other disciplines will become commonplace. In addition, the inclusion of the family, the community, and other available resources will need to occur.

DEFINITION OF HOME HEALTH CARE NURSING

Home health care nursing refers to the practice of nursing applied to a client with a health deficit in the client's place of residence. Clients and their designated caregivers are the focus of home health nursing practice. The goal of care is to initiate, manage, and evaluate the resources needed to promote the client's optimal level of well-being. Nursing activities necessary to achieve this goal may warrant preventive, maintenance, and restorative emphasis to avoid potential

deficits from developing (American Nurses' Association, 1992, p. 7).

Although the provision of home health care has been altered dramatically over the last decade, the nurse remains the primary giver and planner of care. Planners of care have been given a set of standards by the American Nurses' Association to assist them in improving and validating the care that they, as individuals, give (see box below).

To further guide and maintain excellence in home care, the National League for Nurses established a Community Health Accreditation Program (CHAP) in 1987 to accredit home- and community-based agencies in the United States.

STANDARDS OF HOME HEALTH CARE NURSING

Standard I: organization of home health services

All home health services are planned, organized, and directed by a master's-prepared professional nurse with experience in community health and administration.

Standard II: theory

The nurse applies theoretical concepts as a basis for decisions in practice.

Standard III: data collection

The nurse continuously collects and records data that are comprehensive, accurate, and systematic.

Standard IV: diagnosis

The nurse uses health assessment data to determine nursing diagnoses.

Standard V: planning

The nurse develops care plans that establish goals. The care plan is based on nursing diagnoses and incorporates therapeutic, preventive, and rehabilitative nursing actions.

Standard VI: intervention

The nurse, guided by the care plan, intervenes to provide comfort; to restore, improve, and promote health; to prevent complications and sequelae of illness; and to effect rehabilitation.

Standard VII: evaluation

The nurse continually evaluates the client's and

family's responses to interventions to determine progress toward goal attainment and to revise the data base, nursing diagnoses, and plan of care.

Standard VIII: continuity of care

The nurse is responsible for the client's appropriate and uninterrupted care along the health care continuum, and therefore uses discharge planning, case management, and coordination of community resources.

Standard IX: interdisciplinary collaboration

The nurse initiates and maintains a liaison relationship with all appropriate health care providers to assure that all efforts effectively complement one another.

Standard X: professional development

The nurse assumes responsibility for professional development and contributes to the professional growth of others.

Standard XI: research

The nurse participates in research activities that contribute to the profession's continuing development of knowledge of home health care.

Standard XII: ethics

The nurse uses the code for nurses established by the American Nurses' Association as a guide for ethical decision making in practice.

CHAP is now the accrediting body for most agencies. A private organization, the Joint Commission of Home Health, also accredits home health agencies on request (see Chapter 1).

DEFINITION OF HOME HEALTH CARE

Home health care as defined by Medicare includes the following items and services:

1. Part-time or intermittent nursing care provided by or under the supervision of a registered professional nurse
2. Physical, occupational, or speech therapy
3. Medical social services under the direction of a physician
4. Part-time or intermittent services of a home health aide as permitted by the regulations
5. Medical supplies (other than drugs and biologicals such as serum and vaccinations), and the use of medical appliances
6. Medical services provided by an intern or resident enrolled in a teaching program in hospitals affiliated or under contract with a home health agency (Home Health Services, 1982, paragraph 1401)

MEDICARE

Medicare is a federally funded program in the United States that is available to most clients who are older than 65 years of age (see Chapter 4). To receive Medicare benefits in the home, a client must be considered homebound. The law defines a homebound individual as "one who cannot leave the home without assistance and for whom physical effort is taxing and difficult." A physician must refer the need for each service and recertify this need at least every 60 days. The services must include the need for skilled nursing care and for intermittent and medically necessary care. Primary skilled services are considered those provided by registered nurses, physical therapists, and speech therapists. If one of these services is provided in the home, so-called secondary services, which are provided by occupational therapists, social workers, home health aides, or nutritionists, may be reimbursed. The new Medicare regulation providing reimbursement for management and evaluation allows the nurse to continue seeing a client who is at risk for exacerbation of an acute or chronic illness. Nurses are recognized as case managers in the home to prevent recurrences of illness (Allan, 1994).

MEDICAID

Medicaid is a federally funded program in the United States that is available to clients with low incomes (see Chapter 4). It pays for skilled nursing services that are provided by a Medicare-certified agency and ordered by a physician. Coverage varies from state to state. Each state has a responsibility to match federal funds by 50%, but some states provide more assistance than others do.

PRIVATE INSURANCE

Private insurance, whether purchased by individuals or provided by employers, generally covers home health care on a yearly deductible basis (see Chapter 4).

THE INTERDISCIPLINARY TEAM
Nurses

Historically, nursing has been the foundation for home care. The nurse focuses on the family unit when coordinating home care, teaching health promotion and maintenance in the home within the framework of the family unit. This focus has not changed. The nurse's responsibilities have expanded, however, to that of a case manager. Nurses are the first to visit a client following a referral. Nurses gather all intake information and complete the paperwork, including medical and social history, medications ordered, insurance data, caregiver status, consent for treatment, and emergency information. When appropriate, the nurse explains "patient advance directives" (May, 1993, p. 28), which require the agency the nurse represents to honor any living will or durable power of attorney. The nurse is primary liaison between the client and the physician. The nurse often makes referrals to other services such as physical therapists, social workers, or occupational therapists, and coordinates the interaction between the disciplines.

Physicians

Most clients are referred to home health care providers by physicians or discharge planners. It is the responsibility of the physician who makes a referral to communicate necessary information to other members of the health care team. In the United States, federal regulations require that a physician certify plans of care for clients in the home before the client is eligible for Medicare third-party payment. Some private insurance companies have similar criteria. The physician must recertify the plan of care every 60 days for the client to receive third-party payment. A nurse may make one visit to assess a client's status if requested to do so by a neighbor or a family member. After an assessment of the client's status, there must be physician approval to develop a follow-up plan of care.

Physical Therapists

Physical therapists evaluate neuromuscular and functional ability. They emphasize restorative therapy, and are frequently involved in home care when clients have difficulty in ambulation or mobility. They also advise clients in gait training, therapeutic exercises, and similar activities. Physical therapists must get their referrals from a physician.

Social Workers

Social workers were among the first professionals to join nurses in home-based care. They help clients with social, intellectual, and emotional factors that affect their well being. They assist clients to contact available community resources, and they provide advocacy in a variety of ways. Some social workers are specifically trained in counseling techniques and health-related problems, and may provide crisis intervention and equipment procurement when the client cannot pay.

Speech Therapists

Speech therapists focus on restorative therapy. They treat clients with communication and swallowing problems related to speech, language, and hearing.

Nutritionists

Nutritionists join the interdisciplinary team both through direct diet counseling to clients and through staff consultations. They frequently are asked to assist in team conferences to prescribe a therapeutic diet for individual clients. Much of the nutritionist's role in the home involves consultation with nurses and other care providers to assist the provider to give nutritional guidance to clients.

Occupational Therapists

Occupational therapists concentrate on the restoration of small motor coordination. They are frequently involved in enabling clients who have lost the use of their hands or the ability to coordinate finer body movements to function in their homes to maintain independence.

Home Health Aide

The **home health aide** is usually supervised by a registered nurse or a physical therapist. This individual may give personal care, assist in activities of daily living, and perform some miscellaneous supportive tasks temporarily while the client attempts to reach independence. The home health aide implements an established plan of care that has been set up by the nurse or the physiotherapist.

Homemaker

Sometimes a homemaker is placed in a home to assist with household chores.

Miscellaneous Providers

Many agencies in the private sector employ paraprofessional aides to care for clients in the home. Some families employ personal caregivers on a private basis, and these aides become part of the family unit for which the nurse is caring.

In addition to these paraprofessionals, many volunteer agencies and services are available to assist clients in the home, such as Meals on Wheels, Friendly Visitors, and transportation services. Their accessibility depends on the local community's ability to provide them.

Vendors of durable medical equipment provide families with items that can withstand repeated use, such as hospital beds, walking aids, ventilators, intravenous (IV) equipment, and wheelchairs. These vendors work with the family and the home care nurse to determine the support necessary for the client who is being maintained in the home (Haddad, 1987).

Community Resources

Nurses need to know what community resources are available to assist clients. Organizations such as the Knights of Columbus, Kiwanis, the Elks, and local church groups are examples. Many support groups specific to a client's needs may be accessible.

COLLABORATIVE INTERDISCIPLINARY CARE

Medicare-**certified home health agencies** must be interdisciplinary. The role of the nurse focuses on the client and family's physiologic, environmental, and social needs within their community. Effective collaborative case management involves proactive planning and a commitment to the interdisciplinary approach. The first goal should be to facilitate the acquisition of knowledge that enables the client and family to manage their health care needs independently. If that is not possible, the goal may become assisting the family to obtain the help they need in an empathetic, nonstressful manner (Deltogno-Armanasco, Hopkin, & Harter, 1993).

HIGH-TECH HOME CARE
The Growth of High-Tech Home Care

Estimates of the growth of **high-tech therapy** in the home range from 15% to 20% per year. Hundreds of conditions previously treated only in the hospital may now be treated effectively at home using technical equipment formerly used only in the clinical setting. Factors that have promoted the growth of this health care field include the following: (1) earlier detection and increased survival of the chronically ill; (2) the growing number of persons with acquired immunodeficiency syndrome (AIDS); (3) the demographic shift of the largest segment of the population from the young to middle-aged and elderly; (4) greater acceptance of home care by physicians; and (5) third party payers' efforts to reduce cost. Also, improved outcomes (fewer nosocomial infections, improved compliance, client satisfaction) and quality of life are major factors in the success of home therapies. Clients generally do better in familiar surroundings, in their home, and around caring loved ones.

The trend for earliest possible discharge from the hospital for all diagnoses continues. Initiated as a cost containment strategy, hospitals are paid an average sum for a particular diagnosis-related group. Whenever a client can be cared for outside the hospital and the average length of stay is reduced, costs decrease for the hospital (see Chapter 25).

TABLE 26-1   Chronic illness requiring high-tech therapies

In advanced stages or periodic exacerbations, the following conditions may require a type of high-tech home care:

Disorder	Type of high-tech home care
Renal disease	Hemodialysis, enteral nutrition
Gastrointestinal disease	Total parenteral nutrition, enteral nutrition
Neurologic disease	Parenteral or enteral nutrition, miscellaneous parenteral medications
Pulmonary disorders	Ventilator support, parenteral antibiotics
Cardiac disease	Parenteral inotropic agents
Immune System disorders	Parenteral antibiotics, immune globulin (IgIV), nutrition support, other parenteral medications
Hematologic disorders	Blood and blood products, parenteral chelating agents
Cancer	Pain management, blood and blood products, chemotherapeutic agents
Infectious diseases	Parenteral antiinfectives

Anything that can be managed safely and cost efficiently outside of the hospital most likely will be. In the future, the hospitals will primarily be critical care units and a source for outpatient services. Indeed, most nurses working in hospitals agree that this is already the case. Table 26-1 lists chronic illnesses that can be managed outside of the hospital with high tech therapies.

Whether the site is a hospital-based outpatient department or home care division, ambulatory clinic, home health agency, surgery center or home infusion company, the needs and responsibilities of high-tech home care are similar. The importance for nurses to have awareness of all aspects of the particular therapy cannot be overemphasized. Knowledge of the types of supportive equipment and materials available specific to the client's situation is critical. This knowledge promotes nurses as client advocates and assists employers or facilities in being cost-efficient providers.

Providing High-Tech Home Care

Providing services for individuals who need high-tech care requires specific training and education of the health care providers to promote optimal outcomes.

Health care providers have an obligation to provide information and services aimed at promoting better health and minimizing disease processes. The box at right lists various providers of high-tech home care.

The nurse is in the ideal position to be a case manager, or essentially, a problem solver who acts with and for the client to assist him or her to function as independently as possible.

It is apparent that the home health nurse must practice not only community health (health promotion and risk reduction), but must be technically skilled in direct care and teaching activities and must have the clinical judgment appropriate to the acuity level of the client (Cary, 1988).

Discharge planning and care coordination are critical for the successful outcome of high-tech therapies. Whenever possible, team conferences with client and family are arranged. Special equipment may be necessary, and drugs or formulas may require time to acquire and prepare. Initial visits may be done by home care nurses

---

PROVIDERS OF HIGH-TECH HOME CARE

Private agencies, such as the Visiting Nurse Association (VNA), have special divisions, such as an "infusion division" or "oncology division" for advanced technology therapies.

Proprietary agencies are for-profit home health agencies that may provide infusion services by contracting for pharmacy services and clinical specialists or by having an in-house pharmacy and clinical staff.

Infusion companies are proprietary businesses, and in some states are licensed as home health agencies. They may offer nursing services or exist as pharmacies only and coordinate with home health agencies for nursing. The trend is for state licensure of these entities. Some infusion companies have specialized in a particular intensive therapy or client group such as AIDS clients, hemophiliac clients, pediatrics, or women's health.

Hospital based agencies may be nonprofit or for-profit separate businesses although administratively controlled by the hospital. They may provide pharmacy, equipment, and nursing services as well as adjunct services.

Hospice These agencies are for the terminally ill client, to promote a comfortable atmosphere, provide palliative care, and support for the client who remains at home. While the focus of care is the least invasive method, some agencies provide or contract for parenteral pain management.

---

while a client is still hospitalized. In some cases advanced-tech therapy may be initiated in the home, which requires accurate and in-depth admission assessments and planning. Working with the discharge planners and other members of the team, the home health nurse must coordinate services to fit the client's needs and physician's orders.

Nursing Implications and Responsibilities

Intravenous therapy has been recognized as an area of specialty practice and is supported by the Intravenous Nurses Society (INS). The credentialling board for intravenous therapy nurses offers the certification, certified registered nurse intravenous therapy (CRNI), through examination twice yearly. Nurses maintain certification by conducting at least 1600 hours a year in intravenous practice or obtaining required recertification through continuing education programs. The areas of focus of intravenous practice include all aspects of intravenous therapy in nutrition support, oncology, blood and blood products, pediatrics, quality improvement, infection control, and standards of practice. The INS organization (1990) published *Intravenous Therapy Standards of Practice,* which are national standards.

Nutrition support nursing has been recognized as a specialty area of practice by the American Nurses' Association and the American Society for Parenteral and Enteral Nutrition. There are approximately 250 board-certified nutrition support nurses (CNSN) in the United States and Canada (ASPEN Membership Service, 1989). Certification is maintained by practice in the field and examination every 5 years. ASPEN publishes *Standards of Practice for Home Nutrition Support and Nutrition Support Nursing,* as well as the standards for nutrition support dietitians and pharmacists. Professional nurses are the largest group of adjunct nutrition educators and deliverers of nutrition care. As a primary care provider, the registered nurse has had to assume a larger role and greater responsibility in the provision of nutrition care (Orr, 1989). Nurses play a primary role in preparing clients for nutrition support therapy and monitoring and managing progress.

Oncology-certified nurses (OCN) are also responsible in many high-tech agencies or companies for improving the quality of care to the oncology client. The OCN nurse may be responsible for chemotherapy administration, unusual routes of access, and complicated infusion devices that are often needed as well as adjunct therapies such as pain management, antiemetic therapies, and other treatments of oncologic complications. These nurses are certified by the Oncology Nursing Society (ONS) through a credentialling board for a period of 4 years.

Other areas of advanced practice that are useful in advanced technology home care include geriatrics, critical care nursing, and administration.

There are several schools now offering Master of Nursing degrees in high-tech home care. The responsibilities of nurses with advanced certification and specialty degrees include not only offering the best care for the client who requires high-tech therapy at home, but also to be a teacher and resource for other home care staff. An additional area of responsibility for all staff and particularly Master's prepared staff is research. Very little quality research exists about home care and even less about high-tech home care. Validating methods and clinical practice to promote favorable client outcomes is essential to the advancement of nursing as a profession.

HOSPICE CARE

A **hospice,** which is a homelike facility that provides supportive care for terminally ill clients, is a concept that denotes a calm vision of death. It provides a time during which the dying spend their final days in the comfort of their home surrounded by friends and relatives (Paradis, 1985). A goal of most hospice programs is to keep the client in the home. A hospice program frequently operates in close association with a hospital that can provide the client with special treatment when needed. This treatment is given by a hospice unit, which may also provide the client's family with respite services.

The hospice concept is fairly new in the United States. It has been in existence in England since the 1800s, and the idea spread to other countries in the United Kingdom. The goal of a hospice program is to keep the terminally ill client free of pain and symptoms. The emphasis is on **palliative care** rather than restorative care. Clients must be aware of their diagnosis and agree to the process before they can be accepted by a hospice.

The Department of Health and Welfare in Canada has defined a clinical core unit for hospice care. The palliative team specialists and the external palliative team members have specific tasks (see Table 26-2).

Regional palliative care centers are suggesting that, for the sake of economy, a total core unit may not be necessary (Murray & Murray, 1992). It is necessary to provide quality care that is sensitive to the needs of the client and still based

TABLE 26-2 Palliative care service: Human resource team

Core clinical unit

1. Palliative care physician
2. Primary care physican
3. Palliative care case manager
4. Visiting palliative care nurse
5. Social worker or counselor
6. Pastoral care or spiritual coordinator

Palliative team specialists

7. Pharmacist
8. Therapists: occupational, physio-, music/art, massage, and respiratory
9. Nutritionist
10. Homemaker

External palliative team members

11. Equipment suppliers
12. Trained volunteers
13. Extended family caregivers

From "Benchmarking: A tool for excellence in palliative care: Front line dispatch" by A. Murray & H. Murray, 1992, *Journal of Palliative Care, 8*(4), p. 42. Reprinted by permission.

within the family's ability to pay. Therefore, the palliative care nurse manager may face some difficult decisions with regard to who essential team members are.

CASELOAD MANAGEMENT

Caseload management is very different from the concept of collaborative interdisciplinary care. It requires the ability to plan care for a given number of clients during a specific time period. The goal of caseload management is to move the client toward independence in the best way possible while assuring a safe and positive recovery, a satisfactory maintenance level, or a peaceful death. In today's faltering economy, it has also become necessary to factor in the cost of the care being provided. Planning caseload management involves a six-step process, according to Anglin (1992):

1. Clarify the agency philosophy
2. Plan
3. Prioritize the caseload
4. Select an approach

5. Monitor services
6. Evaluate results

The philosophy of the home health agency provides a framework in which to determine the plan for the caseload to be managed. It is often helpful to conduct appropriate inservice sessions for new employees in terms of specific problems that may occur during time allotted for an assigned caseload. For example, weather conditions in some geographic areas may be unpredictable. Some home care companies are located in snowbelt areas that require staff members to have 4-wheel drive vehicles or to be able to cross-country ski. Horseback riding skills may be needed in some remote areas. A boat or a ferry may be required for transportation to islands off the coast.

In urban areas, the nurse must be aware in advance of such community events as a street fair or a sporting event. The nurse must pay attention to road closings, police activities, protests and demonstrations, and traffic accidents, each of which can interrupt the travel time and subsequently the entire caseload.

Safety considerations require additional preparation strategies. Safety guidelines are simple and easy to follow. Expensive jewelry or watches should not be worn. Purses should be carried in the trunk of the car. Credit cards and large sums of money should not be carried. Automobiles should be maintained in good condition. If an area looks unsafe, it is wise not to enter without an escort or other necessary assistance.

Most importantly, the nurse must know the area well. Many factors should be taken into account to make a plan that is predictable and reasonable.

Prioritize the Caseload

Historically, nurses have been rescuers, giving assistance where needed. Most nurses have not had to deal with the management of the finances that are necessary to provide the service. Nurses must begin to take part in developing a plan of action to meet the financial needs of service demands rather than simply responding to society's demands for service. Home care agencies are struggling to maintain service within reimburse-

━━━━━━━━━━ RESEARCH ❦ HIGHLIGHT ━━━━━━━━━━

Adaptation of Family Members in Caregiving Role

Roy's (1984) adaptation model provided the conceptual framework within which to assess how family members adapt to the assumption of the caregiving role, the effect of this role on the psychologic and physiologic health of the caregiver, and the issues associated with interdependence as identified by caregivers of adults dependent on total parenteral nutrition (TPN) home care. The sample of convenience, provided by three accredited home nursing agencies that used similar teaching and TPN home care protocols, consisted of 20 subjects, one of whom served as his own primary caregiver. The subjects (16 spouses, 1 sister, and 2 parents of adult children) ranged in age from 30 to 76 years and the recipients of their care ranged in age from 32 to 78 years. Most of the patients had received TPN for less than 4 years, and the time spent by caregivers averaged approximately 10 hours per day.

Seven subjects, four of whom had been caring for their relatives before the introduction of TPN, indicated that there was no change in the caregiver role with the initiation of TPN. It had been the only change, and nurses provided the care 2 to 3 times or 24 hours per day. Changes in role responsibilities and interdependence evolved around TPN management, increased dependence of the patient with decreased time to themselves, and assistance of family members with increased physical care, decreased visitation or invitation, financial dependence, and role reversal. The health of caregivers remained essentially unchanged and coincided with the complexity of their relative's care, which required nursing support services for relief or initial fatigue or exhaustion until they achieved a routine. There were positive and negative emotional descriptors; the one most often mentioned was depression. Caregiver strength was reflected in success with the provision of home care, and increased independence, confidence, and family unity. Self-sufficiency with infusion administration and its associated responsibility and judgment for required assistance permeated this study.

Although nursing support services were used by all to varying degrees, services were minimal for most, and little assistance from the extended family was evident. While nurses provided encouragement (self-concept support) and essential information about TPN management (role mastery support), they need to intervene by assisting caregivers with the identification of situations in which external support would maintain adaptation. In addition, "families with extensive caregiving demands need encouragement and education about how to incorporate friends and activities into their lives in order to enhance their overall adaptation."

From "Responsibilities and Reactions of Family Caregivers of Patients Dependent on Total Parenteral Nutrition at Home" by C.E. Smith, L. Moushey, J.A. Ross, & C. Gieffer, 1993, *Public Health Nursing, 10*(2), 122-128.

──

ment constraints in the United States. It takes time to prioritize service by analyzing the clients' needs and available resources within the families and services within the community. It may be frustrating to assess the client's desire to progress toward an agreed-upon outcome (Anglin, 1992).

Time spent in the home must be consistent with the amount of time the agency can provide and still remain in business. One study recommends 4.9 visits in one day with an ideal time allotment of 47 minutes per visit (Spollstra, 1986). If the nurse is scheduled to work an 8-hour day, this ideal time allotment would leave 51 minutes of travel time between clients. In a rural area this schedule might not be possible. Particularly, this would not be possible if some clients could only be reached by boat, as in the coastal region of Labrador or on the island of Kodiak in Alaska. In addition, the ideal of 4.9 clients in an 8-hour day is less than the expectations of most agencies. Prioritizing must include the answers to such questions as: What geographic limitations are necessary? How many cases can the agency service and still maintain a desired quality of care? Some of these decisions have to be made on an administrative level. Nurses need to be involved in the planning process (Anglin, 1992).

Monitoring Services

Nurses are not accustomed to placing a price on every action or service given. To assure the survival of individual agencies, fiscal responsibility must become a part of the planning process. One activity that has contributed significantly to the mortality of many home care agencies has been an overextension of services. Client education, referral to community services, and family involvement can maximize the time spent by the skilled nurse. Placement of home health aides and paraprofessionals in maintenance situations may help the nurse to make the most efficient use of time.

Education

Nurses must do their own evaluations of caseload management rather than allow administrators to do it. An understanding of the data on the costs of delivered service, costs of travel time, and the costs of revisits would give them the tools to do their own evaluations. Travel time, telephone time, the actual time in the home, and planning time, should all be documented. Reasonable schedules, quality care, and cost containment should be the goals of caseload management.

The Nurse's Initial Visit

The nurse's role in the home should reflect the health agency's philosophy and mission statement and should include the nurse's personal philosophy and theory base. It also should be consistent with the American Nurses' Association's Standards of Home Health Nursing. Most agencies use the nursing process as a framework for practice. On the first visit to a client's home, the nurse collects the necessary data to assess the client's needs and the appropriateness of the referral. This referral may be from a neighbor, a family member, or a social worker. Most commonly, the referral comes from a physician or a hospital discharge planner. Supervisors or intake nurses usually take referrals. Most agencies have a standard referral form (Figure 26-1). Many referrals are taken in by FAX and may or may not be transferred to a referral form. Intake nurses in the United States must be careful that elderly individuals fit Medicare's definition of homebound. Medicare does not provide funding if an elderly client is not homebound. Answers to appropriate questions may necessitate referral to another agency.

If the client has a telephone, a call made before a visit is wise. The nurse's initial visit does not require a physician's signature; however, a physician referral must be signed on a timely basis. This policy will vary from state to state and from province to province. The nurse should carefully review the referral to make necessary decisions about how it fits into the present caseload (Huebner & Harrison, 1991).

On the initial visit to an adult client's home, the nurse must conduct a physical assessment, a psychosocial assessment, and complete a mental status report. Most agencies insist on a complete review of systems, a family profile, and documentation of the client's financial status and source of payment.

FUTURE TRENDS

The National Association for Home Care (NAHC), which represents home care agencies in the United States, has made the following recommendations to the Clinton administration:

- Acute-care basic benefit packages must include home care and hospice packages
- Any reform plan enacted must include a long-term component
- In-home services provided under both acute care and long term benefits must be designed to ensure individuals' access based on need and not age or other arbitrary conditions, such as prior institutionalization
- Mechanisms for eligibility determination and client management must recognize the importance of provider participation
- Safeguards should exist for quality assurance and cost containment
- Financing for the health reform plan must be progressive and broadly based (Conner, 1993, p. 4).

Research has proven that home care compared with extended hospital care is less costly and preferred by most people. For example, Aetna Life & Casualty Company has reported a $78,000 per-case savings from its individual care management program by using home care for victims of catastrophic accidents (Conner, 1993).

NAHC is pointing out the need to expand many health care services. The government is

Referred by: _____
Title _____ Ph _____
Hospital _____
Dates from _____ to _____

REFERRAL FORM

Patient _____ Date of Birth _____ Lives Alone _____

Address _____ Ph _____

Medicare # _____ Medicaid # _____ Ph _____

Insurance # _____ Group # _____ ID # _____ Ph _____

Emergency Contact _____ Ph _____

Address _____ Ph _____

Physician _____ Add _____ Ph _____

Primary Dx _____

Secondary Dx _____ Surgical Procedure _____
Allergies _____ Homebound Status _____
Medications _____

_____

_____

_____ RN   FREQ _____   _____ PT Evaluation _____

_____ VS/Monitor _____   ___ ROM ___ Active ___ Passive ___ Increase Strength
_____ Instruct Med. Regimen _____   ___ Wt. Bearing ___ Full ___ Partial ___ None
_____ Instruct _____ Diet   ___ Gait Training ___ Transfers ___ Stairs
_____ Catheter _____ FR _____ cc _____   _____
_____ Dressings _____   _____ ST Evaluation _____
_____ Lab _____   _____ OT Evaluation _____

_____ HHA Frequency _____   _____ MSW Evaluation _____
_____ Personal Care _____   _____
_____ Catheter Care _____   _____
_____ Comfort Measures _____
Comments _____

_____

_____

Directions _____

V/O Taken by _____ Date/Time _____

Disposition _____ Admit Visit _____

FIGURE 26-1   Sample referral form of a home health agency.

demanding that costs of health care go down. Research has proven that home care is less costly than inpatient care. Clearly, nurses in the United States must be ready to meet the challenge.

The Baylor HomeCare Agency in Dallas, Texas makes approximately 85,000 visits per year by using a combination of hourly staff and per-visit staff. Hourly registered nurses are paid a salary for 40 hours per week. Per-visit, registered nurses are paid on a fee-for-service basis. The case manager is salaried and is responsible for coordinating all care. The case manager is the person who makes all visits from Monday to Friday and schedules the weekend and evening visits with a fee-for-service registered nurse. Fee-for-service staff are not full-time employees. They are expected to make at least 27 visits per week, however. Baylor compensates for overtime and provides a monetary bonus for performance evaluations that are rated as outstanding. Baylor maintains that the use of full-time hourly staff provides continuity of care. The use of per-visit staff keeps overall costs to the agency down. Incentive rewards and overtime pay keep the employees feeling treated fairly and happy in their work (Whitaker, 1993). This type of innovative planning may be necessary to meet the increased need for home care while keeping the overall costs down.

In Canada, the recession is worsening and there have been more reductions in Federal transfer payments (see Chapter 4). Innovations such as community health centers are increasingly being used. Health care workers who are not necessarily professionals are being called into service to keep costs down.

The province of Manitoba has created a system that divides the province into eight regional offices. Within each region there is a continuing care coordinator responsible for the overall program. Case coordinators are assigned. This may be a nurse or a social worker, depending on the dominant needs of the client. Resource coordinators are responsible for home health staff. Services are provided free of charge but must not exceed the cost of institutionalization (Connor, 1993).

Keeping the costs down and providing quality care in both countries will constitute the challenge of the future for home health care services. Most certainly the Clinton administration is going to affect the manner in which home care is implemented and paid for. Canada, too, has a new administration with a clear mandate to cure a faltering economy.

Chapter Highlights

- Home health nursing refers to the practice of nursing applied to a client with a health deficit in the client's place of residence. Clients and their designated caregivers are the focus of home health nursing practice, according to the American Nurse's Association.

- The Standards of Home Health Nursing Practice establish guidelines to assure quality of care in home health nursing.

- Medicare defines home health care as care that is provided under the supervision of a registered professional nurse. Certified agencies must provide interdisciplinary services.

- Clients who require care in the home include those who are acutely ill, those who are chronically ill, those who are elderly, and/or those who are in need of palliative care.

- Professionals involved in providing home care include nurses, physicians, physical therapists, occupational therapists, social workers, speech pathologists, nutritionists, and home health aides.

- The nurse usually functions as the coordinator of the home care team.

- Hospice care provides palliative care in the home to terminally ill clients.

- Home care may be financed through private insurance, Medicare, Medicaid, and the client's private insurance payments in the United States. In Canada, the federal government finances home care through regional offices.

The nurse assesses the client's ability to pay for services and helps to locate additional sources of funding if necessary.

▪ It is possible that, in the future, a different program for third-party payment will evolve in the United States.

 ## CRITICAL THINKING EXERCISE

The following is the information received by one VNA 1 day before the hospital was to discharge a person who had a cerebrovascular accident.

Name of client: Mrs. R. Jones (lives alone)
Address: 23 Peach Street
Telephone: 832-6468
Birth date: 5/1/25
Referred by: Dorothy Kline, discharge planner from St. Joseph's hospital
Type of reimbursement: Medicare
Nearest relative: Janice Jones (lives out of town)
    Telephone: (203) 922-3800
Medical diagnosis: Cerebral vascular accident, with resulting hemiplegia (left sided), and hypertension

Allergies: penicillin
Medications: Furosemide PO 40 mg qd, Neferpidine 10 mg PO tid
Physician's order: Skilled nursing care, home health aide, physiotherapy twice weekly, occupational therapy, nutritionist consultation

1. Formulate a preliminary plan of care for your visit with the client the next day.
2. Fill out the agency referral form contained in Figure 26-1.
3. List support services needed and referrals to be made.

REFERENCES

Allan, S. (1994). Medicare case management—Philadelphia, PA. *Home Healthcare Nurse, 12*(3), 21-27.

American Nurses' Association. (1986). *Standards of home health nursing practice.* Washington, DC: Author.

American Nurses' Association. (1992). *A statement on the scope of home health practice, Council of Community Health Nurses.* Washington, DC: Author.

Anglin, L. (1992). Caseload management: A model for agencies and staff nurses. *Home Healthcare Nurse, 10*(3), 26-31.

Cary, A. (1988). Preparation for professional practice: What do we need? *Nursing Clinics of North America, 23*(2), 251-341.

Conner, C. (Ed.). (1993, March). Toward meaningful reform. *Caring Magazine,* 4-10.

Deltogno-Armanasco, V., Hopkin, L.A., & Harter, S. (1993). *Collaborative nursing case management: A handbook for development and implementation.* New York: Springer.

Haddad, A. (1987). *High tech home care: A practical guide.* Rockville, MD: Aspen.

Home Health Services. (1982). *Commerce clearinghouse Medicare and Medicaid guide, paragraph 1401.* Washington, DC: U.S. Department of Health and Human Services.

Huebner, E., & Harrison, P. (1991). *The homecare and documentation guide: An orientation and resource manual for home care practitioners* (Suppl. 1). Rockville, MD: Aspen.

May, B.J. (1993). *Home health and rehabilitation: Concepts of care.* Philadelphia: Davis.

Moore, F. (1988). *Homemaker—home health aid to services: Script policies and practices.* Owings Mills, MD: National Health.

Murray, A., & Murray, H. (1992). Benchmarking: A tool for excellence in palliative care: Front line dispatch. *Journal of Palliative Care, 8*(4), 41-45.

Orr, M. (1989). Nutritional support in home care. *Nursing Clinics of North America, 24*(2), 437-445.

Paradis, L. (1985). *Hospice handbook: A guide for managers and planners.* Rockville, MD: Aspen.

Spollstra, S.L. (1986). *Productivity expectations of registered nurses in the home health care setting: A Michigan study.* Unpublished Thesis: Northern Michigan University, Marquette, MI.

Stanhope, M., & Lancaster, J. (1992). *Community health nursing: Process and practice for promoting health* (3rd ed.). St. Louis: Mosby.

Toffler, A. (1970). *Future shock.* New York: Random House.

Whitaker, R. (1993). A home health agency's operational model utilizing per visit and hourly staff. *Journal of Home Health Care Practice, 5*(5), 38-43.

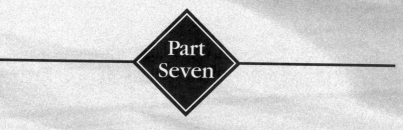

Part Seven

Special Roles and Settings

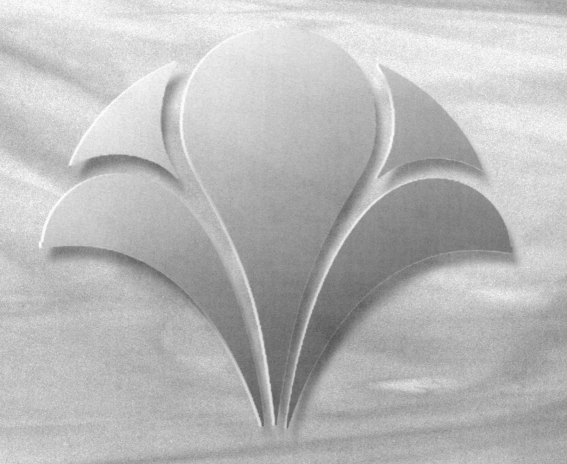

Part VII deals with two important special roles of the community health nurse: occupational health nursing and school health nursing. These nursing disciplines are often practiced in settings in which the nurse is the only health professional on the site. In addition to a strong knowledge base, the nurse must be able to function autonomously and with appropriate assertiveness.

Chapter 27 identifies particular hazards in the workplace, the role of government agencies, and the most frequent types of health hazards experienced by the worker. A model is provided to assist the student to visualize the factors that need to be taken into account when analyzing and solving work site problems.

Chapter 28 provides a description of the problems that might be encountered by a school nurse. Some guidelines are given for solutions to common problems. An overall view of the responsibilities of the school nurse is presented with particular focus on primary prevention of illness.

27

OCCUPATIONAL HEALTH NURSING

Mary K. Salazar ◆ William E. Wilkinson
◆ Christine L. Rubadue

This act is passed to assure so far as possible every working man and woman in the nation safe and healthful working conditions and to preserve our human resources.

(Occupational Safety and Health Administration, 1970)

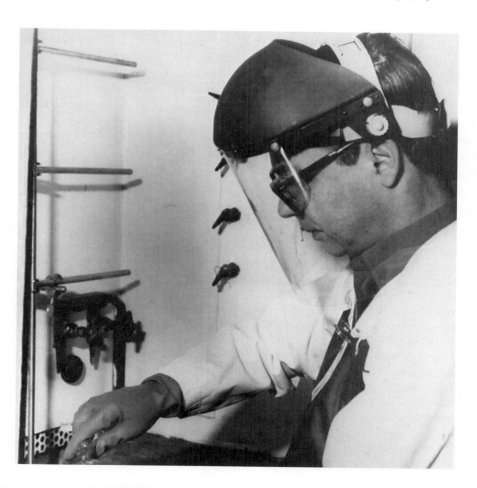

OBJECTIVES

At the conclusion of this chapter the student will be able to:

1. Define the key terms listed.
2. List types of health and safety hazards that exist in the occupational setting.
3. Relate the importance of considering the client's work environment to the implementation of the nursing process.
4. Discuss some of the major governmental groups that affect health and safety legislation.
5. Outline the major occupational hazards to health care workers.
6. Describe a conceptual model of occupational health nursing as a specialty area of community health nursing practice.

KEY TERMS

American Association of
   Occupational Health
   Nurses (AAOHN)
Americans with Disabilities Act
Biologic hazards
Chemical hazards
Educational resource centers
Ergonomics
Hazard Communication Standard

National Institute of Occupational
   Safety and Health (NIOSH)
Occupational health history
Occupational health nursing
Occupational illness
Occupational injury
Occupational Safety and Health
   Act

Occupational Safety and Health
   Administration (OSHA)
Physical hazards
Psychologic hazards
Teratologic effects
Toxicology
Worker's compensation

Occupational health nursing is an area of practice and research within the field of community health nursing. It has a specialized interest in the health and safety of the adult working population. Working adults are essentially the backbone of the world's economy, because through the organization and management of their labor, they produce and distribute virtually all goods and services. Indeed, the years spent working cover the major portion of most life spans. Occupational health nursing focuses on workers of all ages by providing continuous and high-quality health care during what often is a 50-year period of a person's life.

To provide comprehensive and targeted health care services within the community, it is imperative that the occupational setting be considered when conducting assessments and developing interventions. Understanding occupational safety and health, therefore, is an essential component of nursing preparation. Clearly, nurses who choose to work in the field of occupational health nursing must be proficient and knowledgeable about this specialty area; but knowledge about occupational health and safety is also important to nurses in other related and diverse practice areas. Inherent hazards to workers in the occupational setting can potentially affect the health of a large portion of our population. To appreciate the potential effects of hazards in the occupational setting, consider that the majority of the adult population in this country is employed, and that unemployed persons are likely to be living with someone who is a worker. Almost every job involves some degree of health hazard. Thus almost every client, whether in the work setting or not, may potentially be affected by occupational injury or illness. A consideration of the various effects of occupational exposure are essential to good nursing practice.

The purposes of this chapter are to introduce the reader to the field of occupational health nursing and to suggest some practical ways that this knowledge can be useful in nursing practice, regardless of the setting. In addition, some discussion about the special hazards that health care workers themselves face in their work setting is included in various sections. This information is intended to help the reader better understand occupational health from a worker's perspective.

HISTORY

Interest in the health of workers was first noted in the early 18th century when an Italian professor of medicine, Bernardino Ramazzini, often considered the "father of occupational medicine," wrote his treatise *Diseases of Workers* (1713, translated by Wright, 1993). Despite Ramazzini's contribution and the ongoing efforts of many other health care providers, much abuse and neglect continued to occur in the workplace. Injuries and illnesses associated with certain types of occupations were (and in many cases continue to be) considered "acceptable" risks, and neither the employee nor the employer may pay much attention when they occur. For example, it is well known and virtually accepted that coal miners eventually acquire black lung disease, that nurses frequently are afflicted with chronic back pain, and that persons who cut down trees may be killed by a falling tree.

A Century of Promoting Worker Health

Occupational health nurses, formerly called industrial nurses, have been a part of the industrial and other occupational settings in both Europe and the United States for more than a century. During this period they have made many valuable contributions to the health of workers. Betty Moulder is generally recognized as the first occupational health nurse (OHN) in the United States.

She was hired by a group of Pennsylvania coalmining companies in 1888 to provide health care for the coal miners and their families. Ada Mayo Stewart, another important OHN from those early years, was hired by the president of the Vermont Marble Company who, unlike many of his colleagues, had an interest in the health of his workers. Like Moulder, Stewart provided health services not only to the workers but also to their families. These early OHNs provided most of their services in the home setting.

The early twentieth century saw a broad expansion of occupational health services by nurses. As early as 1900 there are records of OHNs being employed in department stores and other retail operations on the West Coast. Of interest is the fact that in 1909 the Milwaukee Visiting Nurse Association "placed the first nurse in a local industrial plant for the purpose of demonstrating to the employer the economic value" of an OHN (Kowalke, 1930, p. 615). With the passage of the first state workers' compensation law in 1911, occupational health nursing began to focus more on workers' injuries in the occupational health setting than on family health services in the home. A significant expansion of occupational health nursing services occurred during World War I. By 1918 there were 1213 OHNs, and by 1930 the Census of Population by Occupation reported that 3189 nurses were employed in industrial settings. Another huge expansion of OHNs occurred during World War II partly because of the industrial expansion that occurred during the war, but also because of an ongoing expansion that resulted when the Social Security Act of 1935 granted federal funds for occupational health services at state levels. By 1943 it was estimated that 11,000 OHNs were working in industrial settings in the United States (Rogers, 1988).

As the number of occupational health nurses increased, interest in forming a national association grew among practicing industrial nurses, and in 1942 the American Association of Industrial Nurses was established. The purposes of the association were to improve occupational health nursing services and to offer opportunities for nurses interested in this area of practice. In 1977 the association changed its name to the **Ameri-**

can **Association of Occupational Health Nurses (AAOHN)** to reflect the expanded role of nurses who work in the occupational setting.

Educational Resource Centers

After World War II there was less interest in occupational health and safety, and the number of injuries in the occupational setting began to rise. Ultimately, this resulted in the passage of the Occupational Safety and Health Act in 1970, which, in turn, resulted in a resurgence of attention to health and safety problems that were occurring in the workplace. After the passage of this act, many businesses introduced occupational health programs for the first time, and the demand for the services of the occupational health nurse greatly increased. Because of the recognized need for more highly trained and skilled occupational health professionals, the **National Institute of Occupational Safety and Health (NIOSH)** developed **educational resource centers** in 1977. One purpose of these centers was to provide graduate-level education for the following professionals: occupational health physicians, occupational health nurses, safety managers, and industrial hygienists. There were also provisions for continuing education, and for research in the field of occupational health. Currently, there are 14 educational resource centers in the continental United States; there is at least one in each federal service region. The University of Washington in Seattle is an example of a NIOSH-sponsored educational resource center, and is called the Northwest Center of Occupational Safety and Health. It has graduate programs in occupational health nursing both at the master's and doctoral levels, an industrial hygiene program leading to a master's and/or a doctoral degree, and an occupational medicine program for practicing physicians. This center also has an active continuing education program.

The number of occupational health nurses in the United States is increasing steadily as the demand for nurses with special knowledge and training in the field of occupational health continues to grow. Today employers are recognizing the importance of protecting the health and safety of their employees. Workers and employ-

ers are now asking occupational health care providers probing questions about exposure, safety, and health issues related to their work environment and about job-related health hazards to themselves and their families. The scope and range of services provided by the OHN today has greatly expanded since the early years.

Government Involvement: Occupational Safety and Health Act

The **Occupational Safety and Health Act** (OSHAct) of 1970 was passed "to assure so far as possible every working man and woman in the nation safe and healthful working conditions and to preserve our human resources." The OSHAct created the **Occupational Safety and Health Administration** (OSHA) and established NIOSH. In the 1990s, there has been a new surge of interest and concern about the limitations of the mandates of the OSHAct and, therefore, a move is underway to institute appropriate reforms (Yorker, 1993).

OSHA, which is part of the Department of Labor, encourages employers and employees to reduce hazards and to improve safety and health programs in the workplace by educating workers and by promulgating and enforcing standards and regulations (McCunney, 1988, p. 47).

It (OSHA) accomplishes its mission by setting health and safety standards, enforcing these standards by the use of intermittent worksite inspections, and assisting employers in solving various worksite problems by offering consultation through state OSHA agencies. Through the onsite consultation program, hazardous conditions can be corrected without OSHA's relying on its enforcement powers.

One of the most recent standards passed by OSHA is called the Bloodborne Pathogens Standard (29 CFR 1910.1030). Bloodborne pathogens are defined as "pathogenic microorganisms present in human blood which can cause disease in humans. These bloodborne pathogens include, but are not limited to, hepatitis B virus (HBV) and human immunodeficiency virus (HIV or AIDS virus)" (U.S. Department of Labor, 1991). This standard mandates that engineering and work practice controls shall be used to eliminate or minimize employee exposure. If occupational exposure remains after institution of these controls, personal protective equipment shall be used. The bloodborne pathogens standard requires that a written exposure control plan for occupational bloodborne pathogens be developed and include the following components: exposure determination, methods of compliance, handling exposure incidents, training, recordkeeping, and biowaste handling.

Another important standard is The **Hazard Communication Standard** (HCS) (29 CFR 1910.1200). This standard was first issued in 1983 and was revised in 1987. The HCS is sometimes referred to as the Worker's Right to Know Act. This standard requires all manufacturers and distributors of hazardous chemicals to provide material safety data sheets that identify the potential effects of the chemicals with which their employees work. It also requires that all employees who handle or are in contact with hazardous chemicals be properly trained and that employers keep a file for each employee that identifies the chemicals to which they are exposed and the dose of the exposure (McCunney, 1988, p. 25).

In addition, under the 1986 amendments reauthorizing the "Superfund" Act (SARA amendments), material safety data sheets or a list of the chemicals for which the company has material safety data sheets must be supplied to local emergency planning committees, state emergency planning committees, fire departments, and state emergency response commissions. In addition, inventories on hazardous chemicals must be submitted to these state and local agencies. Any citizen who requests that information from the state or local authorities is entitled to receive it with certain trade secret exceptions.

The NIOSH was established as a branch of the United States Public Health Service's Centers for Disease Control and Prevention (USPHS/CDCP) within the United States Department of Health and Human Services (U.S. DHHS). NIOSH was created to carry out the following tasks (U.S. DHHS, 1992): (1) respond to requests for investigation of workplace hazards, (2) conduct research to prevent work-related health and safety problems, (3) recommend appropriate regulatory

actions to OSHA, and (4) train occupational safety and health professionals. In keeping with these functions, NIOSH has greatly expanded epidemiologic and laboratory research of the causes of occupational disease and injuries and the methods of preventing them. NIOSH publishes many reports and materials detailing occupational hazards and ways of preventing or controlling them, and it makes recommendations to the Department of Labor regarding emerging problems.

Other Mandates

Workers' compensation laws comprise an array of state and federal laws established to shift some of the costs of occupational injuries and illnesses from the worker to the employer. These laws generally require employers or their insurance companies to reimburse a portion of injured workers' lost wages and all of their medical care. Some states pay for worker retraining and some do not. Workers' compensation laws include both federal and state statutes. In either case, these laws ensure workers who suffer occupational injuries or illnesses prompt, though limited, benefits; additionally, it provides employers with a liability system by requiring employers to carry compensation insurance. Workers' compensation laws currently are under scrutiny for revisions in their application and administration (Wilkinson, 1994).

The federal Coal and Mine Safety Act of 1969 was passed to establish coal mine health standards, to provide benefit payments to coal miners disabled by black lung disease, and to initiate research. This legislation was initiated by the death of 78 miners in a coal mine explosion in Farmington, West Virginia, in 1968. In 1976 the Toxic Substances Control Act (TOSCA) was established to regulate commerce and to protect human health and the environment. This Act, legislated in an attempt to control some of the chemical hazards in industry, requires testing and restricts the use of certain chemical substances.

In 1990 a federal legislation of broad scope proscribing discrimination against persons with disabilities was passed under the **Americans with Disabilities Act** (ADA). According to estimates, as many as 43 million Americans have been segregated from society because of one or more physical or mental disabilities (Cross, 1993). The ADA regulates activities under five titles: employment, public services provided by government entities, public accommodations and services operated by private entities, telecommunications, and miscellaneous (Anfield, 1992). Title I, which is the employment title of this act, requires employers to make *reasonable accommodations* in the workplace; that is, they must make reasonable efforts to assure that the workplace is accessible and usable for employees who have disabilities. Furthermore, employers are prohibited from conducting pre-employment physical examinations for the purpose of determining if an individual has a disability. The employment requirements of the ADA are enforced by the Equal Employment Opportunity Commission (EEOC). EEOC requires employers to post a notice in the workplace that summarizes the provisions of the act and informs employees how to file a complaint if violations occur (Cross, 1993).

WORK-RELATED INJURIES AND ILLNESS
Statistics

According to the most recent data available from the Bureau of Labor Statistics (U.S. Department of Labor, 1993), the total number of reported cases of injury and illnesses in 1991 was slightly more than 6,300,000. (This figure was obtained from the private sector, which represents approximately 75% of the total working population.) Work-related injuries were reported at the rate of 7.9 per 100 full-time workers, with the rates ranging from 2.3 for industries such as finance and insurance to 16.5 for workers in the metal manufacturing industry. Nearly half of these injuries involved lost work days (U.S. Department of Labor, 1993). In the same year, 368,300 new cases of occupational illnesses were reported, 60% of which were related to repeated trauma, such as noise-induced hearing loss and carpal tunnel syndrome. Approximately 2800 work-related fatalities were reported in 1991.

According to several estimates, the actual numbers of occupational injuries, illnesses, and fatalities are greatly underreported (Fingars, Hop-

kins, & Nelson, 1992; Weeks, Levy, & Wagner, 1991). For example, while 2800 fatalities were reported in 1991, it has been estimated that 100,000 deaths occur annually as a result of cancer, lung conditions, or other diseases related to long-term work exposure. On the basis of such discrepancies as these, it is easy to see that the current statistical information may be inadequate. The reason for the discrepancies is twofold: First, many occupational health problems do not come to the attention of the health care provider or employer and therefore are not included in the record keeping of occupational injuries and illnesses. Second, many occupational health problems that come to the attention of the health care provider or employer are not recognized as work-related. Despite difficulties in determining the precise frequency of their occurrence, it is clear from either report or estimated information that occupational-related injuries and illnesses may pose a serious threat to the population.

Definitions

The terms *occupational injury* and *occupational illness* require definition. **Occupational injury** is an injury that results from an acute episode and usually is easily identifiable in terms of its cause and effects. It includes such incidents as cuts, fractures, and sprains that result from an accident in the work environment. Injuries constitute approximately 95% of all compensable accidents in the workplace. **Occupational illness,** on the other hand, is often difficult to diagnose because it tends to be subtle and frequently manifests as a long-term condition that is indistinguishable from chronic conditions of a nonoccupational origin. Occupational illnesses include abnormal conditions or disorders that are caused by exposures to environmental factors associated with employment. These illnesses can result from inhalation, absorption, ingestion, or direct contact.

The results of many long-term exposures to chemical or biologic substances at the work site may be unclear. Often when an illness occurs, the connection to the occupational exposure is overlooked. The following are examples of adverse effects resulting from exposures to occupational hazards:

1. Reproductive and **teratological effects,** including sterility (both men and women), spontaneous abortion, and birth defects. (Teratogens are chemical, physical, or biologic agents that cause harm to fetuses);
2. Cancers, including respiratory and skin cancer and leukemia;
3. Cardiovascular disease, including coronary heart disease;
4. Infectious disease, including Hepatitis A, B, and others; tuberculosis; childhood diseases among health care workers; and bacteria (i.e., brucellosis) and viruses (i.e., rabies), which may occur among nonhealth workers.

Impact

The effects of occupational injury or illness on the employee, the employee's family, the employer, and on society may vary, but in all cases, it has the potential to be significant. The employee and the employee's family may suffer both tangible and intangible consequences of work-related injuries and illnesses. The injury or illness may disrupt family life and in some instances may be responsible for the breakup of families. The loss of earnings plus expenses for care related to the incident can cause problems far beyond those noted at work. Stress may be a direct or an indirect result of the multiple problems, such as the loss of wages and concern about future employment, that are associated with the actual injury or illness. Stress is likely to be especially profound if the employee is the sole wage earner in the family. Other important considerations to both employee and family include the pain and suffering that may accompany the injury or illness.

The employer may experience a turnover in staff, high absenteeism, and possibly a lowered employee morale level as a result of workplace incidents. Ultimately, this leads to a loss of worker productivity. Society pays for the extra costs involved in workers' compensation and other employer losses by paying higher prices for goods and services. Also, society loses revenue from taxes that are not being paid by an unemployed person, as well as the loss of that employee's contribution to society.

MAINTENANCE OF HEALTH IN THE WORKPLACE
Effects of Environment

To determine the relationship between work and health, it is important to understand the type and nature of hazards in the work environment. Approximately one fourth to one third of the working individual's day is spent at the workplace. Adults in this country are likely to spend 40 years or longer in their work environment, which affects their health and their attitudes about health during a large portion of their lives. The health and safety of the worker in the workplace is the central theme of occupational health care. Measuring and evaluating occupational exposures must be considered in terms of their effects on workers. Among the greatest challenges to occupational health professionals is the continual delineation and identification of occupational health risks as new technological advances and new work hazards emerge. The identification of risk factors involves constant surveillance and monitoring of the work environment.

Attitudes Toward Health

The work environment is profoundly affected by attitudes about occupational health. To create successful occupational health programs, both employer and employee must be actively interested and involved in health, safety, and education. Employers, especially those at the highest levels of management, must be interested in a healthy and safe work environment; they must communicate that health is a high priority; and they must enforce policies regarding employee health at lower levels of management. Enforcement may include mandatory participation in health and safety activities, with evaluation of participation to be included in performance appraisals. Employees must want to stay healthy and must take an active role in maintaining a healthy work environment. They must also feel that management is concerned and supportive of their efforts to maintain an optimal level of health. Health and safety professionals in the occupational setting are an essential part of any good occupational health program. These individuals must be committed to working with the various members of the health team, with the management, and with the employees to maintain a healthy work force. In many cases, occupational injuries and illnesses are preventable. Implementing engineering and administrative controls, providing safer materials, identifying health hazards, and educating the work force will inevitably lead to a healthier and safer environment. The occupational health professional must be constantly aware of the hazards that may jeopardize the well-being of the worker.

MAJOR CATEGORIES OF HAZARDS IN THE WORKPLACE

A tremendous array of occupations is represented by the more than 120 million people working in the United States, and American workers are exposed to a variety of potential health hazards in the course of their workday. The injuries and illnesses that result from worksite exposure may cause pain and hardship for these employees. Most hazards that occur in the occupational setting can be classified as physical, ergonomic, chemical, biologic, or psychologic.

Physical

The majority of reported occupational injuries are a result of **physical hazards** that result in injuries with a wide range of causes and effects. Physical factors that contribute to the occurrence of injury include the structure of the work space, the equipment used, the temperature in the work environment, the presence of radiation, the lighting, and noise levels. The most commonly reported injuries include strains and sprains, lacerations, contusions, scratches, and abrasions. By far the most commonly reported type of injury that occurs in work settings is musculoskeletal, particularly back injury.

The physical factors of noise and radiation have received much attention in recent years. Both of these factors are more insidious in nature than many other physical factors, and the health effects that result from prolonged exposure can be devastating. Noise-induced hearing loss is in-

curable and irreversible. It is estimated that about 1 million Americans suffer noise-induced hearing loss annually (Weeks et al, 1991). The most common cause of occupational hearing loss is unprotected exposure to loud noise over an extended period of time. In view of the disabling effects of occupational hearing loss, the importance of prevention cannot be overemphasized.

As with noise, injury because of radiation is most frequently a result of unprotected exposure over an extended period of time. Some radiation generates unstable, highly reactive ions as the energy from this radiation moves through living tissue. This condition is called ionizing radiation. The most serious damage from ionizing radiation occurs within the nuclei of living cells, where chemical changes to deoxyribonucleic acid (DNA), the heredity unit of the cell, may occur. Low doses of radiation over prolonged periods can eventually lead to cancers, tumors, fetal birth defects, and mutations in offspring. Recently there has been concern about the ionizing radiation emitted from video display terminals (VDTs). Reports indicate an increase in incidences of spontaneous abortions among VDT users. Follow-up investigations of these reports, however, have failed to confirm an association (Rudolph & Forest, 1990). Many studies on VDTs are currently in progress. In addition to the effects of exposure to ionizing radiation, there is concern about muscle strain and ocular effects associated with VDT use. Recent data suggest that more than 7 million Americans are exposed to some level of ionizing radiation in their workplaces (Weeks et al, 1991).

The biologic effects of nonionizing radiation are different from those of ionizing radiation. Nonionizing radiation includes ultraviolet, infrared, and laser radiation, as well as microwave radiation. Exposure to ultraviolet, infrared, and laser radiation may cause burns, and ultraviolet radiation is regarded as a cause of skin cancer. The primary effect of exposure to microwave radiation is tissue heating. Some studies suggest that exposure to microwave radiation can result in cataract formation, testicular degeneration, and other reproductive sequelae. Effects on behavior and on immune cell function have been noted with chronic exposure to low levels of microwave radiation (Weeks et al, 1991). There continues to be disagreement among investigators about both thermal and nonthermal effects of nonionizing radiation; therefore, additional studies are necessary to establish safe exposure levels.

Ergonomic

Many injuries that occur in the work setting are the result of the poor use of the principles of ergonomics. The word **ergonomics** is derived from the Greek words, *ergo,* which means work, and *nomos,* which means law. Occupational ergonomics is a discipline that attempts to establish the best fit between the human and the imposed job conditions to maximize the health and well-being, as well as the productivity, of the worker. The guiding principle of ergonomics is to adapt the work site to the worker rather than the worker to the work site. Inadequate attention to ergonomics can result in stress to two major body systems, the musculoskeletal and the peripheral nervous systems. The most common musculoskeletal complaint that results from an inadequate "fit" between the human and the work environment is muscle strain and fatigue, which are frequent results of static muscle work.

Ergonomic problems are commonly experienced by office workers who are required to spend many hours in front of a computer terminal. An inappropriately positioned chair, a poorly designed work station, or prolonged static or awkward posture are examples of situations that may lead to a variety of health and/or safety problems. The determination of the nature of ergonomic problems depends on a complete and accurate assessment of the work station, the work equipment, and an evaluation of equipment designed to reduce ergonomic problems (Pravikoff & Simonowitz, 1994). Recent efforts have focused on the redesign of work stations and the equipment, such as VDTs, and keyboards, as a means of preventing trauma from occurring. Providing employees with adjustable chairs and armboards to support their arms while working on keyboards, and making simple adjustments of the VDTs is likely to reduce the occurrence of common injuries such as cumulative trauma disorders.

Cumulative trauma disorders frequently affect the peripheral nervous systems. Examples of this type of disorder include carpal tunnel syndrome, radial nerve entrapment, and digital neuritis. These conditions are associated with tasks that require repetitive motions. Primary risk factors for these disorders are the frequency with which the tasks are performed and the force and posture required when performing the tasks (Figure 27-1) (Frederick, 1984).

Chemical

More than 60,000 chemicals were commonly used in industry in the 1980s (Omenn, 1986), and approximately 1000 new synthetic chemicals are introduced each year. Determining the hazards associated with these chemicals poses a major challenge to the scientific community. Based on current knowledge, it has been estimated that one in four American workers may be exposed to any of 8000 **chemical hazards** that have been identified by OSHA (DiBenedetto, Harris, & McCunney, 1993). Chemicals in the workplace exist in the form of gases, dusts, mists, vapors, and solvents. Effects from chemicals range from acute, such as chemical burns, to chronic, such as occupational asthma precipitated by chemical exposure. In addition to carcinogenic effects, teratogenic effects, which cause incomplete or improper fetal development, have been attributed to chemical exposure in the workplace. Examples of some common chemical exposures and related diseases are listed in Table 27-1.

The three primary routes of exposure to chemical agents are through inhalation, ingestion, and skin absorption. Inhalation is the major route of entry for gases, vapors, mists, and airborne particulate matter. One disease caused by inhalation of a chemical is chronic bronchitis resulting from exposures to agents such as sulfur dioxide or chlorine. Ingestion is a less common route of exposure. However, it can occur; a chemical on the hands, such as malathion (an insecticide used in agriculture), may be ingested when an employee eats or smokes. Skin absorption most frequently occurs through epidermal cells or through hair follicles and sebaceous glands; a number of factors affect percutaneous absorp-

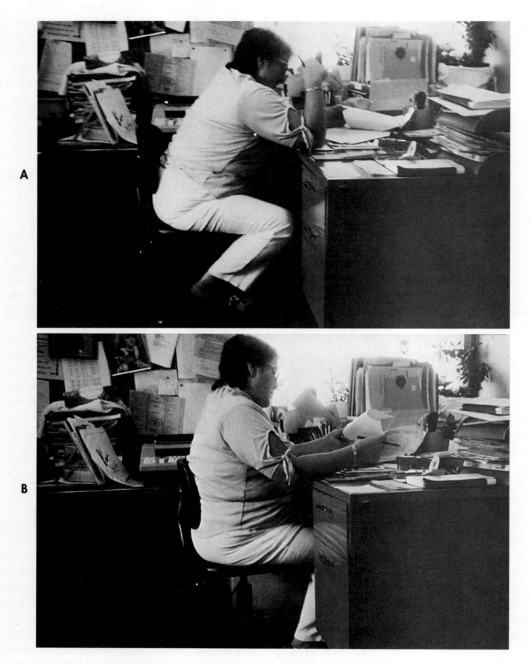

FIGURE 27-1   The fit between the worker and the environment can affect the musculoskeletal system. **A,** Example of poor body alignment; **B,** Example of good body alignment.

TABLE 27-1   Some diseases caused by exposure to chemicals

Chemical	Occupation	Disease
Gasoline	Filling station attendant	Chemical pneumonitis
	Motor transport worker	Pulmonary edema
	Refinery worker	
Coal tar derivatives	Dry cleaners	Leukopenia
	Refinery workers	Leukemia
	Varnish makers	
	Stainers	
	Painters	
Asbestos	Textile makers	Mesothelioma
	Auto brake repairers	Asbestosis
	Construction workers	
	Insulation workers	
Chromium/chromates	Copper etchers	Lung cancer
	Electroplaters	Squamous cell cancer
	Photoengravers	
	Stainless steel workers	
Ethylene oxide	Detergent makers	Dermatitis
	Grain elevator workers	Pulmonary edema
	Hospital workers (CS)	
Vinyl chloride	Resin makers	Raynaud's disease
	Rubber makers	Hepatic damage
	Organic chemical synthesizers	Angiosarcoma
Trichloroethylene	Dry cleaners	CNS depression
	Perfume makers	Peripheral neuropathy
	Textile cleaners	Liver tumors
	Printers	
Carbon disulfide	Degreasers	Behavioral disorders
	Electroplaters	Polyneuritis
	Painters	Atherosclerosis
	Rayon makers	Heart disease
	Wax processors	

From *Occupational diseases: A guide to their recognition* by USPHS/CDC, NIOSH, DHEW, 1977.

tion of chemicals, including the condition of the skin and the nature of the chemical. The effects from skin absorption may be local or systemic. An example of a local effect is an eczema-like syndrome among film developers that results from exposure to color developing solutions. Liver disease is a potential systemic effect of skin absorption of polychlorinated biphenyls.

Toxicology is the science that studies the harmful biologic effects of chemicals. Currently very few of the 60,000 chemicals being used

have been scrutinized by scientists. What scientists have discovered over recent years, however, is that when taken into the body in sufficient amounts, most chemicals, even the most insignificant, can lead to undesirable health effects. Conversely, even the most harmful substance, when taken in a sufficiently minute amount, will be harmless. In other words, the harmfulness or safety of a chemical compound is related to the amount of that compound that is present in the body. Toxicologists attempt to determine the amount of a chemical to which one can be exposed without suffering any harmful effects (Becker & Rosenberg, 1990). It must also be noted, however, that even low levels of exposure to a chemical over extended periods of time can result in serious health effects.

To protect the health of workers, standards related to exposures to chemicals have been established. The American Conference of Governmental Industrial Hygienists (ACGIH) developed guidelines intended to protect the "average" worker from 450 chemicals in 1968 (Levy & Wegman, 1988). These guidelines, which are called threshold limit values, were adopted as recommendations by OSHA when the OSHAct was passed in 1970. Additionally, OSHA has set formal standards for a limited number of chemicals that have been determined to pose substantial threats to workers. (As of 1988, only 24 substances were regulated by OSHA.) Setting standards is an arduous and lengthy task that makes the passage of standards very difficult; therefore, many hazardous substances remain unregulated.

There is great concern in the occupational health community about the lack of specific knowledge about so many chemicals. Although it is known that many chemicals are harmful to humans, the link between exposure and occurrence of disease is ambiguous. One reason is that the disease process is often slow and insidious. Another reason is that many of the diseases that are related to chemical exposure have multifactorial causes. It is next to impossible to identify a single exposure or cause. The problems associated with occupational diseases are discussed in further detail in a later section in this chapter.

Biologic

Biologic hazards result from infection-producing organisms that are found in the workplace. Examples of biologic agents are bacteria, viruses, molds, fungi, and parasites. Biologic hazards vary, depending on the work site. Agricultural workers, for example, are sometimes exposed to fungi-contaminated grain dust, which may cause a hypersensitivity pneumonitis that is commonly known as farmer's lung (Ehlers, Connon, Themann, Myers, & Ballard, 1993); cotton mill workers are susceptible to a fungus disease, coccid-

ioidomycosis; animal trappers may be exposed to rabies, which is a virus; and the bacterium that causes salmonellosis can infect food processing workers (Levy & Wegman, 1988).

It is well documented that health care workers are especially vulnerable to infectious disease (Clever & Omenn, 1988; Levy & Wegman, 1988; Wilkinson et al, 1992). Hospital employees are exposed to staphylococcal and streptococcal infections, hepatitis, tuberculosis, viral infections, and many other infectious diseases. Of recent concern are health care workers' exposure to the human immunodeficiency virus (HIV) that causes acquired immunodeficiency syndrome (AIDS), cytomegalovirus, herpes virus, and scabies. Physicians, nurses, dentists, and laboratory workers are at particularly high risk for viral hepatitis, type B, which probably is the most common and most fatal work-related infectious disease in the United States. It is spread primarily through contact with blood products, often as a result of an accidental puncture with a contaminated needle or other medical instruments. Like hepatitis B, the main source of the HIV virus (for which there is no vaccine), is blood or blood products. Fortunately, an excellent vaccine for the hepatitis B virus is available and should be administered to health care workers who come into contact with blood or blood products. To maximize protection from these and other infectious diseases, the Centers for Disease Control and Prevention (CDCP) developed guidelines for universal precautions among hospital employees. Universal precautions include any precaution a health care worker should take when caring for a client, such as the use of gloves in handling blood or body fluids and adequate hand washing after contact with a client. The difference between universal precautions and the routine precautions nurses take in the course of their work when a known communicable disease is present is that universal precautions are used with all clients regardless of known pathogens because the presence of infectious disease is not always apparent (Barlow & Handeman, 1992). The Bloodborne Pathogens Standard, which was discussed earlier in this chapter, was promulgated by OSHA in 1991 to regulate worker exposure to bloodborne pathogens and to require, among other things, that universal precautions be implemented among all workers who may be exposed to blood or body fluids.

Health care workers represent a substantial portion of the American work force. There has been a particularly rapid growth of these workers in both hospitals and community settings in the last two decades. In the last 10 years much has been written about the many hazards to which workers are exposed. Thus, increasing attention has been given to their health and safety. Guidelines for safe work practices have been established by the American Hospital Association (AHA), by NIOSH, and now by OSHA. There is a continuing need for more research in this area, however, so that compliance with recommendations can be assessed and even more definitive guidelines can be established.

Psychologic

Psychologic hazards are the most difficult to identify because they are the least tangible. They include stress and fatigue, muscular tension, apathy, and depression. Psychologic conditions result from the worker's response to the work environment. Work that depends on meeting deadlines or that conflicts with one's personal values can cause a great deal of stress. Loneliness and boredom have been associated with monotonous tasks. Work sites that have some type of monitoring system may cause workers to feel angry and resentful because of the implication that their integrity is in question. Anger and resentment may result in feelings of alienation, social isolation, and lack of privacy (Karasek & Theorell, 1990). Other conditions that may result in psychologic hazards are shift work, high workload, an unstable work environment (as may be present with corporate takeovers), job rotation, and poor leadership. The emotional energy required in caring for ill people and in meeting the emotional needs of clients and families poses an additional occupational hazard for members of the nursing profession.

Frequently, manifestations of stress are not recognized as being related to the individual's occupation. Family disharmony or marital problems can be a result of poor working conditions. Low self-esteem because of feelings of inadequacy related to the job may lead to self-destructive behaviors such as substance abuse or overeating. Subtle destructive changes in attitudes and behavior that diminish the general quality of life may be an indirect although powerful consequence of an unsatisfactory work environment.

Clearly, occupational stress is a diffuse and complex phenomenon. It is often difficult if not impossible to identify and quantify exposure to stress. It is known, however, that in addition to the psychologic conditions already identified, physical conditions often result from excessive stress. These include coronary disease, hypertension, ulcers, and a variety of nervous conditions. Furthermore, many existing conditions, such as diabetes mellitus and arthritis, may be aggravated by stress. Frequently, studies approach stress from the worker's perspective, and they may suggest that the attitudes and behaviors of the worker must change to decrease stress. A shift of emphasis from the worker to the workplace conditions may, in fact, be more beneficial to the mental health of the employees. Research to identify workplace stressors is an important step toward designing modifications of the workplace so that these stressors can be reduced or eliminated.

Each of these hazards in the work environment can result in a variety of injuries or illnesses. Frequently an overlap exists among the five identified categories; for example, many physical injuries may be by-products of psychologic problems in the workplace. As mentioned in an earlier section, the most commonly reported and recorded health events in the occupational health setting are related to injury. Insidious occupational illnesses generally represent 5% or less of workers' compensation claims received by the Department of Labor and Industries. Obviously, injuries, which account for the other 95%, usually result from an acute episode and are easily identifiable, whereas illnesses are often the result of chronic exposures, and the manifestations are more subtle. Despite the fact that their main mission is to care for others, health care workers are at a particularly high risk for both occupational injury and occupational illness. The box on p. 594 provides an overview of some of the

OCCUPATIONAL HEALTH HAZARDS TO HOSPITAL EMPLOYEES

Physical

Physical hazards have a wide range of causes and effects. Statistics indicate that this category poses the greatest threat to hospital employees, with the most common injuries as follows:

- Puncture wounds from needles and sharps
- Burns and scalds
- Abrasions, lacerations, and contusions
- Hearing loss from overexposure to noise
- Possible genetic damage from exposure to radiation

Ergonomic

An inadequate "fit" between the individual and the work environment is creating an increasing number of hazards for hospital employees. The most common injury in this category is sprain and strain, particularly to the back.

Chemical

The potential for exposure to chemical hazards exists in many parts of the hospital. Chemicals themselves are present in a variety of forms and can manifest toxicity in a number of ways. Among the most common chemicals in the hospital setting are ethylene oxide, anesthetic gases, mercury, and various drugs, detergents, and disinfectants. The most common effect of chemical exposure is a dermatologic reaction. Other potential effects are chromosomal aberration, miscarriages, sterility, and cancer.

Biologic

Biologic hazards are the most obvious and, therefore, the most studied class of hazards to hospital personnel. Among the most common biologic hazards are the following:

- Respiratory viral infections
- Streptococcal, staphylococcal, and enteric infections
- Childhood infections such as rubella, varicella, or mumps
- Hepatitis B or AIDS (rare) via needlestick
- Cytomegalovirus (CMV)
- Tuberculosis

Psychologic

Although stress sometimes is less tangible than other hazards, it is a very real and important factor in the consideration of work-related health problems among hospital employees. The impact of stress can be manifested in a number of ways.

Physiologic manifestations

- Headaches
- Fatigue, muscular tension
- Ulcers
- Coronary heart disease

Psychologic manifestations

- Apathy
- Depression
- Inability to concentrate
- Suicide

occupational health hazards to which hospital employees are exposed.

ROLES AND FUNCTIONS OF THE OCCUPATIONAL HEALTH NURSE

Occupational health nursing is the application of nursing principles to help workers achieve and maintain the highest level of wellness throughout their lives. This specialized practice area is devoted to promoting health in the workplace by preventing employee injury and illness. The emphasis of occupational health is wellness, lifestyle change, and risk reduction, whereas the practice of occupational health nursing involves primary, secondary, and tertiary prevention.

Although the primary focus of occupational health nursing is the worker, the target population also includes the family of the worker, which in many situations is also affected by workplace hazards of the employee. For example, persons who work with lead may bring lead dust home on their clothes, thus exposing their family members to this heavy metal toxin, which could result in the illness of family members as a result of lead poisoning. The consequent effects of this work-related exposure to the family are not likely to be recorded as work-related.

The occupational health nurse has a body of knowledge different from that of other nursing specialists. Special skills required by the OHN include training in safety hazards, disaster planning, familiarity with safety equipment, and accurate and up-to-date knowledge of current legal standards and laws that affect the working population. The OHN has specialized knowledge in the areas of toxicology, epidemiology, occupational health laws, and the environmental sciences.

Occupational health nursing has several other unique features. The OHN often works in isolation from other registered nurses and frequently from other health care personnel. In addition, the OHN frequently is the only health care provider in an organization. Many OHNs create their own jobs and job descriptions. Although they perform according to some set of predetermined guidelines established by the profession itself and by the management of the company, the OHN determines the priorities appropriate to the situation, establishes goals and objectives, and determines the appropriate course of action. In contrast to many other nursing specialties, the focus of occu-

pational health nursing is frequently primary prevention, although secondary and tertiary prevention may also constitute part of the OHN's practice.

A strong relationship between community and occupational health has always existed. Figure 27-2 illustrates how occupational health nursing fits within general nursing practice and community health nursing. Although the OHN's "community" is primarily the workers, she or he also influences the health of the family and the extended community. The OHN serves as a consultant to community health agencies, and some health departments have OHNs on their staff. Ensuring the health of the community frequently requires collaboration among many members of the health community.

Wilkinson (1990) has developed a conceptual model of occupational health nursing (the Wilkinson windmill model), which uses a windmill (Figure 27-3) to describe how occupational health nursing is implemented in the occupational setting. The model has five main components. The core of this windmill is composed of the workers in the organization; the hub represents the OHN; the four blades represent the work environment, the management group in the organization, the other members of the health team, and the occupational health programs. These blades are propelled by the external

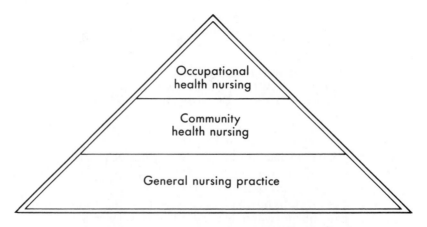

FIGURE 27-2 Relationship among general nursing practice, community health nursing, and occupational health nursing.

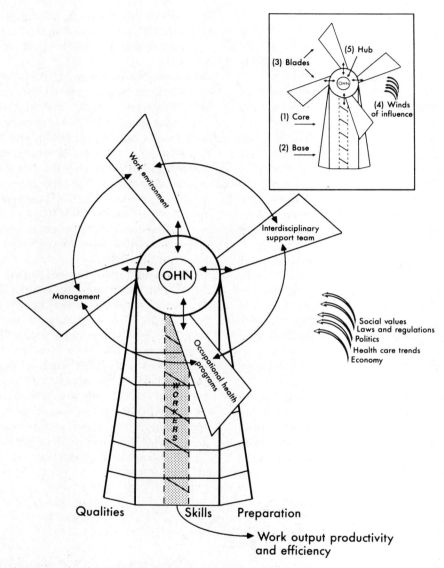

FIGURE 27-3   The Wilkinson model of occupational health nursing. (From "A Conceptual Model of Occupational Health Nursing" by W.E. Wilkinson, 1990, *American Association of Occupational Health Nurses Journal, 38*(2), p. 71. Copyright William E. Wilkinson. Reprinted by permission.)

"winds of influence," which have an impact on the workings of the organization. The winds of influence include social values, laws and regulations, political influences, health care trends, and economic influences. The base of the windmill consists of bricks, which represent the knowl-

edge, the special qualities and skills, and the professional preparation of the OHN.

The roles and functions of the OHN include the duties described in the following section.

Primary care provider. The OHN is a primary care provider for occupational illnesses that are evaluated by means of nursing assessments and diagnoses. This role includes health screening and early detection of disease. The OHN may provide emergency services, preplacement and routine physical examinations, return-to-work assessments, and medical monitoring. Such monitoring includes audiometric testing, vision testing, pulmonary function testing, and any other testing appropriate to specific workplace conditions.

Counselor. The OHN counsels distressed employees and assists in personal and emotional problems. The OHN may be required to provide mental health and crises intervention for employees.

Advocate/liaison. The OHN is frequently a middleman between the employer and management. He or she brings worker problems to the attention of management and works with management to bring about solutions. Although the OHN is hired by management and works for management, his or her primary responsibility is to the employee. The professional objectives of the OHN may be different from those of management.

Manager/administrator. The OHN designs and implements a nursing service within the company that will ensure quality service to the employees. This service requires that the OHN have skills in decision making, problem solving, and independent judgment and communication regarding nursing practices. The OHN often participates in periodic interdisciplinary meetings to coordinate program activities and promote communication. The OHN determines the priorities appropriate to the situation, establishes his or her own goals and objectives, and determines the appropriate course of action.

Teacher/educator. The OHN teaches employees about good health and safety and motivates individuals to improve their health and safety practices. He or she educates the community and the workers about occupational health and safety issues.

Assessor/monitor. The OHN assesses and monitors workers who are exposed to potentially harmful substances or procedures, assesses and monitors the workplace for potential health or safety problems, and develops strategies to minimize the risk to the workers.

Professional member of the health team. The health team in the occupational setting includes the safety manager, the industrial hygienist, and the physician. The OHN collaborates with these members of the health team in exploring ways to promote environmental surveillance, to solve problems, and to advise management about the health and safety needs of the employees.

Researcher. The OHN systematically and continuously collects data concerning the health status of the worker and the real or potential health hazards in the work environment.

The OHN may function in all or only some of the capacities summarized here. The actual job description of any OHN varies, depending on the particular work site. In most smaller industries, the OHN may be the only health professional at the site. Further, the composition of the health team depends on the individual company's perceived and actual need for occupational health services. Because OHNs are revenue saving and not revenue producing, they frequently are required to "prove" their cost effectiveness to convince management that their services are beneficial to the company.

THE OCCUPATIONAL HEALTH HISTORY

It is not unusual for clients' symptoms to be related to workplace exposures. Each health history, therefore, should have an occupational health component. The goal of the U.S. Department of Health and Human Services (1991) is that by the year 2000, at least 75% of primary health care providers should routinely elicit occupational health exposures as part of the client's health history. The **occupational health history** is an excellent means of obtaining information about the possible relationship of an individual's health to workplace conditions. Through the occupational health history, the health care professional may be able to identify actual or potential hazards in the work setting and counsel the client regarding measures that may be taken to minimize any health risk.

In evaluating a health problem, the health care provider should always consider the symptoms in the context of the client's work. At the least, information about each of the following items should be included in the occupational health history: (Levy & Wegman, 1988):

> Description of all jobs held
> Known work exposures and protection from them
> Nonwork environmental exposures
> Presence of symptoms and relation to work
> Patterns of symptoms or illnesses among other workers

The occupational health history can be used at four levels. The basic level identifies the employee's current occupation and the possible health implications; for example, how a diagnosis of laryngitis may affect a teacher's return to work. At the diagnostic level there is an investigation of the possible link between the client's job and a current illness. For example, an occupational health nurse might question if a warehouse worker's back pain is caused by lifting heavy items at the work site. At the next level a client is regularly evaluated for the occurrence of symptoms related to known workplace exposures; for example, employees exposed to a high noise level will be given a regular hearing test. Finally, on the comprehensive level, occupational health history is used for the investigation of complex medical problems. Researchers might explore the possible relationship between the work environment and a client's diagnosis of bladder cancer (Occupational and Environmental Health Committee, 1983).

It is not unusual for the occupational health history to be entirely omitted from a health history. However, few clinicians would omit information about the client's family history. Because the client may spend one third of a lifetime in the job setting, the health implications of occupational exposures cannot be overlooked. The relationship between many chronic conditions and exposures at the workplace is becoming increasingly apparent, but all too often this connection is missed by the health professional. Although physical findings and laboratory tests may raise suspicions that a condition is occupationally re-

lated, it is the occupational health history that ultimately will prove the work relatedness of a medical problem. Figure 27-4 provides an example of a form that can be used to obtain an employee's health history, and Figure 27-5 shows an acute episode form for use when a single incident occurs at the work site. These both show how an occupational health history can furnish a health care provider with invaluable information.

OCCUPATIONAL DISEASE: DIFFICULTIES IN DETERMINATION

Traditionally, occupational health programs have emphasized the prevention of injury, with little or no concern about the prevention of occupational disease. As was pointed out in the section on the occupational health history, it is vitally important that clinicians be aware of the possible relationships between workplace exposures and the occurrence of disease. Four primary reasons are responsible for this missed relationship:

1. The lag time between exposure to an agent and the onset of symptoms
2. The multifactorial origin of many diseases
3. The additive effect of some workplace conditions in conjunction with other exposures or lifestyle behaviors
4. Difficulty in evaluating the contributing role of the workplace

In addition, problems are often inherent in the reporting systems. Frequently, employers, health care providers, or even the employees themselves fail to recognize the occupational relationship of a disease. Many primary care physicians have inadequate training in occupational medicine. Further, an effort to restrict the cost of workers' compensation may lead to a failure to connect a disease with conditions in the workplace.

Although more and more data are being accumulated that demonstrate the relationship between occupational exposures and human diseases, studies are still sparse and inconclusive. An important defense against the occurrence of occupational illness is continued epidemiologic re-

Text continues on p. 602.

Date:_____

Interviewer:_____

EMPLOYEE HEALTH HISTORY

Name:_____ Sex: M ☐ F ☐

Address:_____

Phone: (Home)_____ (Work)_____

SS Number:_____ Occupation:_____

Marital status: S ☐ M ☐ D ☐ W ☐ Date of birth:_____ Race:_____

Allergies: Y ☐ N ☐ If yes, describe:_____

Physician's name:_____

        Address:_____

Date of last physical exam:_____

In case of emergency, please contact:_____

        Address:_____ Phone:_____

MEDICAL HISTORY

A. Hospitalizations (date, surgeries, illnesses, accidents, etc.):_____

_____

B. Past illnesses:_____

C. Current state of health:_____

D. Current medications (name and dose if known):_____

_____

FAMILY HISTORY

Describe any hereditary illnesses among parents or siblings:_____

_____

_____

FIGURE 27-4 Employee health history form.

HEALTH HABITS (do you use the following?)

A. Tobacco? Y ☐ N ☐ Type_____ Amt/day_____

B. Alcohol? Y ☐ N ☐ Type_____ Amt/day_____

C. Caffeine? Y ☐ N ☐ Type_____ Amt/day_____

D. Sleep pattern_____ Amt/24 hours_____

OCCUPATIONAL HISTORY

Job title:_____

Description of duties:_____

Date of hire:_____ How long in current position?_____

A. Do you feel that there are any health risks or hazards associated with your job?   Y ☐ N ☐

If yes, please describe (include symptoms): _____

B. Do you wear protective equipment on the job? Y ☐ N ☐ If yes, please indicate which of

the following: ☐ Gloves ☐ Coveralls/apron ☐ Safety glasses ☐ Mask ☐Respirator

☐ Hearing protection ☐ Other:_____

C. In the past, have you ever experienced an illness or an injury that you think may have

related to your job? Y ☐ N ☐ If yes, please describe:_____

_____

ENVIRONMENTAL HISTORY

A. Have you ever been required to change your residence because
of health problems? Y ☐ N ☐

B. Do you have a hobby or craft that may expose you to chemicals, metals, or other substances?

Y ☐ N ☐ Describe:_____

C. Do you live near any type of industrial plant? Y ☐ N ☐

D. Does your spouse or any other member of your household have contact with dusts or
chemicals at work or during leisure activities? Y ☐ N ☐

E. Do you use pesticides around your home or garden? Y ☐ N ☐

F. Are there any other work, recreational, or domestic exposures that you feel are potentially
hazardous? Y ☐ N ☐ If yes, please describe:_____

_____

FIG. 27-4, cont'd.

Date: _____

Interviewer: _____

ACUTE EPISODE FORM

Name: _____ Sex: M ☐ F ☐

Address: _____

Phone: (Home) _____ (Work) _____

SS Number: _____ Department: _____

Reason for visit (include complete description of symptoms): _____

_____

Date of onset of symptoms: _____

Have these symptoms occurred in the past? Y ☐ N ☐ If yes, describe circumstances: _____

_____

How long have you worked in your current position? _____

Do you feel that your job duties contributed to your symptoms? Y ☐ N ☐

If yes, describe: _____

If you use any protective equipment, does it fit and work properly? Y ☐ N ☐

If no, explain: _____

Are there any other employees in your department experiencing similar symptoms? Y ☐ N ☐

If yes, please describe as completely as possible: _____

_____

Have there been any changes in your work environment in the last year? Yes ☐ No ☐

If yes, please explain when the changes occurred and what they were: _____

_____

Does your condition change when you are away from the work site? Y ☐ N ☐ How? _____

_____

Any other comments? _____

FIGURE 27-5 Acute episode form.

search that explores the relationship of illnesses to exposures and conditions in the work environment. On the basis of resultant findings, work sites can be altered to decrease the risks to the employee. In addition, health care professionals need to be taught to recognize occupational disease. Again, the occupational health history is an invaluable tool that allows primary care providers to make the connection between the disease process and the client's occupational exposures.

THE NURSING PROCESS IN THE OCCUPATIONAL SETTING

The occupational community, in contrast with many other communities of interest to the health professional, consists of an essentially well population. The primary objective of occupational health nursing is to maintain and enhance the health of the workers and to prevent injury and illness that could occur as a result of occupational exposures. The community health nursing process described in Chapter 3 provides an excellent framework for accomplishing this objective. The case study below illustrates how this nursing process might be used in the occupational setting.

OCCUPATIONAL SAFETY AND HEALTH PROGRAMS

Phenomenal growth has occurred in occupational health and safety programs in the last two decades, partly as a result of a national movement toward primary and secondary prevention. This trend is reflected by the publication of the surgeon general's reports, Healthy People (U.S. DHHS, 1979), Promoting Health/Preventing Disease: Objectives for the Nation (U.S. DHHS,

■ CASE STUDY

Earl is the chief occupational health nurse for a busy telephone company. It is a typical Friday morning in the health unit. Earl is reviewing the health unit logs for the past month. These logs summarize all employee visits to the health unit, including the reason for the visit and the action taken. A certain pattern over this last month captures Earl's attention. He notices that eight employees from the North office have visited the health unit complaining of a headache during this period. Some of them visited the unit twice. Earl checks the previous month's log and notes that there were five similar visits during that month. A further check reveals that during the two previous months, there were no visits. Earl decides that a thorough investigation of the situation is warranted. He calls the administrator of the North office to tell him that he will visit that building early this afternoon.

Assessment

For the assessment phase of the community health nursing process, Earl will perform the following actions:

1. Review the charts of the employees who visited the health unit with the complaint of a headache to determine the exact job responsibilities of the employee and to obtain a more detailed description of the visit.
2. Interview the administrator of the North office to determine if there have been any changes in office equipment, procedures, or other during the last 2 months.
3. Walk around the work environment to identify any potential risk factors.
4. Interview a sampling of the employees with headache to determine if the symptoms persist.
5. Interview employees who work in the same environment who did not visit the health unit to determine if any of them had similar symptoms.
6. Confer with the industrial hygienist, occupational physician, and safety manager to determine if they have any information to contribute to Earl's assessment.

Through this assessment the following facts were revealed. In addition to the headache, several of the employees complained of blurred vision. This office building, which is only 6 months old, has no windows that open and it faces the afternoon sun. A check with the building engineer indicates that no ventilation problems have been identified. The entire office was equipped with new video display terminals (VDTs) a little more than 2 months ago. The employees who visited the health unit continue to have the headaches and occasional blurred vision, but they have managed to keep them at a tolerable level through the use of over-the-counter analgesics such as acetaminophen or aspirin. It was discovered that several employees with similar symptoms had not reported them to the health unit. In all cases the headaches are less pronounced or disappear altogether on the weekends. All affected employees are regular VDT users and work on the west side of the building near the windows. The employees generally agreed that their work is fast paced and relatively demanding.

Nursing diagnosis

The community health nurse considers the following three components: the health problem, the population characteristics, and the environmental characteristics. In this case the health problem is the regular occurrence of headache and blurred vision during the working week. The population consists of adult persons who are otherwise healthy and who spend more than half their workday using VDTs. The environment in which the health problem occurs is on the west side of the North office, near a bank of windows that cannot be opened. In addition, it was determined that although this area has sufficient lighting for general work, glares on the VDT screen and otherwise inadequate lighting make close work and the reading of the screen difficult. In view of these findings, Earl makes the following diagnosis: risk of decreased quality of work life, decreased productivity, and lowered employee morale among VDT operators in the North office of the Ring-a-Ding Telephone Company related to the regular use of VDT equipment, inadequate lighting and screen glare, and a fast-paced work environment, as demonstrated by the regular occurrence of headaches and blurred vision. Earl considers that the symptoms may be related to the physical environment or to stress that results from the demands of this job.

Planning and implementation

Earl's primary goal for this population is to decrease the occurrence of headache and blurred vision through the alteration of the environment. He discusses his findings and his diagnosis with the administrator in the North office and the safety engineer, and together they plan appropriate strategies to address the identified problems. As a result of this meeting, the following changes were implemented:

1. Antiglare screens were purchased for all VDT operators.
2. The lighting system was assessed and revised so that close work and screen reading could be accomplished without eye strain.
3. All VDT operators were encouraged to break up their work day so that they never spent more than 1 hour at the screen during a single sitting.
4. Shades were placed on the windows to prevent direct sunlight from entering the west section of the building.
5. A stress management class was developed and offered to all employees in this office. The administrator, recognizing the significance of the problem, agreed to allow employees to participate in the class during work hours.

Evaluation

Earl will carefully monitor this population to determine if there is a decrease of symptoms as a result of the changes that were made. He will not rely on health unit visits. He will make periodic visits to the North office so that he can interview the employees, particularly those who work on the west side of the building. He will ask the administrator to inform him if he becomes aware of any other complaints.

1980), and Healthy People 2000 (U.S. DHHS, 1991). In addition, the passage of the Occupational Safety and Health Act in 1970 focused attention on the need to improve the health and safety of the working population in this country.

Because of the great variation of work sites and the diversity of jobs, the potential hazards and the type of programs are also considerably varied. Safety and health programs in the occupational setting can be broadly divided into two categories: those that focus on occupational safety and health issues and those that focus on health promotion outside the workplace. The first group of programs includes safety education, health surveillance such as hearing-conservation training in handling materials, and communication about hazards. The programs include, of course, treatment of occupational injuries and illnesses. Programs that are not occupationally related may or may not be a part of a company's total health program. In addition to treatment of injuries or illnesses unrelated to the work site, programs can include a variety of health promotion activities, such as hypertension screening and follow-up, cancer screening and education, cholesterol screening, smoking cessation, automobile safety, and substance abuse programs. The purposes of any safety and health program are to provide a safe and healthy work environment and to promote the personal health behaviors of employees so they can help to maintain a healthy and productive work force.

Occupational health programs generally include preventive health care and health maintenance. Professional services that may be included in a comprehensive program are preplacement examinations, medical surveillance, treatment of occupational injuries and illnesses, consultation services, and in some cases primary care (DiBenedetto et al, 1993). Health and safety programs at the work site can make a significant contribution to the overall health of the adult population of this country. In addition to the direct health effects, these programs often result in increased job performance and job satisfaction of workers. Studies have indicated that well-planned health and safety programs increase productivity and decrease absenteeism and turnover among employees. Ongoing research in this area will assist occupational health providers in developing effective and efficient programs that will provide the maximum benefit to the working population.

Chapter Highlights

- Occupational health nurses have worked in industrial settings in the United States and Europe for more than 100 years and have made many valuable contributions to the health of workers.

- Educational resource centers, of which there are 14 in the continental United States, provide education and research in the field of occupational health nursing.

- The actual number of illnesses and injuries with occupational causes is difficult to estimate because many do not come to the attention of occupational health professionals or are not recognized as work related. An occupational injury is an injury that results from an acute episode and is usually easily identifiable in cause and effect.

- An occupational illness is an abnormal condition or disorder caused by exposure to environmental factors associated with employment.

- In many cases occupational injury and illness are preventable. Governmental involvement in improving safety in the workplace includes the passage of the Occupational Safety and Health Act and the establishment of the Occupational Safety and Health Administration and the National Institute of Occupational Safety and Health.

- Most hazards that occur in the workplace may be classified as physical, ergonomic, chemical, biologic, or psychologic.

- Health care workers, who represent a large portion of the work force, are particularly vulnerable to occupational illness as a result of exposure to infectious diseases.

- The OHN, whose focus tends to be on primary prevention, is frequently the only health professional in the work setting.

- The roles and functions of the occupational health nurse include primary care provider, counselor, advocate/liaison, manager/administrator, teacher/educator, assessor/monitor, professional member of the health team, and researcher.

- All health care providers should include an occupational health component as part of a general health history by obtaining information such as the following: a description of all jobs held, known work exposures and protection from them, environmental exposures unrelated to the workplace, the presence of symptoms and their relation to work, and patterns of symptoms or illnesses among other workers.

- Occupational illnesses are often difficult to diagnose because the cause and effect may not be closely related.

- As a result of a national movement toward primary and secondary prevention, the number of occupational health and safety programs has grown dramatically.

- Occupational health and safety programs can contribute greatly to the general health of the adult population, and increase job satisfaction and productivity.

 CRITICAL THINKING EXERCISE

A large construction company has had an increase in injuries reported and an increase in musculoskeletal problems among the workers. Work has slowed and the cost of liability insurance has risen. OSHA has sent an occupational health nurse as a consultant to help the company correct their problems. The company is attempting to build a large office building in Nome, Alaska. The season is summer, and the company has scheduled work shifts around the clock because of the 24 hours of daylight available to them. Most of the managers have been brought from the home company in Ohio. Laborers have been recruited from a nearby town where many of the Eskimo residents are willing to work for minimum wage. They are willing workers, but unskilled. They need much direction.

1. Using the Wilkinson windmill model, list some of the things that may be causing trouble for the company.
2. The occupational health nurse sent by OSHA is the only health professional on the site. What should he/she suggest to the company management with respect to accident prevention and musculoskeletal injury?

REFERENCES

Anfield, R.N. (1992). Americans with Disabilities Act of 1990: A primer of Title I provisions for occupational health care professionals. *Journal of Occupational Medicine, 34*(5), 503-509.

Barlow, R., & Handeman, E. (1992). OSHA's final bloodborne pathogens standard: Part I. *American Association of Occupational Health Nurses Journal, 40*(12), 562-567.

Becker, C.E., & Rosenberg, J. (1990). Clinical toxicology. In J. LaDou (Ed.), *Occupational medicine.* Norwalk, Connecticut: Appleton and Lange.

Clever, L.H., & Omenn, G.S. (1988). Hazards for health care workers: *Annual Review of Public Health, 9,* 273-303.

Cross, L.L. (1993). Americans with Disabilities Act: Meeting the requirements. *American Association of Occupational Health Nurses Journal, 40*(6), 284-286.

DiBenedetto, D.V., Harris, J.S., & McCunney, R.J. (1993). *Occupational health and safety manual.* Boston: OEM Press.

Ehlers, J.K., Connon, C., Themann, C.L., Myers, J.R., & Ballard, T. (1993). Health and safety hazards associated with farming. *American Association of Occupational Health Nurses Journal, 41*(9), 414-421.

Fingar, A.R., Hopkins, R.S., & Nelson, M. (1992). Work-related injuries in Athens County 1982 to 1986: A comparison of emergency department and workers' compensation data. *Journal of Occupational Medicine, 34*(8), 779-787.

Frederick, L. (1984). An introduction to the principles of occupational ergonomics. *Occupational Health Nursing, 32*(12), 643-645.

Karasek, R., & Theorell, T. (1990). *Health work: Stress, produc-*

tivity, and reconstruction of working life. New York: Basic Books, Inc.

Kowalke, E. (1930). Industrial nursing service provided by public health nursing association. *The Public Health Nurse, 22,* 615-617.

Levy, B.S., & Wegman, D.H. (1988). *Occupational health: Recognizing and preventing work-related disease.* Boston: Little, Brown & Co.

McCunney, R.J. (1988). *Handbook of occupational medicine.* Boston: Little, Brown & Co.

Occupational and Environmental Health Committee. (1983). Taking the occupational history. *Annals of Internal Medicine, 99,* 641-651.

Omenn, G.S. (1986). A framework for risk assessment for environmental chemicals. *Washington Public Health, 6*(Summer), 2-6.

Pravikoff, D.S., & Simonowitz, J.A. (1994). Cumulative trauma disorders: Developing a framework for prevention. *American Association of Occupational Health Nurses Journal, 42*(4), 164-170.

Rogers, B. (1988). Perspectives in occupational health nursing. *American Association of Occupational Health Nurses Journal, 36*(4), 151-155.

Rudolph, L., & Forest, C.S. (1990). Female reproductive toxicology. In J. LaDou (Ed.), *Occupational medicine.* Norwalk, Connecticut: Appleton and Lange.

U.S. Department of Health and Human Services. (1991). *Healthy people: National health promotion and disease prevention objectives* (DHHS Publication No. 91-50212). Washington, DC: U.S. Government Printing Office.

U.S. Department of Health and Human Services. (1992). *NIOSH: Health hazard evaluation program.* (DHHS Publication No. 648-004/40829). Washington, DC: U.S. Government Printing Office.

U.S. Department of Health, Education, and Welfare. (1979). *Healthy people: The Surgeon General's report on health promotion and disease prevention.* (PHS Publication No. 79-55071). Washington, DC: U.S. Government Printing Office.

U.S. Department of Health, Education, and Welfare. (1980). *Preventing disease/promoting health: Objectives for the nation.* (DHHS Publication No. 1980-640-185.3679). Washington, DC: U.S. Government Printing Office.

U.S. Department of Labor/OSHA. (1991). *Occupational exposure to bloodborne pathogens: Final rule.* (Federal Register, 56(235),64004-64182; Docket No. H-370). Washington, DC: U.S. Government Printing Office.

U.S. Department of Labor. (1993). *Occupational injuries and illnesses in the United States by industry, 1991.* (Bureau of Labor Statistics Bulletin 2424). Washington, DC: U.S. Government Printing Office.

Weeks, J.L., Levy, B.S., & Wegman, G.R. (1991). *Preventing occupational disease and injury.* Washington, DC: American Public Health Association.

Wilkinson, W.E., Salazar, M.K., Uhl, J.E., Koepsell, T.D., DeRoos, R.L., & Long, R.J. (1992). *Occupational injuries: A study of health care workers at a Northwestern Health Science Center and teaching hospital. American Association of Occupational Health Nurses Journal, 40*(6), 287-293.

Wilkinson, W.E. (1990). A conceptual model of occupational health nursing. *American Association of Occupational Health Nurses Journal, 38*(2), 71-75.

Wilkinson, W.E. (1994). Therapeutic jurisprudence and workers' compensation. *Arizona Attorney,* March, 1994.

Wright, W.C. (1993). *Diseases of Workers* (B. Ramizzini, Trans.). Thunder Bay, Canada: OH&S Press. (Original work published 1713).

Yorker, B. (1993). Occupational safety and health reform: An interview with Patrick Tyson. *American Association of Occupational Health Nurses Journal, 41*(8), 396-410.

SCHOOL HEALTH NURSING

Mary Rea

He who has health has hope; and he who has hope, has everything.

Arabian Proverb

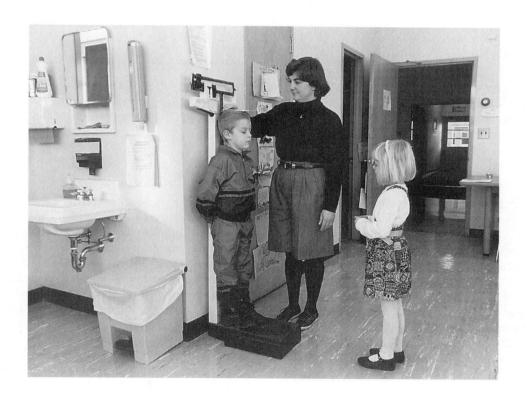

OBJECTIVES

At the conclusion of this chapter the student will be able to:

1. Define the key terms listed.
2. Discuss the historical and current role and functions of the school nurse.
3. Identify key areas of health promotion and education.
4. Identify factors influencing nursing interventions for implementation in relation to the needs of a specific school population.
5. Identify primary, secondary, and tertiary levels of prevention within the school community.

KEY TERMS

Accepting environment
Child advocacy
Health education
Individual Education Plan (IEP)

Individual Placement and Review
    Committee (IPRC)
Immunization programs
Needs assessment

School nursing
Suicide prevention programs
Substance abuse programs

A child who is at an optimal level of health is able to learn. Learning will foster opportunities, hopes, and the fulfillment of dreams. The school nurse helps to promote the highest level of wellness for children in the school setting. Comprehensive school health services are being developed to assist in meeting the needs of each community's population of children. Intervention at primary, secondary, and tertiary prevention levels are incorporated through collaboration with a diverse group of educational personnel and health care providers in the community who have fewer financial resources (Nader, 1990; Sullivan & Bogden, 1993). The school nurse can be a central person in coordinating services.

According to the American Association of Nurses (1990), "the purpose of **school nursing** is to enhance the educational process by the modification or removal of health-related barriers to learning by promotion of an optimal level of vellness." School health programs promote

health by focusing on prevention, early identification and intervention, providing first aid, counselling, health instruction, and dealing with the needs of physically and developmentally challenged students (Allensworth & Kolbe, 1987). Nursing interventions involve preventing disease, lowering the risks of acute or chronic health conditions, minimizing the effects of health problems, and preparing children and youth to make decisions and act in ways that positively affect their future health.

The health of our youth is a continuously changing challenge. Social, cultural, and economic factors, geographic location, technological advances, and the level of education of parents, all have contributed to this change. Many children live in poverty and do not have access to health care services. These elements have necessitated the expansion of both health services and the nurse's role in the school and have led to a maturation of the role (Thurber, Berry, Cameron, 1991).

HISTORICAL PERSPECTIVE

Mandatory school attendance at the end of the 19th century contributed to an increase of communicable diseases. Health care programs stressed hygiene, communicable disease control, and assessment for identification of signs of disease or abnormal health (Smith, Redican, & Olsen, 1992). The first school health services were medical inspections that took place in Boston schools in 1894. The purpose of these inspections was to identify children with communicable diseases such as scarlet fever, diphtheria, pertussis, chickenpox, and mumps, and eventually parasitic diseases including scabies, impetigo, and ringworm (Wold, 1981). No follow-up was provided, and children were excluded from school sometimes longer than was necessary. Deaths occurred as a result of communicable diseases, which had an impact on intervention.

Lillian Wald and Mary Brewster introduced the concept of what is known as Public Health Nursing, in the late 1800's (see Chapter 1). Their methods included advocating for public policy change to improve health education and public health standards. Wald viewed education as an important aspect of public health nursing. The first nurses involved with children and schools were public health nurses (Thurber, Berry, & Cameron, 1991). Lina Rogers Struthers was appointed to serve four schools in New York City in 1902. Her involvement with families of sick children included teaching them how to prevent further illness and decrease school absences. Positive outcomes of her intervention led to the hiring of 25 more nurses by the school board in New York City (Wold, 1981).

Education about communicable diseases, health examinations, and immunization of children were key components of intervention by public health nurses. Identification of physical problems and providing home follow-up demonstrated a broader approach to correct, for example, poor vision or difficulty hearing. Finally, nurses were hired to work primarily in the schools. Disease prevention was the primary focus rather than wellness maintenance. First aid and record keeping were other aspects of the role of the school nurse (Wold, 1981).

The role of the school nurse expanded in the 1930's, which caused school nurses to be overextended and to face divided allegiance to health in the schools and health education. Delegation of health service tasks to teachers allowed nurses to redirect their time. As resources became more available in the 1950's and 1960's, counselling, coordination of community services, and assessment of the environment became responsibilities of the school nurse (White, 1985; Wold, 1981). Role confusion became more apparent as other professionals such as social workers and psychologists, who also addressed psychosocial and health needs, became involved.

By the 1970's the position of the school nurse was unclear. On one hand nurses were encouraged to expand their roles, improve educational preparation, and increase community involvement. At the same time budgetary cutbacks caused loss of job security, role confusion, and role reduction. The needs of students were changing, thereby requiring a change in priorities. Lack of tangible outcomes and outcomes that were primarily long range, led to elimination of school nurse positions and the hiring of health clerks and aides, who were nonprofessionals. This meant that addressing total health needs of the child was limited and fragmented. (Wold, 1981). This fragmented care marked the beginning of the need for school nurses who could develop child-focused outcomes, and the need for these nurses to demonstrate accountability and value of their contributions.

CURRENT ISSUES

School nurses have played a significant part in school health programs. They need to be flexible, creative, and involved in revising their role to fit with new directions; otherwise, the role of the school nurse may be jeopardized. Economic justification for services is necessary and therefore, the value of the school nurse must be ascertained (Kozlak, 1992).

Historically the issue of responsibility has not been resolved between the departments of health and education. (Hill-White & Christansen, 1987). An interactive relationship has occurred, which has caused much inconsistency in the continuity of administering mandated programs and services. Administration of the program by non–health-care administrators or by health care administrators out of the school system, poses a set of problems that affect how services provided by the school nurse are offered (Hill-White & Christansen, 1987). Since the presence of a school nurse is not mandatory, the quality and quantity of the service are not legislated. As a result, the tasks of determining appropriate services and qualifications of school nurses and evaluating performance are often at the discretion of school district administrators.

National health objectives for the year 2000 seek to increase school-based education to prevent human immunodeficiency virus (HIV) infection, alcohol and other drug use, tobacco use, injury, and sexually transmitted diseases. The objectives also advocate changes to promote an increase in education regarding nutrition, human sexuality, and nonviolent conflict resolution. Expansion of immunization laws for schools, and reducing the risks for multiple problem behaviors and poor mental health have also been included in identified priorities for the direction of health care (United States Department of Health and Human Services [U.S. DHHS], 1991). The school nurse can play a significant role in the creation expansion of existing services. Health education plays a significant role in each of the health objectives for the year 2000 (see box on page 611).

Health education has proven to be effective at reducing risk behaviors associated with the leading causes of death; that is, heart diseases, cancer, stroke, chronic obstructive pulmonary diseases, unintentional injuries, pneumonia and flu, diabetes mellitus, suicide, acquired immunodeficiency syndrome (AIDS), and homicide. The school nurse can continue to contribute valuable knowledge and skills in an attempt to meet the objectives relating to school health. Responsibility needs to be a fundamental component of health care reform. This means sharing of responsibility by the health care system, schools, and the community. Prevention includes health education, which in turn helps to create supportive environments for healthy lifestyle choices (Jorgensen, 1994).

Nursing will be directly affected by the outcome of health care reform. Nurses need to network with other professionals involved in school health programs to become better informed about successful models of care for school children. Becoming involved at a policy level and exploring funding sources will help to strengthen support for school health programs. Investing in children is a cost-effective means of promoting well-being. School-based clinics may be one method of reaching more children who presently do not have access to health care because of economic circumstances (Baker, 1994).

EDUCATIONAL PREPARATION AND CLASSIFICATION

Educational preparation of the school nurse ranges from the associate degree or diploma-prepared nurse to a nurse who holds a master's degree. School nurses can be classified into the following three categories: 1) the nurse with generic nursing education; 2) the licensed registered nurse; or 3) the licensed practical nurse. The noncertified nurse is required only to have state licensure as a registered nurse. The second category includes nurses who have obtained additional education in school health or a related field at a master's level and are granted certification to practice in schools by the state. In the state of New York, for example, the school nurse as defined by the Department of Education is a certified School Nurse Teacher (SNT). These nurses generally have focused their continuing education on counseling or health education. The third category of nurses is school nurse practitioners who have completed continuing education programs of varying length. They may also be certified by the American Nurses' Association. These nurses receive their education from schools of nursing and focus on clinical nursing skills such as assessment and management of children's health. Certified nurses' responsibilities include the mandated services along with counseling and classroom teaching activities. No uniform practice expectations exist other than mandated screening for vision, hearing, and scoliosis, and first aid intervention.

In Canada, school nurses are hired by public health units or departments and have a minimum of a baccalaureate degree. Some diploma-pre-

NATIONAL HEALTH OBJECTIVES FOR THE YEAR 2000 RELATED TO SCHOOL HEALTH

1.8 Increase to at least 50% the proportion of children and adolescents in first through twelfth grade who participate in daily school physical education.

1.9 Increase to at least 50% the portion of school physical education class time that students spend being physically active, preferably in lifetime physical activities.

2.17 Increase to at least 90% the proportion of school lunch and breakfast services and child care food services with menus that are consistent with the nutrition principles in the *Dietary Guidelines for Americans.*

2.19 Increase to at least 75% the proportion of the nation's schools that provide nutrition education from preschool through twelfth grade, preferably as part of quality school health education.

3.10 Establish tobacco-free environments and include tobacco-use prevention in the curricula of all elementary, middle, and secondary schools, preferably as part of quality school health education.

4.13 Provide to children in all school districts and private schools primary- and secondary-school educational programs on alcohol and other drugs, preferably as part of quality school health education.

5.8 Increase to at least 85% the proportion of people ages 10 through 18 who have discussed human sexuality, including values surrounding sexuality, with their parents, and/or received information through other parentally endorsed sources, such as school and religious or youth programs.

7.16 Increase to at least 50% the proportion of elementary and secondary schools that teach nonviolent conflict resolution skills, preferably as part of quality school health education.

8.2 Increase the high school graduation rate to at least 90%, thereby reducing risks for multiple problem behaviors and poor mental and physical health.

8.4 Increase to at least 75% the proportion of the nation's elementary and secondary schools that provide planned and sequential quality school health education from kindergarten through twelfth grade.

9.18 Provide academic instruction on injury prevention and control, preferably as part of quality school health education, in at least 50% of public school systems (grades K through 12).

13.12 Increase to at least 90% the proportion of all children entering school programs for the first time who have received an oral health screening, referral, and follow-up for necessary diagnostic, preventive, and treatment services.

18.10 Increase to at least 95% the proportion of schools that have age-appropriate HIV education curricula for students in fourth through twelfth grade, preferably as part of quality school health education.

19.12 Include instruction in preventing transmission of sexually transmitted diseases in the curricula of all middle and secondary schools, preferably as part of quality school health education.

20.13 Expand immunization laws for schools, preschools, and day care settings to all states for all antigens.

From *Healthy people 2000: National health promotion and disease prevention objectives: Full report, with commentary* (DHHS Publication No. [PHS] 91-50212), by U.S. DHHS, 1991, Washington, DC: U.S. Government Printing Office.

pared nurses have obtained community health qualifications through continuing education programs from a college or university. It is not uncommon for health units to employ a small number of registered nurses without university nursing qualifications to provide immunization, hearing, and vision screening programs.

The American Nurses' Association, the Colleges of Nurses in Canada, and the professional nursing associations have developed philosophies and standards of practice for community nurses that would be applicable to nurses practicing in the school setting. (See box on page 612.)

STANDARDS OF SCHOOL NURSING PRACTICE

Standard I: theory

The school nurse applies appropriate theory as basis for decision making in nursing practice.

Standard II: program management

The school nurse establishes and maintains a comprehensive school health program.

Standard III: nursing process

The nursing process includes individualized health plans, which are developed by the school nurse.

Standard IV: interdisciplinary collaboration

The school nurse collaborates with other professionals in assessing, planning, implementing, and evaluating programs and other school health activities.

Standard V: health education

The nurse assists students, families, and groups to achieve optimal levels of wellness through health education.

Standard VI: professional development

The school nurse participates in peer review and other means of evaluation to assure quality of nursing care provided for students. The nurse assumes responsibility for continuing education and professional development and contributes to the professional growth of others.

Standard VII: community health systems

The school nurse participates with other key members of the community who are responsible for assessing, planning, implementing, and evaluating school health services and community services that include the broad continuum of promotion of primary, secondary, and tertiary prevention.

Standard VIII: research

The school nurse contributes to nursing and school health through innovations in theory and practice and participation in research.

From *Standards of School Nursing Practice,* by American Nurses Association, Washington, DC: Author. Copyright 1983 by American Nurses' Association. Reprinted by permission.

OUTLINES AND STANDARDS DEVELOPED BY THE AMERICAN NURSES' ASSOCIATION

School nurses need a range of knowledge and skills to provide essential services. Health assessment skills are an important requirement. The school nurse is having to recognize and intervene when children present with minor ailments, offer counseling and guidance, detect potential health-related problems, make appropriate medical referrals, and act as an extension for other involved medical services. School nurses must sharpen their diagnostic and technical skills because more students are coming to school with complex physical and medical health problems. Up-to-date information about services available within the catchment area must be maintained. Therefore, ongoing education is essential.

To function as a school nurse, prioritizing, ordering, delegating, planning, and evaluating are necessary skills. Management of information is a basic necessity, and computerization of student records is the direction for the future. If the school nurse is to be an integral part of the future health care system within the school system, it will be an asset to have the knowledge and skills in computer literacy, information systems, leadership, administrative theories, and models (Oda, 1992). There are a variety of programs in both Canada and the United States that offer continuing education and certification courses for additional skill development and for this specialized area of nursing.

ROLE AND FUNCTIONS OF THE SCHOOL NURSE

In essence the role of the school nurse encompasses a number of different responsibilities relative to the school environment. This role depends on time the nurse spends at school and with administrative requirements. Being visible and establishing relationships with pupils and teachers will enhance appropriate use of services offered. The box on p. 613 identifies the

RANGE OF ACTIVITIES IN WHICH A SCHOOL NURSE MAY BE INVOLVED

Physical care

Emergency/first aid
Health appraisal; assessing health complaints
Developmental assessment
Providing treatment such as tracheostomy care
Assisting in screening programs
Obtaining health history
Communicable disease control
Dispensing of routine medicine

Psychosocial care

Counseling individual students
Obtaining social/emotional history
Crisis management
Leading support groups

Facilitative actions

Referring to other resources
Coordinating services, such as those for physically and developmentally challenged students
Home visits/counseling parents
Follow-up for attendance problems
Participating on school teams (health, placement)
Consulting physicians
Participating in development of IEPs (Individualized education programs)

Teaching/instructive

Health promotion programs; program development
Teaching classes
Inservice programs for teachers
Resource to educational staff, students, parents

Administrative

Health coordination related activities; records
Organizing screening programs
Environmental safety assessment
Policy development
Program evaluation
Budget preparation and justification
Research, such as evaluating health service effectiveness
Peer evaluation

range of activities carried out by the school nurse. Services provided by the school nurse include health promotion, health surveillance, direct care, information resource, case management, administration, and research.

Health Promotion

As a health educator, the school nurse must be an expert on matters of health in school settings, and must be able to transfer knowledge and skills to facilitate the education process. Health promotion includes education that occurs informally at opportunistic times, on a one-to-one basis, with groups, in the form of organized classroom instruction, and through visual displays. The nurse, along with school personnel, should do a **needs assessment** to determine appropriate health promotion programs. This assessment includes identifying high-risk groups of children.

Lifestyle behaviors and attitudes are most susceptible to influence during childhood. Developmentally specific curricula that build on existing knowledge and current topics need to begin as early as kindergarten. Health promotion intervention is most effectively offered at school because the school is the most efficient point of access to large numbers of children, and school exerts a profound influence on children becoming part of a society. Early intervention will yield high returns in terms of improved health (Bartfay, 1994).

Socioeconomic variables have been linked to the use of health services (Stephenson, 1983). Children raised by parents who have not accessed the health care system because of financial limitations or as a result of attitudes, may adapt the same patterns and behaviors modelled in their home environments. The school nurse identifies the behavior patterns of the children of a particular school environment and defines problem areas that need to be addressed (Stephenson, 1983). Optimal health is the highest level of functioning that an individual is capable of attaining within the limitations of his or her internal or external environment. The external environment includes the physical surroundings and the internal environment includes the individual's physical, mental, and social characteristics (Neuman, 1989). The process of health promotion enables people to take on more responsibility and includes protecting their environment (Underwood, Van Berkel, Scott, Siracusa, & Gibson, 1993). School nurses can teach children to adopt a prudent lifestyle that will increase their level of wellness for years to come.

Health Surveillance

The school nurse may have the first contact with a child and thus is in a good position to identify concerns and intervene as necessary. A health interview provides an opportunity for children and parents to consider their health, their worries, and to identify specific health needs. The interview is also an opportunity for the school nurse to identify previous health problems, confirm that they have been resolved, and identify remaining needs (Mattock, 1991). This interview may be done as part of the initial registration process or upon request. It is worthwhile for the nurse to teach school personnel what to observe; signs, symptoms, behavior, complaints; and how to make referrals to the school nurse (Chen, Rose, & Chen, 1987). Case finding, which is the basis of interventions to enhance healthy mind, body, and spirit, is a significant component of the nurse's function.

Direct Care

In schools where the nurse is present on a very regular basis, direct care in the form of first aid, providing emergency services, and doing specific medical procedures such as catheterization, giving medications, tracheostomy care, and gastric tube feeding may be provided. Inclusion of children with complex needs has increased this direct care function. The school nurse may also be responsible for teaching and supervising identified school personnel who are involved in carrying out certain procedures required to maintain a child's health in the school environment.

Information Resource

The school nurse who practices in some ways as a generalist can be a significant resource to both students and teachers. Being available to provide information and recommendations will help prevent unnecessary crises related to special needs children and children who may be in a compromised state of health. The school nurse is a valu-

able resource person because he or she can inform about medication side effects, screening procedures to be performed, and treatment modalities for specific problems and health conditions. School health nurses are also involved in making referrals to a variety of services for medical attention and for behavioral and emotional concerns.

Teachers and other school personnel often seek information regarding their own personal health concerns. As a health promoter and health educator, offering support becomes second nature for the community-based nurse. Assisting teachers in dealing with stress and symptoms of burnout (Belcastro & Gold, 1983), recommending appropriate health services, and providing counseling related to health-enhancing health behavior, are valuable services that need to be included when clarifying the nurse's role within the school setting. The box below outlines possible strategies to promote the role of the school nurse within the school environment.

HOW SCHOOL NURSES CAN INFORM TEACHERS ABOUT THE NURSE'S ROLE

1) Explain to teachers what can be offered and how it will be done.
2) Reassure teachers that interventions and programs are not intended to take over their classroom activities.
3) Work with the teachers who are receptive to involvement, and their support will be passed on to their colleagues.
4) Assist with health education by developing programs with the teachers. Whether or not the teacher or the school nurse actually provides the educational program when both are involved, each will feel part of the team and each has significant skills and experience to offer.
5) Be visible and offer incidental health teaching in a nonpreaching, nonthreatening way to encourage approachability in the future.
6) Demonstrate what can be offered by participating on educational planning and policy development committees.
7) Offer support and reassurance to teachers when they deal with special needs children.

Case Management

The school nurse is an ideal person to manage the care of chronically ill, physically disabled, developmentally disabled, and other high-risk children in the regular school system (Joachim, 1989; Rustia, Hartley, Hansen, Schulte, & Spielman, 1984). Case management involves coordination of services and liaison between home, school, the primary health care team, and other involved support agencies. The purpose of integrating, coordinating, and advocating for individuals is to enhance quality of client care and cost effectiveness (Smith, 1993). Collaboration with medical and social services working in the context of the team approach is imperative. As an effective liaison, the nurse promotes an environment in which parents feel at ease when participating in decision making about their child's health and educational needs (Collis & Dukes, 1989).

An essential part of the case management role includes **child advocacy.** The school nurse is involved to protect, improve, and maintain the health of children because health and learning go hand in hand. As an advocate, the school nurse identifies areas of concern and assists in seeking out the best possible way of approaching a given situation through school-based, community-based, or hospital-based services. Activism has affected child health and welfare issues over the years. This will continue to be an area where school nurses advocate for the changing needs of children in their schools. This may involve providing information and recommendations for the development or modification of school health policies. For example, this kind of action would be beneficial in setting up protocols for medication administration and handling of certain equipment. As a member of school planning committees, the nurse can influence decisions and programs to ensure that realistic goals are set for a specific child.

Administration

A variety of administrative and clerical activities may be expected of the school nurse. Record keeping related to the health status of students continues to be a regular function. This includes noting exemptions from immunization programs or health assessments because of religious or philosophical reasons, obtaining necessary consents, and attendance monitoring in some cases. Confidentiality of school records is an important issue that must be addressed. Some nurses may be involved in planning, implementing, and evaluation of existing school health programs and their own and other nurses' performance.

Research

School nurses are becoming more knowledgeable and aware of the need for research. This is an important method of documenting the effects of services and a means of improving clinical practice. In addition, research will help to prove the worth of school nursing. Theory-based practice affirms the value of nurses' unique contributions to health care. Goals will focus on promoting quality of life, health, and client-directed healing (Smith, 1993). Research will provide the credibility for nurses to influence health policy, which is also a part of the role of the school nurse (Oda, 1991).

Jacobson (1994) carried out a qualitative study with the purpose of developing an understanding of the meaning of stressful life experiences. More studies of this kind enable more reliable assessment mechanisms for identifying children at risk. Appropriate prevention intervention strategies can then be implemented to better meet the needs of specific populations and age groups.

PRIMARY PREVENTION

Primary prevention includes prevention of both physical and psychosocial health problems. Intervention is indicated when a stressor that is known to be damaging is a risk, but a reaction is not yet evident (Neuman, 1989). Primary prevention involves health promotion and disease protection (Kobokovich & Bonovich, 1992). Programs that are focused on wellness and health promotion prepare children so they will be equipped to make wise health-related decisions in adult life. Providing education at school will give those children who do not have good role models at home a chance to be exposed to facts and information about healthy behaviors and risk factors that may affect their own lives in the future.

—————— RESEARCH 🌿 HIGHLIGHT ——————

Stressful life experiences and their meaning to older children

Jacobson (1994) explored the meaning of stressful life experience in the Chicago metropolitan area. Fourteen children between the ages of nine and 11 were interviewed. Three principal dimensions emerged once data were categorized. They included feelings of loss, feelings of threat to self, and feelings of being hassled. In all cases the children identified experiences occurring in the first two dimensions to be more troublesome than the third. Responses relayed experiences of losses of significant persons not only through occurrences of death but also through other situations. Relocation was one example. Feelings of threat to self included areas concerning interpersonal loss exemplified by loss of approval of a significant adult, lack of respect or regard for feeling, loss of self-esteem, feelings of being blamed unfairly, situations leading to feelings of fear, aggression, or anger. Feelings of being hassled were typically presented in a matter-of-fact manner implying that they were to be expected. These scenarios associated with hassles were the basis of children's descriptions of good versus bad days. The study reinforced previous documentation in the literature that children's perceptions of life events may be quite different from adult's perceptions.

From "The meaning of stressful life experiences in nine-to-eleven-year-old children: A phenomenological study, by G. Jacobson, 1994, *Nursing Research, 43*(2), pp. 95-99.

For many years nurses have been involved in identifying effective and ineffective means of promoting health and preventing disease in healthy populations. The new direction of public health involves instructional programs directed at promoting healthy behavior in relation to safety, nutrition, exercise, use of alcohol, drugs, tobacco, and the like. School health programs are addressing needs of school-age children, who make up 25% of the American population. This has an impact not only on the current health of children but also on their future health status (Pigg, 1989).

The school nurse will be directly or indirectly involved in educational programs. Outside agencies may also become active participants in the programs for promoting healthy behaviors. Areas of primary prevention intervention for the school nurse include immunization, health education, suicide prevention, prevention of substance abuse, and accident prevention.

Immunization

School nurses are involved in various capacities with **immunization programs.** In many cases the school nurse oversees immunization for communicable diseases that are common to school-age children. This involves record keeping and follow-up with parents when a child requires updated immunization. Parents are responsible for taking their child to a physician or to a health care clinic. In school districts where the population tends to be transient, close monitoring is essential. There are still many children who are not adequately immunized; however, in some areas immunization clinics are held at the school. Mandatory immunization clinics are a thing of the past (Igoe & Goodwin, 1991).

Health Education

Schools today are going beyond the typical health education curriculum followed in past years. Special programs for at-risk children and adolescents are being provided. Because of their knowledge base, school nurses are invaluable in assisting schools in developing and carrying out programs. Areas of **health education** that a school nurse may be involved in directly or indirectly include the following: nutrition and diet; exercise and fitness; sex education/family planning/adolescent pregnancy, and sexually transmitted disease prevention; substance abuse; and programs to reduce mental health disorders, accidents, and the incidence of cancer. To integrate basic information effectively, the nurse and school personnel cannot lose sight of the cultural factors that may influence healthy and unhealthy habits.

Education about nutrition and healthy lifestyle practices can play a major role in decreasing the incidence of premature heart disease, cardiovascular disorders, cancer, and a variety of other illnesses. Diet education to decrease risk factors relating to cardiovascular disease include recommendations such as low salt, low fat, low sugar, and high fiber intake, and weight control, along with the endorsement of a regular exercise program (Carmon, Hauber, Howell, & Rice, 1990; Perry et al., 1990).

The establishment of programs that encourage the development of good problem-solving skills among students in high-risk groups is one strategy that will enhance education programs. This approach involves the learner in identifying factors that influence their health behavior (positive and negative), alternative behavior options, barriers, and positive and negative outcomes of behavior. This educational approach also helps in the implementation and modification of behavior that is based on certain circumstances encountered (Singleton, 1994).

Cancer continues to be one of the greatest causes of potential years of life lost from disease before age 65 (Seffrin, 1989). It is well documented that some cancers are preventable. Many cancers are related to lifestyle. With the vast amount of research that has occurred to date, individuals have a better chance of conducting their lives in such a way that they may not have to experience the devastation of cancer. Educating students to empower them to create and change their own destiny is an essential principal of educational programs that promote health. Influencing children at an early age about dietary practices and the consequences of tobacco use will enhance a positive, long-term effect because the children will have a basis from which to make decisions and choices. For example,

"Reach For Health," a cancer prevention project, developed "The Fun and Fit Friends Want to be Popular," which was a puppet show presented to students in kindergarten to grade three. Students in grades four to six present the program, which encourages the eating of fruits and vegetables. The underlying intention of the simple, relevant message is to decrease cancer risk by decreasing fat intake and increasing fiber intake. The program involves the students and encourages action (Henry, Standley, Sarason, & Anthony, 1994).

Education relating to HIV and AIDS needs to take place both in and outside of the classroom. Educational programs vary in each school district. Programs dealing with aspects of promoting positive behaviors begin as early as grade four and go up to grade 12. Teaching about risk-reduction, communication skills, decision-making skills, and about sexuality as a positive component of human development rather than attaching judgemental attitudes and fear encourages the adoption of positive behaviors. Education of students, parents, and school personnel promote the greatest success for communicating facts and changing behaviors. Safer sex education programs are integrated into various aspects of the health curriculums offered in the schools.

HIV prevention programs should recognize that progressive substance abuse may be an important indicator of risk for HIV infection and AIDS. Discouragement of all substance abuse, therefore, must be emphasized not only with respect to injection drug use but also through its association with unsafe sexual behaviors (Lowry et al, 1994).

Suicide Prevention Programs

School nurses are in a good position to initiate and be involved in **suicide prevention programs.** Suicide prevention programs would include training of teachers and school staff regarding suicide awareness, identification of potential suicide victims, and knowledge of community resources available. For example, an individual may indicate the presence of "termination behaviors" evidenced by withdrawal from family and friends, giving verbal cues, exhibiting loss of interest in usual activities, or acting out of character (Finch & Robins-Holm, 1994). Parent workshops would focus on symptom awareness and available community resources. Student workshops and programs would concentrate on dealing with stressful life issues, where to receive help, resources available in the community, and peer support and counseling services within the school environment.

Programs may involve self-evaluation of emotional status and teaching coping skills and stress management options. Preparing students to have effective methods of dealing with potentially stressful life situations will hopefully alleviate illness situations that would require more involved intervention at a later date.

Substance Abuse Prevention

Programs related to substance abuse are often incorporated into the health curriculum. School nurses may be involved as resource persons for up-to-date information. **Substance abuse programs** need to include not only information about tobacco and drugs such as cocaine, marijuana, and the like, but also information about over-the-counter drug abuse and use of anabolic steroids among athletes. The approach to alcohol use and abuse prevention programs implemented by school nurses must include intervention directed at stress control, social integration, and success in school (Thombs & Beck, 1994).

School-based smoking prevention programs continue to be high on the school nurse's priority list. Cigarette smoking has been linked to the causes of lung cancer, cancer of the larynx, and cancer of the oral cavities and esophagus. It is also a factor associated with cancers of the bladder, pancreas, and kidney. Youths who live in environments where tobacco and alcohol use is widespread are less likely to develop negative attitudes about using these substances unless they receive consistent messages from adult family members and community members that using these substances is unacceptable (Singleton, 1994). Effective programs will delay the onset of smoking among adolescents, thereby reducing the incidence of taking up the habit as adults

SUMMARY OF ESSENTIAL ELEMENTS FOR A SMOKING PREVENTION PROGRAM

1) Programs need to include information about social consequences; social influences on tobacco use; peer, parent, and media influences; short-term physiologic effects; and training in refusal skills, which would involve modeling and practice at resisting.

2) Length of the program should be 2 five-session units focusing on smoking prevention in at least two of the years between grades six and nine, if not each year.

3) It would be ideal to include some aspect of tobacco-use prevention in all grades, initiating the program in grade six or seven.

4) Peer involvement in the delivery of a smoking prevention program at school has proved to have greater weight in influencing attitudes.

5) Parental support of such programs is imperative for their effectiveness. Actual parental involvement may enhance positive effects, particularly in the elementary grades. Support from school staff may also have an effect on influencing attitudes through modeling.

6) Teacher training for implementation of a smoking prevention program is necessary. Including demonstration and experiential activities, such as role playing and refusal skills, for example, will maintain consistency in the message and direction of the curriculum set-up.

7) For the program to be implemented successfully, community norms and relevant needs need to be taken into consideration. Existing policies, costs, ease of implementation, and the interests of the school community, including administrators, parents, and students, must be addressed and incorporated (Glynn, 1989, pp. 181-188).

(Glynn, 1989). Smoking prevention efforts directed at high school students need to include refusal skills and smoking cessation messages that are culturally and developmentally relevant (Kelder, Perry, Klepp, & Lytle, 1994; Elder et al., 1994). The box above offers suggestions for components of a smoking prevention program.

Accident Prevention

Today children and adolescents are endangered by their own choices and behavior. Present-day technology has allowed children and adolescents to survive traumatic situations that in the past would have ended their lives. The outcome today, however, may be that a child is left with residual cognitive and/or physical deficits. Drinking and driving, use of drugs, ignoring bicycle safety, practicing unprotected sex, use of tobacco, poor diet, and lack of exercise puts our youth at risk for chronic disease and disability. Programs geared at awareness, problem solving, and taking on responsibility for self and actions can be presented in many forms. It is imperative to incorporate factors characteristic of the population of children to promote successful outcomes evidenced by attitude and behavior change.

The school nurse is instrumental in identifying safety hazards within the school environment for both able-bodied children and those with disabilities. The school nurse works in conjunction with other professionals to identify problems, determine high-risk groups of children, and to develop solutions.

SECONDARY PREVENTION

Secondary prevention involves a screening of health conditions, referral, and counseling and treatment. Intervention at a secondary level involves management of existing symptoms and attempting to strengthen the client's own line of defense. According to Neuman (1989), at the secondary level, a reaction to a stressor has occurred. It includes early and immediate treatment of a disability and or limitation (Kobokovich & Bonovich, 1992). In some school districts, school nursing is moving away from individualized screening and health care and into working more with groups. Health issues relating to the population of children as a whole based on demographics and specific characteristics of the school population are driving intervention to a much greater extent. Areas of intervention include health screening; communicable disease monitor-

ing; preschool visitation/assessment; addressing mental health needs, eating disorders, adolescent reproductive health; and providing HIV/AIDS support services.

Health Screening

The underlying premise of health screening programs involves the value that certain health conditions can be identified and corrected at the earliest possible time. Screening programs that are typically provided include vision, hearing, scoliosis, speech and language development, and motor disturbances. The nurse in the school may conduct the screening tests or may make arrangements for the screening to occur. Often, vision and hearing screening occurs at the kindergarten level and on request for older children. Follow-up by the school nurse involves interpreting of results, contacting students and parents, and making arrangements for further diagnostic assessment or treatment.

Communicable Diseases Monitoring

In many localities the school nurse has taken on less of a role in the screening of pediculosis (head lice). Alternative programs have been instituted to deal with this ongoing issue (Clore & Longyear, 1990). In some localities, community volunteers are recruited to provide the screening program. Once a child is identified as having head lice, the school nurse may be involved in verification and communicating with parents either verbally or with written material about how to deal with pediculosis effectively. Follow-up telephone intervention to reinforce treatment, proper handling of personal belongings, and cleaning of the environment is beneficial for chronically infested children.

Involvement with regard to identifying other contagious diseases, such as chicken pox and conjunctivitis, includes identification and follow-up based on specific procedures outlined by health departments and communicable disease control centers. Procedures for exclusion from school and required medical follow-up, and immediate treatment while the child is at school will all be clearly outlined in a handbook of school policies. School nurses maintain current knowledge regarding follow-up care and are involved in regularly updating school personnel regarding these policies.

Preschool Visitation/Assessment

Some health departments and school boards continue to provide preschool assessment intervention. Screening children for hearing, vision, and physical developmental problems is a beneficial secondary prevention strategy to ensure that children are able to succeed in the school setting and that realistic expectations are placed on them. Often a full physical examination by a physician is required before school entry.

Early detection allows time for follow-up to occur before the child is expected to function in the learning environment. At this time of intervention, the school nurse also provides health teaching to parents accompanying the child regarding health matters such as immunization, nutrition, hygiene, and an introduction to the school nurse and his or her role (Marino, 1991). Any issues or concerns that parents may have relating to their child's attendance at school is also dealt with at this opportune time.

Addressing Mental Health Needs

Direct contact with children may not be solely for physical health needs. More and more children are exhibiting the signs and symptoms of emotional disturbances, a fact that affects their abilities to function successfully within the school environment. Many more children are having to deal with family situations that are stressful and lack security and consistency related to both parents working, family breakdown, living with a chronic illness or disability, a family member facing unemployment or relocation, and increasing social pressures. The school nurse must be prepared to identify psychopathology and provide crisis intervention to the students in their care, as well as to reach out to families. Suicide, particularly among teenagers, is prevalent, and it is not uncommon for young children to contemplate this as a means of ending their pain and suffering.

Schools offer a very accessible setting to detect problems related to mental health. Supports within the community are insufficient to deal with all the children who require professional intervention. Stigma associated with mental illness and problems related to parents' ability to transport their children are additional barriers to access. Even at young ages, children may find confiding in the school nurse and talking about some of their daily problems helpful in making them feel better. Attention is required to identify children with special needs who are at risk for social and emotional problems as a result of stressors faced within an integrated setting. Schools have a growing need for consultation services about mental health issues (Puskar, Lamb, & Norton, 1990). The school nurse is a nonthreatening source of support who has no connection to the grading process and discipline protocols, and therefore can be available to a student who wishes to seek advice without worrying about approval.

Regular support groups for children to attend, for example at lunch time, may be a means of reaching children and providing support to those facing stressful situations associated with divorce, death and dying, and socialization (Nash, 1987). Teaching children specific skills along with providing a safe avenue to vent feelings offers a valuable means of dealing with the stressors related to family breakdown, living with a disability or illness, and facing other unfortunate life experiences. The use of imagery (Winn, 1988) or relaxation can be effective in coping with pain and stress management. Teaching children strategies to cope at various stages of their lives might involve such things as being able to say no, developing appropriate social skills, adopting safe behavior, making decisions, and dealing with a whole gamut of issues caused by peer pressure that may involve risk-taking rather than health-enhancing behaviors.

Signs and symptoms that may be observed by the nurse or reported to the nurse may include such things as the following: difficulties with learning; perfectionism; difficulties with socialization; mood swings; unhappiness; depression; psychosomatic symptoms such as headaches and stomach aches; refusing to attend school; verbal and physical aggression; defiant behaviors; and attention-seeking behaviors. More and more, classroom teachers are expressing the frustration of having to spend more time on behavior issues with children in class, which takes away from the actual focus of learning.

Eating Disorders

Obesity is a controllable health problem. It is a prevalent nutritional disease that requires addressing by school health support personnel (Sherman, Alexander, Gomez, Kim, & Marole, 1992). Anorexia nervosa and bulimia, which are frequently seen in adolescents, are other eating disorders that have serious medical, social, and emotional consequences.

Eating disorders are influenced by the cultural background of the student, family practices, parents' knowledge about nutrition, values toward food, physical activity, genetic predisposition, and emotional status. Canadian and American statistics indicate that iron deficiency is widespread among certain disadvantaged children and adolescent girls. Nutrition education and interventions should target specific subgroups at risk (Gibson, 1994). School nurses are in a good position to become involved in early detection and intervention programs for children with eating disorders. Risk factors that may lead to eating disorders include the following: 1) over achievement; 2) perfectionist or obsessional personality; 3) chaotic family system; 4) a recent family or personal crisis; 5) a friend with an eating disorder; 6) participation in body-conscious sports; 7) low self-esteem; and 8) impulsivity (Connolly & Corbett-Dick, 1990).

Educational programs need to include such topics as basic nutrition knowledge, assertiveness, promoting self-worth, and balancing one's life, as well as enhancing communication between parents and their children, and information relating to specific eating disorders. Preparing teachers to identify symptoms related to behavior and social interactions will assist the school nurse in preliminary case finding. It is necessary for the school nurse to take a relevant health history including physical status, nutritional status, eating habits, medications, and an assessment of a student's emotional status. Involving parents and referring to outside medical or social services will be indicated based on the initial findings. As a case manager, the school nurse helps to facilitate a support network that will increase the likelihood that students will complete the treatment program arranged. Working to establish commitment on the part of the student and family may be a challenge, but is an essential component for success. Figure 28-1 exhibits a school conference that takes place for a variety of reasons, with the purpose of ensuring that team members, consisting of school personnel and community-based personnel, work together to provide a unified approach for supporting students.

Adolescent Reproductive Health

It is imperative for the school nurse to work in collaboration with school support personnel to endorse a comprehensive approach to the area of adolescent reproductive health (Santelli & Coyle, 1992; Kobokovich & Bonovich, 1992). Adolescent pregnancy continues to be a prevalent issue. Studies have shown that within the last two decades young women are becoming sexually active at an earlier age (Newcomer & Baldwin, 1992). Providing an atmosphere of trust will enable students to openly discuss concerns and will promote early identification and intervention.

The range of activities carried out by the school nurse associated with adolescent pregnancy prevention involves counseling and referring for the following: pregnancy testing, counseling, contraception, treatment of suspected sexually transmitted disease, providing inservices to school personnel regarding sexuality, and teaching students about sexually transmitted disease (STD), family life/human sexuality, and decision-making techniques. As an advocate, the nurse at school is a resource person for curriculum development and other community-based pregnancy prevention programs.

To develop relevant programs and support for a particular population of adolescents within a school community, the school nurse, school personnel, and affiliated support services identify risk factors and characteristics of the population within their school community. Cultural backgrounds, educational levels of parents, socioeconomic status, and religious background are some factors that will have an effect on the sexual behavior of the students.

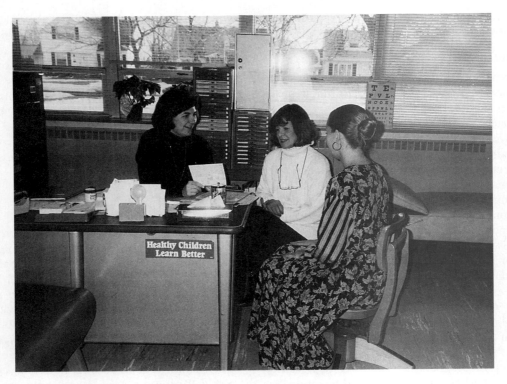

FIGURE 28-1   School nurses need to be members of school-based teams. They have valuable knowledge and skills to assist in accessing appropriate resources. They are in a good position to be a liaison with home, school, and community agencies.

School-based care providers offer support to students and may be a liaison with hospital-based professionals who are involved in providing prenatal and postnatal care for adolescents. Education and support at school may induce compliance. The school nurse provides psychosocial support to adolescent parents and their families regarding the various stressful difficulties associated with pregnancy and parenthood. Education for this population of clients includes not only aspects specifically related to care of the baby, but also addresses coping with the ensuing responsibilities of parenthood, nutrition, contraception, and developmental issues. When outside services are not being accessed, the school nurse may offer a component of the prenatal care. By monitoring blood pressure, weight gain, and screening for possible complications of pregnancy, the school nurse functions as a significant member of the health care team involved in providing

both prenatal and postnatal care (Stevens-Simon & Beach, 1992).

HIV/AIDS Support Services

School nurses, school counselors, psychologists, teachers, and administrators all need to be involved in implementing a program that helps students fully comprehend the effects of the HIV epidemic on their lives. Essential components of an HIV/AIDS support service include preventive education, health monitoring, counseling and support, HIV test counseling and support, referral to outside services, and a policy-making mechanism (American Association for Counseling and Development et al., 1990; Flaskerud, 1989).

Specifically, the school nurse takes on the role of planner, manager, and change agent (Brainerd, 1989). Developing a health care plan that will specify who will be involved with HIV-related issues at the school and to what extent, will be supportive to students. Counseling for students who may be at high risk, before and after testing, must also be available. Having a faculty or staff member who has AIDS may also pose some concerns that need to be dealt with.

School staff, health care professionals, psychologists, social workers, and other support staff need to be included in developing policies to address the needs of HIV-infected students. Issues concerning confidentiality, the implementation of universal precautions for handling body fluids, and the development and implementation of the educational programs at school will have to be dealt with (American Association for Counselling and Development et al., 1990).

TERTIARY PREVENTION

Tertiary intervention involves preventing a recurrence of a problem or illness or to limit the extent of the negative effects of an existing problem. Nursing actions at this level of intervention are guided by an intention to prevent complications, minimize limitations associated with a condition, and enhance optimal functioning guide nursing actions. Tertiary interventions, according to Neuman (1989), maintain a reconstituted state of wellness once the client's resources have been mobilized. Nursing actions addressing tertiary prevention focus on aspects of rehabilitation and limiting altered health (Kobokovich & Bonovich, 1992; Rustia et al., 1984). Prevention of recurrence of an acute or chronic health condition and involvement with special needs children will be included.

Prevention of Recurrence of An Acute or Chronic Condition

Terminally ill children, medically fragile children, and children with chronic illnesses are being integrated among their peers. Supporting the teacher, the child, and peers, as well as being a resource to parents, is another aspect of the role of the school nurse. Any factors that may cause exacerbation of an existing condition need to be eliminated. This action would involve health teaching so that the child, school personnel, and parents work together in eliminating risk factors. The nurse must monitor activities that ensure

that treatment, therapy, and daily routines are carried out to maintain an optimal level of wellness. Anticipating possible problems so they are dealt with in advance is an important strategy to maintain a child's dignity and to prevent major crises from occurring.

Involvement With Special Needs Children

Physically and cognitively challenged children have a full range of academic opportunities available to them. The elimination of barriers to education began in 1975 when the Education for All Handicapped Children Act, Public Law 94-142, came into effect. As a result, children are offered education in the least restrictive environment. An **Individualized Education Plan (IEP)** is formulated for each student identified. Combinations of special education programs range from general education with intervention for specific learning disabilities, to special education on a part-time or a full-time basis. By offering a variety of options, children with varying degrees of learning difficulties receive appropriate educational support, thus minimizing the stigma associated with labelling (Repetto & Hoeman 1991).

A multidisciplinary team makes recommendations for school programming. School nurses are included under the term *related services*. The nurse is involved in the identification process as part of the school-based team, and assists in identifying strengths and weaknesses and health care needs to determine appropriate services to be put into place, and in establishing realistic goals and expectations. Identification of children involves reviewing of records, observing the student in the school setting, and seeking out additional information as necessary.

In Canada comparable legislation has been passed. In Ontario, for example, Bill 82 was passed in 1980 to amend the Education Act of 1974. The act ensured that as of September 1, 1985, all school boards would be responsible for providing special education for students. Once a child is identified as exceptional, a special education **Identification Placement and Review Committee** (IPRC) determines an appropriate educational program and placement that meets the child's needs. Current educational, medical, and psychologic assessments are used to identify

■ CASE STUDY

Mariah K. was an 8-year-old-girl who was returning to school after sustaining a severe closed-head injury as a result of a car accident. Mariah had been a passenger in the car driven by her aunt. She was in a coma for 2½ weeks and remained in hospital for another six weeks until she was medically stable. Mariah was then admitted to an acute rehabilitation facility for six weeks, during which time she made significant gains. Mariah was discharged to go home and continued to receive outpatient physical therapy, occupational therapy, and speech and language therapy three times per week. She had been in grade three before the accident, which occurred in January.

Upon discharge from the rehabilitation facility, Mariah was able to dress herself, eat, and go to the bathroom with minimal assistance. She required some supervision and assistance, particularly at the end of the day when she was more tired. Mariah continued to have an ataxic gait but required no aids. Her balance was off, particularly when she was fatigued. She had coordination difficulty with her right arm (dominant side); however, she was very motivated to do as much as she could with it in spite of residual limitations. Cognitive functioning was impaired as evidenced by memory difficulties, information processing difficulties, and a significant attention deficit. A neuropsychologic assessment was to take place six months after the injury. Mariah's speech was slower but very understandable. Mariah tended to be impulsive at times, and when she became frustrated she would cry easily. However, overall Mariah was demonstrating obvious improvements in all areas.

The school nurse contacted Mrs. K. when she learned from the principal that Mariah would be returning to school. She obtained updated information about Mariah's present level of functioning, services in place, and concerns that Mrs. K. had regarding Mariah's school reentry. Information about family members, their levels of coping, and any concerns about their understanding of the situation were explored as well. The family was involved with a social worker from the treatment center. Mrs. K. suggested that perhaps having a tutor until Mariah was back to the way she used to be might make her return to school easier. The benefits of having Mariah amongst her peers and getting used to a routine were offered. Reassurance that her physical and cognitive needs could be met in the school environment was given as well. Information about supports available through the school and the process of developing an individualized school program were explained to Mrs. K. It was also suggested that a meeting be arranged with all involved professionals, with the parents, and with school personnel to discuss the necessary arrangements for Mariah's reentry.

Nursing Diagnosis

1) Knowledge deficit related to recovery from a brain injury
2) Safety concerns related to altered level of functioning.

Plan of Action

1) Facilitate a meeting at the school with school personnel, parents, therapists, social worker, and other involved support services.
2) Obtain up-to-date information from attending physicians.
3) Facilitate a visit to the school for Mariah before her first day of attendance.
4) Provide a disability awareness program for classmates (and for the whole school population if warranted) regarding implications of recovering from a brain injury. (Include information about how to appropriately help an individual, what the individual may be feeling/experiencing as a result of absences because of therapy appointments, fatigue, difficulty understanding directions, concentration difficulties.) The purpose of the program is to sensitize the children in the class, to alleviate fears, and to teach them how they can be supportive and accepting. Visual aids, experiential activities, and role modeling are possible techniques that may be helpful to the students to enhance better understanding.
5) Provide an inservice to teachers regarding recovery from a head injury and implications within the classroom setting. Explain that Mariah will con-

tinue to demonstrate obvious physical and cognitive recovery for two to three years postinjury; however, Mariah will not be the same little girl that she was before the accident. Present possible strategies to use in situations such as distractibility, impulsivity, frustration, memory deficits, which may be difficult for both Mariah and her teachers.

6) Maintain regular contact with parents and involved professionals regarding Mariah's adjustment, progress, and problems. Explore the need for additional supports and facilitate referrals as necessary.

7) Be available to teachers to deal with coping issues; it is sometimes difficult to deal with a child exhibiting dramatic differences in academic and behavioral performance. Some teachers, in essence, will go through a grieving process when a child returns to school with residual deficits after a severe brain injury.

The conference took place before Mariah started school. Issues discussed involved safety, dressing, toiletting, involvement in physical education, transportation, academic programming, socialization, and communication. All members in attendance were clear about expectations and who to contact in the event of a problem. The importance of maintaining a consistent routine was emphasized. It was decided that Mariah would attend school half days in the morning for the core subjects. She would continue to receive therapy in the afternoon. A recreation therapist would be contacted by the school nurse to assist with setting up possible programs such as swimming for the afternoon or evening. When fatigue became less of a problem, Mariah would attend full days. Therapy suggestions that could be implemented into the regular program would be offered on an ongoing basis. A daily log book would be used by all persons involved to maintain consistency in communication. The school agreed to provide an aide to assist the teacher in the classroom for the first three months. After that time the situation would be reevaluated, and appropriate supports would be determined.

The teacher appeared to be quite anxious about having Mariah in her class, given that she had other students in her class with special needs ranging from behavioral to physical. Plans were made to provide additional information by the school nurse and the therapists. The school nurse agreed to spend time in the classroom to observe and provide additional support as necessary until the teacher felt more confident in her skills.

A meeting was planned to develop an IEP by school personnel and parents within the next two weeks. Adjustment to school would be the initial primary focus. Another meeting date was set to be held in three months, to be attended by all team members involved in Mariah's case (multidisciplinary; involving school personnel and outside agencies involved) to review Mariah's progress and to determine the need for any changes.

Mariah adjusted well to the grade three program and seemed to make even greater gains once she was with her peers. Issues came up relating to safety, seizure medication, and social expectations. Team members and medical professionals were contacted by the school nurse to resolve concerns by both parents and school personnel. Ongoing involvement for the school nurse included case management, education regarding recovery from a brain injury, and being a resource person. Documentation and obtaining appropriate consents were important administrative responsibilities as well. The grade four teacher was provided with education and information before Mariah started school the following September.

---

the child's needs and abilities. The IPRC is made up of the principal of the school or a supervisory officer, and at least two other members, such as the classroom teacher and resource/special education teacher (Government of Ontario 1985a, 1985b, 1987).

Salend and Mahoney (1982) stressed the importance of maintaining appropriate hygiene habits for successful mainstreaming to occur. For example, nurses in the school promote changes and support the child who may have difficulty with bowel and bladder control, dressing, and social skills. Involvement from outside services may be indicated.

As an advocate, the school nurse clarifies misconceptions that prevent acceptance of students with disabilities. Experiences at school have major implications for the development of every school-aged child. Every child needs to have a sense of belonging to a peer group, which influences a child's feelings of self-worth. Physically disabled children are faced with additional barriers that able-bodied students do not have to overcome. Adults involved in the child's school environment help shape healthy and accepting attitudes towards the disabled and intervene to remove both physical and psychosocial barriers. The school nurse assists by emphasizing the uniqueness of the child as opposed to the disability.

Nurses in the school assist at a tertiary prevention level by limiting the alteration of health, taking corrective and restorative measures, and promoting maximal adaptation (Logan & Dawkins, 1986). Supporting teachers involved with the special needs child and contributing suggestions will prevent problems related to safety issues and acceptance.

Activities that a community-based nurse offers to promote an **accepting environment** include the following: 1) interpreting the background medical history and present medical and therapy involvement for school personnel, and educating about the implications of the child's abilities and limitations within the classroom setting; 2) assisting in the development of procedures and training to meet the health care needs of the child; 3) monitoring health care services provided by other school personnel and outside agencies; 4) assisting in making recommendations for modifications to the child's school program; 5) providing emotional support to school personnel directly working with the disabled child; and 6) acting as a liaison between school, community, health care providers, parents, and child.

FUTURE CONSIDERATIONS

It is becoming more and more evident that financial restraint is greatly affecting the direction of health care. School nurses offer a significant contribution to child health care. Advocating and demonstrating the value of interventions offered at primary, secondary, and tertiary prevention levels will be imperative. Research will provide a sound basis to justify the value of this specialized area of nursing. Routine types of programs have no place in the school anymore. Each school community must evaluate needs on an ongoing basis to determine priorities directly related to the children in their district. Nurses must clarify their role or other persons will.

Chapter Highlights

- The school nurse is involved to promote an environment that allows an optimal level of wellness for the school-age child. The school nurse may oversee or present programs that focus on preventing disease, lowering the risks of acute or chronic conditions, minimizing the effects of existing health problems, early identification and intervention, and promoting healthy lifestyle choices.

- The role of the school nurse is varied as a result of a lack of uniform guidelines and differing approaches to the administration of school health services. The range of functions includes health promotion, health surveillance, direct care, information resource, case management, administration, and research.

- School nurses need to revise their role to fit new directions of health care. The health care objectives for the year 2000 strongly advocate for expansion of health education programs that are supportive of the role of the school nurse.

- School nurses need to maintain up-to-date knowledge about issues relating to the school age population to be resourceful and supportive to school personnel.

- The case management aspect of the role of the school nurse is a significant component that contributes to the success of integration for special needs children and the provision of services for children experiencing a compromised state of health.

- School nurses are involved directly and indirectly in implementing educational health-promotion programs. Topics include safety, nutrition, substance abuse, human sexuality, and addressing of mental health needs. The process of health promotion enables people to take on more responsibility for themselves and includes protecting their environment. Education to instill this value is beneficial at an early age.

- School nurses collaborate with school personnel, other existing professionals, and agencies to provide a comprehensive health service to address the needs of the school-age population. Identifying high-risk groups will help to direct resources appropriately.

 CRITICAL THINKING EXERCISE

The superintendent of the school district requests that the primary school nurse educator write a set of guidelines to be given to parents when they register their children. The guidelines are to help parents understand what the school will ask of them if the following health problems should occur:

1. Head lice
2. Chicken pox
3. Conjunctivitis
4. Problems such as hearing loss or visual acuity deficits
5. Inadequate immunization

Using information found in the chapter, write a set of guidelines for the superintendent.

REFERENCES

Allensworth, D.D., & Kolbe, L.J. (1987). The comprehensive school health program: Exploring an expanded concept. *Journal of School Health, 57*(10), 409-411.

American Association for Counseling and Development, American School Health Association, National Association of School Nurses, National Association of School Psychologists, National Association of Social Workers, Education Commission, National Association of State School Nurse Consultants, National Coalition of Advocates for Students. (1990). Guidelines for HIV and AIDS student support services. *Journal of School Health, 60*(6), 249-255.

Baker, C. (1994). School health: Policy issues. *Nursing and Health Care, 15*(4), 178-184.

Bartfay, W. (1994). Reading, writing and health. *The Canadian Nurse, 90*(2), 29-32.

Belcastro, P.A., & Gold, R.S. (1983). Teacher stress and burnout: Implications for school health personnel. *Journal of School Health, 53*(7), 404-407.

Brainerd, E.F. (1989). HIV in the school setting: The school nurse's role. *Journal of School Health, 59*(7), 316-317.

Carmon, M., Hauber, R.P., Howell, C., & Rice, M. (1990). Cardiovascular screening programs: Implications for school nurses. *Pediatric Nursing, 16*(5), 509-511.

Chen, S.C., Rose, D.A., & Chen, E.H. (1987). A health-awareness program for elementary school teachers. *Public Health Nursing, 4*(2), 105-110.

Clore, E.R., & Longyear, L.A. (1990). Comprehensive pediculo-sis screening programs for elementary schools. *Journal of School Health, 60*(5), 212-214.

Collis, J.L., & Dukes, C.A. (1989). Toward principles of school nursing. *Journal of School Health, 59*(3), 109-111.

Connolly, C., & Corbett-Dick, P. (1990). Eating disorders: A framework for school nursing initiatives. *Journal of School Health, 60*(8), 401-405.

Elder, J., Woodruff, S., Sallis, J., de Moor, C., Edwards, C., & Wildey, M. (1994). Effects of health facilitator performance and attendance at training sessions on the acquisition of tobacco refusal skills among multiethnic, high-risk adolescents. *Health Education Research, 9*(2), 225-233.

Finch, E., & Robins-Holm, E. (1994). Patients at risk of suicide. *The Canadian Nurse, 90*(7), 31-34.

Flaskerud, J. (1989). *AIDS/HIV infection: A reference guide for nursing professionals.* Philadelphia: W.B. Saunders.

Gibson, R. (1994). Iron concerns in Canada. *The Canadian Nurse, 90*(6), 11-13.

Glynn, T.J. (1989). Essential elements of school-based smoking prevention programs. *Journal of School Health, 59*(5), 181-188.

Government of Ontario. (1985a). *Education Act* (Ontario Regulation 554/81). Toronto, Ontario, Canada: Adam Gordon, Queen's Printer.

Government of Ontario. (1985b). *Education Act* (Ontario Regulation 274). Toronto, Ontario, Canada: Adam Gordon, Queen's Printer.

Government of Ontario. (1987). *Education Act.* Toronto, Ontario, Canada: Adam Gordon, Queen's Printer.

Henry, H., Standley, J., Sarason, B., & Anthony, C. (1994). The fun and fit friends want to be popular; Puppets in nutrition education for children. *Journal of Nutrition Education, 26*(4), 205A.

Hill-White, D., & Christansen, T. (1987). The declining status of school nurses in New York. *Journal of School Health, 57*(4), 137-143.

Igoe, J.B., & Goodwin, L.D. (1991). Meeting the challenge of immunizing the nation's children. *Pediatric Nursing, 17*(6), 583-585.

Jacobson, G. (1994). The meaning of stressful life experiences in nine-to-eleven-year-old children: A phenomenological study. *Nursing Research, 43*(2), 95-99.

Joachim, G. (1989). The school nurse as case manager for chronically ill children. *Journal of School Health, 59*(9), 406-407.

Jorgensen, C. (1994). Health education: What can it look like after health care reform? 1993 SOPHE presidential address. *Health Education Quarterly, 21,* 11-26.

Kelder, S., Perry, C., Klepp, K., & Lytle, L. (1994). Longitudinal tracking of adolescent smoking, physical activity, and food choice behaviors. *American Journal of Public Health, 84*(7), 1121-1126.

Kobokovich, L.J., & Bonovich, L.K. (1992). Adolescent pregnancy prevention strategies used by school nurses. *Journal of School Health, 62,* 11-14.

Kozlak, L.A. (1992). Comprehensive school health programs: The challenge for nurses. *Journal of School Health, 62*(10), 475-477.

Logan, B., & Dawkins, C. (1986). *Family-centered nursing in the community.* Reading, MA: Addison-Wesley.

Lowry, R., Holtzman, D., Truman, B., Kann, L., Collins, J., & Kolbe, L. (1994). Substance use and HIV-related sexual behaviors among U.S. high school students: Are they related? *American Journal of Public Health, 84*(7), 116-1120.

Marino, L. (1991). Pre-kindergarten health visitation day in Boardman, Ohio Schools. *Journal of School Health, 61*(6), 269-271.

Mattock, C. (1991). Stepping off the medical treadmill. *Health Visitor, 64*(5), 154-156.

Nader, P.R. (1990). The concept of "comprehensiveness" in the design and implementation of school health programs. *Journal of School Health, 60*(4), 133-138.

Nash, W.E. (1987). School children as consumers-What are their health needs? *Health Visitor, 60,* 387-388.

Neuman, B. (1989). *The Neuman Systems Model* (2nd ed.). Norwalk, CT: Appleton & Lange.

Newcomer, S., & Baldwin, W. (1992). Demographics of sexual behavior, contraception, pregnancy and sexually transmitted diseases. *Journal of School Health, 62*(7), 265-270.

Oda, D.S. (1992). Is school nursing really the "invisible practice?" *Journal of School Health, 62*(3), 112-113.

Oda, D.S. (1991). The invisible nursing practice. *Nursing Outlook, 39,* 26-29.

Perry, C.L., Stone, E.J., Parcel, G.S., Ellison, R.C., Nader, P.R., Webber, L.S., & Luepker, R.V. (1990). School-based cardiovascular health promotion: The child and adolescent trial for cardiovascular health (CATCH). *Journal of School Health, 60*(8), 406-413.

Pigg, R.M. (1989). The contribution of school health programs to the broader goals of public health: The American experience. *Journal of School Health, 59,* 25-30.

Puskar, K., Lamb, J., & Norton, M. (1990). Adolescent mental health: Collaboration among psychiatric mental health nurses and school nurses. *Journal of School Health, 60*(2), 69-71.

Repetto, M.A., & Hoeman, S. (1991). A legislative perspective on the school nurse and education for children with disabilities in New Jersey. *Journal of School Health, 61*(9), 388-391.

Rustia, J., Hartley, R., Hansen, G., Schulte, D., & Spielman, L. (1984). Redefinition of school nursing practice: Integrating the developmentally disabled. *Journal of School Health, 54*(2), 58-62.

Salend, S.J., & Mahoney, S. (1982). Teaching proper health habits to mainstreamed students through positive reinforcement. *The Journal of School Health, 52*(9), 539-542.

Santelli, J.S., & Coyle, K. (1992). Adolescent reproductive health: Roles for school personnel in prevention and early intervention. *Journal of School Health, 62*(7), 294-297.

Seffrin, J.R. (1989). Multiple school health interventions: A key to successful cancer education and prevention. *Journal of School Health, 59*(5), 179-180.

Sherman, J.B., Alexander, M.A., Gomez, D., Kim, M., & Marole, P. (1992). Intervention program for obese school children. *Journal of Community Health Nursing, 9*(3), 183-190.

Singleton, J. (1994). Nutrition and health education for limited income, high-risk groups: Implication for nutrition educators. *Journal of Nutrition Education, 26*(3), 153-155.

Smith, D.W., Redican, K.J., & Olsen, L.K. (1992). The longevity of growing healthy: an analysis of eight original sites implementing the school health curriculum project. *Journal of School Health, 62*(3), 83-87.

Smith, M. (1993). Case management and nursing theory-based practice. *Nursing Science Quarterly, 6,* 8-9.

Stephenson, C. (1983). Visits by elementary school children to the school nurse. *Journal of School Health, 53*(10), 594-599.

Stevens-Simon, C., & Beach, R.K. (1992). School-based prenatal and postpartum care: Strategies for meeting the medical and educational needs of pregnant and parenting students. *Journal of School Health, 62*(7), 304-309.

Sullivan, C., & Bogden, J.F. (1993). Today's education environment. *Journal of School Health, 63,* 28-32.

Thombs, D., & Beck, K. (1994). The social context of four adolescent drinking problems. *Health Education Research, 9,* 13-22.

Thurber, F., Berry, B., & Cameron, M.E. (1991). The role of

school nursing in the United States. *Journal of Pediatric Health Care, 5*(3), 135-140.

Underwood, E., Van Berkel, C., Scott, F., Siracusa, L., & Gibson, B. (1993). The environmental connection. *The Canadian Nurse, 89*(11), 33-35.

U.S. Department of Health and Human Services (U.S. DHHS). (1991). *Healthy people 2000: National promotion and disease prevention objectives: Full report, with commentary* (DHHS Publication No. (PHS) 91-50212). Washington, DC: U.S. Government Printing Office.

White, D.H. (1985). A study of current school nurse practice activities. *Journal of School Health, 55*(2), 52-56.

Winn, M.F. (1988). Imagery and the school nurse. *Journal of School Health, 58*(3), 112-114.

Wold, S. (1981). *School nursing: A framework for practice.* St. Louis: Mosby.

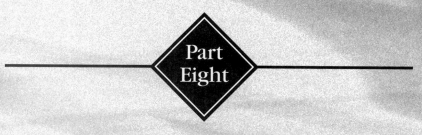

Issues and Concerns in Community Health Nursing

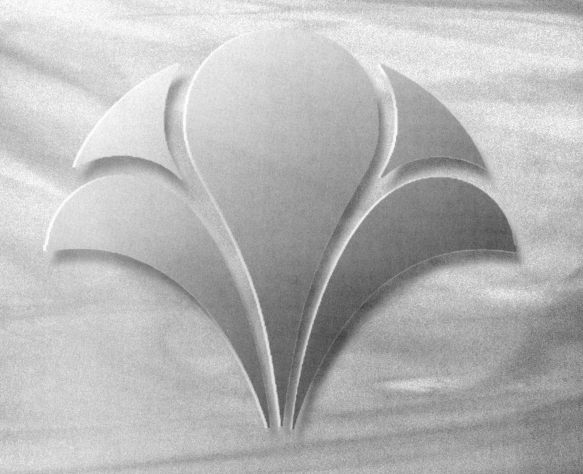

Community health nurses need to be concerned with the total community as they endeavor to prevent illness and maintain wellness. The environment plays an important role in the overall well-being of clients. Pollution, in many forms, can adversely affect health. Nurses need to be aware of this. Advocacy requires a familiarity with the laws affecting the community and its residents. Also important is a knowledge of the political structure within which the nurse must advocate.

Chapter 29 deals with some of the problems associated with today's environment and describes ways the nurse can educate clients to the actions they can take to remain healthy when pollution becomes a threat to their health.

Law and ethics are an inherent part of community health nursing practice. Chapter 30 addresses the legal and ethical issues facing community health nurses today. The chapter also demonstrates how nurses can communicate ethical caring to their clients and participate in the legal process on behalf of the communities they serve.

Chapter 31 outlines many health policy issues and describes the actions needed in community health nursing as a result of future trends in the health care delivery system, consumer action, nursing, research, and political action.

ENVIRONMENTAL CONCERNS

Arthur S. Cookfair

. . . this most excellent canopy, the air, look you, this brave o'erhanging firmament, this majestical roof fretted with golden fire, why, it appears no other thing to me than a foul and pestilent congregation of vapors.

Shakespeare *(Hamlet)*

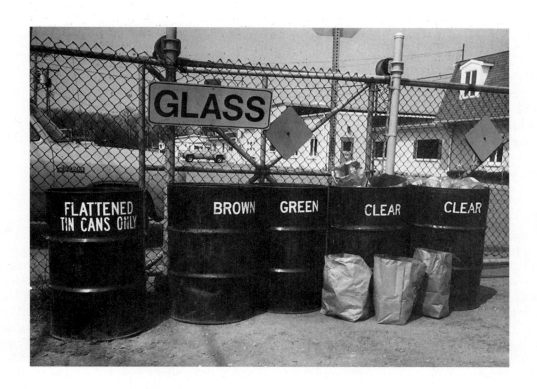

OBJECTIVES

At the conclusion of this chapter the student will be able to:

1. Describe the evolution of environmental issues from a historical perspective.
2. Describe the effect of increasing population on the environment.
3. Describe the effect of solid waste on the health of the community.
4. Describe the problems of hazardous wastes and their harmful effect on the health of the community.
5. Describe the hazards of water pollution on the health of the community.
6. Describe the effect of noise pollution on the health of the community.
7. Describe the problem of air pollution in the community.
8. Identify the common sources of radiation hazards in the community.
9. Describe appropriate nursing interventions at primary, secondary, and tertiary levels to protect the community from environmental hazards and to rehabilitate the victims of such hazards.

KEY TERMS

Air pollution
Biomagnification
Chemical waste
Formaldehyde
Hazardous wastes
Incineration
Ionizing radiation

Landfill
Lead poisoning
Noise pollution
Open dump
Pollutant
Polychlorinated biphenyls
  (PCBs)

Population effect
Radioactive waste
Radon
Recycling
Smog
Solid waste
Water pollution

Human concern about the environment and actions to protect it can be traced to the earliest recorded civilizations. The concept of burying human wastes and maintaining a sanitary environment can be found in the Law of Moses (Deuteronomy 23:12-13). As early as 3000 to 1000 BC, the Minoan civilization on the island of Crete disposed of solid wastes by burial in large pits, with layers of earth at intervals.

In a primitive society, on a sparsely populated Earth, the solutions were relatively simple. Nature's purification systems normally could maintain a suitable environment. Water was purified by distillation (evaporation), and the vapors were condensed and returned as rain, cleansing the air as it fell. Ground waters were cleaned by percolation through the soil. Plants and animals died, were decomposed by the action of microorganisms, and eventually returned to the soil to provide nutrients for new life. The elements of this dynamic purification and recycling system maintained a balance. As human population increased and technology advanced, however, nature's purification systems became overloaded. The problem of properly disposing of the products — especially the waste products — of human activity increased in magnitude as well as complexity.

With the advent of industrial societies, not only did the output of human activities increase with population growth (as one might expect), but because of the "progress" of technology, the output per person became greater. The increase in human productivity began to outpace even the dramatic increase in population. To complicate things still further, it has become increasingly apparent that advances in technology are a two-edged sword. On the one hand, useful products of modern technology have resulted in an increase in the standard of living of people throughout the world. On the other hand, that same technology has allowed human beings to use the Earth's resources in the creation of new and sometimes hazardous chemicals.

When the products of human activity enter the environment and affect it adversely, those products are referred to as **pollutants,** and we say that the environment has been polluted. Pollution can be defined as an undesirable change in the physical, chemical, or biological characteristics of the air, water, or land that can adversely affect the health, survival, or well-being of human beings or other organisms. The pollution or adverse environmental condition does not have to be one that causes direct physical harm. Excessive or unwanted noise can be considered pollution even though it may cause no physical injury and the most likely harm will be psychological stress. Similarly, a foul odor can be considered pollution even if its major offense is to the senses.

THE POPULATION EFFECT

It takes little imagination to visualize a correlation between population and the total amount of waste produced by all human activities. The greater the number of people, the greater the amount of waste. Human waste products — biological, chemical, or physical — if present in too great a quantity to be acceptably assimilated by the environment, become pollutants and affect our health or general well-being. As a result, any consideration of environmental issues that may impinge on the health of a community should take into account the **population effect.**

World population currently is estimated at a record level of about five billion. The population of the United States accounts for about one twentieth of the total. Both U.S. and world populations are growing but at substantially different rates. Changes in population depend on births, deaths, and migration (immigration and emigration). Numerical changes in total world population occur only as a result of the difference between births and deaths, whereas changes in population of a country (or city or any other unit of population) are also influenced by immigration and emigration as people move from place to place.

The average number of babies born (live births) worldwide is estimated to be about 249 per minute, or about 358,000 per day. Deducting the average number of deaths (100 per minute or 146,000 per day) leaves a net increase in human population of 212,000 persons per day. To illustrate the enormity of such a growth rate, it has been estimated that it takes fewer than five days to replace a number of persons equal to all Americans killed in U.S. wars and fewer than 12 months to replace the more than 75 million persons killed in the world's largest disaster — the bubonic plague epidemic of the fourteenth century (Miller, 1986).

As frightening as the magnitude of world population growth is, it is further complicated by the fact that the growth is occurring exponentially, or geometrically. The phenomenon of exponential growth can be dramatically illustrated in graphic form, plotting population versus time. The resulting graph is characterized by a distinctive shape that, for obvious reasons, is often referred to as a "J" curve (see Figure 29-1).

It took from the dim beginnings of human life until 1830 AD for the human population of the earth to reach one billion. Within 1 century the population doubled, reaching the 2 billion mark about 1930. Just 30 years later (1960), despite the devastating effect of a world war, the number of people reached 3 billion. The 4 billion mark was reached 15 years later (1975) and by 1987 the human population of the earth had reached 5 billion (Population Institute, 1991).

The 6 billion mark will probably be reached in 1995-96, as the words on this page are being read.

The dramatic growth in world population over the last century was due, not to a rise in

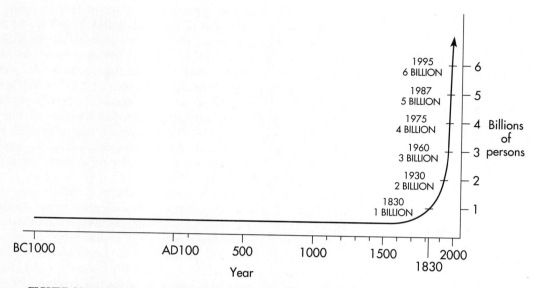

FIGURE 29-1   World population growth. The human population of the world is growing at a rate of about a quarter of a million people a day — and this rate is accelerating. (*Adapted from* The Population Institute's Annual Report *1991.*)

birth rates but rather to a decline in death rates, especially in the less developed countries. The reasons for the decline in death rates include the following (Miller, 1986):

1. An increase in food supplies because of improved agricultural production (partially attributable to the use of chemical pesticides — an environmental two-edged sword)

2. Better food distribution as a result of improved transportation

3. Better nutrition

4. Reduction of diseases associated with crowding — such as tuberculosis — because of better housing

5. Improved personal hygiene, including the use of soap, which reduces the spread of disease

6. Improved sanitation and water supplies, which reduce death rates from plague, cholera, typhus, dysentery, diphtheria, and other fatal diseases

7. Improvements in medical care and public health technology through the use of antibiotics, immunization, and insecticides

Concern for the effect of population growth on the environment usually focuses on the quantity of pollutants produced, that is, the more peo-

ple, the more pollution. There is, however, another dimension to the environmental effect of people. When the number of persons in a given space, whether it is a city or a planet or a meeting hall, reaches some undefined level of density, the environment becomes less desirable and is referred to in terms such as "crowded" or "congested," which have negative connotations.

A high-population density thus can produce a psychological, if not physiological, stress. In terms of the definitions of pollution and pollutants presented earlier, when population density is high enough, people per se become pollutants.

WASTE DISPOSAL AND DISPERSAL
Solid Waste

The disposal of solid waste probably is the earliest recognized form of environmental problem. Nowhere is the environmental maxim that "everything must go somewhere" more evident on a daily basis than in the simple act of carrying out the garbage. When this individual daily ritual is multiplied by the number of persons in a population center, the result can be a logistics problem of staggering proportions. New York City generates 27,750 tons of garbage a day. As staggering as that amount is, it represents but a small fraction of the total commercial, industrial, and domestic waste produced in the United States — estimated at more than 6 billion tons per year.

For regulatory purposes, the U.S. Congress (Resource Conservation and Recovery Act of 1976) has defined **solid waste** as any garbage, refuse, sludge (e.g., from a waste treatment plant), and other discarded material — including solid, liquid, semisolid, or contained gaseous materials resulting from industrial, commercial, mining, and agricultural operations — as well as waste from community activities (Hall, Watson, Davidson, Case, & Bryson, 1986). Within this broad definition, subcategories of hazardous waste and nonhazardous waste also have been defined.

The traditional methods of solid waste disposal include the open dump, the landfill, ocean dumping, and incineration, or some combination of these.

Open dump. The **open dump** is simply what the name implies, a land area in which garbage and other waste materials are deposited, and little consideration is given to the sanitary conditions of the site. Typically, such dump sites provide a breeding ground for rats, flies, roaches, and other scavengers. The action of such pests as vectors in transmitting communicable disease is well known. Air pollution and water pollution problems associated with open dumps have been common. The Resource Conservation and Recovery Act (1976), which requires that open dumps be closed or upgraded to landfills, prohibits the establishment of new open dumps.

Landfill. The **landfill** is an improved version of the open dump, in which wastes are covered intermittently with layers of earth to minimize air pollution and accessibility to rats, flies, and other vectors. If care is not taken in the location of a landfill, the potential exists for contamination of ground water and/or surface water because of run-off and leaching. In recent years the term *sanitary landfill* has been applied to landfills that have been located carefully so that the potential for ground water or surface water contamination is minimized and in which the waste typically is spread in thin layers and frequently compacted and covered with a layer of earth.

Modern landfills often incorporate systems to prevent ground water contamination and to monitor ground water quality. In the United States the landfill now is the major method of permanent disposal for nonhazardous wastes. Most of New York City's tremendous daily output of garbage is disposed of in a 3000-acre site — the world's largest landfill — on Staten Island. The Staten Island site, known as Fresh Kills, is not without its problems, however, and its future is uncertain. It rapidly is becoming a symbol of the problem of municipal garbage. It has been estimated that, within a dozen years or so, the piling of wastes at Fresh Kills will result in its becoming the highest point on the eastern seaboard south of Maine. It will rise 500 feet above the New York Harbor, half as high as the Chrysler Building and half again as high as the Statue of Liberty. Similar situations are found in most of the larger landfills around the country. They are becoming saturated.

Ocean dumping. Throughout much of history the oceans have been viewed as the ultimate sink, capable of absorbing an infinite amount of waste. The nations of the world have used the oceans as a disposal site for everything from garbage and sewage to toxic chemicals and radioactive waste. In the early part of this century the ocean dumping of municipal wastes was common in the coastal areas of the United States. In 1933 a U.S. Supreme Court decision, involving New York City, resulted in a prohibition of ocean dumping of municipal waste. However, ocean dumping of other forms of waste continued. The United States took another step forward in 1972 with the passage of the U.S. Ocean Dumping Act. Over the two decades since then, the volume of industrial wastes dumped into U.S. ocean waters has been reduced dramatically. The ocean dumping of sewage sludge (the effluent of sewage treatment plants) continues to increase. In 1973, according to the Environmental Protection Agency (EPA), about 7.9 million tons were dumped into U.S. waters (EPA, 1988).

Recent years have seen an increasing worldwide concern for the potentially harmful effects of indiscriminate ocean dumping. By 1975 some 54 nations, including all the major maritime nations, had agreed to stop the dumping of certain types of chemical, biological, and nuclear wastes into the ocean.

Despite the increasing concern and regulation, unacceptably high quantities of slowly degradable and nondegradable plastic products, toxic chemicals, and other potentially harmful substances still find their way to the ocean. The "safe" level, above which pollutants will cause serious harm to the oceanic food chain and to human beings who depend on it, is difficult to determine. It is known that some pollutants, such as polychlorinated biphenyls (PCBs) and certain toxic mercury compounds, can be biologically magnified in marine or fresh water food chains (see Figure 29-6). Considerable research into the complexities of ocean systems is necessary before an environmentally sound ocean dumping program will be possible. Nevertheless, future waste management strategies, in the United States and internationally, no doubt will include carefully regulated ocean dumping as one of several waste disposal options.

Incineration.   Until recently the open burning of wastes at home was commonplace. Typically it was carried out in fireplaces, leaf piles, rubbish heaps, and even crude backyard incinerators. Increasing concerns about air pollution have led to the banning of such backyard burning in many areas. The result, of course, has been an increase in the quantity of waste that must be collected and disposed of. The effect varies with location. In 1970 an ordinance banning backyard burning in Sacramento, California, was followed over the next year by a nearly 50% increase in solid waste collected (Tchobanoglous, Theisen, & Eliassen, 1977). Although crude, open burning, whether in the backyard or in an open dump (Figure 29-2), generally is banned, many metropolitan areas, as well as individual businesses, now use modern, highly efficient incineration

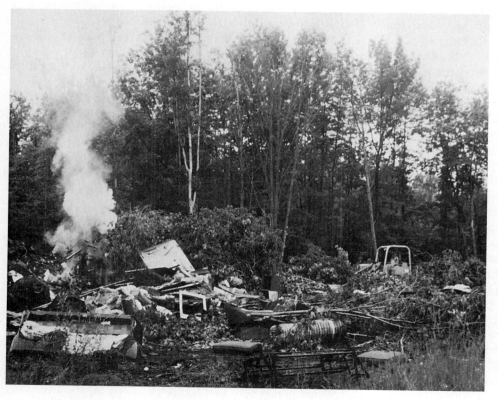

FIGURE 29-2   Burning of wastes in an open dump is banned in many communities.

techniques as an alternative or as a supplement to landfill disposal. **Incineration,** used as an adjunct to landfill, can reduce the volume of refuse by 90% or more and, as a result, considerably extend the useful life of a landfill. A modern incinerator is an efficient and a carefully engineered unit designed to maximize the combustion of solid waste while minimizing the emission of pollutants. A modern efficient incinerator, however, requires a high initial investment and is expensive to operate.

The high costs of incineration have led to the development and use of units that use the heat produced from the burning of refuse to generate steam and/or electricity that can be sold to nearby industries or to the local electrical utility (Figure 29-3). Critics of disposal by incineration have raised questions about environmental hazards associated with the emission of pollutants such as dioxins. Although zero emission of pollutants is not possible, many believe that incineration is the best available technology for disposing of many waste products.

The disposal of waste is further complicated by the difficulty of locating an acceptable site. Whether it is an incinerator or a landfill, "NIMBY" (not in my back yard) is a common community response. No one wants to live near a waste disposal facility, yet everyone needs to dispose of waste.

Recycling. Recycling is an environmental alternative to disposal. Most environmentalists advocate **recycling** as an environmentally acceptable method of reducing the disposal problem. It is becoming an increasingly attractive alternative as landfills become saturated. Many of the materials that currently are exhausting the capacity of our landfills can be recycled. Among them are paper, textiles, aluminum, glass, scrap iron and steel, rubber, and lubricating oils. A few states have passed mandatory recycling laws that require residents to separate their recyclable materials for collection at the curb, much like regular garbage collection. Thousands of smaller localities have started their own recycling programs. Nine states have enacted "bottle bills" that require pur-

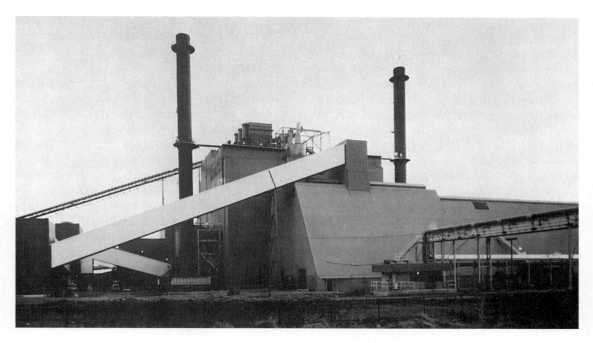

FIGURE 29-3 A modern energy from municipal waste facility. This plant has the capacity to incinerate more than 600,000 tons of municipal and household waste per year from which a steady supply of steam and electricity are produced.

chasers to pay a deposit on cans and bottles, to be refunded to them when the empty container is returned. The distributor then collects them and facilitates recycling. The aluminum industry recycles about 50% of the cans it produces. Recycled aluminum accounts for about a third of the raw material used.

Recycling has another major advantage. In most instances it takes considerably more energy to extract and refine virgin materials than to process recycled materials. For example, the use of recycled aluminum in cans results in a 96% energy savings.

Hazardous Waste

As though the sheer volume of waste produced by an affluent and growing U.S. population were not enough of an environmental problem, modern technology has provided a further complication — the production (and ultimately, the disposal) of **hazardous wastes.**

Radioactive waste. The advent of the nuclear era brought with it the production of nuclear power, nuclear weapons, and a new form of medicine, nuclear medicine. All these activities generated **radioactive waste** that must be processed and safely disposed of and stored. Much of the existing radioactive waste is stored temporarily in deep pools at nuclear plants or in underground tanks. Serious proposals for long-term disposal have included such locations as outer space, underground salt mines, on land beneath the Antarctic ice cap, and in the sediments of the deep ocean floor. As with other hazardous wastes, everyone wants it safely disposed of — somewhere else. Scientists continue to search for the best disposal plan, but the final solution is likely to be as strongly influenced by political as by scientific considerations.

Chemical waste. At the turn of the century the United States was heavily dependent on the importation of chemicals from Germany. The first World War broke that dependency, and a fledgling American chemical industry was spurred into growth. The second growth spurt came with World War II. The postwar period saw the emergence of the United States as a world leader in the manufacture of chemicals and in the creation of new chemicals and new materials. New pesticides, plastics, drugs, synthetic fabrics, coatings, detergents, and a host of other products appeared on the scene and became a part of everyday life. The chemical industry has helped to make possible the highest standard of living the world has known.

That is the good news. The bad news is that with every new pesticide, every new plastic, and every new chemical product comes a potential environmental health hazard from the product itself and from the chemical by-products of its production, from its disposal as **chemical waste,** and even from the use of the new product itself. By the late 1950s a few voices could be heard raising concerns about the potential environmental pollution from pesticides.

In 1962 Rachel Carson added her voice to the growing concern about our environment. Her book, *Silent Spring,* focused a nation's attention on the environment and, probably more than any other single event, triggered the environmental movement and an environmental awareness that continues to this day. In the years since, "Love Canal" and "Bhopal" have become a part of our vocabulary, and PCBs and methyl mercury have taken their place alongside *Streptobacillus* organisms and the poliomyelitis virus as disease-causing agents.

More than 4 million chemical compounds are known. Of these, it is estimated that more than 60,000 are produced commercially, with about 1000 new compounds being introduced each year (Department of Health, Education and Welfare, 1979). This output of the chemical industry produces the major portion of hazardous wastes. More than 90% of the hazardous wastes produced in the United States come from the chemical, petroleum, and metal-related industries (Miller, 1986).

Since World War II an estimated six billion tons of hazardous wastes have been generated in the United States. The improper and often illegal disposal of much of these hazardous wastes has created a series of what many environmentalists refer to as "chemical time bombs" — sites where improperly protected toxic wastes present a very real present or potential health hazard. The EPA

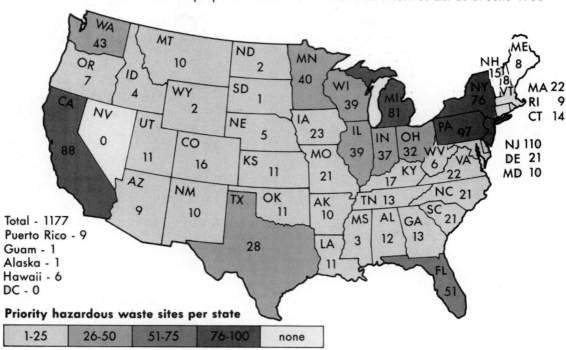

Numbers are actual and proposed sites on EPA's National Priorities List as of June 1988

Total - 1177
Puerto Rico - 9
Guam - 1
Alaska - 1
Hawaii - 6
DC - 0

Priority hazardous waste sites per state

| 1-25 | 26-50 | 51-75 | 76-100 | none |

FIGURE 29-4 Priority hazardous waste sites per state. Numbers represent actual and proposed sites on EPA's national priority list as of June 1988. *(From* National priority list, supplementary lists and supporting materials, *June 1988, by the Office of Emergency and Remedial Response (Superfund), 1988, Washington DC: U.S. Environmental Protection Agency.)*

has identified nearly 1200 sites as especially hazardous and has placed them on a national priorities list (Figure 29-4).

Hazardous wastes can become a threat to human health in various ways: direct exposure of persons at or near the disposal site or as a result of accidents during transport to the site; exposure to polluted air resulting from improperly controlled incineration; use of ground water or surface water that has become contaminated by leaching or run-off from waste-disposal sites; and consumption of food contaminated through biological magnification of toxic chemicals (see discussion later in this chapter).

The time interval between the disposal of a chemical in a waste-disposal site and the manifestation of adverse health effects can be divided into three phases (Grisham, 1986):

1. The time required for release across the site boundary

2. The time required for transport through the environment to the site where human exposure occurs

3. The latency period for the manifestation of human health effects

For some chemicals, in some situations, the time period may be extremely brief and may be measured in minutes or hours. In other instances, the time interval may be measured in years or decades — the "chemical time bomb." The following hypothetical "worst case" scenarios illustrate the difference between the two (Grisham, 1986):

1. The driver of a tank truck filled with waste acid arrives at the disposal site and inadvertently

drains the acid into a previously dumped cyanide salt mixture, which immediately reacts to form cyanide gas. In a few minutes the gas would be rapidly released into the air; the driver and others in the immediate area then might inhale significant quantities and become immediately, and possibly fatally, ill.

2. A buried drum containing hazardous chemical waste could, over a period of years, rust through, releasing the chemical into the ground, where it would then begin a slow process of migrating through the soil, beyond the disposal site, ultimately percolating into the ground water. If the chemical were not readily degradable and ground water flow rates were low, the chemical would migrate in the ground water for decades before being pumped out of the ground in drinking water. The latency period between human exposure and manifestation of disease might be extensive, such as for cancer or chronic liver or kidney damage.

The immediate harmful effects of many common chemicals have been long recognized. Arsenic and cyanides are poisonous; strong acids such as sulfuric or hydrochloric acid will burn human tissue, as will strong alkalis, such as sodium hydroxide (lye); ammonia gas will irritate the lungs. Recently, however, there has been a growing concern about the longer-range, and sometimes more subtle, effects of many chemicals. Some effects are difficult to detect or to measure, such as mental depression, birth defects, lowering of intelligence, or depressed immunity, which can, in turn, lead to other health effects that are still more difficult to relate to a source.

A chemical health hazard may not be apparent until substantial damage has occurred over a long period. In the area of a fishing village on Japan's Minamata Bay, between 1953 and 1960, a strange illness developed and spread among the population. More than 100 persons exhibited symptoms of brain and nerve damage; 19 babies were born with congenital defects; and more than 40 people died. The victims had been eating methyl mercury–contaminated fish from the bay; a plastics manufacturer had been dumping mercury wastes into the bay. Mercury poisoning

is now known as Minamata disease and has been diagnosed in other exposed populations.

The health hazards presented by many chemicals are by no means limited to the potential contact resulting from waste disposal. A very real health hazard may be encountered from chemicals contacted in a variety of ways: during the use of a common chemical for the purpose for which it was intended in the home, on the street, and in the workplace or in other environments that are a part of our everyday life. Solvents present in paints and varnishes, pesticide residues on fresh fruits and vegetables, and chemical food additives are but a few of the ways in which we are brought into contact with chemicals — often toxic chemicals — on a daily basis.

Some chemicals are resistant to degradation and will persist and spread throughout the environment until it is virtually impossible to avoid long-term, low-level exposure. The harmful effects of such exposure often are difficult to assess and are controversial even when acute effects from exposure to high concentrations are well known. The saga of PCBs probably is one of the best examples.

PCBs first were manufactured in the United States in 1929. They are a group of toxic, oily, synthetic organic chemical compounds that have been used in the production of plastics, paints, adhesives, hydraulic and heat transfer fluids, dust-control agents on roads, and a host of other industrial uses. Because of their particular electrical properties, they were used extensively as insulating and cooling fluids in electrical transformers and capacitors.

PCBs played a useful role, with little controversy or question about health effects for nearly 40 years. Then, in 1969, they were identified as the causative agent in an outbreak of a disease that afflicted some 1000 persons in southern Japan. The victims exhibited skin discoloration and scaling, severe acne, numbness, neuralgic pains, edema of the eyelids, and marked general weakness. Children born of mothers affected by the PCBs had PCBs in their blood, and some exhibited the same dark pigmentation and eye discharge that had been observed in adult victims. Of 13 recorded births to exposed mothers, 2 were stillborn and 10 showed the aforementioned symptoms. The victims of what has come to be known as the Yusho disease had eaten food cooked with a rice oil contaminated with PCBs.

In the early 1970s PCBs were found in cow's milk (and subsequently in human milk), many inland and ocean fish, most meats, and in the bodies of human beings. With the Toxic Substances Control Act (TSCA) of 1976, Congress banned the manufacture, processing, and distribution of PCBs except in totally enclosed electrical equipment. Since that time, although the total level of PCBs in food, human beings, and the environment has declined, the actual number of persons with at least trace levels of PCBs has increased. The EPA believes that virtually *all* Americans have PCBs in their bodies (Figure 29-5).

Despite environmental legislation the story of PCBs is by no means over. The EPA estimates that

sealed electrical transformers and capacitors still in use by utility companies contain some 750 million pounds of PCBs. Each year some will be released into the environment from leaking or exploding equipment. More than 250 million pounds have been disposed of in dumps and landfills or have been dispersed, often illegally on roadsides or other areas.

PCBs have been described as the "universal pollutant" (Holum, 1977). They are found in the tissue of marine microorganisms and have migrated upwardly through the food chain to fish and predatory birds, becoming concentrated in the process. Although they are relatively insoluble in water, they are soluble in fats and thus accumulate or are stored in fatty tissue, including human fat tissue. Fish feeding in PCB-contaminated waters often have levels of PCB 1000 to 100,000 times the level of that found in the sur-

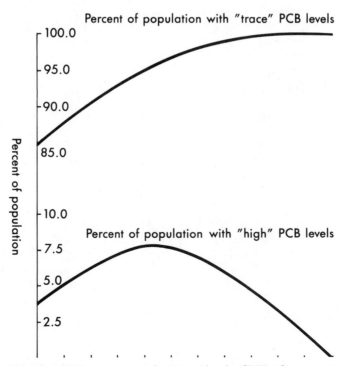

FIGURE 29-5   Although nearly everyone now has "trace" levels of PCBs, the percentage of population with "high" levels has gone down. *(From Office of Toxic Substances, 1988, Washington DC: U.S. Environmental Protection Agency.)*

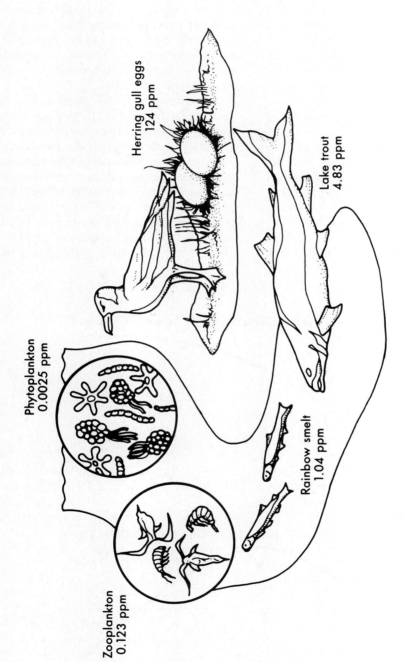

Phytoplankton
0.0025 ppm

Zooplankton
0.123 ppm

Herring gull eggs
124 ppm

Rainbow smelt
1.04 ppm

Lake trout
4.83 ppm

FIGURE 29-6 Persistent organic chemicals such as PCBs bioaccumulate and are magnified in the food chain. This diagram shows the degree of concentration in each level of the Great Lakes aquatic food chain for PCBs (in parts per million [ppm]). The highest levels are reached in the eggs of fish-eating birds such as gulls. *(From The Great Lakes, an environmental atlas and resource book, 1987, jointly produced by Environment Canada and the U.S. Environmental Protection Agency, Toronto and Chicago.)*

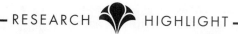

RESEARCH ✦ HIGHLIGHT

The Effect of Prenatal PCB Exposure on Visual Recognition Memory

A sample of 123 white, predominantly middle-class infants (69 males and 54 females) from Grand Rapids, Michigan, was selected for this study. The mothers were screened regarding their fish consumption habits, with 92 being fish eaters and 31 nonfish eaters. The fish eaters had consumed at least 11.8 kg of PCB-contaminated Lake Michigan fish over the six previous years. (PCBs accumulate in the body over time, exposing the fetus to risk from PCBs acquired both before and during pregnancy.) Data on infant feeding patterns were collected at two, four, five, and seven months, and infants were classified into five categories ranging from exclusively breast-fed to exclusively bottle fed.

At age seven months, each infant was tested in the laboratory while seated on the mother's lap in front of an observation chamber containing a pivoting stimulus presentation "stage" and administered Fagan's test of visual recognition memory (*Journal of Experimental Child Psychology, 16,* 1973, 424-

450). The test was administered by one of three examiners, who was blind with respect to fish consumption and biological measure of PCB exposure. Each infant was first exposed to a target photo simultaneously in left and right positions. After the infant fixated the target for a total of 20 seconds, the familiar target was paired with a novel target for two five-second recognition periods, reversing the left-right positions from one period to the next. Visual recognition was defined as the percent of total fixation paid to the novel target for each of the three pairs of targets.

The study suggests a possible relationship between prenatal PCB exposure and deficits in visual recognition memory at seven months in infants who appeared clinically normal at birth. The authors suggest that further research is needed to determine the potential of the test to predict long-term damage.

From "The effect of intrauterine PCB exposure on visual recognition memory" by S.W. Jacobson, G.G. Fein, J.L. Jacobson, P.M. Schwartz, & J.K. Dowler, 1985, *Child Development, 56,* pp. 853-860.

---

rounding water. This **biomagnification** continues upward through the food chain (Figure 29-6). Consumption of Great Lakes coho salmon caught in sport fishing has been noted as a significant source of chronic exposure to PCBs (Cordle, Locke, & Springer, 1982). Consumption of Lake Michigan fish has been correlated with PCB levels in human maternal serum and milk (Schwartz, Jacobson, Fein, Jacobson, & Price, 1983).

The long-term human health effects associated with chronic low-level exposure to chemical pollutants such as PCBs are difficult to assess. Recently, a new multiple-effects model has been proposed that emphasizes subtle behavioral alteration as an early sign of toxicity and as evidence that a particular chemical agent may produce long-term impairment in susceptible

persons (Fein, Schwartz, Jacobson, & Jacobson, 1983). In another study (Fein, Jacobson, Jacobson, Schwartz, & Dowler, 1984) it was found that babies born to women who consumed moderate quantities of PCB-contaminated Lake Michigan salmon or trout were smaller than infants in a controlled group.

WATER POLLUTION

Historically, the most serious community health problems associated with water supplies have been waterborne diseases such as typhoid, infectious hepatitis, cholera, and dysentery. In the United States, deaths from these diseases no longer are considered major health problems, but they still are common in many parts of the world. **Water pollution,** the entry of disease-causing bacteria and viruses into a water supply, most commonly occurs through human or animal feces. In the United States and other more developed countries, waterborne diseases are controlled by the purification of sewage in septic tanks or waste treatment plants before being released into the water supply. Although the level of treatment varies depending on the sophistication of the sewage plant, treatment typically includes removal of solids by filtration and sedimentation (primary treatment) and biological processing (secondary treatment). A few sewage plants add a highly sophisticated tertiary treatment stage to remove most of the remaining contaminants. Regardless of how many stages of treatment are employed, the final step is a disinfection process — treating the effluent with chlorine gas before its final discharge.

Measurements of water quality commonly rely on three indicators: (1) the concentration of dissolved oxygen (DO), (2) the biological oxygen demand (BOD), and (3) the fecal coliform bacteria count. Most aquatic animals and plants require oxygen. The DO is the amount of dissolved oxygen gas in a quantity of water at a particular temperature (20° C). At that temperature, at normal atmospheric pressure, the maximum concentration of DO is nine ppm, that is, nine parts of oxygen per million parts of water.

Organic matter in water is broken down by bacterial action. The amount of DO required for bacterial decomposition is expressed as the BOD as parts per million of DO consumed over a five-day period at 20° C and normal atmospheric pressure. When the BOD causes the DO content to fall below five ppm, the water is considered to be seriously polluted.

The water quality, for drinking and swimming purposes, is indicated by the number of colonies of fecal coliform bacteria present in a 100 ml sample of water. Water generally is considered safe to drink if it contains fewer than 10 coliforms per liter. In the United States water qualities are mandated by the Clean Water Act (for recreational waters) and the Safe Drinking Act.

Although the sewage treatment and purification may be carried to the point of producing drinkable water, the treated water is not sent directly into the immediate water supply. Instead it generally is discharged into a river, lake, or the water table and once again becomes a part of the natural water supply. When drinking water is taken from some new location, a further purification, which includes chlorination, takes place.

As a result of sewage treatment and drinking water treatment procedures commonly employed in the United States, the incidence of waterborne disease is low. There is concern, however, about the possible contamination of water supplies with some of the 60,000 commercially produced chemicals. Hundreds of synthetic organic chemicals have been identified in drinking water supplies around the United States. Even the chlorination of drinking water, which purifies the water by killing bacteria, may, at the same time, create another environmental hazard. It has been found that the chlorine reacts with organic compounds present in the water to form chloroform, a chemical known to be toxic in concentrated form (Grisham, 1986).

About half of all Americans rely on ground water as their source of drinking water; the remainder rely on surface water, that is, streams, rivers, lakes, and reservoirs as their source.

NOISE POLLUTION

Noise can be defined as any sound that is unwanted, disagreeable, or harmful to our well-being. It is a physiologic or psychologic stress. Noise is sound that has become a pollutant, making it **noise pollution.**

Sound consists of oscillations of atmospheric pressure that are caused by a vibrating object (sound source). It can be characterized or qualified in terms of frequency (pitch), measured in cycles per second or herz (Hz), and in terms of intensity on a scale called a decibel (dB) scale. On the decibel scale the softest sound that can be heard by human beings is given a value of 0 dB. Figure 29-7 shows the level of intensity (dB) of various common sounds. Because the scale is logarithmic, each 10-dB increase represents a tenfold increase in intensity. Thus a rise in intensity from 10 dB (rustle of leaves) to 40 dB (quiet radio) represents a thousandfold increase.

Noise pollution can be a physiologic or a psychologic stressor, or both, and can elicit a response ranging from mild irritation to pain or permanent hearing loss. Pain occurs at intensities

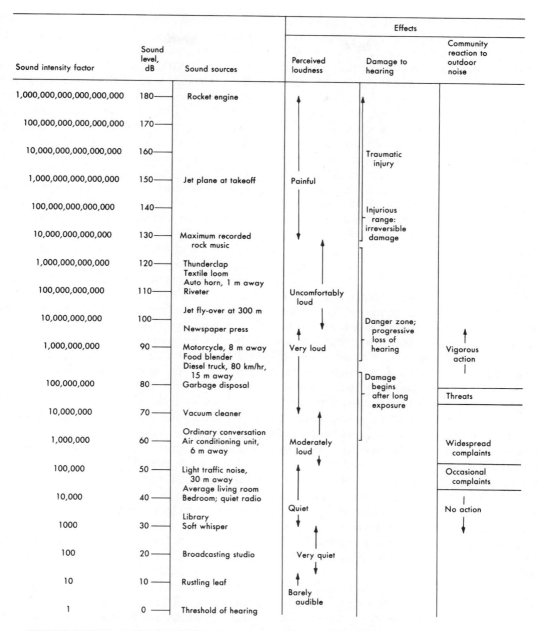

Sound intensity factor	Sound level, dB	Sound sources	Effects		
			Perceived loudness	Damage to hearing	Community reaction to outdoor noise
1,000,000,000,000,000,000	180	Rocket engine			
100,000,000,000,000,000	170				
10,000,000,000,000,000	160			Traumatic injury	
1,000,000,000,000,000	150	Jet plane at takeoff	Painful		
100,000,000,000,000	140			Injurious range: irreversible damage	
10,000,000,000,000	130	Maximum recorded rock music			
1,000,000,000,000	120	Thunderclap Textile loom Auto horn, 1 m away			
100,000,000,000	110	Riveter	Uncomfortably loud		
		Jet fly-over at 300 m			
10,000,000,000	100	Newspaper press		Danger zone; progressive loss of hearing	
1,000,000,000	90	Motorcycle, 8 m away Food blender Diesel truck, 80 km/hr, 15 m away	Very loud		Vigorous action
100,000,000	80	Garbage disposal		Damage begins after long exposure	Threats
10,000,000	70	Vacuum cleaner			
1,000,000	60	Ordinary conversation Air conditioning unit, 6 m away	Moderately loud		Widespread complaints
100,000	50	Light traffic noise, 30 m away Average living room			Occasional complaints
10,000	40	Bedroom; quiet radio	Quiet		No action
1000	30	Library Soft whisper			
100	20	Broadcasting studio	Very quiet		
10	10	Rustling leaf			
1	0	Threshold of hearing	Barely audible		

FIGURE 29-7 Sound levels and human responses. (*From* Environmental science *(pp. 536-37) by J. Turk & A. Turk, 1988, Philadelphia: W.B. Saunders. Copyright 1988 by W.B. Saunders Co. Reprinted by permission.)*

above approximately 120 dB and hearing loss from prolonged exposure at about 90 dB or above. Hearing loss may occur at lower decibel levels if exposure to the noise is continuous over a very long period.

Moderate levels of noise can cause irritability, fatigue, and a reduced ability to cope. Quantifying lower-intensity noise as a psychological stressor is difficult because the response is highly subjective. Cultural, social, and personal differences can affect an individual's perception of sound. What is music to one person may be noise (and thus a stressor) to another.

It is unlikely that, under normal circumstances, noise can be totally eliminated from one's environment. However, much can be done in the community and in the home to minimize or control noise. Noisy machinery often can be replaced by newer, quieter machinery. If this is not possible or practical, ear protection should be used. Traffic noise reaching a home from a busy highway can be lessened by an appropriately placed barrier of trees or shrubs. Noise transmission within a home can be minimized by the use of carpets and draperies and acoustical materials of construction.

AIR POLLUTION

The earliest form of human-induced **air pollution** probably came into existence when the first human beings learned to start a fire. However, the Earth was sparsely populated, and human ability to affect the quality and composition of the atmosphere was limited. It was not until human beings developed sufficient technology to give rise to the Industrial Revolution that large-scale air pollution from human activities became a problem. The advent of another technological triumph—the internal combustion engine—ushered in the age of the automobile, a new source of air pollution. In the United States, England, and other industrialized nations, laws and regulations limiting the discharge of soot and smoke into the atmosphere came into existence. Although the initial attempts at regulation were of limited effectiveness, they were an indication of a growing concern.

The United States experienced its first major air pollution disaster in 1948 when emissions from steel mills and other industrial facilities became trapped by a combination of topographic and weather factors (temperature inversion) in a stagnant air mass over Donora, Pennsylvania. The heavily polluted air remained stationary for 5 days, resulting in at least 20 deaths and more than 6000 illnesses.

In London, in 1952, an even more deadly air pollution disaster occurred, resulting in the death of some 4000 persons. These and other devastat-

ing episodes served to focus attention on the serious nature of air pollution and triggered efforts in the industrialized nations to find a solution.

In the United States a growing concern about the environment throughout the 1960s and specific concern about the health threat from air pollution resulted in the passage of the Clean Air Act of 1970. Under this act the EPA set air-quality standards for those common pollutants that posed the greatest overall threat to air quality across the country. Under the Clean Air Act, these pollutants, termed *criteria pollutants,* include ozone, carbon monoxide, airborne particulates, sulfur dioxide, lead, and nitrogen oxides (Table 29-1). Under the Clean Air Act the EPA also is required to set National Emission Standards for Hazardous Pollutants (NESHAPs). Hazardous pollutants are defined as those that can contribute to an increase in mortality or serious illness. Standards have been set for asbestos, beryllium, mercury, vinyl chloride, arsenic, radionuclides, benzene, and coke oven emissions (Table 29-1). Other air pollutants are being analyzed to determine whether they are hazardous and require regulation.

Between 1975 and 1986, federal air pollution control laws in the United States were a major factor in the reduction of the average levels of airborne particulates by 23%, sulfur dioxide by 37%, carbon monoxide by 32%, ozones by 13%, nitrogen dioxide by 14%, and lead by 87%.

As shown by the previous discussion, weather conditions can be critically important in the formation of a smog. Smogs (and fogs) commonly are associated with, or even caused by, an atmospheric condition known as a temperature inversion. The term refers to an "upside down" atmospheric condition. Normally, the atmosphere becomes colder with increasing altitude. In the case of a temperature inversion, a warm air layer forms aloft so that the air is colder at ground level. If there is no wind, the air mass is stationary and the warm air layer acts like a lid on the lower atmosphere, sealing in the cooler, lower air and preventing its escape by convection. The pollutants then are trapped near the ground level.

To alert the public to air quality and air pollution conditions, the EPA and other government

TABLE 29-1   Health effects of the regulated air pollutants

Criteria pollutants*	Health concerns
Ozone	Respiratory tract problems such as difficult breathing and reduced lung function
	Asthma, eye irritation, nasal congestion, reduced resistance to infection, and possibly premature aging of lung tissue
Particulate matter	Eye and throat irritation, bronchitis, lung damage, and impaired visibility
Carbon monoxide	Ability of blood to carry oxygen impaired
	Cardiovascular, nervous, and pulmonary systems affected
Sulfur dioxide	Respiratory tract problems; permanent harm to lung tissue
Lead	Retardation and brain damage, especially in children
Nitrogen dioxide	Respiratory illness and lung damage

Hazardous air pollutants†

Asbestos	A variety of lung diseases, particularly lung cancer
Beryllium	Primary lung disease, although also affects liver, spleen, kidneys, and lymph glands
Mercury	Several areas of the brain as well as the kidneys and bowels affected
Vinyl chloride	Lung and liver cancer
Arsenic	Causes cancer
Radionuclides	Causes cancer
Benzene	Leukemia
Coke oven emissions	Respiratory cancer

From *Environmental progress and challenges: EPA's update* (p. 13) by the Environmental Protection Agency, 1988, Washington, DC: Author.

* Criteria pollutants — those pollutants commonly found throughout the country that pose the greatest overall threat to air quality.

† Hazardous air pollutants — those pollutants that can contribute to an increase in mortality or serious illness.

agencies have developed a pollution standards index (PSI). The index (Table 29-2) uses a scale of 0 to 50 correlated with descriptive terms for air quality, expected health effects, and warnings.

The concentration of air-polluting sources in large cities, such as automobiles, trucks, airplanes, and factories, often in combination with the effect of local topography and weather, can create an extreme air pollution problem referred to as **smog** (derived from the words smoke and fog). Simply stated, smog refers to a situation in which the pollutants are present in such concentrations that visibility is reduced and eye and lung irritation is experienced. Despite the derivation of the word, neither smoke nor fog is a necessary ingredient but either or both may be present. Episodes of smog are a common phenomenon in large cities and highly industrialized areas.

The immediate health effects of smog are generally recognized and have been experienced by millions of city dwellers around the world. It is particularly harmful to elderly persons and to those who suffer from respiratory ailments. The fastest-growing cause of death in New York City in the late 1960s was emphysema. Its incidence rose 500% during that decade. During the same period the incidence of bronchitis rose 200% (Holum, 1977).

Children are especially vulnerable to air pollution. Children's airways are narrower than those of adults. As a result, air pollution that might produce only a slight response in an adult may cause a potentially significant obstruction in the airways of a small child. In addition, in response to a substantially higher need for oxygen relative to their size, children breathe more rapidly than adults. The result is the inhalation of more pollutants per pound of body mass than is the case with adults (Committee on Environmental Health, 1993).

As a concerned health professional, the community health nurse should (1) become informed about the specific air pollution problems of his or her community, (2) assume the role of environmental risk communicator, making clients

TABLE 29-2   Pollutant standards index—health effects information and cautionary statements

Psi	Air quality	Health effects	Warnings
0-50	Good		
51-100	Moderate		
101-200	Unhealthful	Mild aggravation of symptoms in suscep-tible persons, irritation symptoms in healthy population	Persons with existing heart or respiratory ailments should reduce physical exertion, outdoor activity.
First stage alert			
201-300	Very unhealthy	Significant aggravation of symptoms, decreased exercise tolerance in persons with heart or lung disease, widespread symptoms in healthy population	Elderly persons with existing heart or lung disease should stay indoors, reduce physical activity.
Second stage alert			
301-400	Hazardous	Premature onset of certain diseases, significant aggravation of symptoms, decreased exercise tolerance in healthy persons	Elderly persons with existing heart or lung disease should stay indoors, avoid physical exertion; general population should avoid outdoor activity.
Third stage alert			
401-500	Significant harm	Premature death of ill and elderly; healthy people experience adverse symptoms that affect normal activity	All persons should remain indoors, windows and doors closed; all persons should minimize physical exertion, avoid traffic.

From *Environmental science* (p. 636) by J. Turk & A. Turk, 1988, Philadelphia: W.B. Saunders. Copyright 1988 by W.B. Saunders Co. Reprinted by permission.

and the community in general aware of the health implications of air pollution, and (3) serve as an informed community advocate by expressing concern about health hazards of community air pollution to the appropriate state and federal legislators and officials.

RADIATION IN THE ENVIRONMENT

Radiation is energy radiated through matter or space in the form of particles or waves. For purposes of discussion and study, it generally is divided into two types: ionizing and nonionizing radiation.

Nonionizing radiation, which includes such forms of radiant energy as visible light, infrared, ultraviolet, microwaves, and radio waves, involves lower energy, which, as the name implies, does not produce ions. Possibly the most serious health threat from nonionizing radiation is from solar ultraviolet radiation, the principal cause of skin cancer in human beings. It is estimated that between 100,000 and 200,000 new cases of skin cancer occur per year in the United States. Notwithstanding such serious health hazards, public concern about radiation has focused primarily on ionizing radiation.

Ionizing radiation, which includes x-rays, gamma rays, alpha particles, and beta particles, is a high-energy radiation capable of dislodging electrons from the atoms it hits to form highly reactive charged particles called ions.

Until Roentgen's discovery of x-rays in 1895, all exposure to ionizing radiation came from natural sources. Scientific and technologic developments since then have resulted in a wide variety of human-induced radiation sources based on the application of x-rays and on the development and applications of nuclear energy. However, despite the advent of human-induced radiation sources, the natural background represents the largest source of radiation exposure, about 73% of the total (Mossman, Thomas, & Dritschilo, 1986). Most of the natural background radiation we are exposed to comes from cosmic rays (from outer space), from terrestrial radioactivity (such as in rocks and soil), and from internal sources (from natural radioactive materials present in our air, water, and food). Cosmic rays are estimated to account for about 15% of the total natural background radiation. These radiations are extraterrestrial; that is, they originate in outer space, primarily from galactic sources. Because they must pass through the Earth's atmosphere, their intensity will depend, in part, on altitude. Thus exposure to such radiation would be higher in Denver (altitude, 5000 feet) than in New York City (sea level). Additional cosmic ray exposure, although slight, will occur during air travel; the dose rate from cosmic rays at 35,000 feet is about 100 times higher than at sea level. The risk associated with flying 6000 miles by jet increases by one part in one million the chances of death as a result of cancer caused by cosmic radiation (Table 29-3).

The principal source of natural background radiation is from **radon,** a radioactive gas formed in rocks and soil. Recently there has been considerable concern over the threat of death from radon-associated lung cancer. Because radon concentration is relatively low in outdoor air and high in indoor air, it is described in the section on indoor pollution.

TABLE 29-3 Risks that increase the chance of death by one part in one million

Activity	Cause of death
Smoking 1.4 cigarettes	Cancer, heart disease
Drinking one-half liter of wine	Cirrhosis of the liver
Spending 1 h in a coal mine	Black lung disease
Spending 3 h in a coal mine	Accident
Living 2 days in New York or Boston	Air pollution
Traveling 6 min by canoe	Accident
Traveling 10 mi by bicycle	Accident
Traveling 300 mi by car	Accident
Flying 1000 mi by jet	Accident
Flying 6000 mi by jet	Cancer caused by cosmic radiation
Living 2 months in Denver on vacation from New York	Cancer caused by cosmic radiation
Living 2 months in average stone or brick building	Cancer caused by natural radioactivity
One chest x-ray taken in a good hospital	Cancer caused by natural radiation
Living 2 months with a cigarette smoker	Cancer, heart disease
Eating 40 tablespoons of peanut butter	Liver cancer caused by aflatoxin B
Drinking Miami drinking water for 1 year	Cancer caused by chloroform
Drinking 30 12-oz cans of diet soda	Cancer caused by saccharin
Living 5 years at site boundary of a typical nuclear power plant in the open	Cancer caused by radiation
Drinking 1000 24-oz soft drinks from recently banned plastic bottles	Cancer from acrylonitrile monomer
Living 20 years near a polyvinyl chloride plant	Cancer caused by vinyl chloride (1976 standard)
Living 150 years within 20 mi of a nuclear power plant	Cancer caused by radiation
Eating 100 charcoal-broiled steaks	Cancer from benzopyrene
Living within 5 mi of a nuclear reactor for 50 years	Cancer caused by radiation

Man-made radiation sources include medical x-rays or medical applications of radioactive substances, fallout from nuclear weapons testing, emissions from nuclear power plants, and a variety of very low-level sources classified as consumer products, including wrist watches, color television receivers, and smoke detectors.

The largest source of human-induced radiation exposure is from medical and dental x-rays used in the diagnosis and treatment of disease. In the United States it is estimated that more than two thirds of the population receive diagnostic medical examinations or dental x-rays or both each year. The health effects of high doses of radiation are well known. The largest single source of data is from studies of the survivors of the atomic bombings of Hiroshima and Nagasaki in World War II. At the high levels of exposure involved, a significant number of excess cancers have been documented. There are, however, considerable difficulties in applying the data from such studies to determine health risks from low-level exposures. Mossman et al. (1986) have estimated that less than 2% of all cancer deaths may be attributable to ionizing radiation, the greatest portion of which (73%) is from natural background radiation. (See Table 29-3 for a comparison of the risk of death associated with several types of radiation exposure with other environmental or lifestyle related risks.)

ENVIRONMENTAL DISASTERS

It takes people to make a disaster. The San Andreas fault became a potential disaster site only after San Francisco and other communities moved toward the fault and built across it. Similarly, a chemical waste site may become a disaster location only when people move to the site. As the population increases, so does the likelihood that a hazardous area will become a disaster site (Cookfair, 1981).

Environmental disasters can be natural or human-induced. They may occur with the suddenness of an explosion or the slow pace of toxic chemicals seeping through soil. A contrast in disaster characteristics may be seen in the comparison of two recent human-induced chemical disasters — Love Canal and Bhopal.

Love Canal is probably the most highly publi-

cized chemical waste site disaster to occur in the United States. It began with the dumping of waste chemicals into an abandoned canal nearly a half century ago. Between 1942 and 1952, 21,800 tons of waste chemicals were dumped into the canal. The site was sealed with a clay cap, and for nearly a quarter of a century the hazards buried there seemed all but forgotten as roads, an elementary school, a children's playground, and hundreds of homes were constructed on and around the site. In the mid-1970s, after unusually heavy precipitation, chemical wastes began to surface and to infiltrate into residential basements (New York State Department of Health, 1981). Among the residents there were complaints of unusually high numbers of birth defects, miscarriages, and cancers. The following months and years brought fear, heightened by reports and studies of migrating toxic chemicals and health hazards, fanned by the media, and compounded by a confused societal response. The fear of toxic chemicals, the disruption of lives, the economic instability as the value of homes in the area plummeted, and the mass relocation of hundreds of people all contributed to what may ultimately be the greatest tragedy of Love Canal — the psychological stress imposed on the victims.

Numerous health studies were undertaken from 1978 to 1984 with varying results and a general lack of coordination. The New York State Department of Health reported a "slight increase" of miscarriages and low birth weight infants associated with one section of the Love Canal neighborhood (New York State Department of Health, 1981). Analysis of blood tests found that residents of some areas, closest to the canal, may face a greater-than-expected risk of liver disease. However, the study also found that none of the individuals with abnormal test results, who subsequently were examined by their physicians, showed any clinical evidence of liver disease. In addition, it was found that the liver functions returned to normal once residents relocated away from the Love Canal neighborhood (Silverman, 1989).

No definitive study has determined the health effects of exposure to chemicals at Love Canal. Those studies that were undertaken have been criticized on various scientific grounds. No deaths appear to be attributable to chemical exposure at Love Canal, and it will take years to determine long-term health effects. Even if the physical health effects to former residents are minimal, the psychological damage still may be great. Those affected will live out their lives in fear of latent chemical effects on them, their children, or their grandchildren.

Other disasters are less subtle in their approach. Late on the evening of Sunday, December 2, 1984, the contents of a chemical storage tank in Bhopal, India, began to rise in temperature, gradually at first. Some time after midnight, driven by a runaway chemical reaction, the tank became dangerously hot and the pressure rose rapidly and uncontrollably. The result was the release of 80,000 pounds of highly volatile, highly toxic methyl isocyanate (MIC) gas. It quickly spread as a foglike cloud over the large, densely populated shanty-town neighborhoods near the plant. Many residents died in their beds while others awoke to choking pain and panic. They tried to run from the cloud but were blinded and choked by the gas and died moments later in the streets. The number of dead still is in question. The Indian government estimates the death toll at about 2300, but other estimates range as high as 10,000. The lower number is based on available records from hospitals and burial grounds; the higher estimate is from such data as the number of death shrouds sold in Bhopal in the days that followed. Estimates of those injured range from 10,000 to 200,000, many of them left with permanent respiratory ailments and vision impairment.

M.N. Nagoo, the Madhya Pradesh director of medical services and one of the many physicians who rushed to the disaster site, described the scene in the following words (Lepkowski, 1985, p. 19):

I tell you, the morning of December 3 was a sight. People running away from Bhopal, volunteers coming in with needed supplies, schoolboys and girls looking after victims, giving them water, tea, bread. I think 70,000 could have died if we hadn't had the right medicines on hand.

Initially 170,000 persons were treated, out of which 11,500 were critically ill and hospitalized. The rest were put in tents or sheds. With the help of volunteer organizations, scouts, students, we organized medical treatment and arranged for water, medicines, and food. There was tremendous cooperation. We have 500 doctors here now, five major hospitals, 22 clinics, and we called 500 more doctors from the outside, plus 200 more nurses and 700 paramedics. Besides the treatment in hospitals, we organized 25 teams of doctors to give treatment in the affected areas.

The state already had enough drugs like cortisone, bronchial dilators, antibiotics, and Lasix (to combat edema). These were the basic ones we used. Then we got a lot of equipment and oxygen from the government of India and neighboring districts. Great Britain, France, and West Germany airlifted respirators and ventilators to us.

We have kept six clinics open around the clock, besides the 35 units already working and the 30-bed hospital we started at the former residence of the police superintendent next to the Union Carbide plant. Seven more clinics have been opened, four of which perform blood and urine tests.

Clinics in Bhopal continue to treat the victims, most of them suffering from lung or eye damage. Among the survivors, possibly thousands are totally or partially blinded.

Love Canal and Bhopal are human-induced disasters, and by hindsight, they may be viewed as tragedies that need not have occurred. Nevertheless, other human-induced disasters will occur, and together with natural disasters, such as floods, tornadoes, earthquakes, and blizzards, they form a part of the environmental health concerns that health professionals can expect to deal with on both a short-term, immediate basis and a long-term basis.

Many communities and many hospitals have considered the possibility of disaster occurrence and have formulated some plan for response. The success of any response to disaster is likely to depend heavily on nursing action. But the disaster itself may disrupt the best laid plans.

Hurricane Andrew reached the Miami area about midnight on Sunday, August 23, 1992. During the hours before, many nursing home residents were moved to hospitals and radio bulletins advised pregnant women who were within 6 weeks of delivery to stay overnight in a hospital. Temporary facilities were set up to handle the overload. Nurses and other hospital person-

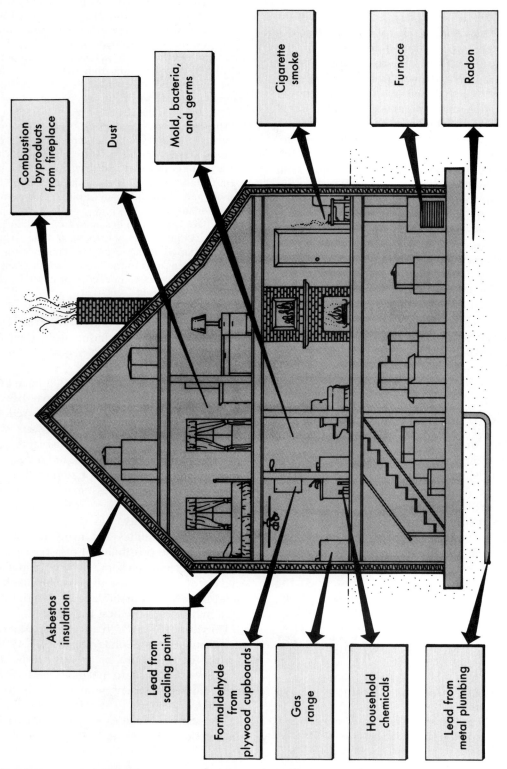

FIGURE 29-8 Sources of pollution in the home.

nel volunteered for hurricane duty, reporting for work with pillows and blankets, prepared to stay as long as needed. The community braced itself for the onslaught; daylight became night and night became nightmare as the hurricane struck.

Throughout the night, winds of up to 160 miles per hour pounded the area, flattening buildings, destroying telephone lines, and disrupting transportation, communication, and power and water supplies. In one hospital, seven babies were delivered by flashlight. In another, with the failure of a backup electrical generator, nurses used breathing bags to manually respirate patients for 12 hours.

The following morning Hurricane Andrew headed west leaving behind crippled or closed hospitals and nursing homes and 250,000 people homeless — many of them nurses and other hospital personnel. One hospital (Baptist Hospital) estimated that at least half of its 3200 employees were among those left homeless.

As devastating as the night was, the worst was yet to come. During the days that followed, many of the facilities normally taken for granted simply were not there. Power outages meant no air-conditioning — during the hottest season of the year — as temperature rose above 90° F. In some areas water was unavailable. Without water, toilets could not be flushed, and nurses could not wash their hands while feeding babies and changing diapers. In one hospital, for 4 days water was brought from nearby swimming pools to be poured down toilets to provide a flushing action. What water was available was declared unsafe for drinking, bathing, or even washing hands (Mallison, 1992). In addition to the devastation of hospitals, hundreds of physician's offices, clinics, pharmacies, dialysis centers, and other health care facilities were demolished. The emergency rooms, still operating, were overloaded with patients experiencing pulmonary and cardiac problems, asthma attacks, and injuries such as chain-saw accidents as people worked under trying conditions to repair ruined houses (American Journal of Nursing, 1992).

Nurses from around the state and across the country came in as volunteers. Twelve tent cities were set up to house the thousands of homeless. Military nurses and medical personnel were brought in to reinforce the Red Cross nurses and other volunteers that were operating clinics in the tent cities. In the weeks that followed, the Red Cross sent out a call for volunteers who could make a 3- to 6-week commitment. A total of 370 professional nurses were brought in as Red Cross volunteers. Hurricane Andrew has since been characterized as the worst natural disaster ever to strike the United States.

When major disaster strikes, the local health services are often strained to the utmost and unable to provide the health services needed. Outside health services, especially nurses, are required to help the disaster victims. The Disaster Health Services (DHS), a component of the American Red Cross Disaster Services, provides a vehicle for organizing health care providers, on a volunteer basis, to respond to the needs of disaster victims. The Red Cross maintains a roster of more than 1100 professional nurses that can be called on as volunteers and provides a sequence of courses in Disaster Health Services to prepare them. In addition, when disaster actually strikes, a call for help will generally result in many more nurses adding their names to the volunteer roles.

POLLUTION IN THE HOME

Because a concerned society has reacted to the need to improve the quality of our environment, factory emissions, toxic wastes, automobile exhaust, and a host of other environmental hazards have been regulated. The quality of the environment we share has been noticeably improved. However, regulatory agencies in the United States are reluctant to intrude into the privacy of citizens' homes in the cause of pollution control.

Even if it were acceptable to regulate the home environment — to set permissible limits on the concentrations of pollutants as is done in occupational settings — it would be next to impossible to monitor and enforce compliance. As a result the health hazards posed by pollution in homes often are in excess of those in the outside environment or even in industrial settings. The problem is compounded by the fact that most people spend most of their time at home. Figure 29-8 shows the source of many indoor pollutants.

Some significant indoor pollutants are included in the following list:

1. *Carbon monoxide* is released by unvented gas stoves, kerosene space heaters, wood stoves, and tobacco smoke. It is a tasteless, colorless, odorless, poisonous gas that can react with hemoglobin in the blood and inhibit the distribution of oxygen by the bloodstream. A smoke-filled room with levels of about 120 ppm of carbon monoxide can cause headaches, dizziness, and a general feeling of dullness. It is known that carbon monoxide can cross the placenta in pregnant women and is believed to be a factor in the lower average birth weight of women who smoke. Approximately 1400 people die annually in the United States from carbon monoxide poisoning, most caused by unvented space heaters.

2. *Asbestos particles* (especially in older homes) are released from fireproofing materials, insulation, ceiling tiles, floor tiles, and other building materials. Asbestos is a generic name for several types of naturally occurring fibrous mineral silicates that were used in industry and construction. All commercial forms have been shown to be carcinogenic to human beings (Leman, Dement, & Wagoner, 1980). Epidemiologic studies have focused strongly on exposures in occupational settings. Asbestos insulation, however, has been used in a large number of residences, as well as in public buildings such as schools. Normal aging and deterioration, as well as demolition or remodeling of these structures, will release asbestos fibers into the air where they can be inhaled into the lungs.

3. *Formaldehyde* is a colorless gas, characterized by a strong, pungent odor. It is released in the home environment from particle boards, fiberboards, plywood, and other wood products, as well as from urea-formaldehyde foam insulation. It is strongly suspected as a carcinogen. Exposure to **formaldehyde** in concentrations in the range of 0.01 to 30 ppm in air has been observed to produce eye, nose, and respiratory tract irritation, headaches, drowsiness, nausea, and diarrhea. An excess of 100 ppm has been characterized as extremely hazardous and possibly fatal. (Committee on Indoor Pollutants, 1981).

4. *Nitrogen oxides* are released indoors from unvented gas stoves and space heaters. At concentrations of 0.05 ppm or higher, not unusual in kitchens where gas is used for cooking, nitrogen dioxide may affect sensory perception and produce eye irritation.

5. *Environmental tobacco smoke* is one of the most familiar indoor pollutants and the major source of indoor airborne particulate matter. In addition to particulates, tobacco smoke contains a variety of other contaminants such as inorganic gases, heavy metals, and various volatile organic compounds, including benzene. It has been well publicized that the person who chooses to smoke greatly increases the risk of the development of heart disease or cancer. Now, however, concern for the health threat of tobacco smoke has been extended to nonsmokers.

   The surgeon general has indicated that environmental tobacco smoke — that is, smoke that nonsmokers are exposed to from smokers — poses a risk of lung cancer to the nonsmoker. The EPA states that published risk estimates of lung cancer deaths among such involuntary smokers range from 500 to 5000 per year.

6. *Radon,* which is a colorless, odorless, radioactive gas, is the most serious health threat of the common indoor pollutants. In a survey of 9600 homes in 10 states, the EPA found that 20% are contaminated by potentially health-threatening levels of radon gas. The EPA estimates that radon is responsible for 5000 to 20,000 deaths from lung cancer each year (Table 29-4). According to one estimate (Nero, 1988) hundreds of thousands of Americans are living in houses that have high radon levels, and they receive as large an exposure of radiation yearly as those people living in the vicinity of Chernobyl nuclear power plant did in 1986, when one of its reactors exploded and released radioactive material into the environment.

   Radon gas decays to form submicroscopic solid particles called *radon daughters* (actually

TABLE 29-4 Radon risk evaluation chart

pCi/1	WL	Estimated lung cancer deaths due to radon exposure (out of 1000)	Comparable exposure levels	Comparable risk
200	1	440-700	1000 times average outdoor level	More than 60 times nonsmoker risk
100	0.5	270-630	100 times average indoor level	4 pack-a-day smoker
40	0.2	120-380		2000 chest x-rays per year
20	0.1	60-210	100 times average outdoor level	2 pack-a-day smoker
10	0.05	30-120	10 times average indoor level	1 pack-a-day smoker
4	0.02	13-50		5 times nonsmoker risk
2	0.01	7-30	10 times average outdoor level	200 chest x-rays per year
1	0.005	3-13	Average indoor level	Nonsmoker risk of dying of lung cancer
0.2	0.001	1-3	Average outdoor level	20 chest x-rays per year

From Office of Air and Radiation Programs, 1987, Washington, DC: U.S. Environmental Protection Agency.

NOTE: Measurement results are reported in one of two ways: measurement of *radon gas* (pCi/1) or measurement of *radon decay products* (WL).

pCi/l, Picocuries per liter; *WL,* working levels.

forms of polonium, a radioactive metal). The solid "daughter" particle, possibly riding piggyback on a dust particle, can become lodged in the lung and continue to emit radiation. Radon is a natural decay product of uranium and is found in limestone, black shale, and phosphate rock. Most indoor radon comes from rocks and soil around a building and may enter through microscopic cracks and joints in the basement walls.

Testing a home for radon can be fairly simple and relatively inexpensive. Do-it-yourself test kits can be purchased for as little as $10 to $25. Homes with elevated radon levels can be made safe by the use of fairly simple procedures, generally involving ventilation, for a moderate sum, generally about $500 to $1000.

7. *Lead,* a useful and easily worked metal that has been mined and used since antiquity, is now high on the list of recognized environmental health hazards found in the home. It has no known physiological benefits, but its recognized toxic effects are considerable (Pruess, 1993). In the home, recognized sources of **lead poisoning** include lead-based paint, dust, soil, food, and drink-

ing water (Weitzman, Aschengrau, Bellinger, Jones, Hamlin, & Beiser, 1993).

Before the 1970s, gasoline vapor containing organo-lead anti-knock additives was a major source of environmental lead. In the United States, in 1975, environmental concern prompted a government mandate that automobile engines be designed to use unleaded gas. Later in that decade, a second major source of environmental lead was attacked. In 1978, the residential use of lead-based paint was prohibited. Despite these major regulatory efforts, which did, in fact, reduce the lead hazard substantially, some of the deleterious effects from these sources remain. Nearly three fourths of all housing built before 1980 contains lead-based paint, and dust and soil in many areas is still heavily contaminated by the residue of lead-based paint or leaded gasoline used in the past (Weitzman et al., 1993).

The toxic effects of lead are a hazard to all age groups. However, as with other toxins, children are particularly vulnerable (see Figure 29-9). Because of their smaller size and body mass, the in-

☐ Effects in children generally occur at lower blood lead levels than in adults.

☐ The developing nervous system in children can be affected adversely at blood lead levels of less than 10 μg/dl.

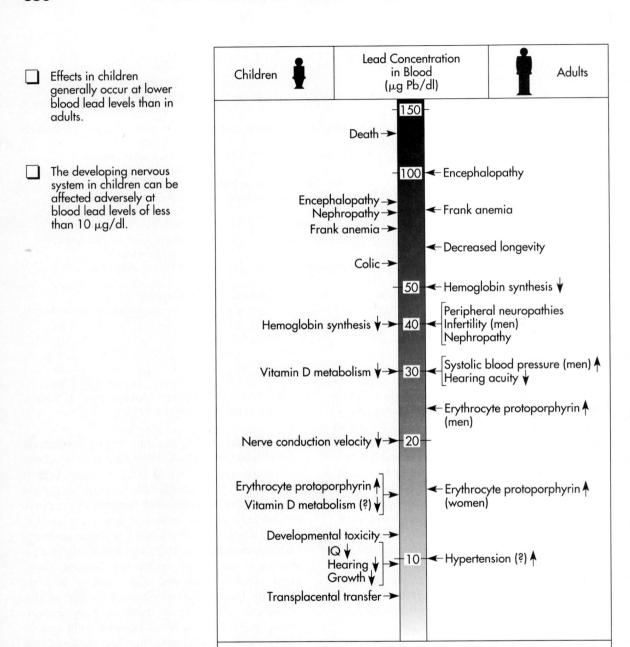

FIGURE 29-9   Effects of inorganic lead on children and adults — lowest observable adverse effect levels. *(From Case studies in environmental medicine: Lead toxicity, 1992, by agency for Toxic Substances and Disease Registry, Public Health Services, U.S. Department of Health and Human Services.)*

gestion of a given amount of lead will result in a higher proportion of lead per unit of body weight than in an adult. Furthermore, by virtue of their activities (crawling, putting objects or materials into their mouths), children are more likely to be exposed through ingestion of paint chips, lead-contaminated soil, and the like.

Despite long-standing concern for the risk of leaded paint, deteriorated housing with accessible leaded paint still causes a significant risk to large numbers of children. Despite considerable effort and education, many people are still unaware of the dangers of exposure to leaded paint (Friedman & Weinberger, 1990). It is a goal of the U.S. Department of Health and Human Services (1992) to eliminate lead poisoning as a public health problem. However, efforts to treat lead poisoning after the fact are controversial. Emphasis should be on a proactive program, for example, educating a community to the hazards and sources of lead to which they and, more importantly, their children, might be exposed. An aggressive program, especially in high-risk populations, should include well-child examinations to determine hemoglobin and blood lead levels. The detection of lead poisoning in such examinations should trigger an immediate response on two levels: first, an evaluation of the need for special treatment of the individual, such as chelation therapy; and second, investigation and elimination of the environmental cause.

NURSING INTERVENTIONS

Community health nurses have as a priority goal the prevention of illness in individuals, families, and groups. An assessment of the stressors in a community that affect the health status of the population must include the environment. The interventions then can be planned that prevent a potential problem from becoming an actual one.

Primary prevention involves anticipating and acting in advance of a health problem. Typically, this includes health education to raise the level of awareness in the community of the potential effect of an environmental stressor.

In a world of increasing concern for environmental hazards, the community health nurse must, when needed, assume the role of environmental risk communicator. The need for such a role was demonstrated when it was found that more than 40% of the persons surveyed in New York State did not know where to go for additional information about indoor radon risks (Boyle & Haltgrave, 1989; Kessler & Levine, 1987). Environmental health education of the individual and the community must stress increased environmental awareness, as well as elimination of unwarranted environmental fears.

Secondary prevention focuses on the detection of existing health problems for the individual and the community and the ability to respond with early treatment. For individual clients it may include screening and early diagnosis of specific environmental health problems. For example, in communities where asbestos insulation of buildings is common, it may include screening of individual clients for lung cancer and asbestosis and providing treatment as needed. On a community level, secondary prevention might be exemplified by a study to seek out the presence of asbestos insulation in buildings and to initiate remedial action where appropriate.

Tertiary prevention emphasizes rehabilitation and help in the development of an optimal level of functioning. For example, in the case of children suffering from mental retardation or brain damage from lead poisoning, tertiary prevention might involve a special education program to maximize the child's intellectual development. On the community level it might involve an abatement program to "delead" the community.

Application of the Nursing Process

The following case study illustrates the use of the nursing process with a child whose diagnosis was lead poisoning.

■ **CASE STUDY**

Assessment. A community health nurse was referred by a lead-screening clinic to make a home visit on a 3-year-old boy who had been tested for lead levels in his blood. His levels had been abnormally high, and he was considered at high risk for lead poisoning (plumbism), as well as a possible candidate for chelating therapy.

The nurse noted that the house was old, situated in a run-down neighborhood, and did not seem well maintained. The child lived in a second-floor apartment with his mother, a single parent. The apartment was clean but sparsely furnished. The mother was 18 years old, having given birth to the boy at the age of 15 years. She stated that she received some help from her mother and sister but that she lived alone and maintained her household with some help from social services.

The nursing assessment included a tour of the home. There was a hole in the wall in the boy's bedroom, approximately 1½ feet in diameter. Plaster was falling on the floor. As the nurse watched, the child picked up a small piece and ate it. The mother told him to stop but did not move to halt the behavior. The mother stated that the child was hyperactive and difficult to discipline. Results of a Denver Developmental Screening Test showed him to be within normal developmental stages. However, he did have difficulty sitting still even if bribed with treats and encouraged to coop-

erate by making a game of the test. A revisit was scheduled for the following week. The mother was asked to sweep up the plaster and call her landlord to fix the wall.

Nursing diagnosis. On the basis of this assessment, the nurse formulated the following nursing diagnosis:

1. Potential for lead poisoning related to unsafe environment
2. Ineffective family coping related to parental knowledge deficit

Planning and implementation. Nursing goals included the following:

1. Arranging for a safe environment for the child
2. Teaching the parent the importance of maintaining a safe environment for the child
3. Teaching the parent appropriate methods of controlling the child's behavior
4. Arranging for follow-up screening to determine the child's lead level

Evaluation. Facilitating the repair of the wall in the child's room became the role of the municipal housing authority. The landlord did not respond to calls from the parent or the nurse. In the meantime the nurse showed the child's mother how to use a plastic paste to repair the wall temporarily.

Chapter Highlights

- The growth of industry in society created a greater number and variety of waste products in the environment.

- The disposal of solid waste may be accomplished through open dumps, landfills, ocean dumping, or incineration.

- Recycling of wastes offers the advantages of reducing the total amount of waste to be disposed of and preserving virgin materials.

- Hazardous wastes include radioactive and chemical wastes. Since these wastes are health hazards, proper disposal is critical.

- The latency period between disposal of hazardous waste and the manifestation of adverse health effects may be extremely short, or it may take many years. The effects of many chemicals may be subtle and difficult to detect.

- Water pollution is a serious community health concern because contaminated water may carry bacteria and viruses associated with diseases such as typhoid, infectious hepatitis, chlorea, and dysentery.

- Excessive noise in the environment can lead to permanent hearing loss, as well as general feelings of stress and fatigue.

- Air pollution is a serious health hazard, especially in large, industrialized cities. Weather conditions also can affect the amount of pollution in the air.

- Environmental accidents may occur quickly or very slowly. They are disasters when they occur in heavily populated areas.

- Pollution in the home is difficult to monitor and regulate. Potential indoor air pollutants include carbon monoxide, asbestos, formaldehyde, nitrogen oxides, tobacco smoke, radon, and lead.

 CRITICAL THINKING EXERCISE

It is a hot day in July in a community where heavy industry is prevalent. A community health nurse becomes concerned when the weather reports tell of a temperature inversion with a resultant strong increase in air pollution.

1. Using the material in the chapter, list the types of clients the nurse should call.
2. Write a list of the guidelines that might be given to those clients. What special advice should the nurse offer to parents of small children?

REFERENCES

Agency for Toxic Substances and Disease Registry. (1992). *Case studies in environmental medicine: Lead toxicity.* Washington, DC: U.S. Department of Health and Human Services. *American Journal of Nursing.* (1992). News: Hurricane Andrew puts Florida's hospitals to the test, October, Author.

Binder, S., & Matte, T. (1993). Childhood lead poisoning: The impact of prevention. *Journal of the American Medical Association, 269*(13), 1679-1681.

Boyle, M., & Holtgrave, D. (1989). Communicating environmental health risks. *Environmental Science and Technology, 23,* 1335-1337.

Committee on Environmental Health (1993). Ambient air pollution: Respiratory hazards to children. *Pediatrics 91*(6), 1210.

Committee on Indoor Pollutants. (1981). *Indoor pollutants.* Washington, DC: National Academy Press.

Cookfair, A.S. (1981). Charles H.V. Ebert: Courting disaster. *SciQuest, 54*(6), 18-20.

Cordle, F., Locke, R., & Springer, J. (1982). Risk assessment in a federal regulatory agency: An assessment of risk associated with the human consumption of some species of fish contaminated with polychlorinated biphenyls (PCBs). *Environmental Health Perspectives 45,* 171-182.

Department of Health, Education and Welfare. (1979). *Healthy people,* Washington, DC: U.S. Government Printing Office.

Environmental Protection Agency. (1988). *Environmental progress and challenges: EPA's update,* Washington, DC: U.S. Environmental Protection Agency.

Fein, G.G., Jacobson, J.L., Jacobson, S.W., Schwartz, P.M., & Dowler, J.K. (1984). Parental exposure to polychorinated biphenyls: Effects on birth size and gestational age. *Journal of Pediatrics, 105*(2), 315-320.

Fein, G.G., Schwartz, P.M., Jacobson, S.W., & Jacobson, J.L. (1983). Environmental toxins and behavioral development. *American Psychologist, 38,* 1188-1196.

Friedman, J.A., & Weinberger, H.L. (1990). Six children with lead poisoning. *American Journal of Diseases of Children, 144*(9), 1039-1044.

Grisham, J.W. (Ed.). (1986). *Health aspects of the disposal of waste chemicals.* New York: Pergamon.

Hall, R.M. Jr., Watson, T., Davidson, J.J., Case, D.R., & Bryson, N.S. (1986). *RCRA hazardous wastes handbook* (7th ed.). Washington DC: Government Institutes.

Hileman, B. (1988, February 8). The Great Lakes cleanup effort. *Chemical & Engineering News, 66*(6), 22-39.

Holum, J.R. (1977). *Topics and terms in environmental problems,* New York: Wiley & Sons.

Jacobson, S.W., Fein, G.G., Jacobson, J.L., Schwartz, P.M., & Dowler, J.K. (1985). The effect of intrauterine PCB exposure on visual recognition memory. *Child Development, 56,* 853-860.

Kessler, S., & Levine, E.K. (1987). Psychological aspects of generic counseling. IV. The subjective assessment of probability. *American Journal of Medical Genetics, 28,* 361-370.

Lemen, R.A., Dement, J.M., & Wagoner, J.K. (1980). Epidemiology of asbestos-related diseases. *Environmental Health Perspectives, 34,* 1-11.

Lepkowski, W. (1985). Bhopal report: People of India struggle toward appropriate response to tragedy. *Chemical & Engineering News, 63*(6), 16-26.

Levine, A.G. (1982). *Love Canal: Science, politics, and people,* Lexington, MA: D.C. Heath.

Mallison, M.B. (1992, October). Editorial: Florida nurses still need help. *American Journal of Nursing, 92*(10), 7.

Miller, T.G. (1986). *Environmental science: An introduction,* Belmont, CA: Wadsworth.

Mossman, K.L., Thomas, D.S., & Dritschilo, A. (1986). Environmental radiation and cancer. *Journal of Environmental Science and Health, 4,* 119-159.

Nero, A.V., Jr. (1988). Controlling indoor air pollution. *Scientific American, 258*(5), 42-48.

New York State Department of Health. (1981). *Love Canal special report to the governor and legislature.* Albany, NY: Author.

Population Institute. (1991). Annual Report 1991, Washington DC: Author.

Pruess, H.D. (1993). Review of persistent, low-grade lead challenge: Neurological and cardiovascular consequences. *Journal of the American College of Nutrition 12* (3), 246-254.

Schwartz, P.M., Jacobson, S.W., Fein, G.G., Jacobson, J.L., & Price, H.A. (1983). Lake Michigan fish consumption as a source of polychlorinated biphenyls in human cord serum, maternal serum, and milk. *American Journal of Public Health, 73*(3), 293-296.

Silverman, G.B. (1989). Love Canal: A retrospective. *Environmental Reporter, 20*(Pt.2), 835-850.

Tchobanoglous, G., Theisen, H., & Eliassen, R. (1977). *Solid Wastes: Engineering principles and management issues.* New York: McGraw-Hill.

Turk, J., & Turk, A. (1988). *Environmental science,* Philadelphia: W.B. Saunders.

Wadden, R.A., & Scheff, P.A. (1983). *Indoor air pollution: Characterization, prediction and control.* New York: Wiley & Sons.

Waldbott, G.L. (1978). *Health effects of environmental pollutants.* St. Louis: Mosby.

Weitzman, M., Aschengrau, A., Bellinger, D., Jones, R., Hamlin, J.S., & Beiser, A. (1993). Lead-contaminated soil abatement and urban children's blood level. *Journal of the American Medical Association, 269*(13), 1647-1654.

Wilson, R. (1979). Analyzing the daily risks of life. *Technology Review, 81*(4), 40-46.

Wilson, R., & Crouch, E.A.C. (1988). Risk assessment and comparisons: An introduction. *Science, 236,* 267-270.

30

LEGAL AND ETHICAL ISSUES

Diane K. Kjervik

In a good society, good laws and good ethics would be congruent. But until that happens, it is important to protect the integrity of ethics because it is a powerful source of criticism of both law and society.

Edmund Pellegrino

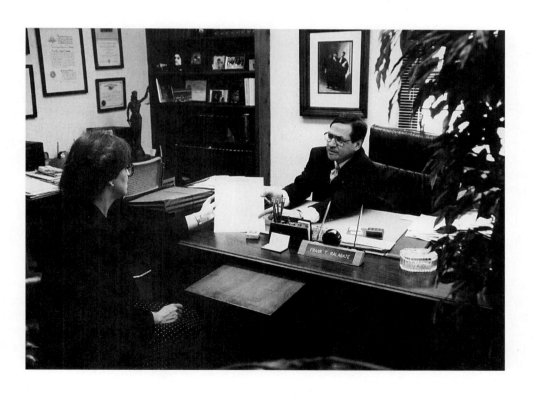

OBJECTIVES

At the conclusion of this chapter the student will be able to:

1. Define the key terms listed.
2. Identify two areas of law and three sources of law relevant to community health nursing practice.
3. Identify three governmental agencies important to community health nursing practice.
4. Describe three elements of a nursing malpractice case.
5. Describe the way in which law and ethics are related to each other.
6. Apply the ethical principle of justice to a community health nursing problem.
7. Distinguish between generalist and specialist community health nurses.
8. Discuss one case in which a community health nurse was sued for malpractice.
9. Describe one policy effort undertaken by community health nurses.
10. Identify three virtues demonstrated by community health nurses.

KEY TERMS

Care-based ethics	Criminal law	Police power
Case law	Deontology	Privileged communication
Categorical imperative	Distributive justice	Standards of care
Civil law	Ethics	Standards of practice
Civil rights	Law	Teleology
Common law	Licensure	Utilitarianism
Confidentiality	Malpractice	Virtue ethics

The interplay between law, ethics, and community health nursing is a complex web of professional values, personal beliefs, and externally imposed societal standards. Community health nurses, who are in close touch with the public, are at the leading edge of change in legal and ethical systems. Opportunities abound to evaluate the quality of ethical standards and legal imperatives and initiate policy changes that exemplify nursing values and beliefs. Health care reform is but one example of policy change that can be ethically grounded and legally implemented (White House Domestic Policy Council, 1993; Brennan, 1993). Community health is a vital part

of successful health care reform, and a clearly conceptualized nursing model of change will be critical in this process. Before examining the role that community health nurses can and do play in the process of policy change, a review of the systems of law and ethics is necessary.

THE LEGAL SYSTEM

Law is a political system that articulates the decisions society makes about its rules of conduct. The purpose of the legal system is to provide an orderly and systematic way of conducting human affairs. The earliest known recorded law existed in around 1700 BC in Babylon where a king estab-

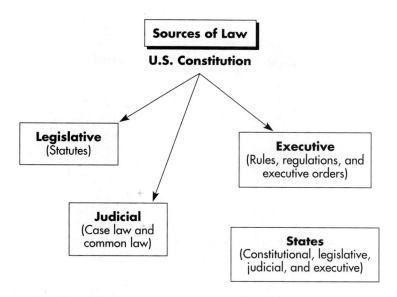

FIGURE 30-1   This figure demonstrates the sources of law that are derived from the U.S. Constitution. Three branches of government (executive, legislative, and judicial) in the federal and state governments are depicted.

lished a code of approximately 280 laws that were imprinted on stone and kept in a temple for the public to see (Loeb, 1992). In the United States, law originates in the United States Constitution, which establishes the three branches of government: the legislative branch, which makes law, the judicial branch, which interprets the law, and the executive branch, which carries out the law. The three branches of government function separately according to their own procedural rules as a reflection of the separation of powers, a principle espoused in the Constitution. Powers are separated so that no one branch will become all-powerful and operate as did the sovereign power in England from which the founders of the United States wanted to be distanced. Each state government is organized in a similar fashion with a state constitution and three branches (legislative, judicial, and executive) that operate separately from one another (see Figure 30-1).

The **common law** is court-made law that is derived from English courts and is changed over time by the judicial system. The goal of the common law is intellectual coherence (Wexler, 1993). Theoretical and philosophical underpinnings of law are to logically build upon and relate to one another. **Case law** refers to judicial cases that build upon common law precedents. Increasingly, in recent years, lawmaking has been done by legislators and administrators rather than judges, and, therefore, the focus of these efforts has been to solve social problems rather than follow the ever-evolving judicial precedent and the ideally coherent structure (Wexler, 1993). The implication that can reasonably be drawn from this is that the community health nurse who strives for policy change may make the most meaningful contribution by seeking change in the legislative and executive branches of government. Congress, state legislatures, and local city councils are examples of legislative bodies. The President, federal agencies such as the Health Care Financing Administration (HCFA) and the National Institutes of Health (NIH), executive orders, governors, and state agencies such as licensing boards and departments of health typify executive branch components. Federal rules and policy take precedence over state laws, but in many areas of the law, the federal government does not act. This is consonant with the tenth amendment of the Constitution, which states that the powers not specifically given to the federal government are reserved to the states. Most public health activity is handled at state and local levels (Pickett & Hanlon, 1990). The government finds its authority in **police power,** the power to regulate the health, safety, and morals in society. Thus, the state can condemn property it wishes to take over, and the federal government can declare drugs or foods unacceptable to the public. Immunization law, tuberculosis control, and Medicare and Medicaid regulations are examples of law specifically affecting community health nursing practice.

Finding the law is a painstaking process and is best handled by an attorney. However, community health nurses should familiarize themselves with the process by which law is made by legislatures, executive agencies, and courts of law. A good review of the process with examples from public health appears in "Law and Public Health," by Pickett and Hanlon (1990). The process of analyzing the law and the methods of finding legal authority have been explicated by nursing law scholars (Weiler & Rhodes, 1991; Kjervik & King, 1990).

Civil Law

The law is generally divided into civil and criminal areas. **Civil law** addresses relationships and resolves disputes among individual persons or among entities such as corporations or hospitals. Types of civil law that affect nursing are tort law, in which the law provides a remedy for a specified wrong such as malpractice (an unintentional act), defamation, assault and battery, and false imprisonment (intentional acts); agency law, in which relationships among principals and agents such as employers and employees are regulated; contract law, which has to do with agreements among people, promises exchanged, and the adequacy of "consideration," or the nature of the exchanged promises, goods, or services; labor law, which regulates employer-employee collective bargaining; and civil rights, which protect given individuals or groups that have suffered discrimination. Community health nurses are most often involved with public health law such as disease prevention policy, child and vulnerable adult abuse enforcement, and school health (Northrop & Kelly, 1987). For example, informed consent for

immunization must be obtained by school health nurses and public health department clinics.

Criminal Law

Criminal law has to do with relationships between a person or entities, such as corporations, and the state. The violation committed by the person or entity is an offense against the state, and the state prosecutes the individual for violating public norms. Examples are murder, assault and battery, fraud, and aiding and abetting suicide. Although few nurses are accused or convicted of criminal acts, their conduct receives a great deal of publicity and thus a disproportionate amount of attention. Criminal law as it relates to community health nursing more commonly appears in situations in which community health nurses are called on to testify in trials in which criminal activities like domestic violence were witnessed by the nurse. Familiarity with the courtroom and legal practice is vital for the community health nurse who wishes to promote positive societal change and to act as an advocate for clients.

ETHICAL THEORIES

Unlike the legal system, which is a political system—a system that decides and exercises power in society—systems of ethics are grounded in philosophy and theology. **Ethics** seeks to answer questions about values, actions, and choices of what is right and wrong (Loeb, 1992). Common theoretical orientations in ethics are deontology, teleology, virtue ethics, and care-based ethics.

Deontology

Deontology is concerned with the rules that govern behavior and the priority of such rules in relation to one another, irrespective of the outcomes of the exercise of such rules. A rule to tell the truth and to not harm a patient are examples of deontological principles. Deontology comes from the Greek word *deon,* which means "that which is binding" (Furrow et al., 1991). Moral obligation and commitment are emphasized in this orientation to ethics (Loeb, 1992). Immanuel Kant and John Rawls typify the theorists who espouse deontology (Beauchamp & Childress,

1994). The **categorical imperative** is a classic rule developed by Kant that means that the rules one chooses to live by as an individual are to be those that can be generalized to all persons. The "Golden Rule" is a simple way to state the categorical imperative. In addition, Kant states that persons are to be treated as ends in and of themselves rather than means to an end (Furrow et al., 1991). The person is to be respected (allowed to determine one's own destiny), and the duty to respect another takes priority over the duty to love the other (Furrow et al., 1991). The emphasis on respect for persons (autonomy) is foundational to such procedures as informed consent to participate in research (Furrow et al., 1991). The most fundamental principle espoused in the nursing code of ethics is respect for persons (Gorlin, 1990).

John Rawls' theory is also typical of the deontological school of thought. Rawls believes that a social contract and view of the "good" could be derived by rational persons acting as if they were ignorant of their particular allocations of personal talents, abilities, and resources (Beauchamp & Childress, 1994). This "veil of ignorance" enables free and rational persons to choose principles of justice (Furrow et al., 1991). The current discussions of justice as fairness are derived from Rawls' beliefs (Lebacqz, 1986). Because of its emphasis on duty to others, deontology is considered by some to be the only theory that makes sense for ethical decision-making in health care (Loeb, 1992). The contractual model underlies a covenantal relationship and a moral reciprocity between health care provider and patient (Furrow et al., 1991). The nursing code of ethics interprets justice as stemming from the fundamental concept of respect for persons (Gorlin, 1990).

Deontology is criticized for its individual rights orientation. Many policy disputes cannot be resolved adequately with a focus on the individual. Collective decisions about where our precious health care resources should be used will not be adequately addressed solely by a concern for individual rights (Furrow et al., 1991). The "veil of ignorance" is criticized as unrealistic and cavalier about class and other forms of power differentials among people (Lebacqz, 1986).

Teleology

Teleology (from the Greek word *telos,* meaning "end") judges the rightness of action by the ends achieved, and is therefore referred to as a consequentialist orientation. **Utilitarianism** is the most common form of teleology and was developed by John Stuart Mill and Jeremy Bentham (Furrow et al., 1991). Utility (or value) is the emphasis on actions that create the greatest balance of value over disvalue (Beauchamp & Childress, 1994). Value is considered by Mill and Bentham to be happiness, and thus the statement of the principle is that happiness means doing the greatest good for the greatest number. More recent utilitarians have expanded the notion of value beyond happiness to include friendship, knowledge, health, certain states of consciousness, and beauty (Beauchamp & Childress, 1994). A problem in utilitarianism is the uncertainty of how to measure happiness and the other values. A distinction is drawn between act and rule utilitarianism. Act utilitarianism examines the acts taken to bring about happiness, and rule utilitarians analyze the rules used to cause happiness. Either approach, however, maintains its focus on the endpoints (Beauchamp & Childress, 1994). The nursing code of ethics states that nurses are to make clinical judgments based on a consideration of the consequences of their actions as well as on rules (Gorlin, 1990).

Virtue Ethics

Virtue is commonly considered a trait of character in a person (Beauchamp & Childress, 1994). Unlike deontology and teleology, virtue ethics addresses intentions and motivations of the moral agent. Aristotle typifies **virtue ethics** in his focus on the person doing the right thing by using contemplative reasoning to understand the problem and then calculative reasoning to decide what to do (Cameron, 1993). Examples of moral virtues are truthfulness, gentleness, and politeness (Beauchamp, 1991). The ends are also important, and, in that sense, Aristotle's description of virtue ethics is similar to teleology. He says that *eudaimonia* (well-being) is a chief good and is manifested in a sense of completeness and self-sufficiency (Gomez-Lobo, 1989).

The physician Edmund Pellegrino (1991) argues that trustworthiness is a virtue to be strived for by health care professionals. He criticizes the use of contracts to supplant a trusting, covenantal relationship between health care professional and patient. He points out that the cardinal virtues (temperance, justice, courage, and prudence) imply a certain degree of self-effacement, and he also notes a criticism of virtue ethics: that it does not tell us how to resolve specific moral problems because it deemphasizes principles, rules, and duties (Pellegrino, 1989). Cameron (1993), a nurse who studied the ethical problems faced by persons with AIDS, found that they used contemplative reasoning (meditating, listening to music, discussing ethical problems with others) and acted with integrity, which to them meant living in harmony with their own beliefs. They also used calculative reasoning in which they balanced deontological concerns (right actions) with teleological ones to make responsible choices so that others would not be hurt.

Care-Based Ethics

In **care-based ethics,** right behavior is motivated by compassion or caring in a sympathetic way for another. One feels what the other person feels as closely as one can and then acts on the other person's behalf (Cameron, 1993). One must be empathetic, intuitive, and receptive. Following rules or maximizing the good are not goals of care-based ethics. In fact, rules are seen to lead to an impartiality or objectivity that care-based ethics rejects, preferring instead an analysis of what the individual in the concrete situation needs in relation to others (subjectivity) (Carse, 1991). Abstract rules, derived from the "objective" world, have led to the notion that the principle of equality, for instance, is something that is achievable, while they have contributed to the overlooking of material inequalities such as power, knowledge, and vulnerability that are experienced more in the subjective realm of the individual (Carse, 1991). Critics point out that as with virtue ethics a lack of rules leads to difficulty in making ethical decisions, and that if caring is the standard for the good, females might have to carry a greater burden of "goodness" than males because of their common actions as caregivers (Cameron, 1993).

Major Ethical Principles Derived from Theories

Autonomy (respect for the person's self-rule), beneficence (doing good), nonmaleficence (not doing harm), justice, compassion, trustworthiness, courage, integrity, truth-telling, fidelity (loyalty), and generosity are principles of moral behavior that can be drawn from ethical theories. A comprehensive moral theory that would be most meaningful for nursing practice would address intent of the moral agent, actions, and outcomes of action. Cameron (1993) proposes such a model that includes both caring and justice in balance with each other and utility and universalizability as endpoints to be sought. For instance, a client living at home who contemplates suicide to end pain associated with a terminal illness may seek the community health nurse's counsel. In this situation, the nurse must consider her own intent (virtues such as compassion and prudence), relevant ethical principles (autonomy and beneficence), and outcomes (relief of pain and death). Intents, principles, and potential outcomes may conflict with one another and should be discussed openly with all involved parties — family members, clergy, the client, close friends, the community health nurse, family physician — to reach consensus about the action to be taken. In situations in which there are no dependent children, the pain is excruciating and intractable, and family and client concur that removal of life-sustaining interventions is the best option, the autonomy interests of the client may prevail. The choice to allow a client to die can, however, be considered in certain circumstances the most humane and beneficent option. Thus, after thorough discussion, the outcome of the analysis may reveal that several principles are served and that the choice to be made is not clearly autonomy versus beneficence.

THE RELATIONSHIP BETWEEN ETHICS AND LAW

The law acts upon only some of the ethical problems that exist in the world. It is only reasonable to believe that ethics sweeps more broadly in its purview than the law, which must make the decision to enforce a given principle or approach. There are some who believe that law and ethics

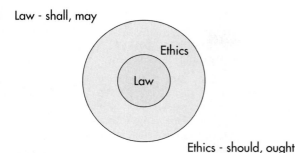

Law - shall, may

Ethics - should, ought

FIGURE 30-2 This figure depicts the relationship between the systems of law and ethics. All matters that are addressed by the law raise ethical questions, but some ethical matters lie beyond the purview of the law. Law is mandatory or permissive, whereas ethics guides individuals and societies in their decisions about what should be done.

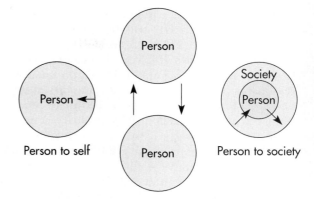

Person to self   Person to society

FIGURE 30-4 Law and ethics both give individuals in society messages about what is desirable behavior. Feedback about rightness can be given by a person to oneself, given by one person to another, and given between persons and society at large.

are mutually exclusive of each other, or, conversely, that they are coextensive with each other (Kjervik, 1990). It seems most reasonable to conceptualize law as either a baseline approach to ethical problems or a consideration that is given to some but not all of the issues tackled by ethical frameworks (see Figure 30-2).

Law varies from ethics because the relationship between law and the individual in most cases is one directional, whereas the system of ethics interacts back and forth with the values of the individual (see Figure 30-3). For instance, law has a system of sanctions that it imposes on persons or entities in a one-way direction whereas the system of ethics cannot be enforced other

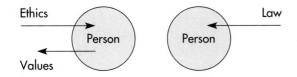

Ethics   Law

Values

FIGURE 30-3 Ethics and law vary in the degree of interchange between their expectations and the persons affected by them. The ethical codes in society are available for scrutiny by members of the community. Personal values are compared by the person to the ethical expectations of society, and choices are made. The law imposes itself upon the members of society with little in the way of interchange.

than through interaction between the person and his or her peers or in a person's exercise of conscience. One aspect of empowerment is to enable nurses, clients, and agencies to make changes in the law proactively, that is, prior to a problem's surfacing. The goal of many nurse-attorneys and nursing lobbyists is to influence the law, thus adding clout to the nursing agenda.

Law and ethics are similar in that they each address a person's relation to himself or herself (messages sent to oneself about the rightness or wrongness of action), a person's relationship to other persons (civil law and ethical codes that speak to the right of privacy, duty of confidentiality, and so on), and a person's relationship to society (criminal law and utilitarianism or social contracts such as a code of ethics) (see Figure 30-4).

ETHICS, LAW, AND COMMUNITY HEALTH NURSING STANDARDS

Both law and ethics achieve maximum influence when they inform the public about what to expect from groups in society that possess the authority of legal and ethical systems. In relation to nursing practice, this means that one who is given licensure by the state and promises to act according to ethical mandates that are part of licensure indicates to the public that the standards expected of the nurse will be demonstrated. **Standards of practice** are professional standards used by courts of law in malpractice cases to decide whether a nurse failed to do what a reasonably prudent nurse in the same or similar circumstances would have done. Boards of nursing faced with a question of disciplinary action against a nurse will also use the standards of practice to decide whether punishment should be given. Community health nursing standards are published by the American Nurses' Association and stress accountability to the client, respect for the client's rights, and advocacy on behalf of the client (*Standards,* 1986). These values reflect the ethical principles of beneficence (accountability), autonomy (respect for client's rights), and justice (advocating for vulnerable populations to balance power relationships). Macklin (1993), a noted bioethicist, has argued that in terms of women's health issues, justice is the primary ethical principle involved since equal respect and access to health care has been denied women, especially women of color and poor women. The same argument can be raised for minorities, older persons, the mentally ill, physically handicapped, and lesbian and gay individuals. Without justice, other ethical aspirations such as autonomy and beneficence or virtues such as courage, temperance, prudence, and trust are meaningless.

Community health nurses are expected to be involved as part of their professional roles in legislative action, social policy development, and other governmental activity. In this way, community health nurses are to influence the law, not merely allow the law to prescribe their own and their clients' behavior.

Historically, nurses, most of whom are women, were reluctant to participate in the political process as it was considered somewhat antithetical to the caring role (Jarvis, 1985). More recently, however, political activity has become part of the role of a nurse who advocates for his or her patients and also for himself or herself. Community health nurses must become comfortable with and knowledgeable about organizational politics (formal and informal), governmental actions, folk politicians in local communities,

---

AGENCIES IMPORTANT TO COMMUNITY HEALTH NURSES

Federal Agencies

Department of Health and Human Services (DHHS)
- Social Security Administration
- Health Care Financing Administration
- Office of Human Development Services
- Public Health Service

Department of Commerce
- Bureau of the Census
- National Oceanic and Atmospheric Administration

Department of Defense
- CHAMPUS (Civilian Health and Medical Program of the Uniformed Services)

Department of Labor
- OSHA (Occupational Safety and Health Administration)
- Mine Safety and Health Administration

Department of Agriculture
- Food and Nutrition Service
- WIC (Supplemental Food Program for Women, Infants and Children)

Department of Justice
- Bureau of Prisons

State Agencies

State Health Departments
- Medical Assistance
- MRDD (Mental Retardation and Developmental Disabilities)
- Mental Health and Addictions
- Licensing Boards
- Health Planning
- Vital Statistics

State Education Departments

State Departments of Corrections

Local Health Departments
- County Level
- City Level

Social Welfare Programs
- Unemployment Compensation
- Social Security Programs
- Welfare Programs

---

and health care organizations in relation to those they serve (Jarvis, 1985). Policy-making is part of the community health nurse's role of caring for the community.

Health care system values held by community

health nurses include accessibility of care at an affordable price. Health care is considered a right rather than a privilege (*Standards,* 1986). These beliefs equate justice with fairness to persons in all classes of society. The law has essentially two functions in public health: to guide procedures fairly (justice) and to assist in the prevention of disease and the promotion of health (beneficence) (Pickett & Hanlon, 1990). Unfortunately, health care students, as other nonlaw students, have not received adequate education in the law despite its importance to public health. In fact, law has been seriously neglected in American education despite the fact that it is changing at the same rate as technology (Pickett & Hanlon, 1990). Remembering that all health care agency actions are based in law can motivate the community health nurse to become familiar with the law. In fact, the nurse may become involved with an agency's role as enforcer of a law (Pickett & Hanlon, 1990). An example is the necessity to report communicable diseases or child abuse. Community health nursing education needs to address application of legal process (Sancier, Stanhope, & Lancaster, 1988). The box on p. 670 shows the federal and state agencies that are involved with community health matters.

MAJOR ETHICAL AND LEGAL ISSUES IN COMMUNITY HEALTH NURSING

The primary purpose of community health nursing is to promote and maintain the health of aggregates (Miller, 1990). Law and ethics play an important role in understanding the concept of aggregates. Law promulgates and implements policy for society at large, and ethics considers the tensions between individual and groups as they are or will be affected by policy. What, for instance, are the boundaries of the aggregates? (What is the community to be served?) Who are the players (stakeholders) in the process of giving care to a community? (Who is the client? Who is the community health nurse?) What roles can caregivers and recipients of care assume? (What is the scope of practice? What are the rights and responsibilities of recipients of care?) What is the environment (context) in which the care is delivered? What is the goal of care? (What is health?) These questions are reminders of the nursing paradigm: nursing, person, context, and

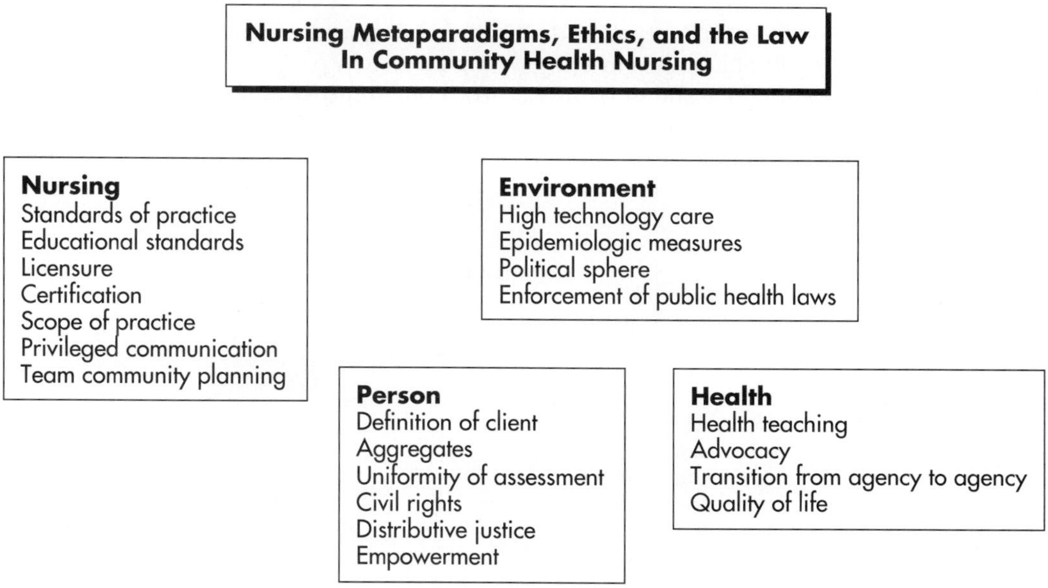

Nursing Metaparadigms, Ethics, and the Law In Community Health Nursing

Nursing
Standards of practice
Educational standards
Licensure
Certification
Scope of practice
Privileged communication
Team community planning

Environment
High technology care
Epidemiologic measures
Political sphere
Enforcement of public health laws

Person
Definition of client
Aggregates
Uniformity of assessment
Civil rights
Distributive justice
Empowerment

Health
Health teaching
Advocacy
Transition from agency to agency
Quality of life

FIGURE 30-5 Nursing paradigms (nursing, person, environment, and health) can be related to legal and ethical issues that arise in community health nursing. This figure shows some of the major issues.

health (Stevenson & Woods, 1986). All are in need of definition in the community health context, and law and ethics address this need. See Figure 30-6 for a depiction of the metaparadigms, ethics, law, and community health nursing issues.

Nursing

To understand community health nursing, both in substance and process, one can review the *Standards of Community Health Nursing Practice* (1986) and the educational standards for both baccalaureate (Hickman, 1992) and master's levels of community health nursing practice (Laffrey, 1991). The generalist is prepared at the baccalaureate level and is expected to provide population-based primary care to individuals, families, and groups. This care includes community-wide assessment, planning, implementation, and evaluation of health programs and services (*Standards*, 1986). Students who expect to enter this level of practice must be taught, among other things, cultural diversity, ethical issues, health policy, the government's role in health care, environmental hazards, and community planning (Hickman, 1992).

The specialist in community health nursing is educated at the master's or doctoral level and, in addition to practicing generalist functions based on even greater informational foundations in epidemiology, demography, biometrics, and community and policy development, formulates health and social policy to affect a community or population, conducts research, and tests theory related to community health practice (*Standards*, 1986). Students who aspire to this level of practice study, among other topics, social and political change theory, theory of justice and ethics, legal issues, public health ethics and policy, economics and politics of health care delivery, quality assurance, and empowerment (Laffrey, 1991).

These statements of standards inform the public of what it can expect when it enters into a contract for community health nursing service. The standard of care will be that which courts of law will scrutinize if a nurse is sued for malpractice. Figure 30-6 outlines the elements that must be shown to win a malpractice case. Failure to perform one's duty as a community health nurse (falling below the standard of care) that through a direct relationship (proximate cause) results in injury to the patient is **malpractice.**

Standards of care can also be established by reference to textbooks on community health nursing practice, policy manuals in public health nursing agencies, and the testimony of expert witnesses (other community health nurses). Because of the importance of the testimony of experts, peer review and consultation by colleagues about one's decision-making process in the clinical area are vital. Attendance at continuing education programs is also helpful in keeping the community health nurse up to date on recent practices in the field.

Community health nurses have rarely been

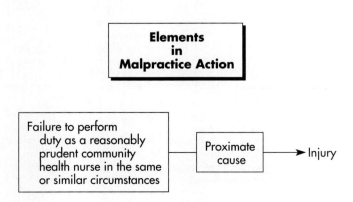

FIGURE 30-6   In a legal action for malpractice, several elements must be proved by the plaintiff (the injured party). A causal relationship must exist between the breach of the legal duty and the injury to the patient.

sued for malpractice, as pointed out by Northrop and Kelly (1987). One area in which they have been sued concerns the duty to warn students who receive vaccinations about serious side effects of the vaccine. In a recent case, *Mazur v. Merck & Co, Inc.,* 964 F.2d 1348, 1992, a federal court of appeals decided that the public health nurse was not a "learned intermediary," a designation that would have required the nurse to weigh the risks and benefits of administering the vaccine and relaying this information to the person to be vaccinated. The description of the nurse's education leaves the impression that the education of community health nurses is somewhat less than would be expected from examination of the Standards. "Nurse Frederick," as she is referred to by the court, was a school nurse who had completed a 1-year nurse practitioner program at the University of Pennsylvania. In spite of this, the court states that "Nurse Frederick stated herself that the 'emphasis' of her formal education was on 'education' rather than 'nursing.' As part of her training to become a registered nurse, she learned how to administer vaccines. But although Nurse Frederick had some classes in medication, she was never trained in weighing the risks and benefits of vaccination in a given instance. In 1980, Nurse Frederick attended a 1-year, nurse practitioner program at the University of Pennsylvania. But this program centered on physical examinations of children and did not include detailed instruction on immunization or pediatric diseases" (*Mazur v. Merck & Co.* [at 1359]). Further testimony by "Nurse Frederick" indicated that she was unaware that subcutaneous sclerosing panencephalitis is a complication of vaccination for measles, that she did not know how a virus passes through the body and causes illness, how a vaccine works, and why a child with a fever should not be vaccinated (*Mazur v. Merck & Co.* [at 1359]). The defendant manufacturer prevailed in the lawsuit by contractually shifting responsibility to the Centers for Disease Control and Prevention. But the nurse was also freed from responsibility by successfully arguing that she was not a "learned intermediary," which is a dubious distinction at best, considering that in a prior case a Licensed Practical Nurse had been determined to be a learned intermediary in a measles, mumps, and reubella-II immunization program (*Walker v. Merck & Co.,* 648 F. Supp. 931 [1986]).

Case law operates by precedent, and nurses must be careful when legal arguments are developed on their behalf by lawyers who are under an ethical obligation to represent their clients zealously within the bounds of the law. Nurses must be prepared to think beyond the immediate circumstances and the wish to defend themselves to the broader application of the precedent. Neither generalist nor specialist community health nurses are helped by presumptions of the court about their inability to understand basic physiologic principles.

Another way that nursing as a discipline is identified is through its licensure by the state. **Licensure** is a mechanism by which a state acknowledges the contribution of a given profession to society. The state offers the opportunity of licensure to the professional who then takes an examination or asks for a waiver based on licensure by another jurisdiction. Licensure is a form of control by the state over the practice of the professional and has been criticized as having provided no benefit to society or the state other than as a source of revenue (Pickett & Hanlon, 1990). When licensure becomes a way of legislating morals, it can be criticized, for example, licensing massage studios to control prostitution (Beauchamp, 1988). But the advantage to professions like nursing is that licensure sanctions the unique contribution that the profession makes to the health care field. Its identity and autonomous practice are sanctioned by the state. Licensure in all states is as a Registered Nurse, but some states allow for special licensure or certification as an advanced practice nurse. Certification from a professional organization is sometimes recognized by the licensure board as evidence of expertise in a specialty area. Specialists in community health nursing can benefit from such policies.

The scope of practice or scope of employment is another mechanism by which nursing defines itself or is defined by others. Scope of practice enables nursing to be distinguished from medicine, pharmacy, social work, and other health care disciplines. Because nursing is so often assumed to be an appendage of medicine, the scope of employment concept is a useful one. Scope of practice is assessed by examining usual custom and practices of the profession and by noting how a profession is defined in legislation (Northrop, 1988). As with the standard of care, the usual and customary practice of community health nursing can be defined by what is written in textbooks and what is stated as professional standards from major organizations and experiences of peers. Community health nursing's scope of practice is considerably broad (Northrop & Kelly, 1987). Understanding dependent and independent functions is critical such as the ability of an advanced practice nurse to prescribe drugs, which is allowed by some states but not in others. Failure to know what constitutes one's profession may result in a charge of practicing another discipline without a license.

Confidentiality of the communications between nurse and client is protected in section two of the Code for Nurses (Gorlin, 1990). Protection of these communications indicates to the public that there is a boundary between the nurse-client relationship and the outside world. Very few exceptions are allowed. Among them are communication with the treatment team for decisions about care, the quality assurance staff, and the court when the patient waives a statutory right of privileged communication (Northrop & Kelly, 1987). **Privileged communication** is the privilege of the client not to disclose treatment information to a court of law. It is granted by some states to certain health care providers, lawyers, clergy, and spouses. Some states recognize this privilege for nurses. Nurses could strengthen their promise to clients not to disclose this information by obtaining the privilege. Lobbying the legislature for this change would be necessary. Exceptions to the privilege are recognized for reporting of child abuse (Northrop & Kelly, 1987).

To some extent, the autonomy of community health nursing must yield when team community planning is contemplated. As opposed to autonomy, interdependence and collaboration are desirable traits and more in line with the ethics of care. Building networks of caring persons is a worthwhile health care and ethical goal. Although case law is oriented to individual as well as corporate responsibility, legislatures and administrative agencies are more accustomed to group efforts (e.g., lobbyists on behalf of groups, coalitions, and the power of the voting public). Politically expressed interdependence among health professionals can be especially significant in confronting difficult environmental problems or funding challenges from the Public Health Service. The Coalition for Health Funding in Washington, D.C., which is composed of nurses, psychologists, and physicians, to name a few, is an example of a coalition devoted to empowerment of health care providers.

Person

The definition of the population to be served (client) by community health nurses is one with both legal and ethical ramifications. Legally, the question of the scope of the responsibility is relevant to the standards of practice as discussed previously. Aggregates are generally seen to be the focus, but the breadth of definition of aggregates is important. For instance, high-risk populations such as abused and neglected children, vulnerable adults, and migrant workers are within the scope of the communities to be served (Northrop & Kelly, 1987). In health promotion roles, community health nurses may also define the person (client) as well adults or well elderly. The legal issue raised by this is to whom is the duty (standard of care) owed? The ethical issue is similar: to whom is the caring, the beneficence, the justice, and professional virtue owed? Without clarity on this point, the contract for services or covenantal relationship cannot be established in any meaningful way.

Documentation for services rendered is as important in Community Health Nursing as in any other area of nursing. Record-keeping is used as evidence of accountability for assessment, planning, implementation, and evaluation of services. Accountability is the other side of the coin from nurses' or clients' rights. These rights may be considered positive (affirmative) or negative such that one may have a right not to have something done (e.g., surgery) without giving informed consent (a negative right), or one can expect to have something done that has been agreed to, such as hyperalimentation (a positive right). The agency's records can indicate whether the duties and actions that correspond to these rights are fulfilled by the nurse. Juries will assume that if an action is not documented, it was not done. The *uniformity of assessment* and subsequent documentation of the assessment indicates that a standard of practice was followed, and thus clients served by the community health nurse can discover what service was provided and are given notice as to what to expect from the nurse in the future. Clarity of this expectation facilitates accountability to the aggregates served by the community health nurse.

Matters of discrimination and the **civil rights** to be protected arise in community health settings because of the diversity of populations served. What responsibilities do the nurse and person have? Groups of persons (aggregates) that are similarly situated are to be treated equally under the law. This expectation parallels the principle of justice in ethics. Some groupings such as racial or ethnic groups are treated with special scrutiny by courts because of a history of discrimination. Other groups such as women or the elderly are provided some scrutiny but not at the same level as racial groupings. The scrutiny provided by courts appears when they say to legislatures or state agencies that one group may be treated differently from another group only if the differentiation is shown to be substantially necessary to meeting the goal of the policy.

Discrimination cases are often difficult to prove. In *Kein v. Commonwealth of Pennsylvania,* 543 A.2d 1261, 1988, the court held that the plaintiff, a community health nurse I, did not allege sufficient facts to prove discrimination in a situation in which she was not promoted. Also, Ms. Kein did not demonstrate that there was a linkage between the job she desired and the skills required in her present position. Like discrimination cases, comparable worth cases are extremely difficult to win, and in Madison, Wisconsin, a group of female public health nurses tried to prove that their work was comparable in skill, effort, and responsibility to sanitarians who were all male and who were paid more than the nurses (*Briggs v. City of Madison,* 536 F. Supp. 435, 1982). The nurses lost the case because (1)

the city argued that the only way to retain the sanitarians was to raise their salaries, and (2) the nurses were unable to show evidence that the city's actions were motivated by discriminatory intent.

Even when a civil rights case is settled in favor of the plaintiff, attorneys fees may be difficult to collect. In *Young v. Kenley,* 641 F2d 192, 1981, Ms. Young, a public health nurse, won a settlement in a discrimination suit that alleged that she was denied a promotion because of her race. Ms. Young asked the district court (initial level court in the federal system) twice for attorneys fees and was turned down. Upon appeal to the circuit court of appeals (the second level court in the federal system), she was granted attorneys fees, the court saying that the settlement agreement reached with the state did not preclude Ms. Young from recovering attorneys fees.

Distributive justice also relates to the person or client cared for by the community health nurse. Whether one segment or type of population will receive certain services that another segment does not raises the issue of distribution of services and fairness of allocation. Community health nurses become involved in these questions when they screen clients for services, deciding whether a certain social service or health care service is necessary for the client. The issue also surfaces when community health nurses advocate for certain populations with state agencies that make allocation decisions, such as those making decisions about Medicaid payments or hospice services. Distributive health policies are those that create nongovernmental benefits, such as the Nurse Education Act under Title VIII of the Public Health Service Act (Miller, 1990). This Act provides funds for training nurses primarily at advanced levels of education to provide for personnel needs for the nation. Redistributive policy allocates resources from one group to another, (Medicare is one example) (Miller, 1990). Analysis for purposes of distribution addresses questions of costs and benefits of a given policy. From the vantage point of ethical theories, this analysis is a utilitarian question. Is happiness for the greatest number of persons generated by the policy? The utilitarian analysis tends to overlook the needs of minorities and thus is criticized an inadequate approach to empowerment of vulnerable populations. However, as Macklin (1993) points out, when women's needs are at issue, a utilitarian approach to justice can be very helpful because women are in the majority numerically, and thus the greatest happiness for women would be the greatest happiness for the majority of society. The needs of other vulnerable groups, the elderly, handicapped, and racial minorities might best be served by Veatch's view of equality of moral worth, opportunity, or outcome (Veatch, 1986). The test of outcome of policy is by far the strongest argument to be made on behalf of vulnerable populations, the question being, "What is the outcome of the policy as it affects each and every person, including those who are most disadvantaged?"

Environment

The context in which care is delivered is critical to a focus on aggregates. Systems theory describes the relationship among elements of a system and the surrounding suprasystem (Bertalanffy, 1968). The primary theoretical stance taken in this theory is that all parts of the system are affected by a change in any one part. Thus because the environment (suprasystem) is the situation in which community health nursing is practiced, it is relevant to the provision of care. The environment is an integrated part of the whole (the system of health care). Changes in the suprasystem affect the system, which subsequently must respond to that change. Systems of law and ethics are components of the suprasystem that relate to persons in the health care system as depicted in Figure 30-3. Legal and ethical policies are often associated with other aspects of the suprasystem such as technology and epidemiology.

A major issue affecting the practice of community health nursing is high-technology care, particularly that occurring in the home. Because of outside forces, namely the diagnosis-related grouping system of health care financing instigated in the 1980s by the Health Care Financing Administration, patients are discharged "sicker and quicker" from hospitals. Community health nurses now find themselves managing high-technology equipment in the homes. Legal liability

and ethical responsibilities have thus changed. The standard of practice expected of community health nurses has incorporated these new technologies. Legally, the expectation of a reasonably prudent community health nurse (Figure 30-6) has altered in practice and would be reflected in the testimony of community health nurse experts who evaluate whether a breach of the standard of care has occurred. Ethically, doing good for clients (beneficence) includes high-quality implementation of the equipment and assessment of its effect on clients and their families. Autonomy needs of clients are greater when dependence on machinery precludes maximum forms of autonomous expression. With greater dependency and vulnerability, loss of autonomy lurks as a predictable possibility (Lidz, Fischer, & Arnold, 1992). Questions of justice emanate from the expense of the equipment, which may not be affordable to all families. The ethics of care may provide the best protection from the impersonality of the environmental pressures, resulting in the continual focus on the unique requirements of the individual and the family.

Epidemiology assists the community health nurse to ascertain the status of the environment in which care is provided. As with high-technology care, epidemiology is a tool that can improve care or create the added burden of recognizing the vast array of needs that, given current health care resources, cannot be met in a just and humane way. Yet to ignore epidemiologic information seems to defy the principle of non-maleficence (doing no harm) in that ignoring available facts ignores the needs of the human community and can result in harm. Both legal and ethical principles mandate attention to all facts that can be obtained using current scientific tools.

Dealing with the political sphere is also imperative for community health nurses (Miller, 1990; Northrop & Kelly, 1987; *Standards,* 1986). Community health nurses act as change agents and as such must face the power structure head-on as lobbyists to congress, as experts providing testimony in legislative hearings, as expert witnesses and parties to cases in which justice is sought, as participants in the rule-making process in health care agencies, and as relentless hounders of political leaders. With limited national resources for defense spending, environment clean-up, entitlement programs, and reduction of the federal debt, community health nurses cannot afford the luxury of passive acceptance of the status quo. They must fight for health care as other power forces, such as insurance companies, fight for their special privileges. The ethics of fighting fairly are worth considering. Exercise of virtues such as benevolence, effacement of self interest, honesty, compassion, and prudence assist the nurse who engages the forces that would remove resources from health care. Remembering the thousands for whom the nurse speaks removes much of the anxiety of speaking as an advocate.

The community health nurse interacts directly with the environment by assisting with the enforcement of public health laws. Child abuse, communicable diseases, gunshot wounds, and abuse of vulnerable adults (elderly and handicapped) are reportable by community health nurses. Reporting requirements serve the interest of the public in the safety of its citizens. Issues of confidentiality, privacy, and informed consent are raised and must be carefully preserved as far as possible in these mandatory reporting situations (Northrop & Kelly, 1987). The community health nurse may also have to testify in court about termination of parental rights (Northrop & Kelly, 1987). It is important not to promise clients total confidentiality when entering into caring relationships with them. A situation might arise in which the nurse must report a client's behavior to a social welfare agency or testify in a court of law, and trust would be compromised if the promise is broken.

Health

Community health nurses are experts in the use of persuasive power. The trend is toward influence and away from use of the coercive power of the state (Pickett & Hanlon, 1990). *Health teaching* situations place the community health nurse in a position to exercise influence. Their definitions of health and strategies to maintain health can be conveyed in terms that people can understand and accept. However, it is important that the community health nurse also attend to the client's definition of health and proposed approaches to the challenges confronted (Gale,

1989). Mutuality in the discussions with shared power between the client and the community health nurse is a laudable goal. Ultimately, the power to decide what path to take lies with the client, and if the client chooses a path that the nurse considers foolish, for example, drinking alcohol again or returning to the battering spouse, the nurse must maintain a respect for the client and the client's choice. Without this respect, ethical principles of autonomy, beneficence, and justice are not served. To remove a client's choice or overcome it with one's own choice shows contempt for the client's self-determination (autonomy) and elevates a nurse-centered conclusion about what is "good" for the patient above the client's own, which amounts to parentalism (beneficence) (Benjamin & Curtis, 1992), and disturbs fairness (justice) by tipping the power balance in favor of the nurse. When clients disagree with what the health care establishment thinks should be done, they are sometimes considered incompetent by the health care professionals. Considering someone to be incompetent for this reason turns the purpose of incompetency on its head and uses it against the patient instead of for the patient. (Informed consent requires competency, information, and volition to be considered valid consent [Kjervik & Grove, 1988].) Determinations of competency can be challenged as biased in favor of the current power structure and are especially inadequate in their evaluation of women (Stefan, 1993). Community health nurses need to be aware of the adequacy of the decision-making ability of clients and also of their own values and conclusions that may stand in the way of respect for the client's decision.

Advocacy is a demonstrable way to exercise respect and caring for the client. Mutuality, facilitation, protection, and coordination are necessary to the role of advocate (Leddy & Pepper, 1989). The Code for Nurses mandates that nurses take action when health care or safety of the client and the public is jeopardized (Gorlin, 1990). Advocacy has also been framed in terms of helping a client to decide (Corcoran, 1988) or assisting the client to know his or her needs and experiences well enough to make decisions (existential advocacy) (Gadow, 1990). Although advocacy for clients and society is well-accepted within nursing literature, the nurse's role as advocate has been criticized as it occurs within the hospital setting. Bernal (1992) argues that patient advocacy exercised by nurses is too often linked to the need for autonomy of nursing roles, and thus the altruistic motives of nursing are lost. While Bernal, a hospital ethicist, does not see the relevancy of professional autonomy to speaking effectively for clients, nurses who have been effectively silenced by loyalties to physicians and hospitals know the importance of the credibility that autonomous practice brings. In fact, nurse autonomy, client autonomy, and advocacy are intertwined, which does not denigrate the need for interdisciplinary collaboration in decision making. Rather, interdisciplinary collaboration is most effective when all voices including the consumer's are heard.

Community health nurses, like nurse attorneys and nurse ethicists, span the boundary between systems. The transition from hospital to home is one of the common system shifts that must be negotiated by community health nurses. A very protective environment, the hospital, which tends toward parentalism, must be left for the more autonomous expectations of the home environment. The community health nurse attends to the effect of the shift on the client emotionally, physically, socially, and ethically. When the shift is from agency to agency (as with nursing home to hospital), the community health nurse must be conversant with the policies of the two institutions so that the client's health needs are managed smoothly. Values of the client are important to assess as the decision about the transfer is made. The shift is more likely to be successful if the client is ready and willing to move.

Although most frequently associated with inpatient settings in which end of life decisions are frequently faced, quality of life issues arise in community health nursing as well. Clients in the community are making difficult decisions about abortion, whether to remove the ventilator or life-sustaining nutrition and hydration from a terminally ill relative, whether to establish a guardianship for a vulnerable relative, or whether to commit suicide. These situations and others evoke questions about the value of life and the quality of life that is lived. Community health nurses sit with families, individuals, and policy makers as they struggle to handle these questions. As the population ages as it will during the next decades, more questions of this sort will arise by virtue of the shear numbers of persons in a vulnerable state. Advance directives such as living wills and durable powers of attorney will become more common, and community health nurses will be asked to assist with the decision making necessary to effectuate these documents. Distributive justice will bear on the resolution of these dilemmas when resource allocation is at issue. Likewise, questions of beneficence and caring will surface as an individual patient's choice is death over life. Autonomy relates as directly to the decision to let go of life as it does to making the decision for surgery. What more intimate decision can a person make than the one to die, how to die, and under what conditions? Society must decide whether such a decision is ethical and legal. The case of Nancy Cruzan demonstrated the U.S. Supreme Court's support of the right to refuse treatment, but it left to the states the question of how this would be regulated (*Cruzan v. Director, Missouri Department of Health,* 110 S.Ct 2841, 1990). Community health nurses with their vast experience of clients who live with dying and make the decision to let go of life can speak clearly in policy forums about the effects of these decisions on individuals, groups, and communities.

Chapter Highlights

- Community health nurses are at the leading edge of change in legal and ethical systems affecting health care.

- Sources of law are the U.S. Constitution and the three branches of government created by the Constitution. Similar sources of law exists on each of the state levels of government.

- Civil law deals with disputes among persons or agencies, and criminal law deals with relations between persons and the state.

- Common theoretical orientations in ethics are deontology, teleology, virtue ethics, and care-based ethics.

- Principles derived from ethical theories are beneficence, non-maleficence, justice, compassion, trustworthiness, courage, integrity, truth-telling, fidelity, and generosity.

- Law and ethics are closely related with ethical matters covering broader matters than the law.

- Ethical and legal issues related to community health nursing can be understood within the nursing paradigm: nursing, health, the person, and context.

- Analysis of the nurse's intent, ethical and legal principles involved, and potential outcomes provides the most comprehensive way to resolve ethical questions that arise in practice.

 ## CRITICAL THINKING EXERCISE

A woman in late middle age is experiencing intractable pain from terminal cancer. She shares with her hospice nurse the fact that she is contemplating suicide. She also asks the nurse's advice.

1. Write a paragraph as a personal response that you think might be given to this woman. Consider compassion, autonomy, beneficence, and outcomes as outlined in the chapter.

2. A nurse aided and abetted suicide might have a problem with criminal law. What are the laws in your state/province regarding this issue?

REFERENCES

American Nurses' Association. (1986). *Standards of Community Health Nursing Practice.* Kansas City: Author.

Beauchamp, D.E. (1988). *The health of the republic: Epidemics, medicine, and moralism as challenges to democracy.* Philadelphia: Temple University Press.

Beauchamp, T.L. (1991). Aristotle and virtue theories. In Beauchamp T.L. (Ed.): *Philosophical ethics: An introduction to moral philosophy.* New York: McGraw-Hill.

Beauchamp, T.L., & Childress, J.F. (1994). *Principles of biomedical ethics,* (4th ed.). New York: Oxford University Press.

Benjamin, M., & Curtis, J. (1992). *Ethics in nursing* (3rd ed.). New York: Oxford University Press.

Bernal, E.W. (1992). The nurse as patient advocate. *Hastings Center Report, 22,* 18-23.

Bertalanffy, L.V. (1968). *General system theory.* New York: George Braziller.

Brennan, T.A. (1993). An ethical perspective on health care insurance reform. *American Journal of Law and Medicine, 19,* 37-74.

Cameron, M.E. (1993). *Living with AIDS: Experiencing ethical problems,* Newbury Park, Calif: Sage.

Carse, A.L. (1991). The "voice of care": Implications for bioethical education. *Journal of Medicine and Philosophy, 16,* 5-28.

Corcoran, S. (1988). Toward operationalizing an advocacy role. *Journal of Professional Nursing, 4,* 242-248.

Furrow, B.R., Johnson, S.H., Jost, T.S., & Schwartz, R.L. (1991). *Bioethics: Health care law and ethics.* St. Paul: West.

Gadow, S. (1990). Existential advocacy: Philosophical foundations of nursing. In Pence, T. (Ed.). *Ethics in nursing: An anthology.* New York: National League for Nursing.

Gale, B.J. (1989). Advocacy for elderly autonomy: A challenge for community health nurses. *Journal of Community Health Nursing, 6*(4), 191-197.

Gomez-Lobo, A. (1989). Aristotle. In Cavelier, R., Guoinlock, J., & Sterba, J. (Eds.). *Ethics in the history of western philosophy.* New York: St. Martin's Press.

Gorlin, R.A. (Ed.). (1990). *Codes of professional responsibility* (2nd ed.). Washington, D.C.: Bureau of National Affairs.

Hickman, M.P. (1992). *Essentials of baccalaureate nursing education for entry level practice in community health nursing.* Lexington, Ky: Association of Community Health Educators.

Jarvis, L.L. (1985). *Community health nursing: Keeping the public healthy* (2nd ed.). Philadelphia: F.A. Davis.

Kjervik, D.K., & Grove, S. (1988). A legal model of consent in unequal power relationships. *Journal of Professional Nursing, 4*(3), 192-204.

Kjervik, D.K. (1988). The connection between law and ethics. *Journal of Professional Nursing, 6*(3), 138, 185.

Kjervik, D.K., & King, F.E. (1990). The legal research method: An approach to enhance nursing science. *Journal of Professional Nursing, 6,* 213-220.

Laffrey, S.C. (1991). *Essentials of master's level nursing education for advanced community health nursing practice,* Louisville, Ky: Association of Community Health Nursing Educators.

Lebacqz, K. (1986). *Six theories of justice.* Minneapolis: Augsburg.

Leddy, S., & Pepper, J.M. (1989). *Conceptual bases of professional nursing.* Philadelphia: J.B. Lippincott.

Lidz, C.W., Fischer, L., & Arnold, R.M. (1992). *The erosion of autonomy in long-term care.* New York: Oxford University Press.

Loeb, S. (Ed.). (1992). *Nurse's handbook of law and ethics,* Springhouse, PA: Springhouse.

Macklin, R. (1993). Women's health: An ethical perspective. *Journal of Law, Medicine, and Ethics, 21,* 23-29.

Miller, T.W. (1990). Political involvement and community health advocacy. In Spradley, B.S. (Ed.). *Community health nursing: Concepts and practice.* Boston: Little, Brown Higher Education.

Northrop, C.E., & Kelly, M.E. (1987). *Legal issues in nursing.* St. Louis: Mosby.

Pellegrino, E.D. (1989). Character, virtue, and self-interest in the ethics of the professions. *Journal of Contemporary Health Law and Policy, 5,* 53-73.

Pellegrino, E.D. (1994). Editorial response to Halevy and Brody. *American Journal of Medicine, 96,* 289-291.

Pellegrino, E.D. (1991). Trust and distrust in professional ethics. In Pellegrino, E.D., Veatch, R.M., & Langan, J. (Eds.). *Ethics, trust, and the professions: Philosophical and cultural aspects.* Washington, DC: Georgetown University Press.

Pickett, G., & Hanlon, J.J. (1990). *Public health: Administration and practice* (9th ed.). St. Louis: Mosby.

Sancier, K.A., Stanhope, M., & Lancaster, J. (1988). *Community health nursing workbook: Process and practice for promoting health.* St. Louis: Mosby.

Stefan, S. (1993). Silencing the different voice: Competence, feminist theory and law. *University of Miami Law Review, 47,* 763-815.

Stevenson, J.S., & Woods, N.F. (1986). *Nursing science and contemporary science: Emerging paradigms. Setting the agenda for the year 2000,* Kansas City: American Academy of Nursing.

Veatch, R.M. (1986). *The foundations of justice: Why the retarded and the rest of us have claims to equality.* New York: Oxford University Press.

Weiler, K., & Rhodes, A.M. (1991). Legal methodology as nursing problem solving. *Image: Journal of Nursing Scholarship, 23,* 241-244.

Wexler, D.B. (1993). Therapeutic jurisprudence and changing conceptions of legal scholarship. *Behavioral Science and the Law, 11,* 117-29.

White House Domestic Policy Council. (1993). *The President's health security plan.* New York: Times Books.

PROFESSIONAL ISSUES

Carol Batra

For us who Nurse, our Nursing is a thing, which, unless in it we are making progress every year, every month, every week, take my word for it, we are going back.

Florence Nightingale

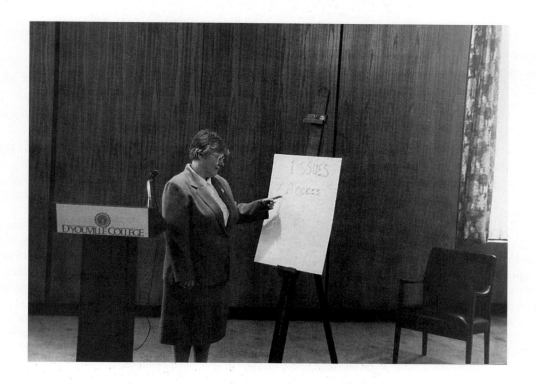

OBJECTIVES

At the conclusion of this chapter the student will be able to:

1. Recognize the strategies for empowerment of community health nurses.
2. Define types and models of change and change agent skills.
3. Identify multipurpose and community health professional nursing organizations and their functions.
4. Contrast levels of political involvement for nurses in the community.
5. Recognize community health nursing issues in each phase of the nursing process.
6. Describe actions needed in community health nursing as a result of future trends in the health care delivery system, consumers, nursing, research, and political action.

KEY TERMS

Advocacy	Empowerment	Restraining forces
Change agent	First order change	Second order change
Driving forces	Refreezing	Unfreezing

As we approach the twenty-first century, we find ourselves living in a time of challenge and change in cultures worldwide, in political and economic conditions, and in professional and philosophical nursing world views. For nurses to move to the center stage of leading health care reform, they need to become empowered to exert the influence of their numbers.

Empowerment is an interactive process that develops, builds, and increases power through cooperation, sharing, and working together (Hawks & Hromek, 1992). Knowledge is a critical component of power. According to Schmieding (1993), nurse empowerment is an evolutionary process. It is influenced by (1) the evolving role of women, (2) societal changes that have increased people's involvement in the decision-making process, (3) increases in the level of education, and (4) economic factors that have forced delegation of decision making to lower organizational levels. Schmieding emphasizes that a vision of nursing is pivotal to all aspects of clinical

and administrative decision making. Furthermore, nurses should view organizational position as a potential empowering factor. Delegation of authority itself is empowering (Schmieding, 1993).

Empowerment can be achieved through an understanding of the change process, through participation in organizations that are important vehicles for community health nurses, and through political activity to foster community advocacy. As nurses position themselves for the year 2000, knowledge of the current community health nursing issues and predicted future trends will further their empowerment.

EMPOWERMENT THROUGH THE CHANGE PROCESS

"The job of leaders is not simply to predict how the world will change, but to create change." So said Jonathon Peck of the Institute for Alternative Futures, at the Annual Conference of the American Academy of Nursing, October 11-12,

1992 (Pender, 1993a). Successful use of the change process requires a knowledge of change theory.

Types of Change

Change can be categorized into different types according to specific characteristics. Duncan (1978) cited change as being either haphazard or planned. Haphazard change is usually random with no effort being made to prepare for the onset of the change cycle. In contrast, planned change results from deliberate and conscious action to modify the activities of a given system to meet the demands of the new force within the system.

Sampson (1971) labeled change as developmental, spontaneous, or planned. Developmental change occurs as an individual, group, or organization progresses from infancy to maturity. As growth occurs, frequent and rapid adjustments take place in physical size, complexity, and the nature of the interrelationships. These modifications generally are transformed in an orderly, progressive fashion. Spontaneous change is a response to natural, uncontrollable events. Often it is unpredictable or unanticipated; hence preplanning is not possible. Planned change is an intentional effort to intervene in the ongoing state to produce a new state.

Archer, Kelly, and Bisch (1984) use the concepts of Watzlawick, Weakland, and Fisch (1974) to apply first-order and second-order change to implementing change in communities. **First-order change** is change brought about in a system without the system itself being changed. The assistance given by the community health nurse to clients to help them to work the system to meet their needs is an example of first-order change. For example, an elderly couple may believe that they are getting the "run around" when dealing with the Social Security and Medicare offices. The nurse may serve as their advocate by contacting a colleague in the office to facilitate the processing of the couple's benefits.

Second-order change, on the other hand, is focused on the system rather than the system's clients. Second-order change seeks new ways to do things, new approaches, structures, and ideas. For this same elderly couple's situation, second-order change would mean changing the Social Security and Medicare processing and office procedures such that they would be streamlined and hence more amenable to helping the couple to receive their benefits.

Historically nurses often reacted to, rather than initiated, change. They increasingly took over techniques formerly performed only by physicians, such as blood pressure measurement, administration of intramuscular and intravenous injections, and more recently, physical assessment techniques. Nurses added to their patient care responsibilities voluminous administrative paper work generated by institutional and health care reimbursement bureaucracies. Now nurses are realizing that initiation of change is both a professional responsibility and an untapped source of power. Planned change is a means of exercising control over one's personal and professional destiny.

Planned change may be defined as "a deliberative and collaborative process involving a change agent and a client system, such as an individual, a group of people, an agency, an organization or a social institution" (Brooten, Hayman, & Naylor, 1978, p. 81). Bennis, Benne, Chin, and Corey (1976, p. 4) describe planned change as "a conscious, deliberate, collaborative effort to improve the operations of a human system, whether it is a self-system, social system, or cultural system, through the utilization of valid knowledge."

Models of Change

Several models have been developed to explain the process of change. These models have many similarities; consequently, it is most helpful for nurses to select the one that is clearest and most relevant for their practice and world view. The following is a discussion of three change models: (1) the Lewin model, (2) the Rogers model, and (3) the Lippitt model.

The Lewin model. The work of Lewin (1951) is considered to be the origin of classical change theory. He named three steps in the change process: unfreezing, moving to a new level, and refreezing (Figure 31-1). In **unfreezing,** participants would be motivated to be ready for change by "thawing them out." They would be helped to recognize a need for change and to work on

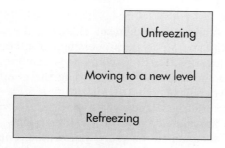

FIGURE 31-1 Lewin's three steps in the change process.

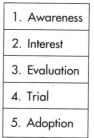

FIGURE 31-2 Rogers' five phases in the change cycle.

identifying or diagnosing the problem and developing a solution by choosing from a number of alternatives. The change agent would have to establish trust and respect with the group. Once the group viewed the change as being in their best interest, they would be ready for the next step.

In the second of Lewin's steps, the actual moving to a new level of behavior occurs. The participants scan a variety of options. They may pretest different change strategies and begin the transition period.

Refreezing is Lewin's final step where the newly acquired behavior is integrated by the participants. They need continuous and intermittent reinforcement for the new behaviors to remain in place. The change agent and leaders in the system need to provide constructive criticism, praise, encouragement, and positive feedback.

Lewin also developed the concepts of driving and restraining forces. **Driving forces** are those that encourage the change process to move in the direction of the desired change. **Restraining forces** hinder or inhibit the desired change. Both forces need to be identified by the change agent to establish support systems to facilitate the dominance of the driving forces over the restraining ones.

The Rogers model. Rogers (1962) expanded on Lewin's model by emphasizing the environment and the background of the participants in the change process (Figure 31-2). He stressed the fluid and reversible qualities of the change process. He identified that each participant might accept the change initially, but then reject it. Alternately, the participant could initially reject the change, but later adopt it. Rogers expanded

Lewin's unfreezing step into awareness, interest, and evaluation phases. The effectiveness of moving to the next phase was dependent on the participants' keen interest in the change and their commitment to working toward its implementation. Rogers used the term trial phase for Lewin's moving to a new level step and the adoption phase for Lewin's refreezing step.

The Lippitt model. Lippitt (1973) contends that no one can escape change. He maintains that the key to dealing with change is to create carefully constructed strategies for intervention (Figure 31-3). During Lewin's unfreezing step, Lippitt identifies the need to diagnose the problem. An open mind to all possibilities is necessary at this point. Key people who have authority and power in the organization must be involved from the beginning of the process. Also, it is necessary to assess both the participants in the change process and the environment of the proposed

1. Diagnosis of the problem
2. Assessment of motivation and capacity for change
3. Assessment of change agent's motivation and resources
4. Selecting progressive change objectives
5. Choosing the appropriate role of the change agent
6. Maintenance of the change once it has been started
7. Termination of a helping relationship

FIGURE 31-3 Lippitt's seven stages in the change process.

change for the capacity for change. Lewin's restraining and driving forces would need to be identified here. Furthermore the change agent's motivation and resources must be honestly and critically assessed. Trusting and respecting the change agent are instrumental in this phase.

The step Lewin identifies as moving to a new level is expanded into two stages by Lippitt: selecting progressive change objectives and choosing the appropriate change agent role. In the former stage, careful step-by-step strategies need to be devised. The change agent role may be that of information gatherer, motivator, expert role model, catalyst, teacher, or group leader. Congruence between the change agent's and the participants' perception of the change agent role greatly facilitates progress at this point.

Lippitt specifies two final steps for Lewin's refreezing step. Maintenance of the change must be accomplished through open lines of communication. Publicity of the change should occur now so that other areas in the organization or in other organizations may become involved in a similar project. Finally, Lippitt describes termination of the helping relationship whereby the change agent withdraws from the situation, following a predetermined plan. The participants increasingly take on the maintenance roles previously performed by the change agent. The change agent may remain in a greatly reduced consultant role until no longer needed.

The Nurse as a Change Agent

The **change agent** generates ideas, introduces the innovation, develops a climate for planned change by overcoming resistance and marshalling forces for acceptance, and implements and evaluates the change (Lancaster, 1982). The change agent may be from inside or outside the organization. Lancaster offers guidelines for nurses to be effective in change-agent roles. The nurse must be accessible to all who are involved in the change process. Trust must be nurtured both ways between the change agent and the participants. The nurse needs to be honest and straightforward about goals, plans, priorities, and problems. The responsibilities of others need to be defined, and they must then be given the freedom to carry out those responsibilities. The nurse needs to develop a balance between lead-

ing and developing the leadership capacities of the participants. Motivation of the change participants will be achieved if they feel that their contributions are invaluable for the outcome of the project. Acknowledgement for what they do right and a private discussion of how their actions may impede progress are imperative. Everyone affected by the change needs to be involved from the beginning. The change must be sanctioned by the people in control of the organization for its legitimization. Careful listening to the knowledge and wisdom of the participants in the organization is of paramount importance.

Hall and Weaver (1985) provide a list of change skills that are needed for nursing practice. Table 31-1 summarizes these skills and their purposes. The change agent in nursing would benefit by a self-examination for personal strengths or weaknesses in these areas.

EMPOWERMENT THROUGH PARTICIPATION IN ORGANIZATIONS

"If the health care system is to be reformed, nurses must participate. Individually and collectively, nurses need to find ways to influence health care policy-making so that their holistic voice is heard" (Murphy, 1992, p. 158). Collective voices available to community health nurses include professional nursing, public health, and community organizations. Nurses traditionally have not communicated directly with associate health professionals, administrators, and politicians. The role that 1.9 million professional nurses can play in the use of health care resources and health-promotion community programs has yet to be fully recognized. With the 1993 election of a president committed to health care reform, nurses have renewed a commitment to their full participation in health care delivery to the nation's diverse populations (Pender, 1993b). The following includes a sampling of the organizations accessible to community health nurses to be heard as a political voice.

Professional Nursing Organizations

Hegyvary (1990) provides a guide to nursing organizations: what they are and how to choose them. She categorizes them into multipurpose or-

TABLE 31-1   Change skills for nursing practice

Skill	Purpose(s)
Inquiry	Ability to think critically, question assumptions to increase knowledge
Helping	Ability to enable clients to cope effectively
Teaching	Ability to impart health-related knowledge, develop skills, instill values in clients
Supervision	Ability to assist others to increase their performance skills
Coordination	Ability to unify the actions of health care providers
Collaboration	Ability to work together to pursue common goals
Consultation	Ability to share specialized expertise in a form usable by those less knowledgeable
Negotiation	Ability to bargain to secure agreement
Confrontation	Ability to increase awareness of differing perceptions through assertive communications
Lobbying	Ability to influence decision making to advance one's goals
Administration	Ability to determine policy to achieve the purposes of the organization
Reconciliation	Ability to use antagonistic views to create constructive alternatives to resolve contradictions

Modified from *Distributive nursing practice: A systems approach to community health* (2nd ed.) (p. 135) by J.E. Hall & B.R. Weaver, 1985, Philadelphia: J.B. Lippincott.

ganizations and clinical specialty organizations. Nurses tend to join professional organizations for a stronger sense of professional identity. Organizations provide a network for nurses to discuss professional concerns, a medium for formalizing action for health care and legislative reforms, and a mechanism for staying on top of professional issues.

Multipurpose organizations.   Two national U.S. nursing organizations are considered to be multipurpose organizations: the American Nurses' Association and the National League for Nursing. The International Council of Nurses is the international nursing organization with a multipurpose function.

The American Nurses' Association (ANA) has a wealth of resources related to their functions: standards of nursing practice, education and nursing services, code of ethics, credentialing, legislation, health policy, evaluation, research, economic and general welfare, professional leadership, professional development of nurses, affirmative action, collective bargaining, communicating with the membership, consumer advocacy, and representation of the profession (ANA, 1983). The ANA accredits continuing education programs, provides for certification of individual nurses (including community health nursing certification), supplies data for research and analysis,

and implements an economic and general welfare program. The ANA is the only U.S. nursing association with official representation in the International Council of Nurses. Although its 200,000 members are not a majority of the 1.9 million nurses, the ANA is still the most visible, active, and comprehensive of all of the American nursing organizations. Its origins can be traced back to 1893.

Annually, the ANA publishes a very useful resource directory (1990), which they label as *Nursing's National Yellow Pages. The American Nurse* is ANA's official newspaper and contains news stories, opinion columns, addresses of many useful offices, nursing supplies and equipment, and features on the effect of forces influencing the profession. The *Capitol Update* is the newsletter from ANA's office in Washington. It analyzes and interprets federal activity that influences nursing and conveys how individuals and groups can shape national policy decisions. Four times a year, the *Nursing and Health Care Events* calendar publishes more than 800 notices for conferences held by nursing and health-related organizations.

Of specific interest to community health nurses is the ANA Council of Community Health Nurses. In the *CHN Communique*, the Council publishes its projects, legislative updates, research results, and commentary of concern to community health nurses. ANA publications of standards of practice specific to community health nurses may be found in the box below. ANA has three guides depicting innovative models for community-based nursing services: *A Conceptual Model of Community Health Nursing* (ANA, 1980), *A Guide for Community-Based Nursing Services* (ANA, 1985), and *Community-Based Nursing Services: Innovative Models* (ANA, 1986).

The National League for Nursing (NLN) was created in 1952 based on a decision made at the 1950 ANA convention. It was the result of a merger of three organizations: the National League for Nursing Education, the Association of Collegiate Schools of Nursing, and the National Association of Public Health Nurses. This organization includes nurses, interested non-nurses, and relevant institutions to strengthen the collaboration between nursing education and nursing service. Unlike the ANA whose membership is only for registered nurses, the NLN is open to both individuals and agencies, and the inclusion of non-nurses has created ongoing controversy. The membership remains small: 1500 individual members and 1700 institutional members.

The NLN has eight designated functions, including strengthening and supporting nursing services, promoting research for the knowledge base of nursing education and practice, maintaining responsiveness to its membership, promoting

---

STANDARDS OF NURSING PRACTICE PUBLISHED BY THE AMERICAN NURSES' ASSOCIATION

Standards of College Health Nursing Practice, 1986

Standards of Commumity Health Nursing Practice, 1986

Standards of Home Health Nursing Practice, 1986

Standards for Nursing Practice in Correctional Facilities, 1985

Standards of Practice for the Primary Health Care Nurse Practitioner, 1987

Standards of School Nursing Practice, 1983

---

public understanding and support of nursing, and exploring new avenues for promoting nursing, such as alternative health care settings (NLN, 1983). NLN regularly reviews and accredits nursing education programs through its appropriate councils. One of the NLN's eight councils is the Council of Community Health Nurses. In conjunction with the American Public Health Association, NLN also conducts an accreditation program for community health services.

The NLN has published two sets of standards specific to community health nursing: *Standards of Excellence for Home Care Organizations* (NLN, 1989) and *Standards of Excellence for Community Health Organizations* (NLN, 1990). It should be noted that the emphasis of these two publications is on agencies rather than the individual community health nurse.

The International Council of Nurses (ICN) is a federation of national nurses' associations in 79 countries, representing about 500,000 nurses. Its stated objective is to provide a medium through which national nurses' associations may share their common interests, working together to develop the contribution of nursing to the promotion of the health of people and care of the sick. The ICN has been concerned with nursing education, nursing service, and nurses' social and economic welfare.

Clinical specialty organizations. Clinical specialty organizations specific to community health nurses include the Public Health Nursing Section of the American Public Health Association and the Association of Community Health Nursing Educators.

The American Public Health Association (APHA) was founded in 1872 and is the oldest and largest professional organization of public health workers in the world. Its 55,000 individual and agency members represent more than 40 different public health disciplines. Its functions include researching health problems and suggesting guidelines based on that research, setting standards for public health, fostering professional advancement through the 25 special interest sections and continuing education, conducting surveys and launching public awareness campaigns, planning and implementing projects to improve health, and providing expert testimony on legislation and health issues. The APHA publishes the *American Journal of Public Health, The Nation's Health,* and the *Washington Newsletter.* The APHA compiled a summary of *Healthy People 2000: National Health Promotion and Disease Prevention Objectives* (APHA, 1990) and *Healthy Communities 2000: Model Standards* (3rd ed.) (APHA, 1991).

The Public Health Nursing Section of the APHA was founded in 1922 and comprises approximately 3000 members. In 1980, the organization developed the *Definition and Role of Public Health Nursing in the Delivery of Health Care,* a statement that was adopted as official policy for the APHA.

The *Association of Community Health Nursing Educators* (ACHNE) was established in 1978. Its goal is to shape public health policy by setting agendas for excellence in community and public health through nursing education by directing consensus building, influencing the political process, establishing criteria for curriculum content, setting the qualifications for faculty, establishing guidelines for preparation for practice, promoting the synthesis of public health and nursing sciences, and promoting knowledge development through research. The ACHNE has published community health nursing research priorities (ACHNE, 1991, 1992), *Essentials of Baccalaureate Nursing Education for Entry Level Community Health Nursing Practice* (ACHNE, 1990), *Essentials of Master's Level Community Health Nursing Education for Advanced Practice* (ACHNE, 1991), *Essentials of Doctoral Education for Community Health Nursing* (ACHNE, 1994), *Differentiated Nursing Practice in Community Health* (ACHNE, 1993), and *State of the Art of Community Health Nursing Education, Research, and Practice* (ACHNE, 1990, 1991, 1992).

Community Organizations

Community health nurses have a wealth of community organizations that provide opportunities to interact with consumers of health care and politically active groups and to become involved with health policy decision making.

The National Association for Public Health Policy (NAPHP) focuses on the development of public health policy. It prepares model legislation, finds legislators to introduce the legislation, and monitors the processing of the bills toward passage. Nine councils target issues of concern for public health policy: Alcohol Policy, The Environment, Health Departments, Inquiry Control, Maternal–Child Health, Medical Care, Mental Health, Occupational Health, and Smoking Prevention.

Political Action Committees (PACs) have developed to provide a mechanism to organize and fund campaign activism. The ANA established N-CAP (Nurses' Coalition for Action in Politics) to solicit funds for political purposes and carry out political education of nurses. Other PACs evolved from business and professional groups, organized labor, and other large community organizations. Lobbying and political education activities may be spearheaded by such groups as the League of Women Voters, National Organization of Women, National Women's Political Caucus, Association of State Democratic Chairs, the Republican National Committee, and the Public Citizen.

A variety of voluntary community organizations provide the community health nurse with educational resources for clients, support and networking functions for specific health problems, and access to national resources. Examples of these include the American Cancer Society, the American Heart Association, the American Diabetes Association, and the United Way, among others.

EMPOWERMENT THROUGH POLITICAL ACTIVITY

As the majority of primary care providers in this country, nurses should be the most influential health care group in grassroots political and economic change. Every day, nurses witness the problems of access, cost, and quality of care. Because of this majority, it would seem that nurses would also be the most qualified group to articulate the country's health care problems. Nurses continue to maintain their ethic of caring. This caring ethic should motivate nurses to work for social change for their communities. Nurses need to be more influential in legislative and policy-making positions. When nurses represent 1.9 million voters, many more nurses should be elected to office.

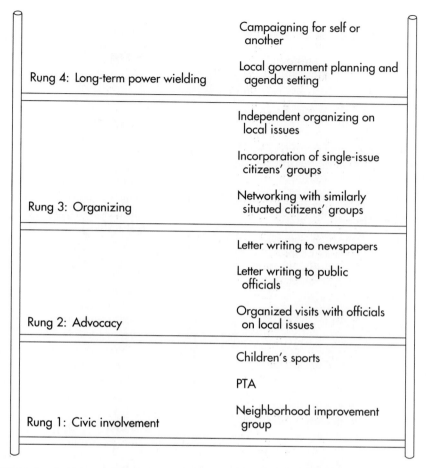

Campaigning for self or another

Local government planning and agenda setting

Rung 4: Long-term power wielding

Independent organizing on local issues

Incorporation of single-issue citizens' groups

Networking with similarly situated citizens' groups

Rung 3: Organizing

Letter writing to newspapers

Letter writing to public officials

Organized visits with officials on local issues

Rung 2: Advocacy

Children's sports

PTA

Neighborhood improvement group

Rung 1: Civic involvement

FIGURE 31-4 Chalich and Smith's model for individual political development. *(From "Nursing at the grassroots" by T. Chalich & L. Smith, 1992,* Nursing and Health Care, 13*(5), 242-244.)*

Chalich and Smith (1992) have proposed a model of political involvement for a nurse activist to follow a path of increasing political sophistication (Figure 31-4). This model is a ladder that has progressive activities at four distinct levels.

Civic Involvement

Kalisch and Kalisch (1982) consider a spectator level of political participation to being exposed to political stimuli. Nurses should seek out information through reading newspapers, viewing political television programming, and reading newsletters and mass media information. The professional nursing journals frequently have legislative columns and updates. The ANA produces a newsletter to keep nurses apprised of the cur-

rent legislation. A second level of spectator political participation is voting. A higher level still is by revealing one's partisanship by political discussions, displaying bumper stickers, and wearing campaign buttons.

Chalich and Smith (1992) portray some case studies of nurse activism at the community level. They describe nurses such as Sharon Malhotra, who is a national leader in efforts to expose the risks of lawn care pesticides. Nurse Terry Swearingen spends 16 hours each day fighting the construction of a hazardous waste incinerator. Shirl Rings, the health and welfare chair of her local PTA, is a nurse who has received national recognition for her efforts to reduce the amount of pesticides applied in local schools.

In describing strategies for nurses to become empowered for professional, political, and health policy involvement, Batra (1992) lists a number of local community branches of national organizations and neighborhood advisory groups that nurses can easily become involved in, according to their areas of interest. Examples of these may be found in the box below. The local community newspapers have a wealth of information on when and where such community groups are meeting and what issues are being discussed.

Advocacy

Historically, according to Sprayberry (1993), organized nursing has experienced a wrenching duality between the roles of professional health care provider and consumer advocate. She states that for grassroots, political awareness and activity, creating health care reform that is equitable for both consumers and providers requires the expertise and active involvement of every nurse. She suggests that nurses need to be better informed to appreciate how their own practice and communities are affected directly by decision-making bodies far removed from the work setting. Implementation of state and federal policies has direct consequences for local delivery of care: staffing, wages, workloads, or policies and procedures. Proactive strategies to prevent detrimental legislation, rather than reactive attempts to repair damage in local implementation, fosters empowerment and control.

Mitty (1991) considers **advocacy** to be a sociopolitical activity. Opportunities for advocacy arise in the personal, occupational, or professional arenas. An advocate is a person or group who pleads the cause of another or defends a cause or proposal. Mitty also points out that the role of nurse advocate demands that we be watchful for the excesses of regulated care and sensitive to the subtle indignities and intrusions of the health care system on human and civil rights. Letter writing and visits to public officials are two political tools that nurses can use.

Letter writing. Writing letters to the editors of newspapers is an excellent way to express reactions to published views. This form of influence allows readers in a community to see different viewpoints. Staff in the local legislators' offices are particularly attentive to letters to the editor for keeping attuned to the daily pulse of the community. Letters are generally brief and to the point. Figure 31-5 shows two examples.

Letters to legislators and politicians produce the greatest impact if they (1) are from individual citizens, as opposed to group efforts, (2) are well-

---

EXAMPLES OF COMMUNITY BOARDS AND COMMITTEES FOR NURSES' POLITICAL INVOLVEMENT

Organizations	Committees
Adult Day-Care Center	Advisory Council
Alzheimers Society	Board of Directors
American Cancer Society	County Chapter Board of Directors
	Diet and Cancer Program Development Task Force
American Red Cross	Healthy Heart Committee
	Obesity Task Force
Big Sisters Association	Board of Directors
Community Health Center	School Health Advisory Board
Federation of Neighborhood Centers	Community Advisory Board
Mayor's Committee on Aging	Elder Abuse Subcommittee
Nursing Home	Board of Directors
Planned Parenthood	Public Affairs Committee
Psychiatric Center	Community Residence Board
	Women's Issues Board
Recreation Center	Advisory Board
Refugee House	Board of Directors
	Education Committee
Regional AIDS Task Force	Nutrition Committee
Regional Network in Aging	Board of Directors
School Board of Education	Drug and Alcohol Abuse Committee

From "Empowering for professional, political, and health policy involvement" by C. Batra, 1992, *Nursing Outlook 40*(4), 170-176.

Although you'd never know it from your article on the nursing shortage, men are nurses too. "Fewer young women are entering nursing..." Really, now.

Bill Brown
Chicago

There is a proposal being considered by Hillary Rodham Clinton's health care task force that deserves a closer look: Loosening the regulations that restrict nurses' work. Permitting nurses to play a more active role in screening patients and treating run-of-the-mill ailments is a cost-effective solution to the shortage of primary-care physicians. At community nursing centers, complete physicals can cost from as low as $30 and vaccinations $6. Weight-control programs, screening for early cancer detection, hypertension, vision and hearing problems, are available at low costs. An economist at Wellesley College last year produced results that the US would save $6.4 to $8.75 billion annually in health costs, if the barriers to nurse practitioners were removed. What a novel idea.

Terry Lee
New York

FIGURE 31-5 Examples of letters to the editor.

written and thoughtful, (3) are limited to one page, and (4) mention any prior action taken by the legislator on the issue (Kalisch & Kalisch, 1982). Appropriate titles and addresses may be found in Figure 31-6.

Spradley (1990) summarizes the following points to consider when writing to a public official:

1. Letters should be neat, brief, and preferably typed.
2. When a bill is being discussed, correspond with all members of the committee, addressing each individually.
3. Include the following content as concisely as possible:
   (a) One sentence stating the issue
   (b) One sentence stating your position on the issue
   (c) A statement on the status of the proposed legislation
   (d) A list of reasons to support or oppose the pending legislation: (1) financial, (2) groups adversely affected, (3) weaknesses of opposing view, (4) benefits that override weaknesses of your view
   (e) Specific data to support the above reasons: (1) dollar amounts, (2) number and names of affected groups, (3) numbers within groups, (4) identification of processes, equipment, and loopholes that have adverse or positive effects
   (f) A final clear, concise statement on what action you wish the legislator to take: (1) vote for or against the legislation, (2) meet with your organization, (3) ask for more information, (4) convey contents of your letter to appropriate people

Organized visits with officials. Lobbyists have great influence on the actions of public officials. The officials in turn appreciate the individ-

President

The President
The White House
Washington, D.C. 20500

  My dear Mr. President:

  Most respectfully yours,

Governor

The Governor
State Capitol
City, State, Zip

  Dear Governor Cuomo:

  Respectfully yours,

U.S. Senator

The Honorable Edward Kennedy
Senate Office Building
Washington, D.C. 20510

  My dear Senator Kennedy:

  Yours very truly,

U.S. Congressperson

The Honorable Richard A. Gephardt
House Office Building
Washington, D.C. 20515

  My dear Mr. Gephardt:

  Yours very truly,

Mayor or City Councilperson

Mayor Joey Brandon (or) Councilperson Joey Brandon
City Hall
City, State, Zip

  Dear Mayor Brandon: (or) Dear Mr. or Ms. Brandon:

  Yours very truly,

FIGURE 31-6   Titles and addresses for letters to political leaders.

ual contact with those knowledgeable about the health care system, particularly nurses, to gain a more accurate perspective on the issue. Visits generally last only 3 to 5 minutes; consequently, a fact sheet or a brief letter of introduction is productive. The legislator's staff members are equally viable contacts. They will have more time to spend and be more knowledgeable about the details of the issue. Generally the staff members are the ones who do all the background work and draft the wording of the bills for the public official. The most effective nurse lobbyists regularly establish contacts with their local legislators. Frequently as a result of this networking, they become resources that the staff members will contact to find out more information on a particular issue.

In addition to visiting public officials' offices, nurses can attend a legislative hearing for a proposed bill or regulation. Legislators listen more carefully when they see, by their physical presence, that a nurse or nurses in their constituency take the time and effort to show concerns about an issue. Preparation would be the same as is described in the contents of a letter to a public official. Legislative committees of the local or state nursing association can provide excellent written material for background information and arguments pertaining to any pending legislation.

Nurses can meet with political candidates and push a nursing point of view on issues. They can get the attention of their peers, in their state and in their community, on behalf of their candidates and *Nursing's Agenda for Health Care Reform* (ANA, 1991). Nurses should exude enthusiasm that politics and nurses are a dynamic mix (Betts, 1992).

Organizing

Pender (1993c) proposes that nurses adopt President Clinton's hosting of town meetings to "meet the people" to discuss national issues that affect their lives. Nurses could hold these town meetings in conjunction with extension services in rural communities, urban leagues, parent-teacher organizations, neighborhood organizations, and service and charitable groups. These meetings could be held in such locations as community centers, religious institutions, and schools, and in such vulnerable population sites as homeless shelters, teen centers, safe centers for those subjected to domestic violence, and senior citizen centers. Questions to be asked should include:

(1) What services are viewed as minimally helpful or as ineffective?

(2) What services or programs are needed to help citizens competently care for themselves and their dependents?

(3) What services, programs, or changes in policy are needed to change health-threatening to health-promoting environments locally?

(4) How can the quality and cultural sensitivity of health care be improved?

Pender (1993a) suggests that nurses become involved in community partnership models. Community-based services should be tailored to meet the needs of persons from diverse backgrounds, and communities should take control of their health and work collaboratively with health care professionals. Figure 31-7 suggests the transformations in health care that should be orchestrated by nurses.

One example of a community partnership model is the collaborative practice project in Spokane, Washington (Barker, Bayne, Higgs, Jenkin, Murphy, & Synoground, 1994). A group of representatives from nursing education, health, social service, and other community agencies meet monthly to address issues of providing care to homeless, low-income, and uninsured persons in Spokane. Their Committee for Health Care of the Poor collectively identified the community problems and issues and community-level interventions. Four community diagnoses were formulated: insufficient database for community-wide planning, inadequate low-income housing, insufficient community resources for low-income clients, and lack of use of existing community services. Their findings were shared with policy makers and individual agencies.

Pender (1993a) further suggests that commu-

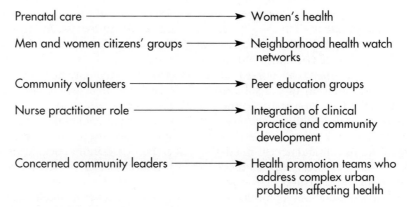

Prenatal care ⟶ Women's health

Men and women citizens' groups ⟶ Neighborhood health watch networks

Community volunteers ⟶ Peer education groups

Nurse practitioner role ⟶ Integration of clinical practice and community development

Concerned community leaders ⟶ Health promotion teams who address complex urban problems affecting health

FIGURE 31-7 Transformations in health care to organize community groups. *(From "Creating change through partnerships" by N.J. Pender, 1993a,* Nursing Outlook, 41*(1), 8-9.)*

nity health nurses are the "hinge-pins" who will recruit, train, and support the peer education groups in the community. She reported on the need for health and business partnerships whereby nurses work with local business leaders to develop an incentive system to use health care services. Mobile health station activities would be positioned at business sites. Donors are recruited for the medical and educational supplies needed for underserved areas.

Long-Term Power Wielding

Public policy internships offer an ideal immersion into Capitol Hill to gain hands-on experience with public policy. Sharp, Biggs, and Wakefield (1991) provide a list of structured programs, including their purposes, eligibility, financial data, duration, and application procedures. They also describe how a nurse could negotiate directly with his or her own congressional office for arranging an individual internship. Brief contact letters should include a résumé that highlights educational and experience backgrounds and experiences with health issues, with any local or state government office, and with policy development. An indication of the time frame and expectations of any financing involved would be included. Contacts with the professional nursing organizations to establish a network would increase the likelihood of being successful in this venture. Finally, they emphasize not to undersell the contributions you could make to the congressional office. The Clinton administration's emphasis on cutting the health care budget and making health care more equitable makes the middle to late 1990s opportune for a nurse's expertise on Capitol Hill.

The Oregon Plan (Capuzzi & Garland, 1990) is an example of the involvement of nurses in every aspect of the collaboration of consumers and health care professionals to reshape the health care system. Nurses provided expert testimony during legislative sessions and hearings where they affirmed the health and access needs of specific populations and emphasized the need for health promotion, prevention, and case management. Nurses participated on committees such as the mental health and chemical dependency subcommittee. They volunteered as com-

munity coordinators and meeting facilitators. The Oregon Nurses' Association monitored the process and kept people informed by writing articles in newsletters and conducting information sessions and continuing education courses.

Kalisch and Kalisch (1982) describe political campaign work as the highest level of political participation. Initially nurses can work in campaigns as a visible nurse in a range of activities, such as duplicating, working phone banks for candidates, stuffing envelopes, ringing doorbells, holding meet-the-candidate sessions, arranging political parties, taking people to the polls, preparing registration lists, working in a voter registration drive, and raising money for candidates. Running for a political office and becoming involved in the party organization are the ultimate in political involvement.

COMMUNITY HEALTH NURSING ISSUES

The professional issues challenging community health nursing have been raised throughout the previous chapters in relation to the topics under discussion. What follows is a summary of these issues viewed from each of the phases of the nursing process. First of all, empowered community health nurses need to be able to address the following questions:

1. Who is assessed by community health nurses: the individual, family, group, or community?
2. What do community health nurses assess?
3. What nursing diagnoses do community health nurses use?
4. What types of nursing interventions do community health nurses use in practice?
5. How do interventions differ with differences in client focus?
6. How is community health nursing evaluated for quality of care, cost effectiveness, and outcomes assessment?
7. How should community health nurses prepared at the following levels be used?
   a. BSN (Bachelor of Science in Nursing)
   b. MSN (Master of Science in Nursing, with a major in Community Health Nursing)
   c. MPH (Master of Public Health, not a nursing degree at the graduate level, but with a BSN prior preparation)

8. What clinical settings are most effective for teaching community health nursing?

Some difficult ethical issues in community health nursing today are faced by Capitol Hill:

1. Who shall be the priority recipients of community health nursing practice?
2. Who shall have access to care?
3. Who shall pay for the care?
4. What should be the level of care?
5. Who determines the cost effectiveness of funded care?

Assessment

The previously listed questions, which challenge community health nurses, suggest that there may be a wide variety of areas that are considered appropriate and necessary for assessment in community health nursing.

It can be concluded from the wealth of assessment tools available that the tool to be selected depends on the client of concern to the community health nurse. Add to the above tools the choice of many more assessment guides according to the particular nursing theoretical framework or model adopted by the community health nurse in practice. Another whole area of tools for client assessment are those required by the reimbursing agency to justify the need for the care given. Needs assessment instruments are used to evaluate the functional capacity of the client, the need for nursing and other health care requirements to meet the client's needs and to assist with functional incapacities, and the resources available to meet those requirements. The issue is clearly one of how organized data collection can be conducted in community health nursing with an endless assortment of structures for that data collection to take place.

Diagnosis

With the lack of clarity in terms of nursing assessment in community health nursing, it follows that nursing diagnosis in community health nursing is equally undeveloped. Hamilton (1983) provides an extensive analysis of community nursing diagnoses. She points out that there may be a difference between the nursing of individuals in the community, nursing of individuals influenced by the community, and nursing of the community directly.

Zink (1994) reviewed home care documentation systems that used nursing diagnoses. The most publicized classification system has been the Omaha Visiting Nurse Service System, which was developed in 1980 and has since been adopted by many states. Client problems, identified by community health nurses, were described by a cluster of signs and symptoms and then organized in a nonexhaustive list.

Muecke (1984) critiques the concept of community health diagnosis and proposes the following steps to identify the community of concern:

1. Identification of the health risk of the community
2. Specification of the characteristics of the community and its environment that are etiologically associated with the risks
3. Specification of the health indicators that verify the risk

Risner (1990) identifies criteria that set community nursing diagnoses apart from individual or family nursing diagnoses:

1. They are generated from assessments not only of the state of individuals but also of the state of the community as a physical, sociocultural, and experiential entity.
2. Relational statements imply intervention not by providing direct client services, although these may be the ultimate result, but by instituting some change in the present community.
3. The implied direct client is the community; the indirect client is the individual.

For example, passing a state law prohibiting smoking in public places may be the result of a community diagnosis of increased number of respiratory diseases related to air pollution. The total community is the direct client targeted for the intervention, while the individual is the indirect client.

The lack of an existing and nationally recognized categorization of the reasons for a visit by a community health nurse points out the lack of development of a common understanding of community nursing diagnosis. Valid and reliable systems for classifying home visits in terms of the presenting problems potentially amenable to the interventions of community health nurses would group patients in an organized and retrievable fashion to facilitate evaluations of interventions and patient outcomes. Measures of case mix and severity of illness are necessary to judge the intensity of needed nursing care. The combination of these measures might lead to the development of diagnosis-related groups for home health practice.

Goals

Goeppinger (1984) examines the principle issues of community health nursing from the perspective of the following questions:

1. What are the goals of community health nursing practice?
2. What are the target systems that community health nurses intend to change?
3. What roles are particularly appropriate for community nurses?
4. In what settings do community health nurses practice?

A variety of position statements articulated the goals of community health nursing practice in the early 1980s. The ANA Division on Community Health Nursing published *A Conceptual Model for Community Health Nursing* (ANA, 1980). The APHA Public Health Nursing Section published the *Definition and Role of Public Health Nursing in the Delivery of Health Care* (APHA, 1982). These statements provided such divergent positions that the question arose: Should the goals be eclectic, extensive, and inclusive; or focused, restrictive, and exclusive?

In September 1984 there was a joint conference of the APHA, the ANA, the NLN, the Association of Graduate Faculty in Community/Public Health Nursing, and the Division of Nursing, Bureau of Health Professions. Consensus was reached on the essentials of and preparation for community/public health nursing practice. "Public health nursing" referred to the health promotion and disease prevention activities associated with the nursing services provided in official health agencies. "Community health nursing" referred to nursing care given by nurses in scattered community settings, including doctors' of-

fices, work sites, schools, street clinics, and other similar community locations. The basic "public health nurse" was prepared in public health nursing at the BSN level. The "public health nurse specialist" was prepared in public health nursing at the graduate level. The "community health nurse" was an umbrella term for any nurse who works in the community (including the public health nurse) or who is not practicing specifically in a health-related institutional setting. The "community health nurse specialist" was a nurse who had graduate preparation in any area of nursing and worked in the community setting (U.S. Department of Health and Human Services, 1985).

Interventions

A major nursing intervention issue is that of the measurement of costs of community health nursing in the home health care setting. Kovner (1989) categorizes alternatives into four models: per visit, acuity of care, hourly, and by diagnosis. She recommends a time-based approach adjusted for differential use of supplies.

The setting for community health nursing practice leads to a question of whether community health nursing is setting-specific. Is it community-oriented simply because of its site or is it community-oriented because it emphasizes the collective need? Three newer and related developments in nursing community settings have been the nursing center concept, nurses in private practice or nursing entrepreneurship, and parish nursing.

Nursing centers may be referred to as community nursing organizations, nurse-managed centers, nursing clinics, or community nursing centers (ANA, 1987). In 1989, the National League for Nursing established the Council for Nursing Centers. Its functions are to provide assistance to individuals, agencies, and educational institutions to develop, improve, and evaluate nursing centers. They provide leadership in setting standards for such centers, promote continuing education programs and publications specific to nursing centers, promote demonstration projects and research, and collaborate with other national groups in achieving quality, cost-effective health care. The Council promotes nursing centers among consumers as sources of affordable, quality health care and promotes nursing centers as clinical sites for students in nursing and other related disciplines (NLN, 1993).

Nursing centers are a relatively new phenomenon in that over half have been established since 1988. These centers give clients direct access to professional nursing services that are holistic and client-centered and are reimbursed at a reasonable fee level. Annual budgets ranged from $1500 to $40,000,000 in 1990 (Barger & Rosenfeld, 1993). Nursing centers are reimbursed for services by private pay, no compensation, Medicaid, private insurance, and Medicare. They may be freestanding businesses, but most are affiliated with universities or other service agencies. The accountability and responsibility for client care remains with the nurse, and the overall accountability for the center remains with a nurse executive. Barger and Rosenfeld (1993) found that nurses employed by nursing centers are significantly better educated than in other health care delivery settings; most have BSN degrees with certifications, and many have master's and doctoral degrees. Client populations cared for by the centers are primarily racial minorities, the very young and very old, and the poor. Their data clearly demonstrate that community nursing centers are serving populations that are typically neglected and underserved. Most nursing centers provide primary care services (ambulatory care, immunizations, outpatient care), assessment and screening services (cancer screening, cholesterol screening, and women's health screening), educational programs (wellness promotion), and counseling (stress management and psychological counseling). The relationship of the nursing center to the other agencies offering community health nursing services is an interesting issue.

The development of private practice in nursing, a new organizational model for nursing services, has led to increased motivation for the acquisition of third-party reimbursement for nursing services. The American Nurses' Foundation (1988) conducted a study on the characteristics, organizational arrangements, and reimbursement policies of nurses in private practice. Nursing centers may be one such setting for nursing entrepreneurs. This movement may be one means of responding to the competition for limited resources and pressures for new ways of delivery of care. On the other hand, this movement contradicts the prediction that nurses would have few chances of creating new fee-for-service programs. Issues continue to be raised on the sources of financing for nursing care, the mechanisms for paying nurses, and the systems of organizing and delivering nursing care.

In 1985, the *Nurse-Entrepreneur's Exchange: The Newsletter for Business-Minded Nurses* was founded and published to update nurses on business opportunities and provide a forum for networking. By 1988, the National Nurses in Business Association (NNBA) was established to foster independent nursing practice. The Association acts as a national communication network, provides information to promote the development of independent practice models, promotes nontraditional career options for nurses, monitors legislation affecting independent nursing practice, markets the image and role of the nurse in business, and conducts research related to independent practice and the delivery of health care (NNBA, 1994). The Association's publications provide a wealth of examples of independent practice and concrete suggestions on how to establish and conduct innovative nursing businesses. Current periodicals published by the NNBA include *Alternatives: NNBA's Non-Traditional Career Opportunities Bulletin, The Exchange,* and the annual *National Nurses in Business Directory.*

Among some of the innovative nursing roles in the community are parish nurses or ministers of health, who are functioning in a variety of church congregations of various denominations. These nurses spend their time in home, hospital, and nursing home visitations, health teaching, telephone time on behalf of parishioners, health screening, and counseling (McDermott & Burke, 1993). Djupe, Olson, and Ryan (1991) found that the parish nurse serves as health educator, personal health counselor, referral source and liaison with community resources, coordinator of volunteers and support groups, and interpreter of the close relationship between faith and health. The parish nurse may be funded by the church, hospital, or foundation sponsorship.

Evaluation

Measurement of the outcomes of community health nursing care leads to a variety of questions and issues:

1. What are the consequences of organizing care around reimbursement guidelines rather than a theory-based approach?

2. What level of focus of community health nursing is most cost-effective: individuals, families, groups, or communities?

3. What are the effects of changes in referral patterns, level of illness of clients referred, intensity of services required, and quality of services delivered?

4. What measures of patient outcomes in terms of behavioral or functional changes can be used to evaluate the interventions of community health nurses?

5. What are the effects of different management procedures for specific types of clients?

6. What is the effect of various management structures and types of agencies on the way home care is delivered?

7. What are the relationships between client assessment, care plans, and client outcomes?

Flynn and Ray (1987) contrast several quality assessment criteria or measurement strategies for a quality assurance program, categorizing them according to environmental, structure, process, or outcome measures. They point out that a major problem with existing criteria is that different agencies use different classification schemes for their client populations, thereby reducing the possibilities of sharing methods or comparing across agencies. Classifications may be organized by diseases or problem categories. Multiple-problem populations present even greater difficulties. Very few of the existing criteria have established either reliability or validity.

THE FUTURE OF COMMUNITY HEALTH NURSING

Conway-Welch (1990) discusses the view of the immediate future (5 to 15 years) as proposed by the 1986 National Commission on Nursing Implementation Project. The major forces for shaping nursing's role in the health care environment are considered to be:

1. Shifting payment systems
2. Increased proportion of the aged population
3. Increased competition among health care providers
4. Increased complexity of client needs and severity of client conditions
5. Government intervention in cost containment

Trends in Health Care Delivery

The health care delivery system will continue to be driven by a business orientation and profit motive. These forces will be fuelled by government intervention to contain costs and will result in structural and delivery changes. This business orientation will demand more precise justification of costs and substantive data on the results of intervention. The emphasis will be on productivity, making the need for the monitoring of quality even more crucial. This trend will necessitate the development of data on the cost–benefit outcomes of nursing care.

The shifting payment system and the explosion of technology will cause client populations to shift away from acute care hospitals. Multi-tiered care systems and the problems of dealing with uncompensated care may increase. To lower the costs of long-term care, services for the management of chronic illness and need for home care services will both increase dramatically (Conway-Welch, 1990).

A major focus in health care reform proposals is community-based primary health care services as a part of any basic health care package for all citizens. Primary health care is not just community health care or primary medical care but refers to a range of programs adapted to the patterns of health and disease of people in a particular setting; a level of care backed by a well-organized referral system; a strategy for reorienting the health system to provide the whole population with effective essential care; and a philosophy based on the principles of social equity, self-reliance, and community development (World Health Organization, 1987). Implications of this goal for the year 2000 include universal coverage with essential health services, which may mean high-cost care will need to be cut back. Services must be effective, efficient, and affordable. Health services must have an integrated focus encompassing disease prevention, health promotion, and curative and rehabilitative services. Individual and community participation must be sought. Health must be viewed as a part of growth and development, rather than as a result of the developmental process (Collado, 1992).

Consumer Trends

The profile of the consumer of health care will shift to an increasing proportion of elderly persons with escalating needs for uncompensated care. The greater numbers of immigrant populations will require larger numbers of nurses who speak a second language and have an understanding of ethnic diversity.

Although self-care and wellness services will increase, consumers may not take advantage of these services. Instead, they will continue to use the health care system for illness care. Futurists predict that consumers will force a more responsive health care system.

With the increasing frequency of decision making by clients, families, and health care providers on extending life through the use of procedures and equipment, the quality of life afterwards will be a major challenge. Ethical issues will be an increasing concern (Conway-Welch, 1990).

Nurses and Nursing

Since the government role in health care is expected to continue, nurses must learn to be adept at influencing public policy. Nursing organizations will have to be involved in the public arena to influence policy. The public arena may be the workplace, the community, the state legislature, or Congress.

The changing settings of health care delivery will necessitate a larger number of nurses practicing outside the hospital setting. At the same time, advanced preparation will be needed to manage the increasingly complex needs of clients in the acute care setting.

In community health nursing, there is and will continue to be a shortage of baccalaureate, master's, and doctorally prepared nurses and an oversupply of associate-degree nurses (Association of Community Health Nursing Educators, 1993). It

is critical that planned change include the shifting of one educational system to another. The increased acuity and level of complexity in community-based illness care requires increased expertise in assessment and clinical judgment. The recent emphasis on community-based primary care requires expertise in assisting clients to make lifestyle changes and to develop health-enhancing behaviors. The future nurse's practice will be based on a greater use of research and scientific data regarding health promotion and disease prevention strategies as a result of lifestyle, environmental, and social issues. These issues will require nursing interventions at both the macro and the micro levels.

The Association of Community Health Nursing Educators (1993) reiterated the 1984 Consensus Conference position in their recommendation that there should be two levels of community/public health nurses: the community health nurse generalist and the community health nurse specialist. The entry level qualification for a generalist position is the BSN, and first-line supervisory positions require a BSN and 2 years of community health nursing experience along with a plan for the completion of a master's degree in community/public health nursing. Middle management positions require nurses with a master's degree in community/public health nursing and 3 years of experience, including 2 years of supervision of professional staff. All consultant and specialty positions also require the master's in nursing degree and appropriate certification.

Because of the changes in ways that health care will be delivered, it is expected that nurses will provide services in a greater diversity of settings, consistent with the business orientation of health care services. Contractual agreements, private practice, professional collaboration, consultation, and other nursing entrepreneurial endeavors will be multiplying (Conway-Welch, 1990).

In February 1991 the ANA adopted *Nursing's Agenda for Health Care Reform.* The plan shifts the emphasis of the health care system from illness and cure to wellness and care. There will be universal access to a standard package of essential services. The ultimate goal will be to merge all government-sponsored health programs into a single public program. Then there will be coverage options accessed through an integration of public and private plans and resources. The plan also specifies cost-effective, quality care that balances individual health needs and self-care responsibilities with provider capabilities. Review mechanisms for outcome and effectiveness measures, managed care, and case management are key concepts here.

The future will be shaped by the degree of acceptance and implementation of nursing's agenda at the policy-making level. A major move in a desirable direction occurred in March 1993 when ANA representatives were called to meet with the First Lady, Hillary Rodham Clinton, and the President's Health Care Reform Team. Key messages delivered to nurses were that (1) universal access, cost containment, and quality of care must be addressed simultaneously; (2) the health care delivery system must be restructured based on consumer need and not on the medical model; (3) primary care, public health, and a continuum of services must be increasingly made available; (4) institutional reimbursement must not compromise quality patient care by limiting nurse–patient ratios; (5) consumers must have access to nursing care, and barriers must be eliminated; and (6) funding for nursing education is a cost-effective public investment (Betts, 1993).

Leadership and Change

Porter-O'Grady (1994) calls for creating whole-systems change and building partnerships among providers, hospitals, and health professionals. Health care is at the limit of its resources. Current service structures must be changed to create links between components. While hospitals will remain the cornerstone of health care service, they need to join in efforts to create truly healthy communities and become involved in coalitions with other public health services. Finally he charges nurses to a political and social vigilance to take advantage of new opportunities. Nurses should pay attention to the political playing field, associate with people in positions of power, and hold political positions. Nursing offers just what the American health consumer hopes for. Local, regional, state, and federal politics are the legitimate territory for health issues and the appropriate work place for nurse leaders.

Maraldo (1990) reinforces these dictates in suggesting that as professionals we must muster nursing's resources in areas that will have the greatest effect on the most people. Nursing must move in the directions of the greatest strategic leverage and invest resources that will yield the greatest power for nursing. She sees nurses functioning as case managers and in private practice arrangements as a strategy for increasing the prestige of nursing in the public's eye. Nurses taking on the authority and responsibility of making decisions about client care is a route easily followed in community health nursing practice. Working for financial independence in the reimbursement of nursing care in and out of hospitals and across settings is an important ingredient to achieving this increased leverage for nursing. Again, political involvement is implied as crucial for providing leadership for changes in community health nursing.

The focus on disease prevention and health promotion in health care reform is a most promising redirection for nursing. Nurses are the only health care professionals who fully understand how family and community resources can be developed and used to substitute for expensive technology and inpatient care. Nursing has enormous possibilities to take the lead in designing and evaluating high-quality measures for community-based care, cross-site care, family care abilities, environmental concerns, and assuring that the patient is educated and empowered to make informed decisions about his or her own health care (Mundinger, 1994).

Chapter Highlights

- Nurse empowerment is an evolutionary process.

- Change may be haphazard, developmental, spontaneous, or planned and may be first order or second order.

- Various models of change processes and change skills need to be used by nurses who wish to become change agents.

- Participation in nursing and community organizations is a means to empowerment.

- Political involvement for a nurse activist can evolve from civic involvement, advocacy, and organizing to long-term power wielding.

- Issues in nursing assessment involve who is the client and what tool will be used to conduct the assessment.

- Community nursing diagnosis is difficult without a standardized classification system.

- Nursing goals are unclear when the target systems in the community are not specified.

- Nursing interventions have new developments with nursing centers, nursing entrepreneurship, and parish nursing.

- Evaluation of nursing care in the community is dependent on the assessment of client outcomes.

- The future trends in community health nursing will be influenced by shifting payment systems, increased elderly and knowledgeable consumers, shortages of BSN and MSN nurses, implementation of *Nursing's Agenda for Health Care Reform*, political action, and nursing leadership.

 CRITICAL THINKING EXERCISE

You have just learned that there are plans to locate a hazardous waste dump near your home and local schools. Draft letters, plan visits with appropriate public officials, and develop some community part-nerships to tackle the proposed action. What professional and community organizations and resources would you seek out to help you?

REFERENCES

American Nurses' Association. (1980). *A conceptual model of community health nursing.* Kansas City: Author.

American Nurses' Association. (1983). *Staff organization, philosophy, and functions.* Kansas City: Author.

American Nurses' Association. (1985). *A guide for community-based nursing services.* Kansas City: Author.

American Nurses' Association. (1986). *Community-based nursing services: Innovative models.* Kansas City: Author.

American Nurses' Association. (1987). *The nursing center: Concept and design.* Kansas City: Author.

American Nurses' Association. (1990). *Nurses resource directory: Nursing's national yellow pages.* Kansas City: Author.

American Nurses' Association. (1991). *Nursing's agenda for health care reform.* Kansas City: Author.

American Nurses' Foundation. (1988). *Nurses in private prac-*

tice: Characteristics, organizational arrangements, and reimbursement policy. Kansas City: Author.

American Public Health Association. (1982). The definition of public health nursing practice in the delivery of health care. *American Journal of Public Health, 72,* 210-212.

American Public Health Association. (1990). *Healthy people 2000: National health promotion and disease prevention objectives.* Washington, DC: Author.

American Public Health Association. (1991). *Healthy communities 2000: Model standards* (3rd ed.). Washington, DC: Author.

Archer, S.E., Kelly, C.D., & Bisch, S.A. (1984). *Implementing change in communities: A collaborative approach.* St. Louis: Mosby.

Association of Community Health Nursing Educators. (1990). *Essentials of baccalaureate nursing education for entry level community health nursing practice.* Lexington, KY: Author.

Association of Community Health Nursing Educators. (1991). *Essentials of master's level community health nursing education for advanced practice.* Lexington, KY: Author.

Association of Community Health Nursing Educators. (1991). *Research agenda for community health nursing.* Lexington, KY: Author.

Association of Community Health Nursing Educators. (1991). *1990 state of the art of community health nursing education, research, and practice.* Lexington, KY: Author.

Association of Community Health Nursing Educators. (1991). *Research priorities.* Lexington, KY: Author.

Association of Community Health Nursing Educators. (1992). *Research priorities for community health nursing: 1992.* Lexington, KY: Author.

Association of Community Health Nursing Educators. (1992). *1991 state of the art of community health nursing education, research, and practice.* Lexington, KY: Author.

Association of Community Health Nursing Educators. (1993). *Differentiated nursing practice in community health.* Lexington, KY: Author.

Association of Community Health Nursing Educators. (1993). *1992 state of the art of community health nursing education, research, and practice.* Lexington, KY: Author.

Association of Community Health Nursing Educators. (1994). *Essentials of doctoral nursing education for community health nursing.* Lexington, KY: Author.

Barger, S., & Rosenfeld, P. (1993). Models in community health care: Findings from a national study of community nursing centers. *Nursing & Health Care, 14*(8), 426-431.

Barker, J.B., Bayne, T., Higgs, Z.R., Jenkin, S.A., Murphy, D., & Synoground, G. (1994). Community analysis: A collaborative community practice project. *Public Health Nursing, 11*(2), 113-118.

Batra, C. (1992). Empowering for professional, political, and health policy involvement. *Nursing Outlook, 40*(4), 170-176.

Bennis, W.G., Benne, K.D., Chin, R., & Corey, K.E. (1976). *The planning of change* (3rd ed.). New York: Holt, Rinehart & Winston.

Betts, V.T. (1992). Achievement through activism: A call for nurses to be political. *American Nurse, 24*(8), 5.

Betts, V.T. (1993). Nurses, the White House and health care reform. *American Nurse, 25*(4), 5.

Brooten, D.A., Hayman, L.L., & Naylor, M.D. (1978). *Leadership for change: A guide for the frustrated nurse.* Philadelphia: J.B. Lippincott.

Capuzzi, C., & Garland, M. (1990). The Oregon plan: Increasing access to health care. *Nursing Outlook, 36*(6), 260-263, 286.

Chalich, T., & Smith, L. (1992). Nursing at the grassroots. *Nursing and Health Care, 13*(5), 242-244.

Collado, C.B. (1992). Primary health care: A continuing challenge. *Nursing and Health Care, 13*(8), 408-413.

Conway-Welch, C. (1990). Emerging models of postbaccalau-

reate nursing education. In J.C. McCloskey & H.K. Grace (Eds.) *Current issues in nursing* (3rd ed.) (pp. 137-144). St. Louis: Mosby.

Djupe, A.M., Olson, H., & Ryan, J. (1991). *An institutionally based model of parish nursing services.* Park Ridge, IL: National Parish Nurse Resource Center.

Duncan, W.J. (1978). *Essentials of management* (2nd ed.). Hinsdale, IL: Dryden Press.

Flynn, B.C., & Ray, D.W. (1987). Current perspectives in quality assurance and community health nursing. *Journal of Community Health Nursing, 4*(4), 187-198.

Goeppinger, J. (1984). Primary health care: An answer to the dilemmas of community nursing. *Public Health Nursing, 1*(3), 129-140.

Hall, J.E., & Weaver, R.R. (1985). *Distributive nursing practice: A systems approach to community health* (2nd ed.). Philadelphia: J.B. Lippincott.

Hamilton, P.A. (1983). Community nursing diagnosis. *Advances in Nursing Science, 5*(3), 21-36.

Hawks, J.H., & Hromek, C. (1992). Nursing practicum: Empowering strategies. *Nursing Outlook, 40*(5), 231-234.

Hegyvary, S.T. (1990). A guide to nursing organizations: What they are and how to choose them. In J.C. McCloskey & H.K. Grace (Eds.). *Current issues in nursing* (3rd ed.) (pp. 316-320). St. Louis: Mosby.

Kalisch, B.J., & Kalisch, P.A. (1982). *Politics of nursing.* Philadelphia: J.B. Lippincott.

Kovner, C. (1989). Public health nursing costs in home care. *Public Health Nursing, 6*(1), 3-7.

Lancaster, J. (1982). Change theory: An essential aspect of nursing practice. In W. Lancaster & J. Lancaster (Eds.). *Concepts for advanced nursing practice: The nurse as a change agent.* St. Louis: Mosby.

Lewin, K. (1951). *Field theory in social science.* New York: Harper & Row.

Lippitt, G.L. (1973). *Visualizing change: Model building and the change process.* LaJolla, CA: University Associates.

Maraldo, P.J. (1990). The aftermath of DRGs: The politics of transformation. In J.C. McCloskey & H.K. Grace (Eds.) *Current issues in nursing* (3rd ed.) (pp. 387-392). St. Louis: Mosby.

McDermott, M.A., & Burke, J. (1993). When the population is a congregation: The emerging role of the parish nurse. *Journal of Community Health Nursing, 10*(3), 179-190.

Mitty, E.L. (1991). The nurse as advocate: Issues in LTC. *Nursing and Health Care, 12*(10), 520-523.

Muecke, M.A. (1984). Community health diagnosis in nursing. *Public Health Nursing, 1*(1), 23-35.

Mundinger, M.O. (1994). Health care reform: Will nursing respond? *Nursing and Health Care, 15*(1), 28-33.

Murphy, N.J. (1992). Nursing leadership in health policy decision-making. *Nursing Outlook, 40*(4), 158-161.

National League for Nursing. (1983). *NLN mission and goals: 1983-1985.* New York: Author.

National League for Nursing. (1990). *Standards of excellence for community health organizations.* New York: Author.

National League for Nursing. (1989). *Standards of excellence for home care organizations.* New York: Author.

National League for Nursing. (1993). *Council for Nursing Centers: Membership directory.* New York: Author.

National Nurses in Business Association. (1994). *NNBA organizational fact sheet.* Petaluma, CA: Author.

Nightingale, F. (1969). *Notes on nursing: What it is and what it is not.* New York: Dover (originally published in 1860).

Pender, N.J. (1993a). Creating change through partnerships. *Nursing Outlook, 41*(1), 8-9.

Pender, N.J. (1993b). Health care reform: One view of the future. *Nursing Outlook, 41*(2), 56-57.

Pender, N.J. (1993c). Reaching out. *Nursing Outlook, 41*(3), 103-104.

Porter-O'Grady, T. (1994). Building partnerships in health care: Creating whole systems change. *Nursing and Health Care, 15*(1), 34-38.

Risner, P.B. (1990). Nursing diagnosis: Diagnostic statements. In J.W. Griffith & P.J. Christiansen (Eds.) *Nursing process: Application of conceptual models* (3rd ed.) (pp. 158-178). St. Louis: Mosby.

Rogers, E. (1962). *Diffusion of innovations.* New York: Free Press of Glencoe.

Sampson, E. (1971). *Social psychology and contemporary society.* New York: Wiley & Sons.

Schmieding, N.J. (1993). Nurse empowerment through context, structure, and process. *Journal of Professional Nursing, 9*(4), 239-245.

Sharp, N., Biggs, S., & Wakefield, M. (1991). Public policy: New opportunities for nurses. *Nursing and Health Care, 12*(1), 16-22.

Spradley, B.W. (1990). *Community health nursing: Concepts and practice* (3rd ed.). Glenview, IL: Scott, Foresman/Little, Brown.

Sprayberry, L.D. (1993). Nursing's dual role in health care policy. *Nursing and Health Care, 14*(5), 250-254.

U.S. Department of Health and Human Services. (1985). *Consensus conference on the essentials of public health nursing practice and education: Report of the conference September 5-7, 1984.* Washington, DC: Author.

Watzlawick, P., Weakland, J.A., & Fisch, R. (1974). *Change: Principles of problem formation and problem resolution.* New York: Norton.

World Health Organization. (1987). *Leadership for health for all: The challenge to nursing: A strategy for action.* (A report of an international conference of leaders in nursing for health for all, Tokyo, Japan). Geneva: Author.

Zink, M.R. (1994). Nursing diagnosis in home care: Audit tool development. *Journal of Community Health Nursing, 11*(1), 51-58.

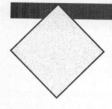

GLOSSARY

A

Abstinence: Total voluntary avoidance of a substance or an activity.

Abuse: Any type of physical or emotional maltreatment of another individual, ranging from violent attacks to passive neglect.

Accelerating change: Quickening of the pace of change in society.

Access to care: The availability of health care, particularly for individuals unable to pay for it.

Accident prevention: A plan of education to reduce unintended injuries.

Accountability: To be answerable to someone for something.

Accreditation: A voluntary system by which agencies are recognized as having met predetermined standards of the acccrediting body.

Acid fast bacilli (AFB): Bacteria that remain stained even after they have been washed in an acid solution. Tubercle bacilliare is one kind of acid fast bacilli. The diagnosis is not confirmed until a culture is grown and identified as M. tuberculosis.

Acne vulgaris: A form of acne characterized by comedomes which may close, forming cysts that can cause permanent scarring. It is a common health problem of adolescents.

Acquired Immune Deficiency Syndrome (AIDS): A disease caused by a virus that effects cell-mediated immunity. It has a long incubation period, follows a protracted and debilitating course, is manifested by various opportunistic infections, and is always fatal at this time.

Active immunity: A long term resistance to disease brought about naturally by infection or artificially by innoculations of the agent itself in killed or modified form.

Activities of daily living (ADLs): Actions such as bathing, dressing, and toileting that are normally performed on a daily basis.

Activity theory: Theory of aging stating that most older adults maintain a high level of activity to promote well-being and satisfaction. The amount of activity is influenced by previous life-style.

Act utilitarianism: The process of examining the acts taken to bring about happiness.

Acute care case management: A management style that is patient-centered and focuses on patient outcomes and nurse accountability.

Adaptive model: A model that views health as the effective functioning of adaptive systems.

Addiction: Compulsive, uncontrollable physical or psychological dependence on a substance or habit.

Adjourning: The fifth and final stage of group development, in which the group terminates its task and comes to some kind of closure.

Admission criteria: Factors to be considered when evaluating a client's suitability for receiving high-technology care in the home.

Adolescence: The period of life between the ages of 13 and 20 years. In Western societies adolescence may be prolonged.

Adolescent kyphosis: A mild curvature of the spine, usually self-limiting and often undiagnosed. It may be precipitated by poor posture during a rapid growth spurt.

Adult day care: Services designed to meet the unique needs of older adults who live in the community but cannot function completely autonomously and may need some supervision. Services include socialization and health promotion.

Advocacy: The act of pleading or supporting the cause or viewpoint of another person. In health care, advocacy is a demonstrable way to exercise respect and caring for the client through the use of mutuality, facilitation, protection, and coordination of care.

Advocate: One who protects and supports a client's right to quality health care.

Affective domain: One of three domains concerning learning behaviors; deals with expression of feeling, interests, attitudes, values, and appreciation.

Agent: A factor, inanimate or animate, whose presence or lack of presence may lead to disease, disability, or death.

Aggregate: Collection of individuals who share similar characteristics or experience common factors.

Aging: The process of growing older.

AIDS: Abbreviation for acquired immune deficiency syndrome.

AIDS related complex: A subclinical form of AIDS.

Air pollution: Concentration of dust, soot, and other particles in the atmosphere that may increase the incidence of illness.

Al-Anon: Support group for family members of alcoholics or other substance abusers.

Alcohol: A central nervous system depressant consumed in liquid form that may impair one's judgment, cause unconsciousness, and damage the liver if consumed in excess.

Alcoholics Anonymous: Self-help groups of recovering alcoholics whose goal is to stay sober.

Alcoholism: The extreme dependence on excessive amounts of alcohol, associated with a cumulative pattern of deviant behaviors.

Alienation: The act or state of being estranged or isolated which may be related to a failure to establish an identity during adolescence.

Altered coping mechanisms: Lack of ability to problem solve in a positive way. May result in acts of subjugation and aggression as a manifestation of anger and frustration by prisoners in a jail.

Altered family processes: A state in which functions of a family unit are chronically disorganized, leading to conflict, ineffective problem solving and self-perpetuating crises.

Altered growth pattern: A lack of steady linear growth and development.

Alternative or complementary treatment modalities: Healing practices traditionally used by nonwestern cultures which include acupuncture, reflexology, and herbalism, among others.

Alzheimer's disease: A progressive dementia of unknown etiology characterized by confusion, memory failure, disorientation, and inability to carry out purposeful movements. The disease may take a few months to 7 years to progress to a complete loss of functioning.

American Association of Occupational Health Nurses (AAOHN): Association formed by nurses practicing in occupational health, to improve nursing services and offer opportunities for nurses interested in this area of practice.

American Association of Retired Persons (AARP): Organization providing information and various benefits to persons over 50 years of age.

American Nurses Association (ANA): The national professional association of registered nurses in the United States.

Americans with Disabilities Act: Federal legislation that prohibits discrimination against persons with a disability.

Amphetamines: Synthetic psychoactive drugs that are available in capsule or tablet form.

Analytical study: A study conducted by formulating and testing a hypothesis.

Anergy: The inability to mount a delayed-type hypersensitivity response to skin test antigens because of immunosuppression, which is caused by disease or immunosuppressive drugs.

Anorexia nervosa: A disorder characterized by a prolonged refusal to eat, emaciation, amenorrhea, and emotional disturbance concerning body image.

Anthropometric measures: Measurement of growth by comparison of height, weight, and age to standardized growth charts.

Antibody: A protein found mostly in serum that is formed in response to exposure to a specific antigen.

Antigen: Substance that stimulates the formation of an antibody.

Antitoxin: Antibody formed in response to a toxin.

Apgar score: A system of scoring an infant's condition on five factors at 1 minute and again at 5 minutes after birth. The maximum score is 10. Those with low scores (less than 4) need immediate attention to survive.

Apnea monitoring: Use of a device that monitors the client's (usually an infant) breathing. An alarm sounds if breathing stops.

Artificial immunity: Immunity acquired by inoculation of the agent in killed or modified form.

Assessment: A systematic collection of data that assists one in identifying the needs, preferences, and abilities of a client.

Association: A relationship between two factors or events that demonstrates that they occur more frequently together than one would expect by chance alone.

Asthma: A respiratory disorder characterized by paroxysmal dyspnea and wheezing caused by constriction of the bronchi.

Autism: A developmental disability characterized by abnormal emotional, social, and language development. The autistic child may engage in repetitive and ritualistic behavior and appears to be unable to progress beyond a fixed developmental stage.

Autocratic leadership: Leadership style in which decisions are made by the leader with little or no input from the group members.

Autoimmune theory: A biologic theory of aging where impaired antibodies react with normal cells of the body and kill the normal cells, causing the body to begin to deteriorate.

Autonomy: The quality of being self-governing, including the right to make one's own decisions.

Autonomy vs. doubt and shame: Stage of development during the toddler period described by Erikson as one when the toddler wishes to gain control of the world.

B

Bacillus: A genus of aeorbic, gram-positive, spore-producing bacteria.

Barbiturates: Synthetic drugs that are classified as sedative-hypnotic agents.

Basic structure: In Neuman's model, all the variables that keep the individual or community functioning as a unit, as well as its unique characteristics.

Beliefs: Statements that one holds to be true, but that may or may not be based on empirical evidence.

Beneficence: The quality or state of being, doing, or producing good.

Biologic hazards: Infection-producing organisms found in the environment, such as bacteria, viruses, molds, fungi, and parasites.

Biomagnification: The concentration of pollutants upwardly through the food chain.

Birth rate: Number of live births per 1000 population.

Blended family: Family resulting when two adults who were part of previous families join together to form a new family.

Blindness: The inability to see. Children who are blind from birth will experience greater developmental delays than those who lose their sight later in childhood.

Body image: The perception of how one sees and feels about his or her body.

Body Mass Index: Expression of the relationship between a person's height and weight.

Breastfeeding: The sucking of milk by an infant from the mother's breast.

Bulimia: Binge eating followed by purging, which involves vomiting, and use of laxatives or diuretics.

C

Calcium: A mineral found in dairy foods and green leafy vegetables, necessary for the formation of healthy teeth and bone mass.

Calorie: The amount of energy needed to raise the temperature of one gram of water, 1°C, used to measure the energy value of food.

Cannabis: Another word for marijuana, a drug derived from the Indian hemp plant.

Candidiasis: Infection caused by a species of Candida, usually *Candida albicans,* characterized by pruritius, a white exudate, peeling, and easy bleeding.

Cardinal virtues: The basic qualities of temperance, justice, courage, and prudence.

Care-based ethics: Moral behavior motivated by compassion and caring in a sympathetic way for others.

Caregiver: One who participates in nursing activity for promoting, maintaining, and restoring women's health status.

Caregiver burden: A perception that the caregiving responsibilities have negative effects on the emotional or physical health of the caregiver.

Carrier: A person who harbors and can pass on a specific disease or infectious agent but who does not present with symptoms of the disease.

Case control study: A retrospective study that identifies a group of persons with a disease or disability and a group of similar persons without the disease or disability. The two groups are compared to determine what possible factor(s) might account for the difference in incidence of disease.

Case law: Law based on court or jury decisions.

Case management: Process of using one person, preferably a nurse, to oversee and coordinate the plan of care designed for a particular client, with the aim of assuring continuity of care and meeting individualized client needs.

Categorical imperative: A classic rule developed by Kant that means that the rules one chooses to live by as an individual are to be those that can be generalized to all persons.

Causality: The relationship between two events in which one precedes the other and the direction of influence and nature of effect are predictable and reproducible.

Causal relationships: The association between risk factor and disease showing cause in temporality, strength of association, biologic plausibility, specificity, consistency, biologic coherence, and effect of intervention.

Cerebral palsy: A motor function disorder affecting movement and muscle coordination caused by a nonprogressive brain defect or lesion present at birth or shortly after.

Certification: Receiving a document of approval from a professional organization. It is sometimes recognized by the licensure board as evidence of expertise in a specialty area.

Certified home health agency: An agency, accredited by the Community Health Accreditation Program or the Joint Commission of Home Health, that provides part-time or intermittent nursing care, physical, occupational, or speech therapy, medical social services, home health aide services, medical supplies, or medical services to a client in the home.

Chain of transmission: A complicated mode of transmission involving a causative agent, a host, and an environment.

Change agent: One who purposefully and systematically implements change.

Chemical dependency: Addiction to drugs and/or alcohol.

Chemical hazards: Chemical agents found in the environment or workplace that may have adverse effects on health.

Chemical wastes: Byproducts created by the manufacture of chemicals; these include hazardous and nonhazardous substances.

Child abuse and neglect: Physical or emotional maltreatment and lack of provision for the needs of a child.

Cholesterol: Fatty substance found in foods of animal origin that is associated with a high risk of cardiovascular disease.

Chronic illness: A condition that has one or more of the following criteria: It is permanent, leaves residual disability, is caused by a nonpathologic alteration, requires special training for rehabilitation, and is expected to require a long period of supervision, observation, or care.

Chronic low self esteem: NANDA-approved nursing diagnosis of long-standing self-evaluation/feelings about self or self-capabilities.

Chronicity: Ongoing disease process that may require intervention to maintain the highest level of wellness possible or restore the highest level of functioning.

Circular communication diagram: A method of illustrating the mutual responsibility borne by two participants in an interaction, in which each one has a thought, feeling, and behavioral response to the other's action.

Civil law: Law that addresses relationships and resolves disputes among individual persons or among entities such as corporations or hospitals.

Civil rights: The legal expectations of persons (aggregates) who are similarly situated to be treated equally under the law.

Client: The recipient of care; may be an individual, family, or a group.

Client education: Health education provided as a basic community health nursing intervention at the primary, secondary, or tertiary level of prevention.

Client eligibility: Client and caregiver factors to assess when determining whether an individual can be admitted to a home care program.

Clinical management: A management strategy wherein the emphasis is on allowing the client to become independent of the clinical provider as soon as it is appropriate and possible.

Clinical model: Health is viewed as the absence of disease.

Cognitive domain: One of three domains concerning learning behaviors; deals with intellectual ability.

Cohesion: A group member's sense of belonging and the degree to which one feels that he or she fits into the group and is included by others.

Cohort: A group of persons who share a common characteristic.

Cohort study: Study of a group of persons over time (a specified period) who share a common characteristic.

Common law: Court-made law that is derived from English courts and is changed over time by the judicial system.

Common vehicle: Contaminated material, product, or substance that serves as an intermediate means by which an infectious agent is transported to two or more susceptible hosts.

Communicable disease: An illness caused by a specific infectious agent that arises through transmission of that agent from an infected person, animal, or inanimate reservoir to a susceptible host.

Communication: The giving or receiving of information or messages.

Community: A practice setting, a target of service, or a small group within a larger population.

Community as client: The entire community as the focus and recipient of nursing care.

Community assessment: The process of describing a community, its patterns of morbidity and mortality, and identifying patterns of disease or potential health problems in the community.

Community development group: Groups that come together to support advocacy.

Community health nurse: A nurse who works to promote and preserve the health of populations and who uses a holistic approach to care for the health of individuals in the community.

Community health nursing: A synthesis of nursing theory and public health practice applied to promoting and preserving the health of populations. Health promotion, health maintenance, health education, and continuity of care are used in holistic approach to the management of the health care of individuals.

Community health nursing diagnosis: Nursing diagnosis that is generated from the state of the community and for whom the direct target of intervention is the community itself.

Community health nursing theory: Nursing theory applicable to community health nursing; it may be adaptedx from generic nursing theory or derived from a unique community health nursing perspective.

Comparison group: Any group compared to a group being studied; a control group.

Complex carbohydrates: Carbohydrates containing a large number of glucose molecules, such as those found in cereals and whole grain foods; starches.

Compliance: Cooperation and participation in the prescribed therapeutic regimen by the client.

Concrete operation: Developmental state of the child theorized by Piaget where all aspects of life are taken literally.

Concurrent audit: Quality assurance audit performed by comparing the chart with predetermined criteria during the episode of care.

Confidentiality: The social or legal contract guaranteeing another's privacy. The privacy of communications between nurse and patient is protected in section two of the Code for Nurses.

Conflict: Antagonistic state or action, as of divergent ideas.

Confounding variable: A factor that causes change in the frequency of disease and also varies systematically with a third causal factor being studied.

Congenital anomaly: An abnormal condition present at birth.

Constitutional law: Law based on federal and state constitutions.

Continuing care: The process of activities between and among patients and providers to coordinate ongoing care.

Continuity of care: Personalized, continuous care that begins at the point of entry into the health care system and continues until the health-related problems and needs are resolved by means of interpersonal, interdisciplinary communication with the focus on the patient and his family.

Continuity theory: Theory of aging stating that many adults maintain lifestyles like those they had in young adulthood.

Continuous Medicaid Eligibility: Practice of guaranteeing Medicaid coverage throughout pregnancy for eligible women even if family income and resources fluctuate.

Continuous Quality Improvement (CQI): The ongoing organized practice of improving work processes and systems through the use of teams and data management tools.

Continuum of care: An integrated, client-oriented system of care composed of both services and integrating mechanisms that guides and tracks clients over time through a comprehensive array of health, mental health, and social services spanning all levels of intensity of care.

Correctional institution: Facility for incarceration of individuals convicted of a crime; includes minimum, medium, and maximum levels of security.

Cost containment: Achieving a given objective with an awareness of and a responsibility to keeping the overall costs of services at an appropriate manageable level.

Cost-effective care: Care provided in the most effective manner in terms of cost and setting.

Counselor: One who gives guidance or assistance with problem solving.

Criminal law: Law dealing with relationships between a person (or entities such as corporations) and the state.

Crisis theory: The concept of offering preventive mental and emotional health care to families during transitional periods.

Crisis: An upset in a steady state.

Criteria: Measurable statements that reflect the intent of a standard.

Critical feminist theory: The theory that gender identity develops and persists as a social, economic, and political category.

Cross-sectional study: A study that determines the presence or absence of causal factors of disease or disability for each member of a population at a single point in time.

Cross tolerance: Use of one substance that increases the user's tolerance for similar substances.

Culture: A distinctive way of life that characterizes an ethnic group and that is passed down from generation to generation; learned patterns of behavior.

Cultural assessment: Systematic appraisal of a client's cultural beliefs, values, and attitudes.

Cultural care: A view of care based on Leininger's Sunrise model where world view, cultural, and social structure dimensions provide the overall context in which the client exists.

Cultural diversity: Differences in values, beliefs, and attitudes among people of different cultures.

Culturally congruent care: Nurse-client intervention where cultural relevance must be validated with the client so that it is meaningful in the context of the client culture.

Culture-bound: The inability to consider another cultural point of view.

Cystic fibrosis: An inherited disorder of the exocrine glands causing abnormally thick secretions of mucus, elevation of sweat electrolytes, increased organic and enzymatic constituents of saliva, and overactivity of the autonomic nervous system beginning in infancy. The glands most affected are those in the pancreas and respiratory system. Treatment is directed at preventing respiratory infections. There is no cure, but the advent of effective antibiotics has prolonged the life span.

Cytomegalovirus (CMV): A member of a group of large species-specific herpes type viruses with a wide variety of disease effects; it may cause serious illness in newborns and individuals with depressed immunity.

D

Day care: Care of infants and children while parents are occupied with work or school.

Day Care Center: A state licensed facility where children ranging from infancy through school-age are cared for while the parents are working or are otherwise unable to care for their children.

Death of permanence: Lack of stability in relationships and material possessions caused by a rapidly changing society.

Defining characteristics: Signs and symptoms identified to describe various states of health.

Deinstitutionalization: The practice of discharging mental patients from institutions to halfway houses and group homes or, in some instances to the streets.

Deliriants: Any chemicals that give off fumes or vapors that, when inhaled, produce symptoms similar to intoxication.

Dementia: A condition of deteriorated mentality.

Democratic leadership: Leadership style in which decisions are made jointly by the group leader and group members.

Denial: A response to chronic illness or disability characterized by lack of acknowledgment of the condition and a perception that family life is normal and social significance of the condition is nil; behavior shows normalcy.

Denial/Appeals: Refusal of third-party payers to provide reimbursement for services and the process of requesting reconsideration.

Dental caries: Progressive decay or destruction of a tooth.

Denver Developmental Screening Test: Test for evaluating the motor, social, and language skills of children 1 month to 6 years of age.

Deotological (formalist) theory: Theory of ethics stating that the rightness or wrongness of an action is determined by the nature of the action or motives behind it, not the results.

Dependence: Physical or psychologic state in which the continuous and prolonged consumption of a substance leads to the user's adaptation to its presence.

Depressant: A substance that slows the functioning of a body system.

Depression: A state of feeling sad.

Descriptive study: The study of patterns of disease occurrence by person, place, or time to develop hypotheses concerning cause or origin of the disease.

Descriptive survey: Collection and analysis of existing information, which may lead to formulation of hypotheses and further study.

Designer drugs: Synthetic-organic compounds that are designed as analogs of illicit drugs, with the same narcotic or other dangerous effects.

Detoxification: Withdrawal of an addicting substance under controlled conditions to minimize side effects.

Developmental disability: A chronic disability caused by emotional or physical impairments that manifests itself before adulthood and interferes with a person's ability to function normally in society.

Developmental model: The belief that developmentally disabled individuals are not ill and development is a lifetime priority.

Developmental task: A stage in Erikson's model of emotional development where the adolescent completes the task of identity versus diffusion (a feeling of not belonging anywhere).

Diagnosis: A clinical judgment about individual, family, or community responses to health problems or life processes.

Diagnosis-related groups (DRG): Classification of medical conditions into 23 major diagnostic categories and 470 diagnostic groups, which are used to determine the payment reimbursable by Medicare and other third-party payors.

Diagnostic category: Classification used to describe various states of health that the nurse can treat.

Diet: The foods eaten by an individual, with regard to nutritional qualities, composition, and effects on health.

Dietition: Individual trained in nutrition who assists clients in improving nutritional status.

Direct transmission: Transmission of a disease that occurs when an agent directly affects a host through an accessible portal of entry.

Disability: The loss, absence, or impairment of the normal range of physical or mental ability.

Disability insurance: Financial assistance given to individuals in some states who have documentation from a physician that they cannot work because of a disability.

Disassociation: A response to chronic illness or disability that is characterized by acknowledgment of the condition and a perception that family life is abnormal and social significance of the condition is great; behavior emphasizes abnormality.

Discharge planning: Assessment of needs and arrangement or coordination of services for patients and clients as they move through the health care system.

Disease: A state of nonhealth in which the body is suffering from a malfunction of one or more parts with visible signs or reported symptoms.

Disease prevention: Activities that prevent or contain the spread of disease.

Disenchantment: A response to health professionals in which the client has realized that personal opinions and experience are disregarded. The client may be angry, demanding of information, or distrustful of professional advice.

Disengagement: Pattern in which rigid, impermeable boundaries separate members of a family.

Disengagement theory: Theory that older adults and society undergo a mutual withdrawal that is an inevitable part of the aging process.

Disinfection: A process that results in the elimination of many or all pathogenic microorganisms on inanimate objects with the exception of bacterial endospores.

Distributive justice: A legal process where one segment or type of population will receive certain services that another segment does not and raises the issue of distribution of services and fairness of allocation.

District nursing: The beginnings of public health nursing, as established in England.

Down syndrome: Developmental disorder resulting from the presence of an extra chromosome on the twenty-first pair causing distinct physical characteristics and mental retardation.

Driving forces: Forces that encourage the change process to move in the direction of the desired change.

Drug abuse: Use of drugs for nontherapeutic reasons.

Drug addiction: Physical or psychologic dependence on a drug.

Dysfunctional family: Family that experiences a severe level of anxiety and responds to a crisis by perceiving it as an overwhelming burden.

E

Early Postpartum Discharge: Discharge of a woman within 24 hours of an uncomplicated vaginal delivery or within 3 days of an uncomplicated cesarian delivery.

Ecomap: A schematic drawing showing interactions between a family and other systems in the community.

Education for All Handicapped Children Act: Public Law 94-142, mandating that a "free and appropriate education" be available for all children, regardless of disability.

Educational group: Group formed for the purpose of providing information and education.

Educational need: Need that can be satisfied by a learning experience.

Educational Resource Centers: Regional facilities offering education in various areas of occupational safety and health.

Ego: That aspect of a personality that defines the person's identity to the self; the conscious organized mediator between a person and reality.

ELISA test: A laboratory technique for detecting specific antigens or antibodies, commonly used in the diagnosis of AIDS.

Emic: A view of behavior in terms of the internal structure or function within a culture.

Empowerment: An interactive process that develops, builds, and increases power through cooperation, sharing and working together.

Enabling: Behavior by one person that encourages another to continue acting in a dysfunctional manner by shielding that person from the consequences of the dysfunctional behavior.

Enculturation: The raising of children within a family to conform to the requirements of the social group in which they were born.

Endemic: The habitual presence of a disease or infectious agent in a defined geographical area or population.

Engineering controls: Equipment, devices, or instruments that remove or isolate a hazard.

Enmeshment: Family pattern in which sharing

among members is extreme and intense and where individuality and independence are viewed negatively.

Environment: The combination of all factors that influence the health of a person.

Environmental factor: In nursing diagnosis, a related factor to be considered for nursing diagnosis statements using the Omaha problem classification scheme. Factors in diagnosis include physiologic, psychologic, spiritual, environmental, and sociocultural.

Environmental sensitivity: The process of becoming aware of the effects of the environment on health and working to improve the quality of the environment to raise the level of health in a community.

Epidemic: An outbreak of disease that is sudden and widespread across many localities, regions, or populations.

Epidemiology: Science concerned with the various factors and conditions that determine the occurrence and distribution of health disease, defect, disability, and death among groups of individuals.

Epidemiologic process: The phases of epidemiologic investigation, starting with descriptive study and progressing to analytical study and experimentation.

Epidemiologic triangle: The relationship between an agent, host, and environment necessary for disease to occur. Elimination of any one of these may eliminate the occurrence of disease.

Ergonomics: The study of humans at work to understand the complex relationships among people, physical and psychologic aspects of the work environment (such as facilities, equipment, and tools), job demands, and work methods.

Error and fidelity theory: A biologic theory of aging where fidelity is the production of the correct proteins from the point of gene transcription and translation of the RNA into the amino acids of the cellular structure. As the ability to transfer messages decreases, errors occur that result in production of altered proteins and, over time, the progressive deterioration of cells.

Ethical dilemma: The problem of choosing between two or more equally undesirable alternatives.

Ethics: The discipline that seeks to answer questions about values, actions, and choices of what is right and wrong.

Ethnicity: Affiliation with a value system and with people who share that system.

Ethnocentrism: The belief that one's culture is the only "correct" view of the world.

Etiologic and contributing factors: Those physiologic, situational, and maturational factors that can cause a health problem or influence its development.

Eudaimonia: Well-being. The theory that well-being is a chief good and is manifested in a sense of completeness and self-sufficiency.

Eudaemonistic conception of health: View of health that includes qualities such as self-actualization, fulfillment, and loving.

Evaluation: A systematic, continuous process of comparing the client's responses with outcomes defined by the plan of care.

Examination stage: Developmental stage described by Robert Havinghurst as occuring during later maturity.

Executive branch: The branch of an organization or government that "carries out" the law.

Existentialism: A chiefly twentieth century philosophy that stresses responsibility and freedom of choice in the individual. It is centered on the analysis of existence and of the way humans find themselves existing in the world. Human existence is regarded as indescribable and incomprehensible in scientific terms.

Expected outcome: A statement of what is expected to be accomplished by a certain time.

Experimental study: The study of a disease where there is a deliberate intervention by the investigator. Participants are randomly assigned to an intervention group at the beginning of the study.

Extended family: Several generations of a family living together.

Extrafamily stressors: Influences on a family from political, social, and cultural issues.

Extrapulmonary TB: TB outside the lungs. In the United States, about 15% of reported cases are extrapulmonary sites, such as the kidney, the pleura, the lymph nodes, or the bones.

Extrinsic motivation: Forces outside the individual that cause one to act; rewards or punishments.

F

Factor: Cause or variable that may produce an effect.

Family: A group of people, including at least one adult, who are related to each other by blood or social contract.

Family day care: Care for up to six children in a neighborhood home.

Family developmental tasks: Responsibilities connected with each particular stage of family life.

Family life cycle: Period beginning with formation of a family and ending with its dissolution.

Family violence: Any act by one family member toward another that causes pain or injury, including physical, emotional, and sexual abuse.

Fertility Rate: Number of live births per 1000 women between the ages of 15 and 44.

Fetal Alcohol Syndrome: A set of congenital psychologic, behavioral, cognitive, and physical abnormalities that tend to appear in infants whose mothers consumed alcoholic beverages during pregnancy.

Fidelity: Ethical principle related to keeping promises.

First order change: Change brought about in a system without the system itself being changed.

Flexible line of defense: In Neuman's model, a protective buffer for preventing stressors from breaking through the solid line of defense.

Fluoride: A mineral that, when incorporated into the tooth structure, helps to prevent tooth decay.

Focus groups: A small group of participants whose goal is to discuss a topic and share experiences and viewpoints thus providing information that can be analyzed and interpreted.

Folk healers: Individuals believed by some cultural groups to have the ability to cure illness.

Formaldehyde: A colorless gas often found in homes and suspected to be a carcinogen.

Forming: The initial stage of group development, in which members assemble and begin to assume a sense of common identity.

Frail elderly: Persons, usually over the age of 75, who have health problems, limited income, and a lack of social resources.

Frontier Nursing Service: An organization founded in 1925 by Mary Breckinridge in Lexington, Kentucky, to provide health care to rural families. It is still in existence today.

Fundamental human rights: Claims recognized by law that are legally enforceable.

G

Gamma globulin: Passive immunizing agents obtained from pooled human plasma.

Gender: Expectations and behaviors that individuals learn about femininity and masculinity.

Gender Identity: A person's inner sense of himself or herself as being masculine or feminine.

Generalist: A person who is prepared at the baccalaureate level and is expected to provide population-based primary care to individuals, families, and groups; practices in community health nursing.

Generativity vs. stagnation: Erickson's developmental task of middle adulthood, in which the individual is concerned with achieving major life goals.

Genogram: An assessment tool resembling a family tree that may be used to depict a family's structure.

Geopolitical community: A community defined by statistics recorded relative to person, place, and time.

Glaucoma: Eye disease characterized by increased intraocular pressure, which can cause progressive loss of sight if untreated.

Goal: An aim or end toward which intervention is directed.

Group: An open system composed of three or more persons held together by a common interest or bond.

Growth and development: General rates of physical growth and cognitive development provide milestones from which the infant and child are assessed.

Guarded alliance: A response to health professionals that emphasizes guarding client interests and needs while forming an alliance with professionals to obtain services required.

H

Habituation: Repeated use of a drug to the point at which psychologic dependence occurs.

Hallucinogens: Drugs, both natural and synthetic, that affect the mind and produce changes in perception and thinking.

Handicap: A disadvantage, resulting from an impairment or disability, that limits or prevents the fulfillment of a normal role.

Hazard: The probability that a substance will produce harm under specific conditions.

Hazard Communication Standard: The Federal standard that requires all manufacturers and distributors of hazardous chemicals to provide material safety data sheets that identify potential effects of the chemicals with which their employees work.

Hazardous wastes: Substances that can threaten health if people are exposed to them.

Health: Optimal system stability that is the best possible state for an individual, group, or community at any given time.

Health behavior contract: A formal, written agreement designed to systematically change a client's behavior to improve health.

Health behavior paradigms: Models to explain clients' health behavior, including the health paradigm and the disease paradigm.

Health Belief Model: Rosenstock's theoretical model stating that an individual's decision to perform a health action is determined by perceptions of susceptibility to an illness, severity of the illness, and personal threat of the illness.

Health care delivery system: An organized interrelated system that provides health care to a population.

Health education: Program directed to the general public that attempts to improve and maintain the health of a community.

Health Maintenance Organization (HMO): A prepaid health cooperative with an emphasis on health maintenance and illness prevention. Members prepay their medical fees and all health care is provided by the HMO.

Health promotion: Activities designed to improve one's health and prevent disease; a component of primary prevention.

Hearing loss: The inability to hear, which may range from very mild to profound (total). If present at birth, hearing loss will cause delays in language acquisition and learning.

Hepatitis A: Communicable disease caused by a virus and spread by the fecal-oral route, causing inflammation of the liver.

Herd immunity: The resistance of a group or community to invasion and spread of an infectious agent.

Herpes simplex: Infection caused by herpes simplex virus that produces small, transient, irritating, and sometimes painful fluid-filled blisters on the skin and mucous membranes.

Hiatal hernia: Herniation of the stomach through the esophagous.

High-level wellness: A concept of optimal health that emphasizes the integration of mind, body, and environment.

High-risk aggregate: A collection of individuals who share similar characteristics or experience common factors that place them at risk for death, disease, or disability.

High-tech therapy: Use of advanced equipment in the provision of nursing care, including infusion therapy, phototherapy, apnea monitoring, and ventilator therapy.

Holistic approach: Approach to nursing emphasizing the interrelationship of the body, mind, spirit, and environment in maintaining a wellness state.

Holistic health: An approach emphasizing the mind-body connection in health and illness.

Home health agency: Agency or organization providing skilled nursing and related services for clients in their homes.

Home health aide: Paraprofessional who assists with a client's personal care in the home.

Home health care: The provision of health care and health related services to persons in their place of residence (e.g. skilled nursing care). Direct care provided by the "laying on of hands", or by teaching or demonstration. It may also include assessment and observation of a client who is medically unstable.

Home health care nursing: The practice of nursing applied to a client with a health deficit in the client's place of residence.

Homeless Person's Survival Act: Act passed by the U.S. Congress in 1986 that made homeless persons eligible to receive food stamps, SSI, Medicaid, AFDC, or VA benefits and to be included in the Job Training Partnership Act.

Homeless population: Those people whose primary nighttime residence is a public or private shelter, emergency lodging, park, car, or abandoned building.

Homophobia: The irrational fear or hatred of homosexual men, lesbians, or bisexuals.

Hopelessness: NANDA-approved nursing diagnosis of "a subjective state in which an individual sees limited or no alternatives or personal choices available and is unable to mobilize energy on own behalf."

Hospice: Treatment for terminally ill clients, with emphasis on palliative rather than restorative care. The goal is to keep the client at home, pain free, and symptom free.

Hospital Insurance and Diagnosis Services Act (1961): One of the laws establishing the Canadian national health insurance system. This act provided for tax-supported insurance for hospital service.

Host: A person or animal susceptible to disease or disability.

Human Immunodeficiency Virus (HIV): A retrovirus that is transmitted directly through body fluids; it is the virus that causes AIDS.

Hypothesis: A supposition provisionally adopted to explain an event and guide investigation.

I

Illness: Perception of a nonhealthy state by an individual experiencing symptoms.

Illness trajectory: The perception over time of each person involved in the illness of a person including the total impact the of illness, and the identification, organization, and performance of tasks related to the illness.

Imaging: A mental picture of something not actually present.

Immunity: The condition of being able to resist a specific disease or disability. Two kinds of immunity are active and passive.

Immunization: Administration of a living modified agent, a suspension of killed organisms, or an inactivated toxin to protect susceptible individuals from infectious disease.

Immunization program: In schools, the systematic immunization of students against communicable diseases, the record keeping and the follow-up with parents of children requiring immunization, all overseen by the school nurse.

Immunosuppressive chemotherapy: The administration of drugs that depress the functioning of the immune system, whether intentionally or unintentionally.

Immunoglobulin: A protein that behaves like an antibody or is formed in response to an antigen.

Impairment: Any disorder in structure or function resulting from anatomic, physiologic, or psychologic abnormalities that interfere with normal activities.

Implementation: The carrying out of a plan of care by the client and nurse to achieve the desired outcomes.

Incidence: The frequency of newly occurring cases of a disease in a specified population during a given time period.

Incineration: The burning of waste products to dispose of them.

Incubation period: The time interval between contact with an infectious agent and appearance of the first sign or symptom of a disease.

Indigent: Lacking in resources to reimburse providers for health care.

Indirect transmission: Transfer of disease via a vehicle (food or water), vector (insect), or through the air.

Individual Education Plan (IEP): An educational plan provided for disabled students to ensure that they are offered education in the least restrictive environment. A team of professionals, including school nurses, designs the plan to provide appropriate services to the student.

Individual Placement and Review Committee (IPRC): In Canada, once a child is identified as exceptional, a special education IPRC determines the appropriate educational program to meet the child's needs.

Individual roles: Specialized roles within a group that serve member's own needs rather than those of the group as a whole.

Industrial hygiene: The environmental science of identifying and evaluating physical, chemical, and biologic hazards in the workplace and devising ways to control or eliminate them.

Industry vs. inferiority: A developmental state theorized by Erikson referring to the school-age child's ability to accomplish tasks and projects.

Ineffective family coping: NANDA-approved nursing diagnosis defined as "the state in which a family demonstrated destructive behavior in response to an inability to manage internal or external stressors due to inadequate resources."

Infant: An individual from birth to 1 year of age.

Infant Mortality Rate (IMR): Number of deaths that occur during the first year of life per 1000 live births.

Infectious disease: A clinically manifest disease of man or animal resulting from an infection.

Informed consent: A client agreement to comply with treatment after receiving sufficient information about the procedure(s), inherent risks, and acceptable alternatives.

Infusion therapy: Administration of medications, fluids, or nutrition via the intravenous route.

In-home care: Care for a child in his or her own

home by a relative, friend, or other babysitter.

Initiative vs. guilt: Stage of development experienced by preschoolers. According to Erikson, this stage is characterized by conflict between a desire for independence and dependence on the parents.

Inner harmony: A component of wellness focusing on relaxation and stress reduction.

Instrumental activities of daily living: Daily activities that include shopping, light housekeeping, taking medication, handling finances, using the telephone, and transportation.

Integrity vs. anxiety and dispair: Erikson's stage of development experienced by older adults, in which one's life and accomplishments are evaluated.

Integument: An enveloping layer of skin.

Interfamily stressors: Factors that influence a family as it interacts with other systems in the environment, such as schools or health care facilities.

Intermediate care facility: A residential facility that allows developmentally disabled individuals with medical problems to live in the community and also obtain treatment necessary for their physical needs.

Intervention: Planned confrontation by individuals who care about an addicted person, done in an attempt to force the individual to receive help.

Intimacy vs. isolation: Erikson's stage of development experienced by young adults, characterized by the need to establish an intimate relationship to achieve a sense of well-being.

Intrafamily stressors: Conflicts within the family itself.

Intrinsic motivation: Forces within the individual that cause one to act, including values, beliefs, attitudes, unmet needs, and emotions.

Ionizing radiation: High-energy radiation, including x-rays, gamma rays, alpha particles, and beta particles.

Iron: A mineral necessary to prevent anemia, fatigue, and impaired wound healing.

Iron deficiency: A disease characterized by a lack of iron in the blood.

J

Judicial branch: The branch of an organization or government that "interprets" the law.

Judicial law: Law based on court or jury decisions.

Jumper's knee: A disorder resulting from repetitive trauma to the knee.

Justice: The distribution, as fairly as possible, of benefits and burdens; treating people fairly.

K

Kaposi's sarcoma: A malignant neoplasm often associated with AIDS.

Kin network family: Nuclear families or unmarried members who live in close proximity and work together to exchange goods and services.

King, Imogene: Developed King's Open Systems and Theory of Goal Attainment in nursing theory where the nurse directs community assessment of personal, interpersonal, and social systems and mutual agreement of problems, goals, and means to achieve the goals.

Knowledge deficit: State in which the individual experiences a deficiency in cognitive knowledge or psychomotor skills that alter health maintenance.

L

L'Arche: Communities for the handicapped based on the attitudes of interdependence and mutual value.

Laisséz-faire leadership: Leadership style in which group members are given little direction and are free to make their own decisions.

Landfill: Area where solid wastes are stored and covered intermittently with layers of earth.

Latchkey child: A child who takes care of himself or herself in the absence of the parent.

Late maturity: The phase of life that begins at about 65 years of age and continues until death.

Law: A binding rule of conduct or action prescribed by the decisions of society.

Lead poisoning: Toxic condition caused by ingestion of lead through lead-based paint or water. If prolonged, it may result in hyperactivity or mental retardation.

Leadership: A process used to move a group toward achieving a goal.

Leadership styles: Ways in which a person influences the activities of a person or group in an effort toward goal achievement in a given situation.

Learning: Process of acquiring new knowledge, skills, or attitudes that are synthesized to produce cognitive or behavioral change in the individual.

Learning disability: A group of disorders that may affect the acquisition and use of speaking, listening, reading, writing, reasoning, or mathematical abilities.

Least restrictive environment: A setting most like that inhabited by people without disabilities; to be used for education of developmentally disabled children.

Legionnaires' disease: An acute bacterial pneumonia caused by infection by *Legionella pneumophila* and characterized by influenza-like symptoms.

Legislation and regulation: Law mandated by state, local, or federal legislative branches of government.

Legislative branch: The branch of an organization or government that "makes" the law.

Levels of care: Classification of health care service levels by the kind of care given, number of people served, and the people providing the care. The levels include acute, subacute, skilled, custodial, and chronic.

Licensure: A legal process assuring the public that an individual has met minimum requirements.

Life course theories: A psychosocial theory of aging where the task of later adulthood is to evaluate one's life and affirm that the life has been positive.

Lifestyle Assessment Questionnaire: A tool that allows clients to objectively assess their health behaviors.

Lines of resistance: In Neuman's model, the internal factors that help a client defend against a stressor.

Little leaguer's elbow: An injury resulting from repetitive stress from over throwing that causes lateral compression and medial traction on the elbow.

Logotherapy: A theory of psychotherapy, described by Victor Frankl, that focuses the individual on the unique meaning of life by striving to find a concrete reason for existence.

Long-term care: The provision of care on a recurring or continuing basis to persons with chronic, physical, or mental disorders.

Low Birth Weight (LBW): A birth weight of less than 2500 gm as a result of preterm birth and/or intrauterine growth retardation (IUGR).

Lymphoma: Neoplasm of the lymphoid tissue.

M

Maintenance roles: Behaviors within a group that are an attempt to keep the group working together harmoniously.

Malpractice: An act performed by a professional that, through a direct relationship or proximate cause, results in injury to the patient.

Maturational crisis: Transitional period that occurs across the life cycle, requiring acquisition of new sets of behavior and psychologic growth.

Mammogram: An x-ray film of the soft tissues of the breast.

Managed care: From a health services perspective managed care involves prepaid arrangements and prior authorization. From a nursing perspective managed care means coordinated care with clinical and financial outcomes.

Management models: Models of conducting or supervising an organization.

Mantoux test: A tuberculin skin test given by injecting a purified protein derivative (PPD) of tubercle bacillus, usually into the forearm. This is the most reliable and best standardized technique for tuberculin testing.

Masculinity: Qualities that society associates with men.

Maternal-infant client: The woman and her child as a client from preconception to the post-partum period.

Maternal mortality rate: Number of maternal deaths related to complications of pregnancy, birth, and the puerperium per 100,000 live births.

Medical Care Act (1968): One of the laws establishing the Canadian national health insurance system for tax-supported medical care.

Medical regimen: Therapeutic measures prescribed for clients by physicians and directed toward the management or cure of illness or disease.

Medical self-care: Actions taken to monitor one's own health, such as monitoring diet and exercise or performing breast self-examination.

Medicaid: Federal health insurance program for poor individuals and families.

Medicaid certified agency: An agency that qualifies and meets the standards of the state government in regard to reimbursement by Medicaid.

Medicare: Federal health insurance program for individuals age 65 years and older or some younger, disabled individuals.

Medicare certified agency: An agency that qualifies and meets the standards of the federal government in regards to reimbursement by Medicare.

Melting-pot approach: Belief that cultural diversity recedes as groups adopt traits from the dominant culture.

Menarche: The onset of menstruation.

Menopause: Cessation of menses.

Mental retardation: Subaverage intellectual functioning existing concurrently with deficits in adaptive behavior, as shown by an IQ of less than 70, and inability to perform the skills needed for personal independence and social responsibility.

Metacommunication: Nonverbal communication; body language.

Metaparadigm of nursing: The specific and unique philosophy of nursing, including the concepts of person, environment, health, and nursing.

Midlife crisis: Feeling of dissonance sometimes experienced in middle age if earlier developmental tasks have not been completed.

Migrant Health Act: An act that established special funding for health programs targeted at migrant laborers.

Migrant laborers: Individuals whose principle employment is in agriculture on a seasonal basis, who have been so employed for the last 24 months, and who, for the purpose of such employment, establish a temporary abode.

Mode of transmission: Any mechanism by which a pathogen is spread.

Molestation: The making of inappropriate sexual advances with injurious effect.

Moral: Of or relating to principles of right or wrong in behavior.

Morbidity: The relative incidence of disease.

Mortality: The relative incidence of death.

Motivation: That which stimulates one toward action or inaction.

Motivational theory: Theory that identifies major "satisfiers" and "dissatisfiers" that affect group productivity.

Multiple risk factors: A web of interacting events that place certain aggregates at risk.

Multiple sclerosis (MS): An inflammatory disease of the central nervous system, causing degeneration of the myelin sheath, and resulting in neurologic dysfunction with periods of exacerbation and recovery.

N

Naive trust: A response to health professionals in which the client expects to have personal opinions regarding diagnosis, treatment, and daily management of illness listened to and respected.

Narcotics: Drugs that are derived from the opium poppy or are produced synthetically and used to lower the perception of pain.

National health insurance system: In Canada, a tax-supported health insurance system allowing access to hospital and medical care on a prepaid basis for all Canadians, regardless of age, health status, or financial means provided by cost-sharing through the federal government and the provinces.

National Institute of Occupational Safety and Health (NIOSH): Branch of the U.S. Public Health Service whose responsibilities include investigating workplace illness and accidents, and the presence of workplace hazards.

National Women's Health Network: A public interest group that monitors health policies affecting women, publishes resources, and distributes information regarding women's health.

Natural history of disease: Stages in the process of development and progression of a disease without intervention by humans.

Natural immunity: Immunity that is present at birth or is caused by acquisition of antibodies as the result of a previous infection.

Needs assessment: In school nursing, the assessment to determine appropriate health promotion programs.

Negligence: Failure to act in a reasonably prudent manner, resulting in harm.

Neonatal mortality rate: Number of infant deaths during the first 28 days of life per 1000 live births.

Neonate: An infant from birth to 4 weeks of age.

Neuman's definition of nursing: A unique profession that is concerned with the variables affecting an individual's response to stress.

Neuman Systems Model: A system of nursing process developed by Betty Neuman that uses a total client approach in considering all of the factors affecting the client's level of wellness, including the physiologic, sociologic, psychologic, or developmental factors.

Neuroendocrine theory: A theory of aging where the gradual deterioration of neurons and hormones adversely affects the body systems.

Nightingale, Florence (1820-1910): The founder of modern nursing.

Noise pollution: Sound that is unwanted, annoying, or harmful; excessive noise exposure that can cause permanent hearing loss.

Noncompliance: Client refusal or inability to comply with the treatment plan.

Nonmalfeasance: The intention to do no wrong.

Normalization: A response to chronic illness or disability that has a pattern of acknowledgment of the condition and a perception that family life is normal, and that social signifi-

cance of the condition is minimal; behavior shows normalcy.

Norming: Third stage of group development in which rules for participation are established and members begin to feel more relaxed.

North American Nursing Diagnosis Association (NANDA): An organization of nurses dedicated to the identification, development, and classification of nursing diagnoses.

Nuclear family: Family consisting of a husband, wife, and one or more children.

Nuclear family dyad: Adult couple without children or whose children have grown and left home.

Nurse: An individual concerned with the diagnosis and treatment of human responses to actual or potential health problems. The nurse's role is to keep the client system stable through accuracy in the assessment of effects and possible effects of environmental stressors and in assisting client adjustments required for an optimal wellness level. The nurse's attitude is one of nurturance and caring.

Nursing center: Community center giving the client direct access to professional nursing care that is holistic and client-focused.

Nursing diagnosis: A clinical judgment about individual, family, or community responses to actual or potential health problems/life processes.

Nursing frameworks: Theories of nursing and structures of nursing processes.

Nursing Intervention Classification (NIC): A system created to assist nurses in documenting nursing care given and to facilitate the development of nursing knowledge through evaluation of patient outcomes.

Nursing paradigm: A systematic nursing model that includes nursing, person, context, and health.

Nursing process: A systematic approach to nursing consisting of assessment, diagnosis, planning (including outcome identification), implementation, and evaluation.

Nursing theory: A systematic body of knowledge that attempts to define the role of the nurse and guides nursing practice.

Nutrition: The science that studies the effects of foods eaten on one's health.

Nutritional assessment: Use of various methods and tools to evaluate an individual's intake of food and nutrients.

Nutritionists: A person who provides direct diet counseling and assists in prescribing therapeutic diets for clients.

O

Obesity: Body weight significantly greater than that recommended for an individual's height.

Objective: Statement of intended outcomes or results to be achieved by the client.

Observational study: One of two major types of study where data is generated through observations of study participants. Observational studies may be descriptive or analytic.

Occupational health: The health of the worker and its effect on his or her ability to function in the workplace.

Occupational health history: Collection of information about a client's past and current employment, to identify actual or potential health hazards the client has or is experiencing.

Occupational health nursing: The application of nursing principles to help workers achieve and maintain the highest level of wellness throughout their lives. This specialized practice is devoted to health promotion in the occupational environment based on prevention of illness and injury.

Occupational illness: Abnormal condition or disorder, other than one resulting from an occupational injury, caused by exposure to environmental factors associated with employment.

Occupational injury: Any injury such as a cut, fracture, sprain, amputation, and so on that results from a work accident or exposure in the work environment.

Occupational Safety and Health Act (OSHA): Government act passed in 1970 to ensure healthful and safe working conditions.

Occupational Safety and Health Administration (OSHA): Agency created by the OSHAct that works to improve health and safety in the workplace by educating workers and establishing standards and regulations.

Occupational therapists: Therapists who concentrate on the restoration of small motor coordination.

Official agency: Agency operated by the government.

Office of Research on Women's Health (ORWH): Agency whose efforts are directed to improve research in women's health issues and inclusion of women in research studies.

Omaha problem classification scheme: A list developed by the Visiting Nurse's Association of Omaha that includes 40 client-focused problems or signs and symptoms that form the basis of nursing diagnosis statement in the community setting.

Omnibus Budget Reconciliation Act: Legislation passed in 1982 that cut funding for many domestic programs and reduced the allowable income for families to qualify for Aid to Families With Dependent Children.

Open dump: A land area where solid wastes are deposited, with little regard for sanitary conditions.

Opportunistic infections: Infection or disease caused by normally nonpathogenic bacteria and viruses when the environment is suitable, (i.e., when the host's resistance is compromised).

Orem, Dorothea E.: Developed the Self-Care Deficit nursing theory, which provides for assessment of requisites of the community and establishment of self-care deficits and nursing implementations.

Organizational management: The way in which an organization operates and the way in which its activities are conducted and supervised.

Osgood Schlatter's disease: An inflammation or partial separation of the tibial tubercle caused by chronic irritation.

Osteoporosis: A disorder characterized by abnormal thinning of the bone, occurring most frequently in post-menopausal women.

Outcome: Results of an action that has been taken.

Overcompensation: A response to chronic illness or disability that has a pattern of acknowledgment of the condition and a perception that family life is normal and that social significance of the condition is great; behavior shows abnormality.

Overdose: High dose of a drug that may be life-threatening; emergency care is often required.

P

Palliative: Serving to relieve without curing.

Palliative care: Care given to moderate the pain and discomfort caused by a disease that is terminal.

Pap smear: A smear obtained during a routine pelvic examination commonly used to detect cancers of the cervix.

Paraprofessional: A trained aide who assists a professional nurse.

Parenting: The process of raising children and passing on one's values, attitudes, and beliefs.

Passive immunity: A short-duration resistance to disease brought about artificially by inoculation of specific protective antibodies (hyperimmune) or serum (immune serum globulin). Natural passive immunity is passed from mother to child through the placental barrier in the last trimester of pregnancy or through breastfeeding.

Pathogen or infectious agent: A biologic agent capable of causing disease.

Pathogenicity: The ability to produce clinically apparent illness.

Pathology: The study of the characteristics, causes, and effects of disease, as observed in the structure and function of the body.

Performing: Fourth stage in group development, in which group members function as a unit to complete the task at hand.

Period of communicability: Time period during which a communicable disease can be transmitted from an infected person.

Personal protective equipment (PPE): Specialized clothing or equipment worn by a health-care worker (HCW) for protection against a hazard.

Phototherapy: Treatment of jaundice caused by excess bilirubin by exposure to intense fluorescent light.

Physical fitness: The ability to carry out daily tasks with alertness and vigor, without undue fatigue, and with enough energy reserve to meet emergencies or to enjoy leisure time pursuits.

Physical hazards: Factors in the workplace such as equipment, lighting, noise, and temperature that contribute to occurrence of injury.

Physical therapist: Therapist whose role is to evaluate neuromuscular and functional ability.

Physiologic factor: In nursing diagnosis, a related factor to be considered for nursing diagnosis statements using the Omaha problem classification scheme. Factors in diagnosis include physiologic, psychologic, spiritual, environmental, and sociocultural.

Place: In epidemiology, a location where a disease is more likely to occur.

Plague: Contagious disease caused by a bacillus that has historically been prevalent in crowded and unsanitary conditions and appears to be transmitted by rodents to fleas to humans. It spread rapidly through Europe in the fourteenth century.

Plan: The development of strategies to reinforce healthy client responses or to prevent, minimize, or correct unhealthy client responses identified in the nursing diagnosis.

Planning: Developing goals and objectives and strategies for achieving goals.

Play: Any spontaneous or organized activity that provides enjoyment, entertainment, amusement, or diversion. It may be structured or unstructured and allows children to express feelings, develop cognitive and motor skills, and socialize.

Plumbism: Lead poisoning. A toxic condition caused by ingestion of lead causing central nervous system damage.

Pneumocystis carinii: A protozoan that is a causative agent of plasma cell pneumonia.

Police power: Official power used to enforce

the laws of and regulate the health, safety, and morals in society.

Political action: The process of becoming involved in community relations and with government officials to bring about change.

Pollutant: Any unwanted substance that enters the environment and affects it adversely.

Polychlorinated biphenyls (PCBs): Toxic chemical compounds that were used in industry and have been found in many humans, animals, and food sources, causing a variety of health effects.

Population effect: Theory that states that as the population increases, so does the amount of waste produced.

Postneonatal mortality rate: Number of infant deaths after the first 28 days of life per 1000 live births.

Poverty: The lack of income and the necessities of life.

Power: The ability to influence and/or control others.

PRECEDE Model: Health education planning model that identifies factors in an individual's environment that motivate the individual to exhibit certain health behaviors.

Preconception care and counseling: Provision of health care in which baseline data is gathered within the year prior to pregnancy to identify and modify health problems, personal behaviors, and environmental hazards that could adversely affect the outcome of pregnancy without the limiting factor of a fetus.

Prematurity: The state of an infant born any time before the thirty-seventh week of gestation regardless of birth weight.

Prenatal care: Health care provided to a woman during her pregnancy.

Preoperational stage: Piaget's stage of development experienced by preschoolers, characterized by the development of representational thought and the ability to solve simple problems.

Presbycusis: Loss of hearing caused by aging, including a lessened ability to understand speech.

Presbyopia: Changes in vision caused by aging, including a loss of ability of the lens to accommodate to near and far vision.

Preschool or nursery school: A facility that may or may not be state licensed, where children aged 3 years to 5 years attend full- or half-day school that prepares them for kindergarten.

Preschooler: A child 3 to 4 years of age.

Presumptive Medicaid eligibility: Practice of providing immediate short-term Medicaid eligibility to pregnant women while full Medicaid eligibility is being determined.

Prevalence: The number of existing cases of a disease or occurrences of an event at a particular point in time.

Prevention: The act of stopping or interrupting the progression of disease.

Primary prevention: Actions taken to prevent the occurrence of disease.

Private sector: The component of the health care delivery system financed by private funds and comprising physicians in private practice, private hospitals, and outpatient services.

Privileged communication: The right of the patient not to disclose treatment information to a court of law.

Process: A series of activities used to deliver care.

Program evaluation: Systematic process of collecting information to determine the worth of a set of activities designed to produce a certain outcome.

Proprietary agency: A privately owned, profit-making organization defined under section 501 of the Internal Revenue Code as ineligible for tax exemption.

Prospective Payment System: Payment for medical conditions is predetermined according to the diagnosis-related group (DRG).

Prospective study: Study that starts with a group (a cohort) all considered to be free of a given disease but who vary in exposure to a factor suspected of causing the disease.

Provider: A person or agency providing health care services to clients.

Psychologic factor: In nursing diagnosis, a related factor to be considered for nursing diagnosis statements using the Omaha problem classification scheme. Factors in diagnosis include physiologic, psychologic, spiritual, environmental, and sociocultural.

Psychologic dependence: The craving for a drug or alcohol.

Psychologic hazards: Factors in the workplace that affect the worker's response to the work environment, often resulting in stress, fatigue, or depression.

Psychomotor domain: One of three domains covering learning behaviors; deals with skills known as motor skills.

Psychotropic drugs: Drugs that affect the recipient's behavior and perception.

Puberty: The condition of becoming able to reproduce sexually, marked by maturing of the sexual organs and development of the secondary sex characteristics.

Public health: The health of the community, with particular regard to areas such as the water supply, waste disposal, air pollution, and food safety.

Public Health Nursing: A field of nursing that synthesizes the body of knowledge from the public health sciences and professional nursing theory for the purpose of improving health in the entire community.

Public Law 94-142: The Education for All Handicapped Children Act, mandating that all disabled infants and children are entitled to a "free and appropriate" education.

Public sector: The component of the health care delivery system financed by taxes and comprising federal, state, and local health departments.

Q

Quality: Conformance to standards leading to a degree of excellence.

Quality Assessment and Improvement (QA&I): The systematic study of quality in health care by monitoring and evaluating selected components of care and correcting the deficiencies that are found. This term is growing in common usage and replacing the traditional term Quality Assurance (QA).

Quality Assurance (QA): The traditional term for systematic approaches used to assess and improve quality in health care, often directed toward the meeting of external regulations necessary for accreditation and/or certification.

R

Race: Specific physical and structural characteristics that are transmitted genetically and distinguish one human type from another.

Radioactive wastes: Waste products that are hazardous and decompose over time, spreading into the environment if not disposed of properly.

Radon: A colorless, odorless, inert radioactive gas that may be found in the home. It is a decay product of radium.

Rate: Ratio of cases of disease or deaths to the total population in a given time period.

Ratio: The relationship between two numbers expressed as a fraction; the value obtained by dividing the numerator of a fraction by the denominator.

Readiness to learn: The state of being both willing and able to make use of instruction.

Reality orientation: Nursing intervention designed to assist a cognitively impaired individual in maintaining awareness of the environment.

Recycling: Methods of reusing waste materials, reducing the total amount of waste, and conserving resources.

Referral: A mechanism for communication, coordination, and collaboration between and among health care settings and disciplines to ensure continuity of care.

Refreezing: The final step in the Lewin model of change where the newly acquired behavior is integrated by the participant.

Refugees: Those individuals who flee to a foreign country to escape persecution.

Regression: A retreat or movement backwards; a return to an earlier, more primitive form of behavior.

Reimbursement: Payment for services by a third party (i.e., someone other than the recipient, such as private insurance, Medicare, or Medicaid).

Relationships: In a group, the bonds between its members.

Relative risk: In statistical analysis of data, relative risk measures the strength of association between a specific factor or exposure and risk of disease.

Repatterning: In nurse-client intervention, cultural care repatterning is applied so as to avoid an ethnocentric intervention when the client's usual pattern of behavior is detrimental.

Research process: The systematic use of scientific process to find answers to questions. Research may be descriptive or analytical and is always objective.

Reservoir: Living organisms or inanimate objects that harbor an infectious agent.

Reservoir of infection: A continuous source of infectious disease.

Resistance: The inherent capacity of a human being to resist untoward circumstances, such as disease, malnutrition, or toxic agents.

Restorative health care: Health services provided to help clients regain a maximum level of health and independence following a debilitating illness or injury.

Restraining forces: Forces that inhibit or hinder the desired change.

Retrospective audit: Comparison of the client's chart with predetermined criteria after the episode of care has been completed.

Retrospective study: A study that looks back for a relationship between one condition occurring in the present and another that occurred in the past, such as comparing people diagnosed as having a disease with those who do not (controls).

Retrovirus: A single piece of RNA surrounded by a protein coat. Instead of flowing from DNA to RNA it reverses the process and makes itself into a piece of DNA. It then infects the nucleus of the cell. HIV is a retrovirus.

Risk: Exposure to a situation that may result in an injury, illness, or other loss.

Risk management: A program designed to eliminate or control health care situations having the potential of injury, danger, or liability to clients.

Risk-specific care: An individualized approach to health care that is based on a holistic assessment of each woman's risk for a complicated pregnancy, birth, or postpartum recovery.

Risk-taking behavior: High-risk behavior that leads to violence and injury in the 12- to 24-year-old age group. Some high-risk behavior includes drug abuse, including alcohol and smoking.

Role model: A person who inspires others to imitate his or her behavior.

Role performance model: View of health stating that healthy individuals must fulfill a role in society.

Roy, Sister Callista: Developed the Adaptation Model of nursing process, which provides for assessment of four modes, assessment of stimuli, and identification of responses that will be the basis of the nurse's management of an illness state.

Rubeola: Acute, contagious viral infection causing fever, rash, upper respiratory symptoms, lay term, measles.

Rule utilitarianism: Analysis of the rules used to bring about happiness.

S

Salmonella: Gram-negative bacilli that produce fever, acute gastroenteritis, bacterimia, and localized infection. The mode of transmission is through water or food.

Sandwich generation: Middle-aged adults who are raising their own children and caring for aging parents at the same time.

Saturated fats: Fats whose molecular structure contains the maximum possible number of hydrogen atoms. They are often linked to an increased incidence of cardiovascular disease.

Scapegoating: Blaming someone else for the problems experienced by an individual or in a family group. One member of a family may be designated the scapegoat. It is usually an unconscious process.

School nursing: Provision of nursing services, including health promotion and disease prevention, to children and adolescents within the school setting.

Scoliosis: An abnormal, S-shaped curve of the spine.

Scope of practice: A mechanism by which nursing defines itself or is defined by others; also called scope of employment.

Screening: Identification of unrecognized disease or disability by mass examination of entire populations or high-risk groups.

Seasonal: Occurring periodically at certain times of the year.

Secondary prevention: Actions taken to detect and treat disease in early stages.

Second order change: Change that affects the system by seeking new ways to do things, new approaches, structures, and ideas.

Self-care: The practice of activities that individuals initiate and perform on their own behalf in maintaining life, health, and well-being.

Self-efficacy model: A useful tool for bringing about desired behavioral changes in a specific area of lifestyle by considering the individual's belief that he or she can perform a specific behavior and that performing the behavior will cause a change in health status.

Self transcendence: Focusing on others as a way to find purpose and meaning in life.

Senecense: The state or process of being old.

Sensorimotor period: Piaget's stage of development experienced from birth to 2 years of age, in which the infant explores the environment through the five senses.

Seroconversion: The appearance of specific antibodies in blood serum that has previously been free of them.

Sex role theory: The theory that masculinity is an inner, psychic process that is tied to an outer web of sex roles and gender expectations.

Sexuality: A lifelong process involving biologic functions (giving and receiving pleasure), psychologic factors (body image), and sociocultural influences (identity of being male or female).

Shared governance: A concept in management based on the premise that workers are generally well-educated and that staff deserve a voice in the decisions that affect them.

Shared leadership: Group situation in which two individuals share the leadership responsibilities.

Sickness: Perception of a nonhealthy state by others through visible signs or reported symptoms.

Significant other: Person considered by an individual to be special; this person may be directly responsible for patient care in the home.

Single parent family: Family consisting of one parent living with one or more children.

Situational crisis: Crisis resulting from unexpected changes, causing disequilibrium in the individual or family.

Skilled services: Services that require the knowledge and skills of a professional to perform or teach.

Smog: Air pollution present in concentrations high enough to reduce visibility and cause irritation in the eyes and lungs.

Social competence and breakdown theory: A psychosocial theory of aging where a negative spiral of feedback can occur if an individual experiences a health-related crisis that can lead to a feeling of dependence and incompetence.

Socialization: The process of learning the social requirements of one's cultural group.

Social vulnerability index: A tool that could be used to determine those populations in greatest need of health services. It takes into account the factors of social pathology, economic well-being, education, access to health care, and health status.

Social worker: A professional who helps clients with social, intellectual, and emotional factors that affect their well-being.

Sociocultural factor: In nursing diagnosis, a related factor to be considered for nursing diagnosis statements using the Omaha problem classification scheme. Factors in diagnosis include physiologic, psychologic, spiritual, environmental, and sociocultural.

Somatic mutation theory: A theory of aging where cumulative exposure to background radiation will gradually result in cell mutations and eventual death.

Sodium: An element contained in salt and necessary in small amounts for the body to maintain a proper fluid balance.

Solid waste: Any garbage, refuse, sludge, or other discarded material resulting from industrial, commercial, mining, agricultural operations, or community activities.

Specialist: In community health nursing, one who is educated at the master's or doctoral level and, in addition to practicing generalist functions, formulates health and social policy, conducts research, and tests theory related to community health practice.

Special rights: Rights accorded to the nurse that arise out of the nurse/client relationship.

Specificity: In screening tests, measurement of the probability of an occurrence of one variable in relation to the extent or occurrence of another variable.

Spermatogenesis: The production of male gametes, including meiosis and transformation of the four resulting spermatids, into protozoa.

Spiritual factor: In nursing diagnosis, a related factor to be considered for nursing diagnosis statements using the Omaha problem classification scheme. Factors in diagnosis include physiologic, psychologic, spiritual, environmental, and sociocultural.

Spiritual nursing: Intervention in which the nurse assists the client to relate positively to his or her deepest inner self and allows the expression of concerns and fears about death and other aspects of the essence of life.

Spirituality: A component of health related to the core of existence, sensitivity, or attachment to religious values relating to the belief system of the individual.

Standard: A broad statement of the agreed-upon level of excellence.

Standard of care: A legal term for the measure of care and skill given by a professional to which the courts of law will apply if a nurse is sued for malpractice.

Standards of clinical nursing practice: Standards published by the American Nurses' Association in 1991 that define the responsibilities of nurses in all clinical settings.

Standards of Community Health Nursing Prac-

tice: Standards developed by the American Nurses' Association that establish criteria for structure, process, and outcome to help the nurse in applying the nursing process to the community setting.

Standards of practice: Professional standards used by courts of law in malpractice cases to determine the "standard of care" in deciding whether a nurse fell below what a reasonably prudent nurse in the same or similar circumstances would have done.

Stereotype: The belief that all members of a cultural group behave in the same way.

Stereotyping: The tendency to ascribe the values, attributes, or behaviors of a small number of people to all members of a group.

Stigma: A perception that someone is not considered normal or not of good character or reputation.

Stimulants: Natural and synthetic drugs that have a strong stimulating effect on the central nervous system and are accompanied by a feeling of alertness and self-confidence.

Strategic management process: The organizational planning for selected goals in service delivery or through fiscal palnning by the community agency.

St. Vincent de Paul: Founder of the Sisters of Charity in the early seventeenth century.

Storming: Second stage of group development in which members bargain for position within the group and conflicts arise.

Stressors: In Neuman's model, environmental forces that may alter system stability.

Substance abuse: Use of drugs or substances for reasons other than to achieve a therapeutic effect.

Suicide: The intentional taking of one's own life, the incidence of which is rising among 12- to 19-year-olds.

Suicide prevention program: In school nursing, a prevention program that includes training teachers and staff to identify potential suicide victims and to gain knowledge of community resources.

Support group: Group in which members assist each other in meeting a common need. Also called self-help group.

Surveillance: The process of monitoring incidence and prevalence of communicable diseases through accurate record keeping and data collection to assist health professionals to monitor dangerous outbreaks of disease. It can also facilitate effective health planning to intervene and control the spread of communicable disease.

Susceptible host: A person or animal lacking effective resistance to a particular infectious agent.

Systemic mycosis: A chronic, malignant neoplasm of the skin which is caused by a fungus.

Systems theory: A theory of organization where the system is a set of interrelated and interdependent parts that form a complex whole, and each of those parts can be viewed as a subsystem with its own interrelated and independent parts. Systems can be viewed as closed or self-contained systems or open systems, which interact with the environment.

T

Task roles: Behaviors within a group that contribute to completion of the group's task.

Teacher: A provider of health-related information based on the client's needs.

Teaching: A process that facilitates learning. It includes activities that are a deliberate action that help the student learn. Health teaching is an act in which a client is assisted to become an active member of the health team and to reach an optimal level of health.

Teaching/learning process: Process in which knowledge, attitudes, and skills are imparted to and integrated by the learner.

Teaching situation: The environment in which teaching will take place. It includes the physical, interpersonal, and external environment.

Team conference: Interdisciplinary case conference where all disciplines involved in a patient's care meet to evaluate and revise the plan of care.

Teleological (consequentialist) theory: Theory of ethics stating that the rightness or wrongness of an action is determined by its results or consequences.

Teratogenic effects: Incomplete or improper fetal development caused by external substances.

Tertiary prevention: Actions taken to limit the spread of disease or disability, improve health, and/or maintain stability.

Testicular cancer: A malignant neoplastic disease of the testis that is the fourth most common cause of death among 15- to 35-year-old males. If detected early, the cure rate is high, indicating the need for regular testicular self-examination.

Theory X: Theory of management where the worker is viewed as a person who avoids responsibility and prefers to be directed by a manager in work efforts.

Theory Y: Theory of management where the worker is viewed as a person who is responsible and cooperative.

Therapeutic or medical play: Play activities where children can dress up as health care staff and can act out medical procedures such as giving "shots" to dolls, giving "anesthesia" to teddy bears, and so on. This helps children learn about and prepare for experiences with the health care system.

Third party reimbursement: Payment by a third party insurer for any claims made by a health care provider for health care services rendered to the insured consumer.

Time: In epidemiology, data is collected regarding when a disease occurs to discover trends in health and disease.

Time management: Planning time toward the goal of productivity in carrying out the work assigned.

Tinea capitus (ringworm): A contagious fungal disease transmitted by direct contact.

Toddler: A child between 1 and 2 years of age.

Tolerance: The ability to endure hardship, pain, or ordinarily injurious substances, such as drugs, without apparent physiologic or psychologic injury.

Total Quality Management (TQM): A top down organizational philosophy or way of thinking directed toward the improvement of the quality throughout an organization to meet consumers' needs.

Toxicology: Study of the adverse effect of certain agents on the biologic system.

Toxin: A poisonous substance usually produced by the invading microorganism.

Toxoid: A toxin that has been treated to alleviate toxic properties but retain its antigenic quality, usually to stimulate antibody production.

Trajectory: A curve or surface that passes through a given set of points or intersects a given set of curves or surfaces at a constant angle.

Trajectory of chronic illness: The course, or predictable path, of an illness over time.

Transmission: Any mechanism by which a pathogen is spread, by a source or reservoir, to a person.

Trust vs. mistrust: Erikson's stage of development experienced in infancy, when the infant develops a bond with parents and/or other caretakers.

Tubercle bacilli: Another name for Mycobacterium tuberculosis.

Tuberculosis: Communicable disease caused by droplet infection which causes fever, fatigue, weight loss, coughing, chest pain, hemoptysis, and hoarseness.

Turner's syndrome: A congenital syndrome in females caused by the absence of one of the two X chromosomes.

U

Unfreezing: The first step in the Lewin model of change. Participants would be motivated to be ready for a change, work on recognizing a need for change, identifying the problem, and developing a solution.

Uniform Needs Assessment Instrument: Assessment tool, currently in development, that was mandated by the Omnibus Budget Reconciliation Act of 1986, and that can be used to evaluate a client's need for continuation of services.

Universal precautions: Use of protective barriers, such as gloves, masks, and protective eyewear, to protect mucous membranes from exposure to blood and body substances. Fundamental to this concept is the practice of treating all patients as if they are infected with a blood-borne disease and taking appropriate protective measures.

U.S. Constitution: Document that, among other things, establishes the three branches of government.

Utilitarianism: The greatest-happiness principle, or the greatest good for the greatest number of people.

Utilization review: A set of activities directed toward reviewing care for its appropriateness for a specific client.

V

Vaccine: Substance developed and administered to produce active immunizations.

Values: Views and beliefs that guide one's behavior.

Values clarification: The process of understanding one's own values and how they guide behavior.

Variable: Any attribute, phenomenon, or event that can have different values.

Varicella: Viral infection causing fever, rash, and malaise, also known as chicken pox.

Vector: Any carrier, particularly one that transports an infectious agent.

Vehicle: An inanimate substance that transports an infectious agent to a susceptible host (e.g., food, water).

Vendors: Distributors of durable medical equipment in the home.

Ventilator care: Use of a mechanical device to assist with breathing in cases of pulmonary failure.

Veracity: The intention to tell the truth.

Very Low Birth Weight (VLBW): A birth weight of less than 1500 gm as a result of preterm birth and/or intrauterine growth retardation (IUGR).

Violence: Acts of aggression toward human beings and objects.

Virtue ethics: The examination of a person's character traits that affect intentions and motivations preceding moral action.

Virulence: The power of a microorganism to produce disease.

Visiting Nurse's Association (VNA): Private, nonprofit agencies originally founded to provide health care and education to the poor, funded by charitable contributions and fees based on clients' ability to pay.

W

Wald, Lillian: A public health nurse who founded the Henry Street Settlement in New York City and worked to improve the health of the city's poor residents.

Water pollution: Presence of disease-causing bacteria and viruses in the water supply, often through human or animal feces or through the dumping of solid wastes in the water supply.

Web of causation: An interrelationship of multiple factors that contribute to disease or disability.

Well-being: An individual's perceived condition of existence, pleasure, and kinds of happiness.

Wellness: A dynamic, fluctuating state of being, encompassing physical, psychologic, and spiritual health.

Western blot test: A laboratory blood test to detect the presence of antibodies to specific antigens.

Wheel model: Epidemiologic model of human-environment interactions that are necessary for disease to occur.

Withdrawal syndrome: The unpleasant and sometimes life-threatening physiologic changes that occur when some drugs are withdrawn after prolonged, regular use.

Women's health care movement: A group of health care activists who banded together to share experiences and knowledge and to identify quality health care.

Women's Health Equity Act: A legislative package designed to improve women's access to health care and women's health care and treatment.

Worker's compensation: Laws requiring employers to be financially responsible for wages lost as a result of occupational illness or injury.

Z

Zoonosis: Disease of animals that is transmissible to humans (e.g., rabies).

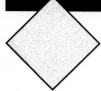

INDEX

A

Abuse
  of alcohol by men, 358-359
  of child, 302-303
  of women, 341-342
Abused women, responses to, facilitative *vs.* inhibitive, *424*
Acceptance in developing cultural sensitivity, 47
Accident prevention
  for children, 290-294
  school health nurse and, 619
Accountability, professional, quality assurance and, 234
Accreditation, quality assurance and, 235-236
Acne in adolescents/young adults, 314-315
Acne vulgaris, 314
Acquired immunodeficiency syndrome (AIDS), 451-460
  case study on, 139-141
  in children, 294-295
  in drug abusers, 526-527
  elimination alteration in, 458
  epidemiology of, 451-452
  in men, 359
  mode of transmission of, 452-453
  nutritional alteration in, 457-458
  palliative care for persons with, 459-460
  pathology of, 455
  psychosocial issues related to, 458-459
  support services for, school health nurse and, 622-623
  treatment of, 456
  universal precautions for, 453-455
Activities of daily living in discharge planning, 555
Activity theory of aging, 371
Acupuncture, 163
Acute care case management, 560
Adaptation in developing cultural sensitivity, 47
Addiction, drug, 523
Adjourning in group development, 221
Administration
  as function of school health nurse, 615
  nursing, culture and, 61-62
Adolescence, 308; *see also* Adolescent(s)
  developmental disabilities in, 501

Adolescent(s), 307-322
  body image and, 335
  chemical dependencies in, 513
  emotional concerns of, 315-316
  emotional development of, 312
  female, menstruation and, 315
  health concerns of, 314-315
  male, health profile of, 352-353
  mortality and morbidity of, causes of, 308-309
  nutritional status of, 309-311
  reproductive health of, school health nurse and, 621-622
  risk taking behavior in, 320
  sexual development in, 316-317
  sexuality and, 338-339
  social concerns relating to, 321
  spiritual development of, 312, 314
  sports and, 317-318
  substance abuse among, 318-320
Adulthood, developmental disabilities in, 501
Adults, young, 307-322; *see also* Young adults
Advocacy, 677-678
  political, empowerment through, 690
Advocate/liaison, occupational health nurse as, 597
Advocates, nurses as, 260
Aerobic exercise for physical fitness, 164
Affective assistance for family with chronically ill member, 489
Affective domain, 180
Affective learning, 180
Affective level of family functioning, 488
African-American males, health profile of, 353-354
Aggregate(s)
  communities as, 20
  definition of, 533
  high-risk, 533
Aging
  characteristics of, *370*
  cognitive changes in, normal, 373
  physical changes in, normal, 372-373
  process of, 367-370
  psychoanalytic theory of, 372
  psychosocial theories of, 370-372

Air pollution, 648-650
Alcohol
    abuse of, 516-517
    abuse of, by men, 358-359
    withdrawal from, disorders associated with, 526-527
Alcoholics Anonymous, 527-528
Alcoholism
    as family stressor, 415
    scope of problem of, 511
Alienation in adolescence and young adulthood, 315
Altered family processes, 414
    characteristics of families with, 417t
Alternative treatment modalities, 162-164
Alzheimer's disease in frail elderly, 380, 383
American Association of Occupational Health Nurses
        (AAOHN), 583-84
American Nurses' Association (ANA)
    outlines and standards developed by, for school
        health nursing, 612
    participation in, 686-687
American Nurses' Association (ANA) model of quality
        assessment and improvement, 242-247
American Public Health Association (APHA), 687-688
Americans with Disabilities Act (ADA), 499t, 585-586
Amphetamines, abuse of, 517-518
Analysis, 179-180
Analytic studies in epidemiologic research, 133-135
Anemia, iron deficiency, in children, 297-298
Anergy, 463
Anorexia nervosa in adolescence and young adult-
        hood, 316
Application, 179
Architectural Barriers Act, 499t
Ardell, Donald, in wellness movement, 147
Aromatherapy, 162-163
Asbestos particles as indoor pollutant, 656
Assessment
    of child growth and development, 286-287
    cultural, enablers of, 48, *50-52,* 53-58t
    standards of community health nursing practice
        and, 87-88
    teaching/learning process and, 185-189
Assessor/monitor, occupational health nurse as, 597
Association, measures of, in epidemiology, 135
*Association of Community Health Nursing Educa-
        tors* (ACHNE), 688
Athletes, male, health profile of, 356-357
Attitude(s)
    readiness to learn and, 188
    toward health, effects of, on health maintenance in
        workplace, 587-588

Attraction power in group, 223
Attributable risk, 135-136
Audiovisual materials, selecting, 192-194
Audit in quality assessment and improvement, 247
Autism, 503
    play and children with, *504*
Autoimmune theory of aging, 368
Automobile accidents, reducing injury from, 292-293
Autonomy *versus* doubt and shame in child develop-
        ment, 287

B

Barbiturates, abuse of, 519
Barton, Clara, in history of community health nursing,
        10
Behavior(s)
    drug-related, *318*
    risk taking, in adolescence, 320
    Theory X and Theory Y of, 201-202
    wellness, assessment of, 158. *159-161,* 162
Behavioral level of family functioning, 488
Bhopal, chemical disaster at, 653
Bicycle accident prevention, 293-294
Biofeedback to achieve inner harmony, 169
Biologic factors, women's body image and, 335-336
Biologic hazards in workplace, 591-592
Biomagnification of PCB effects, 645
Birth rate, 264
    formula used for, 132t
Birth weight, infant mortality and, 262, 263-264
Bisexual men, health profile of, 354-355
Blended family, 395
Bloodborne diseases, occupational exposure to, re-
        search on, *460*
Blue Cross, 72
Blue Shield, 72
Body image, women's health and, 335-337
    biologic factors impacting on, 335-336
    cultural factors affecting, 336-337
    social factors affecting, 336-337
Bone mineral density, menopause and, research on,
        380
Breast cancer risk, mammographic screening and,
        334
Breckinridge, Mary, 12-14
Budgets in financial planning, 207
Bulimia in adolescence and young adulthood, 316

C

Caffeine, abuse of, 518-519
Canada, health care system of, 74-78

Cancer
in frail elderly, 378
testicular, 357-358
Cannabis, abuse of, 520-521
Carbon monoxide as indoor pollutant, 656
Care, direct, as function of school health nurse, 614
Care plan in continuity of care, 557
Care-based ethics, 668
Caregiver burden in family with chronically ill member, 481-483
vulnerability for, *484*
Caregivers, nurses as, 261
Case law, 665
Case management as function of school health nurse, 615
Case managers, nurses as, 261
Case-control studies in epidemiologic research, 135
Caseload management, 211
district nurses and, research on, *212*
for home care, 573-575
Categorical imperative, 667
Causality, 137-138
Cerebral palsy, 502-503
Certification, quality assurance and, 234-235
Change
first-order, 683
leadership and, 700
models of, 683-685
nurse as agent of, 685
process of, empowerment through, 682-685
second-order, 683
types of, 683
Chemical dependency(ies), 509-530
assessment in, 523
in babies of addicted mothers, 514-515
causation theories on, 512
culture and, 512-513
diagnosis in, 523-524
drug addiction and, 523
drug habituation and, 522-523
dual diagnosis in, 523
in elderly, 515-516
evaluation in, 528-529
factors placing populations at risk for, 512-516
family patterns and, 514
in homeless, 512
implementation in, 524-528
issues and trends in, 510-511
in nurses, 516
nursing process in, 523-529
physical, 522

Chemical dependency(ies) — cont'd
poverty and, 512
psychologic, 522
scope of problem of, 511
substances involved in, 516-522
in women, 515
in youth, 513
Chemical hazards in workplace, 589, 591-592
Chemical waste disposal, 640-645
Chemicals, diseases caused by exposure to, 591t
Chicken pox, 449t
Child(ren), 285-304
abuse/neglect of, 302-303
accidents/accident prevention for, 290-294
acquired immunodeficiency syndrome in, 294-295
dental problems in, 294
growth and development of, 286-289
immunizations for, 289-290
iron deficiency anemia in, 297-298
lead poisoning in, 298-300
nutrition for, 296-297
poverty and, 303-304
sensorimotor development of, 287
special needs, school health nurse and, 623-626
violence and, 300-302
Child advocacy, school nurse in, 615
Childhood, developmental disability in, 498-499
Chlamydia, 449t
Cholera immunization, dosing schedule for, 450t
Christianity, roots of community health nursing in, 5
Chromosomal abnormalities, 502
Chronic illness(es), 472-494
care for, evaluation of, 491-493
challenges faced by families with members having, 476-478
definition of, 474
family assessment in, 476-489
prevalence of, 474-475
stigma from, 476
trajectory of, 475-476
Circular communication cycle, 490-491
Civic involvement in political activity, empowerment through, 689-690
Civil law, 666
Civil rights, community health nursing and, 675
Client
education of, 178
in continuity of care, 557
satisfaction of, in quality assessment and improvement, 248
Clinical management, 212-213

Clinical nursing practice, standards of, 87
Cocaine abuse, 518
Coercive power in group, 223
Cognitive changes
  in aging, normal, 373
  in frail elderly, 383-384
Cognitive domain, 179
Cognitive impairments, 502
Cognitive learning, 179-180
Cognitive level of family functioning, 488-489
Cohesion, group, 224
Cohort studies in epidemiologic research, 134-135
Collaborative interdisciplinary care, 570
Common law, 665
Communicable disease(s), 439-470
  control of, 466-469
    engineering controls in, 466-468
    personal protective equipment in, 469
    work practice controls in, 468-469
  definition of, 440
  immunity to, 443-444
  incubation period for, 443
  monitoring of, school health nurse in, 619-620
  period of communicability of, 443
  prevention of, 445
  problematic, 445, 451-466
    hepatitis as, 445, 451
    hepatitis B as, 460-461
    HIV/AIDS as, 451-460
    tuberculosis as, 461-466
  surveillance of, 445
  transmission of
    direct, 442
    indirect, 441
    modes of, 440-442
Communication
  definition of, 397
  in multicultural society, 43-44
  privileged, 674
Communication cycle, circular, 490-491
Communication theory of family coping, 397
Communicators, nurses as, 260-261
Community
  as client, 19-37
    case studies on, 28-36
  definitions of, 20-21
  geopolitical, 20
  wellness in, assessing level of, 28
Community assessment, 22
Community development groups, 225
Community health nursing

Community health nursing — cont'd
  definition of, 16-17
  future of, 698-700
  issues related to, 694-698
  in multicultural society, 38-63
Community health nursing practice, standards of, 87
Community nursing diagnosis statements, guidelines
    for writing, 89
Community nursing services, organizing, 208-209
Community resources in home health care, 570
Community Wellness Program, 157-158
Complementary treatment modalities, 162-164
Comprehension, 179
Comprehensive Health Services amendment of 1966,
    67
Conceptual framework, 21
Concrete operations phase of child development, 287
Confidentiality, 674
Conflict, group, 223-224
Consumer trends, 699
Consumerism as family response to health profession-
    als, 492-493
Continuing care, 553
Continuity of care
  components for providing, 557-558
  discharge planning and, 553
Continuity theory of aging, 372
Continuous quality improvement, 237
Continuum of care, discharge planning and, 553
Contract development in planning process, 191-192
Contracting, health behavior, 152, *153*
Coronary artery disease in frail elderly, 378
Coronary heart disease (CHD) in men, 361
Correlation coefficient, 135
Cost-effective care, discharge planning and, 553
Counseling preconception, 271
Counselor, occupational health nurse as, 597
Criminal law, 666
Crisis theory of family coping, 396-397
Criteria mapping in quality assessment and improve-
    ment, 248
Critical feminist theory, gender identity and, 351-352
Critical thinking by group leader, 222-223
Cross-sectional studies in epidemiologic research, 134
Cultural assessment, 48
  tools for conducting, *50-52, 53-58t*
Cultural care accommodation, 59
Cultural care preservation, 59
Cultural care repatterning, 59
Cultural categorization, issues in, 41-42
Cultural diversification of North America, 39-40

Cultural factors, women's body image and, 336-337
Cultural imposition, 44
Cultural sensitivity, developing, 45-47
Culturally congruent care, 59
Culture
  chemical dependencies and, 512-513
  definitions of, 40-41
  link between health and illness and, 41
  nursing education, administration and research and,
    61-62

D

Death rates, formulas used for, 132t
Defense
  in developing cultural sensitivity, 46-47
  flexible lines of, in immunity, 443
  normal line of, in immunity, 443-444
Delano, Jane, in history of community health nursing,
  10
Deliriants, abuse of, 521
Delirium tremens (DTs), 526
Dementia in frail elderly, 383-384
Denial
  in developing cultural sensitivity, 46
  in family with chronically ill member, 479-481
Dental problems in children, 294
Denver Developmental Screening Test (DDST),
  288
Deontology, 666-667
Dependence in substance abuse, 418
Depression in frail elderly, 382-383
Descriptive studies in epidemiologic research, 133
Desert Shield/Desert Storm in history of community
  health nursing, 15
Designer drugs, abuse of, 521-522
Detoxification, 525
Development, sensorimotor, 287
Developmental Disabilities Act, 499t
Developmental Disabilities Assistance and Bill of
  Rights Act, 499t
Developmental disability(ies), 496-508
  in adolescence, 501
  in adulthood, 501
  autism as, 503
  cerebral palsy as, 502-503
  in childhood, 498-499
  chromosomal abnormalities as, 502
  cognitive, 502
  communication skills in nursing care for, 507
  definition of, 498
  Down syndrome as, 502

Developmental disability(ies) — cont'd
  evaluation of, 507
  health promotion and, 504
  in infancy, 498-499
  learning disabilities as, 503
  mental retardation as, 502
  nursing diagnoses in, 506
  nursing process and, 504-507
  planning for, 506
  prevention of, 504
  in school-age children, 499-501
Developmental framework for studying family, 397-398
Developmental task of adolescents, 312
Developmental variables in assessing family coping
  with multiple stressors, 425
Diabetes mellitus in frail elderly, 378
Diagnosis
  of child growth and development problems, 287-288
  standards of community health nursing practice
    and, 88-89
  teaching/learning process and, 189
Diagnosis-related groupings (DRGs), 68
Diphtheria, 446t
Direct observation in quality assessment and improvement, 247
Disability(ies)
  definition of, 474, 497
  developmental, 496-508
    definition of, 498
  deviance of, response to, 476
  etiquette for, *505*
  learning, 503
  terminology preferred for, 506t
Disability movement, history of, 498
Discharge planning, 551-563
  assessment in, 554-555
  case studies on, *561-563*
  current perspectives on, 553-554
  definitions of, 553
  diagnosis in, 554-555
  evaluation in, 557
  historical perspective on, 551-552
  home care coordinator in, 559
  implementation in, 555-557
  legislation affecting, 553
  outcome identification in, 555
  planning in, 555-557
  primary nurse and, 559-560
  process of, 554-557
  recent changes affecting health care delivery and,
    554

Discharge planning—cont'd
   review of critical process information in, 558-559
   teaching and referral in, 555-557
Disease
   definition of, 474
   frequency of, measures of, 131-133
   natural history of, 128, *129, 130*
   new, investigating, 138-139
   prevention of, in wellness movement, 148
Disenchantment as family response to health professionals, 492
Disengagement, 425
Disengagement theory of aging, 371
Disorganized families, 415
Dissociation in family with chronically ill member, 479
Distributive justice, 675-676
District Nursing Service, 10
Down syndrome, 502
Driving forces in change process, 684
Drowning
   hazards for, *292*
   prevention of, 291
Drug(s)
   addiction to, 523
   designer, abuse of, 521-522
   habituation to, 522-523
   illegal use of, in adolescence, 318-320
Drug abuse; *see also* Chemical dependency(ies)
   in youth, 513
Dump, open, for solid waste disposal, 637
Dumping, ocean, of solid waste, 637-638
Dunn, Halpert L., in wellness/health movement, 146
Dysfunctional families, 415

E

Eating disorders
   in adolescence and young adulthood, 316
   school health nurse and, 621
Ecologic studies in epidemiologic research, 133
Ecomap in family assessment, 402, *403*
Economic causes of homelessness, 535
Education
   of client, 178
      and family in continuity of care, 557
   health, school health nurse and, 616-617
   nursing, culture and, 61-62
Educational groups, 226-227
Educational needs, 185-187
Educational resource centers for occupational health nurses, 584
Educators, nurses as, 261

Efficacy expectations in self-efficacy model of wellness, 151
Egyptians, roots of community health nursing among, 4-5, 7t
Elbow, little leaguer's, 317
Elderly, 366-387
   chemical dependencies among, 515-516
   disability prevention in, 374-376t
   environmental hazards to, *381*
   frail, 377-384
      benign prostatic hypertrophy in, 380
      cancer in, 378
      chronic lung disease in, 378
      cognitive changes in, 383-384
      common health problems of, 378-384
      coronary artery disease in, 378
      depression in, 382-383
      diabetes mellitus in, 378
      neurologic diseases in, 380
      nutrition for, 381
      osteoporosis in, 378, 380
      peripheral vascular disease in, 378
      safety for, 381-382
      skin disorders in, 380-381
   projected demographic trends in, *369-370*
   social concerns for, 385-386
   spiritual nursing care for, 384-385
   suicide in, research on, *382*
Emotional balance, preservation of, with chronically ill family member, 476-477
Emotional concerns of adolescents/young adults, 315-316
Emotional development in puberty, 312
Empowerment, 682
   through change process, 682-685
   through participation in organizations, 685-688
   through political activity, 688-694
Enabling, 425
Encephalitis
   Japanese, immunization for, dosing schedule for, 450t
   tickborne, immunization for, dosing schedule for, 450t
Enmeshment, 424-425
Entrepreneurs, nurses as, 261
Environment
   effects of, on health maintenance in workplace, 587
   ethical and legal issues relating to, 676-677
Environmental concerns, 633-661
   case study on, *660*
   environmental disasters as, 652-655
   nursing interventions and, 659

Environmental concerns — cont'd
    pollution in home as, *654, 655-659*
    population effect and, 635-636
    radiation as, 650-652
    waste disposal/dispersal as, 636-645
        for hazardous waste, 640-645
        for solid waste, 636-640
    water pollution as, 645-646
Environmental sensitivity as component of wellness,
    169-171
Enzyme-linked immunosorbent assay (ELISA) for HIV,
    455
Epidemiologic triangle, 130
Epidemiology, 125-141
    case study in, 139-141
    causality in, 137-138
    concepts of, applications of, to community health
        nursing, 139
    data sources for, 133
    historical evolution of, 127-128
    research in
        analytic studies in, 133-134
        descriptive studies in, 133
        experimental studies in, 135
        methods used in, 133-135
        observational studies in, 133-135
    screening tests in, 136
    statistical concepts in, 135-137
Ergonomic hazards in workplace, 589, *590*
Error and fidelity theory of aging, 367-368
Erythema infectiosum, 446t
Escherichia coli, 446t
Ethical issues in community health nursing, 671-678
Ethical principles derived from theories, 668
Ethical theories, 666-668
Ethics, 666
    care-based, 668
    and law
        community health nursing standards and, 669-671
        relationship between, 668-669
    virtue, 667-668
Ethnocentrism, 44
Evaluation, 180
    of child growth and development, 289
    formative, 209
        guidelines for, *241*
    of organization, 209-210
    performance, 209
    program, 209-210
    summative, 209
        guidelines for, *241*

Evaluation — cont'd
    supervisory, in quality assessment and improvement,
        247
    teaching/learning process and, 197
Examination stage, later maturity as, 371-372
Exchange theory of aging, 372
Exercise(s)
    aerobic, for physical fitness, 164
    isokinetic, 164
    isometric, for physical fitness, 164
    isotonic, 164
    stretching, 164
Experimental studies in epidemiologic research, 135
Expert power in group, 223-224
Extended family, 393
Extrafamily stressors, 426
Extrinsic motivation, 188

F

Family(ies), 389-435
    assessment of, 399-406
    blended, 395
    with chronically ill member
        adjustment tasks for, 477
        assessment of, 476-489
        assessment questions as intervention with, 483-485
            catastrophic expectation, 484-485
            exploring differences, 484, *485*
            hypothetical, 484, *485*
            triadic, 484, *485*
        caregiver burden in, 481-483
        challenges faced by, 476-478
        denial in, 479-481
        dissociation in, 479
        implementation for, 489-491
        normalization in, 478-479
        overcompensation in, 481
        planning for, 485-489
            attitudes toward being helped in, 486-487
            legitimacy of helper in, 485-486
            point of entry in, 486
            priority nursing diagnoses in, 489
            timing of nursing actions in, 487-489
        resources of, 481
        responses of
            to health professionals, 492-493
            to illness or disability, 478-481
    community system including, 407
    conceptual frameworks for studying, 397-399
    coping patterns of, adaptive, 396-397
    coping with multiple stressors, 413-435

Family(ies) — cont'd
  assessment of, 416-426
    developmental variables in, 425
    physiologic variables in, 417-422
    psychologic variables in, 422-423
    sociocultural variables in, 424-425
    spiritual variables in, 423
  capitalizing on strengths of, 427
  case study on, 433-434
  characteristics of, 414-416
  empathizing with predicament of, 427
  encouraging acceptance of three primary rules by, 427
  encouraging realistic goal setting for, 427
  engaging of, in care, 426-427
  evaluation of, 432-433
  implementation for, 428-432
  ineffective coping in
    related to family violence, 429-432
    related to hopelessness, 432
    related to substance abuse, 428-429
  influence of lines of defense and lines of resistance on, 426
  intervention for, 426-428
  nursing concerns for, 416
  planning for, 426-428
  relabeling all members of, as victims, 428
  definition of, 393
  disorganized, 415
  dysfunctional, 415
  education of, in continuity of care, 557
  extended, 393
  functional, 395-396
  health of, 399
  kin network, 393
  nuclear, 393
  nursing care of, 399-406
  nursing care plan for, 409t
  nursing diagnosis for, 406-407
  patterns of, chemical dependencies and, 514
  preserving relationships with, with chronically ill family member, 477
  roles within, 395
  single-parent, 393
  structure of, evolving, 393-395
  types of, 393
  as unit of service, 391-411
  violence within
    assessment for, 419, 420-422t, 422
    ineffective family coping related to, 429-432
Family developmental tasks, 397-398

Family life cycle, 397-398
Federal government in health services system, 68-71
Fertility rate, 264
Fetal alcohol syndrome, 515
Fifth disease, 446t
Fliedner, Theodur, in history of community health nursing, 6
Focus groups, 227
Food Guide Pyramid, 166
Formaldehyde as indoor pollutant, 656
Formative evaluation, 209
  guidelines for, 241
Forming in group development, 220
Frail elderly, 377-384
Frontier Nursing Service (FNS), 12-14
Functional family, 395-396

G

Gender
  definition of, 347
  men's health and illness and, 350-351
  study of, men's health and, 347-348
Gender identity, 347
  critical feminist theory and, 351-352
Gender order, 346
General systems theory, 207-208
Generality of efficacy expectations, 151
Genogram in family assessment, 399-400, 401
Geopolitical community, 20
German measles, 447t
Goal setting
  by group leader, 222
  in multicultural nursing, 48, 59-60
Goal-expected outcome in planning process, 189-191
Gonorrhea, 449t
Government
  federal, in health services system, 68-71
  local, in health services system, 71, 72
  in occupational health nursing, 584-585
  state, in health services system, 71
Greece, ancient, roots of community health nursing in, 5, 7t
Group(s)
  characteristics of, 220
  cohesion of, 224
  community development, 225
  conflict in, 223-224
  definition of, 218-219
  development of, 220-221
  educational, 226-227
  focus, 227

Group(s) — cont'd
  functions of, 219-220
  leader of, 221-223
  motivational theory and, 224-225
  relationships within, 218-219
  role differentiation in, 221, *222*
  self-help, 225-226
  shared leadership in, 223
  small, initiating, 227-229
  social power and, 223-224
  support, 225-226
  types of, 225-227
  working with, 217-229
Growth, altered pattern of, in adolescence, 310
Guarded alliance as family response to health professionals, 492

H

Habituation, drug, 522-523
Hallucinogens, abuse of, 519-520
Handicap, definition of, 474
Harmony, inner, as component of wellness, 167-169
Harvey, William, in history of community health nursing, 8
Hazard Communication Standard (HCS), 585
Hazardous waste disposal, 640-645
  chemical, 640-645
  radioactive, 640
Health
  definitions of, in wellness movement, 147-148
  ethical and legal issues relating to, 677-678
  holistic, 148-149
  and illness, link between culture and, 41
  maintenance of, in workplace, 587-588
  promotion of, as function of school health nurse, 613-614
  surveillance of, as function of school health nurse, 614
Health behavior contract model of wellness, 152, *153*
Health belief model of wellness, 149-150
Health care, financing of, 72
Health care delivery, trends in, 698-699
Health care delivery systems, 65-83
  Blue Cross in, 72
  Blue Shield in, 72
  Canadian, 74-78
  components of, 68, *70*, 71-72
  definition of, 66
  evaluation of, 73-74
  federal government in, 68, *70*, 71
  financing health care in, 72-73

Health care delivery systems — cont'd
  health maintenance organizations in, 72
  independent insurance plans in, 73
  local health departments in, 71
  Medicare/Medicaid in, 72
  Norwegian, 78
  outpatient services in, 71-72
  physicians in, 71
  private hospitals in, 71
  private sector in, 71-72
  public sector in, 68, *70*, 71
  state governments in, 71
  in United Kingdom, 78
  in United States, 67-74
    legislation affecting, 67-68, 69t
  World Health Organization as, 78-81
Health concerns of adolescents/young adults, 314-315
Health education
  school health nurse and, 616-617
  in wellness movement, 148
Health Maintenance Act (1973), 68
Health maintenance organization (HMO), 72
Health promotion
  in senior citizen center, 373, 377
  in wellness movement, 148
Health screening, school health nurse in, 619
Health teaching in community, 175-198
  historical background on, 176-178
  legal issues in, 178
  PRECEDE model of, 181
  teaching/learning theories and, 178-179
Health team, professional member of, occupational health nurse as, 597
Hearing, disabilities of, in elderly, prevention of, 374t
Heart disease, coronary, in men, 361
Hebrews, roots of community health nursing among, 5, 7t
Hepatitis, 445, 451
Hepatitis A, 449t
Hepatitis B, 449t, 460-461
Hero worship as family response to health professionals, 492
Herpes, 449t
Hettler, William, in wellness movement, 147
High-risk aggregate(s)
  homeless as, 534-537
  migrant agricultural workers as, 537-543
  refugees as, 543
High-tech home care, 570-572
Hill-Burton Act of 1946, 67
History, 3-18

HIV, 449t
HIV infection in men, 359
Holistic health, 148-149
Holistic nursing model of wellness, *157*, 158
Home, pollution in, *654*, 655-659
Home care
  caseload management for, 573-575
  collaborative interdisciplinary, 570
  family members in caregiving role in, research on, *574*
  future trends in, 575, 577
  high-tech, 570-572
  hospice, 572-573
Home health aide in home health care, 569
Home health care, 549-578
  community resources in, 570
  definition of, 568
  discharge planning and, 551-563; *see also* Discharge planning
  home health aide in, 569
  homemaker in, 569
  interdisciplinary team for, 568-570
  Medicare/Medicaid and, 568
  miscellaneous providers in, 569-570
  nurses in, 568
  nutritionists in, 569
  occupational therapists in, 569
  physical therapists in, 569
  physicians in, 569
  private insurance and, 568
  social workers in, 569
  speech therapists in, 569
Home health care nursing
  definition of, 567-568
  standards of, *567*
Home safety in accident prevention, 291-292
Home visit, organizing, 213-214
Homeless
  chemical dependencies among, 512
  as high-risk aggregate, 534-537
Homeless Assistance Act, 536
Homelessness
  causes of, 535-536
  proposed solutions for, 526-527
Homemaker in home health care, 569
Homophobia, 354
Homosexual men, health profile of, 354-355
Hopelessness, ineffective family coping related to, 432
Hospice care, 572-573
Hospital Insurance and Diagnostic Services Act, 74

Hospitals, private, in health services system, 71
Host, susceptible, in chain of infection, 442
Human immunodeficiency virus (HIV)
  infection with
    case study on, *459*
    elimination alteration in, 458
    nutritional alteration in, 457-458
    palliative care for persons with, 459-460
    psychosocial issues related to, 458-459
    treatment of, 456
  spectrum of disease with, 455-456
  support services on, school health nurse and, 622-623
  testing for, 455
Humor
  to achieve inner harmony, 169
  older adult and, research on, *171*
Hurricane Andrew, 653, 655
Hygiene factors in motivation maintenance theory, 202
  for groups, 224
Hypnosis to achieve inner harmony, 169

I

Identification Placement and Review Committee (IPRC), 623, 625
Illness
  chronic; *see also* Chronic illness(es)
    definition of, 474
  definition of, 474
  and health, link between culture and, 41
  work-related, 586-587
Imagery to achieve inner harmony, 169
Immigration Reform and Control Act (IRCA), 539
Immune globulin, dosing schedule for, 450t
Immunity, 131, 443-444
  disabilities of, in elderly, prevention of, 376t
Immunization(s)
  for children, 289-290
  school health nurse and, 616
  travel, dosing schedules for, 450t
Impairment, definition of, 474
Impetigo, 446t
Implementation
  barriers to, 195
  of interventions for child growth/development problems, 288-289
  problems with, 195, 197
  teaching/learning process and, 194-197
Incapacitation, dealing with, with chronically ill family member, 477-478

Incidence rate, 131
Incineration of solid waste, 638-639
Incubation period of disease, 441
Individualized Education Plan (IEP), 623
Industry *versus* inferiority in child development, 287
Infancy, developmental disability in, 498-499
Infant(s); *see also* Maternal-infant client(s)
  of addicted mothers, 514-515
Infant mortality rate, 261-264
  in Canada, 264
Infection(s)
  chain of, 441-442
  recurrent, young adults and, 315
  reservoirs of, 130-131
Influenza, 446t
Information resource as function of school health nurse, 614
Initiative *versus* guilt in child development, 287
Injuries, work-related, 586-587
Inner harmony as component of wellness, 167-169
Instrumental activities of daily living in discharge planning, 555
Instrumental assistance for family with chronically ill member, 489
Insurance
  national health insurance system for, 74
  plans for, independent, 73
Integration in developing cultural sensitivity, 47
Interfamily stressors, 425-426
International Council of Nurses (ICN), 687
Intervention(s)
  in chemical dependencies, 525
  in multicultural nursing, 48, 59-60
Intrafamily stressors, 425
Intrinsic motivation, 188
Ionizing radiation, 650-651, 652
Iowa Intervention Project, 99, 101, *103-105*
Iron deficiency anemia in children, 297-298
Islam, roots of community health nursing in, 5
Isokinetic exercises, 164
Isometric exercise for physical fitness, 164
Isotonic exercises, 164

J

Japanese encephalitis, immunization for, dosing schedule for, 450t
Jenner, Edward, in history of community health nursing, 8
Joint Commission model of quality assessment and improvement, 238-239

Jumper's knee, 317-318
Justice, distributive, 675-676

K

Kin network family, 393
King, Imogene, open systems and theory of goal attainment of, 102, *107,* 108-110t
Knee, jumper's, 317-318
Knowledge, 179
Korean War in history of community health nursing, 14
Kyphosis, adolescent, 315

L

Landfill for solid waste disposal, 637
Late maturity, 367
  nursing diagnoses related to, *384*
Law
  case, 665
  civil, 666
  common, 665
  criminal, 666
  definition of, 664
  and ethics
    community health nursing standards and, 669-671
    relationship between, 668-669
  sources of, *665*
Lead as indoor pollutant, 657-659
Lead poisoning in children, 298-300
Leader, group, 221-223
Leadership, 204-205
  change and, 700
  shared, in group, 223
  style of, 204-205
Learn, readiness to, 187-188
Learner in teaching/learning process, 187-188
Learning
  affective, 180
  cognitive, 179-180
  definition of, 178
  developmental capacities for, 184-185t
  principles of, 182, 183t
  process of
    assessment and, 185-189
    evaluation and, 197
    implementation and, 194-197
    mistakes in, 196t, 197
    nursing process and, 182, 185-197
  psychomotor, 180

Learning — cont'd
   theories of, 178-179
   types of, 179-182
Learning disabilities, 502
Legal issues
   in community health nursing, 671-678
   in health teaching, 178
Legal system, 664-666
Legislation affecting discharge planning, 553
Legitimate power in group, 223
Letter writing, political, empowerment through, 690-691
Level of care, discharge planning and, 553
Lewin model of change, 683-684
Licensure, 673
   quality assurance and, 234
Life course theories of aging, 371
Lifestyle assessment questionnaire, 158, *159-161*
Lippitt model of change, 684-685
Little leaguer's elbow, 317
Local health departments in health services system, 71, *72*
Love Canal, 652-653
Low birth weight, infant mortality and, 262, 263-264
Lungs, chronic disease of, in frail elderly, 378
Lyme disease, 446t

M

Magnitude of efficacy expectations, 151
Malpractice, 672-673
Mammographic screening, breast cancer risk and, *334*
Management
   caseload, 211
      district nurses and, research on, *212*
   clinical, 212-213
   concepts of, 200-215
      application of, 210-213
   models of, 202-204
   organization and, 207-210
   organizational, 214
   theory of, developing, 201-207
      leadership in, 204-205
      management models in, 202-204
      planning in, 205-207
   time, 210-211
   total quality, 237
   utilization, in quality assessment and improvement, 249
Manager/administrator, occupational health nurse as, 597
Mantoux tuberculin skin test, 463

Marijuana, abuse of, 520-521
Masculinity(ies), 351
   men's health and, 352-357
Massage techniques, 162
MATCH model of wellness, 155-157
Maternal mortality rate, 264
   in Canada, 264-265
Maternal-infant client(s), 257-282; *see also* Infant(s); Mother(s)
   biostatistical data related to, 261-265
   care of, community health nurse roles in, 260-261
   health care services for, in community, 265-282
      for early postpartum discharge, 273-276
      for home care, 272-273
      for prenatal care, 265-272
      for primary prevention, 265-276
      for secondary prevention, 276-279
      for tertiary prevention, 279-282
   health of, research topics on, *260*
   Healthy people 2000 objectives for, *259*
Maturational crises, 396
Maturity, late, 367
Measles
   German, 447t
   red, 448t
Medicaid, 67, 72, 73t, 568
Medical Care Act, 74
Medical self-care, definition of, 149
Medicare, 67, 72, 73t, 568
Medicare Catastrophic Coverage Act, 68
Meditation to achieve inner harmony, 169
Men
   adolescent, health profile of, 352-353
   as athletes, health profile of, 356-357
   bisexual, health profile of, 354-355
   of color, health profile of, 353-354
   health care for, 345-362
   health issues for, 357-361
      alcohol abuse as, 358-359
      coronary heart disease as, 361
      HIV/AIDS as, 359
      prostate disease as, 358
      suicide as, 360
      testicular cancer as, 357-358
      violence as, 360-361
   health of
      emerging focus on, 348
      study of gender and, 347-348
   health status of, 348-350
   homosexual, health profile of, 354-355
   imprisoned, health profile of, 355-356

Men — cont'd
  morbidity of, 350
  mortality of, 348-350
  theories of health and illness in, 350-352
Menarche, 313-312
Meningococcus, immunization for, dosing schedule for, 450t
Menopause, 339
  bone mineral density and, research on, *380*
  women's health concerns during, *336*
Menstruation, adolescent girls and, 315
Mental health needs, addressing, school health nurse in, 620-621
Mental illness as cause of homelessness, 535-536
Mental retardation, 502
Methadone maintenance, 526
Middle Ages, roots of community health nursing in, 5-6, 7t
Midlife
  body image and, 336
  health maintenance activities promoting wellness in, *337*
  women in, sexuality and, 339-340
Migrant agricultural workers as high-risk aggregate, 537-543
Migrant Health Act, 539, 540-542t
Military service in history of community health nursing, 14-15
Minimization in developing cultural sensitivity, 47
Mistecs, 538-539
Morbidity, 127
  in adolescence, 308-309
  maternal, 264
  of men, 350
Mortality, 127
  in adolescence, 308-309
  of men, 348-350
Mortality rate(s)
  formulas used for, 132t
  infant, 261-264
    in Canada, 264
  maternal, 264
    in Canada, 264-265
  neonatal, 262
  postneonatal, 262
Mother(s); *see also* Maternal-infant client(s)
  mortality rates for, 264
    in Canada, 264-265
Motivation
  in assessment of wellness behaviors, 162
  extrinsic, 188

Motivation — cont'd
  by group leader, 223
  intrinsic, 188
  readiness to learn and, 188
Motivation maintenance theory, 202
Motivational theory, groups and, 224-225
Motivators in motivation maintenance theory, 202
  for groups, 224
Multicultural society
  communication in, 43-44
  community health nursing in, 38-62
    assessment enablers for, 48, *50-52,* 53-58t
    barriers to effective care in, 44-45
    case studies on, 47, 59-60
    goal setting in, 48, 59-60
    interventions in, 48, 59-60
    Leininger's model of, 48
    Sunrise model of, 48, *49*
  using nursing process in, 48, *49-52,* 53-58t, 59
Mumps, 447t
Musculoskeletal system, disabilities of, in elderly, prevention of, 375-376t
Mutual support as group function, 219

N

Naive trust as family response to health professionals, 492
Narcotics, abuse of, 520
National health insurance system, 74
National Health Planning and Resources Act (1974), 68
National Institute of Occupational Safety and Health (NIOSH), 584
National League for Nursing (NLN), participation in, 687
National Women's Health Network, 326
Natural history of disease, 128, *129,* 130
Nature *versus* nurture, men's health and illness and, 350-351
Needs assessment
  as function of school health nurse, 613
  guidelines for, *240*
Neglect, child, 302-303
Neolithic age, roots of community health nursing in, 4
Neonatal mortality rate, 262
Nervous system, disabilities of, in elderly, prevention of, 376t
Networking as group function, 219
Neuman, Betty, nursing process format of, 21
Neuman Systems Model, 21-22
  application(s) of, 22, *23-24,* 25-27t, 27-28
    to concept of immunity, 443-444

Neuroendocrine theory of aging, 368
Neurologic diseases in frail elderly, 380
Nicotine abuse, 519
Nightingale, Florence
    in history of community health nursing, 8-9
    nursing process framework of, 102, 105, 111-112t
Nitrogen oxides as indoor pollutant, 656
Noise pollution, 646-648
Noncompliance as obstacle to implementation, 195, 197
Normalization in family with chronically ill member, 478-479
Norming in group development, 221
North America, cultural diversification of, 39-40
North American Nursing Diagnosis System (NANDA), 89
    nursing diagnoses approved by, *90*
    nursing diagnostic categories approved by, *91-92*
Norwegian health care system, 78
Nuclear family, 393
Nuclear family dyad, 393
Null hypothesis, 137
Nurse(s)
    as change agent, 685
    chemical dependencies among, 516
    in home health care, 568
    nursing and, 699-700
Nurse practitioner performance, factors influencing, 77
Nurse Training Act, 67
Nursing
    contribution of, to Canadian health care system development, 76-77
    ethical and legal issues in, 672-674
    occupational health, 581-565; *see also* Occupational health nursing
    school health, 607-627; *see also* School health nursing
Nursing administration, culture and, 61-62
Nursing education, culture and, 61-62
Nursing frameworks, 87
Nursing Intervention Classification (NIC), 99, 101, *103-105*
Nursing process
    frameworks for, 102, 105-118
    standards of community health nursing practice and, 87-89
    teaching/learning process and, 182, 185-197
    use of, in multicultural society, 48, *49-52,* 53-58, 59
    women's health care and, 329-330

Nursing process format, Neuman's, 21
Nursing research, culture and, 61-62
Nursing theory, community health nursing and, 15-17
Nutrition
    in adolescence, 309-311
    in chemical dependency management, 526
    for children, 296-297
    as component of wellness, 165-167
    in frail elderly, 381
Nutritionists in home health care, 569

O

Objectives, writing, in planning process, 189-191
Observation, direct, in quality assessment and improvement, 247
Observational studies in epidemiologic research, 133-135
Occupational disease, difficulties in determination of, 598, 602
Occupational health history, 597-598, *599-601*
Occupational health nursing, 581-605
    history of, 583-586
    in maintenance of health in workplace, 587-588
    in promoting worker health, 583-584
    roles and functions of, 594-597
    work-related injuries/illness and, 586-587
Occupational illness, definition of, 586-587
Occupational injury, definition of, 586
Occupational Safety and Hazards Administration (OSHA)
    migrant agricultural workers and, 539
Occupational Safety and Health Act (OSHAct), 67, 584-585
Occupational Safety and Health Administration (OSHA), 67-68
    communicable disease precautions required by, *468*
    creation of, 584
    tuberculosis program required by, *468*
Occupational safety and health programs, 602-604
Occupational setting, nursing process in, 602
Occupational therapists in home health care, 569
Ocean dumping of solid waste, 637-638
Office of Research On Women's Health (ORWH), 326-327
Officials, organized visits to, empowerment through, 691-693
Omnibus Budget Reconciliation Act, 68
Operation Restore Hope in history of community health nursing, 15

Orem, Dorothea, self-care model of, 105-106, 113-115t
Organization(s), 207-210
  clinical specialty, 687-688
community, participation in, 688
  of community nursing services, 208-209
  evaluation of, 209-210
  general systems theory of, 207-208
  of home visit, 213-214
  multipurpose, participation in, 686-687
  participation in, empowerment through, 685-688
  professional nursing, participation in, 685-688
Organizational management, 214
Organizing, political, empowerment through, 693-694
Osgood-Schlatter's disease, 317
Osteoporosis
  in frail elderly, 378, 380
  menopause and, research on, *380*
Outcome as assessment measure, 244
Outpatient services in health services system, 71-72
Overcompensation in family with chronically ill member, 481

P

Pain, dealing with, with chronically ill family member, 477
Palliative care, hospice programs for, 572-573
Pathogen, 441
PCBs
  disposal problems from, 643-645
  health problems from, 642-643
  prenatal exposure to, visual recognition memory and, research on, *645*
Peer review in quality assessment and improvement, 247
Performing in group development, 221
Peripheral vascular disease in frail elderly, 378
Person, ethical and legal issues relating to, 674-676
Personal crisis as cause of homelessness, 535
Peru, health service issues in, 81
Physical abuse among runaways, research on, *418*
Physical dependence, 522
Physical fitness as component of wellness, 164-165
Physical hazards in workplace, 588-589
Physical therapists in home health care, 569
Physicians
  in health services system, 71
  in home health care, 569
Physiologic variables in assessing family coping with multiple stressors, 417-422

Plague, immunization for, dosing schedule for, 450t
Planning
  in developing management theory, 205-207
  financial, 206-207
  of interventions for child growth/development problems, 288
  staff, 207
  strategic, 206
  teaching/learning process and, 189-194
  writing objectives in, 189-191
Play, therapeutic, for children, 288
Playground accidents, prevention of, 292
Plumbism in children, 298-300
Poison control interventions, 291
Poisoning, lead, 657
Police power, 665
Poliomyelitis, 447t
Political activity, empowerment through, 688-694
Pollutants, 635
Pollution
  air, 648-650
  in home, *654,* 655-659
  noise, 646-648
  water, 645-646
Population effect, 635-636
Portal of entry into person in chain of infection, 442
Postneonatal mortality rate, 262
Postpartum discharge, early, 273-276
  interventions for, 281
Poverty
  chemical dependencies and, 512
  children and, 303-304
Power
  police, 665
  social, in group, 223-224
PRECEDE model of health teaching, 181
Preconception care and counseling, 271
Pregnancy
  body image and, 335-336
  care during, 265-272; *see also* Prenatal care
Prenatal care, 265-272
  barriers to, 265-270
    client, 267-270
    financial, 266-267
    system, 267
  beneficial outcomes of, 265
  components and content of, 270-271
  health promotion activities in, 270-271
  risk status assessment in, 270
  scheduling, 271-272

Pre-operational phase child development, 287

Presbycusis, 373

Presbyopia, 373

Preschool visitation/assessment, school health nurse in, 620

Prevalence rate, 131-132
formula used for, 132t

Prevention
levels of, 27-28
primary, 128
secondary, 128
tertiary, 128

Primary care provider, occupational health nurse as, 596-597

Primary prevention, 27-28, 128

Prison inmates, health profile of, 355-356

Privileged communication, 674

Problem Classification Scheme, 89, 93-98

Process as assessment measure, 244

Productivity, key concepts of, *210*

Professional accountability, quality assurance and, 234

Professional issues, 681-701

Professional nursing organizations, participation in, 685-688

Program evaluation model of quality assessment and improvement, 239-242

Progressive relaxation to achieve inner harmony, 167

Prostate gland
disease of, 358
hypertrophy of, benign, in frail elderly, 380

Psychoanalytic theory of aging, 372

Psychologic dependence, 522

Psychologic hazards in workplace, 593-594

Psychologic variables in assessing family coping with multiple stressors, 422-423

Psychomotor domain, 180

Psychomotor learning, 180

Psychosocial theories of aging, 370-372

Puberty, 311-314

Public health nursing, 15

P-value, 137

Q

Quality, 236

Quality assessment and improvement, 231-252
accreditation and, 235-236
certification and, 234-235
data sources and methods in, 247-249
environmental context of, 233-234
in health care, 236-237
licensure and, 234

Quality assessment and improvement — cont'd
management roles in, 249-250
models of, 238-247
American Nurses' Association, 242-247
Joint Commission, 238-239
program evaluation, 239-242
outcome in, 237
process in, 237
professional accountability and, 234
research on, 250
social context of, 234-236
structure in, 237

Quality improvement, continuous, 237

Quality improvement movement, 237-238

Quality management roles, 249-250

R

Rabies immunization, dosing schedule for, 450t

Radiation in environment, 650-652

Radioactive waste disposal, 640

Radon, 651
as indoor pollutant, 656-657

Radon daughters, 656-657

Readiness to learn, 187-188

Recycling of solid waste, 639-640

Referral in continuity of care, 558

Refreezing in change process, 684

Refugees as high-risk aggregate, 543
case study on, *544-546*

Regression in altered families, 425

Rehabilitation Act of 1973, 499t

Rehabilitation Amendment, 499t

Relationships
causal, 137-138
within groups, 218-219

Relative risk, 135

Relaxation, progressive, to achieve inner harmony, 167

Renaissance, roots of community health nursing in, 6, 7t

Reproductive hazards, 340-341

Research
as function of school health nurse, 615
nursing, culture and, 61-62

Researcher(s)
nurses as, 260
occupational health nurse as, 597

Reservoir of infection, 441-442
means of exit from, 442

Resignation as family response to health professionals, 492

Resistance, lines of, in immunity, 444

Resources
    family, in family with chronically ill member, 481
    helping group become aware of, leader in, 223
Restraining in change process, 684
Retardation, mental, 502
Reward power in group, 223
Ringworm, 449t
Risk
    attributable, 135-136
    clients at, 437-547
        aggregated of, in community; *see also* High-risk
            aggregate(s)
        aggregates of, in community, 532-547
        from chemical dependencies, 509-530; *see also*
            Chemical dependency(ies)
        from chronic illnesses, 472-494; *see also* Chronic
            illness(es)
        from communicable diseases, 439-470
        from developmental disabilities, 496-508; *see also*
            Developmental disability(ies)
    relative, 135
Risk taking behavior in adolescence, 320
Rocky Mountain spotted fever, 447t
Rogers model of change, 684
Rome, roots of community health nursing in, 5, 7t
Roy, Sr. Callista, adaptation model of, 106, 110, 115, 116-
    118t
Rubella, 447t
Rubeola, 448t

S

Safety for frail elderly, 381-382
Safety/security as group function, 219
Ste. D'Youville in history of community health nursing,
    6, 8
St. Francis of Assisi in history of community health
    nursing, 6
St. Vincent de Paul in history of community health
    nursing, 6
Scabies, 448t
Scapegoating, 425
Scarlet fever, 448t
School health nursing, 607-627
    classification of, 610-611
    current issues related to, 609-610
    educational preparation for, 610-611
    future considerations on, 626
    historical perspective on, 609
    outlines and standards developed by American
        Nurses' Association for, 612
    in primary prevention, 615-619

School health nursing — cont'd
    purpose of, 608
    role and functions of, 612-615
    in secondary prevention, 619-623
    in tertiary prevention, 623-626
School-age children, developmental disabilities in, 499-
    501
Screening tests, 136
Seat belts in injury prevention, 292-293
Secondary prevention, 27, 28, 128
Self reliance model of wellness, 152
Self-care, medical, definition of, 149
Self-concept, nurse's role in promoting, 337
Self-efficacy model of wellness, 150-152
Self-evaluation in quality assessment and improve-
    ment, 247-248
Self-help groups, 225-226
Self-image, satisfactory, preservation of, with chroni-
    cally ill family member, 477
Self-managing work teams (SMWT), 203
Senior citizen center, health promotion in, 373, 377
Sense of belonging as group function, 219
Sensitivity
    cultural, developing, 45-47
    environmental, as component of wellness, 169-171
    of screening test, 136
Sensorimotor development, 287
Sentinel in quality assessment and improvement, 248-
    249
Sex, definition of, 346-347
Sex role theory, 351
Sexual abuse among runaways, research on, *418*
Sexual development, adolescent, 316-317
Sexuality, 337-341
    adolescence and, 338-339
    disabilities of, in elderly, prevention of, 376t
    midlife women and, 339-340
Shared governance, 203-204
Shigellosis, 448t
Sickness, definition of, 474
Single-parent family, 393
Situational crises, 396
Skin disorders in frail elderly, 380-381
Smell, disabilities of, in elderly, prevention of, 374t
Smoke, tobacco, as indoor pollutant, 656
Social competence and breakdown theory of aging,
    372
Social concerns
    for elderly, 385-386
    relating to adolescents/young adults, 321
Social factors, women's body image and, 336-337

Social power in group, 223-224
Social Readjustment Rating Scale, 167, *168*
Social support model of wellness, 152, 154-155
Social workers in home health care, 569
Socialization as group function, 219
Society, multicultural; *see also* Multicultural society
    communication in, 43-44
    community health nursing in, 38-62
Sociocultural variables in assessing family coping with
        multiple stressors, 424-425
Solid waste disposal, 636-640
    incineration for, 638-639
    landfill for, 637
    ocean dumping for, 637-638
    open dump for, 637
    recycling for, 639-640
Somalia, health service issues in, 81
Somatic mutation theory of aging, 368
Specificity of screening test, 136
Speech therapists in home health care, 569
Spiritual development in adolescence/young adult-
        hood, 312, 314
Spiritual nursing care for elderly, 384-385
Spiritual variables in assessing family coping with mul-
        tiple stressors, 423
Sports, adolescents and, 317-318
Staging in quality assessment and improvement, 248
Standards, 243-244
    of care, 672-673
    of clinical nursing practice of ANA, *249*
    community health nursing, ethics and law and, 669-
        671
    of practice, 670
State governments in health services system, 71
Statistical analysis, 20
Statistical significance, 137
Stereotyping, 45
Stimulants, abuse of, 517
Storming in group development, 220-221
Strength of efficacy expectations, 151
Streptococcal sore throat, 448t
Stress, occupational, 593
Stressors, 425-426
    extrafamily, 426
    interfamily, 425-426
    intrafamily, 425
    multiple, family coping with, 413-435
        characteristics of, 414-416
Stretching exercises, 164
Structural-functional framework for studying family,
        398

Structure
    as assessment measure, 244
    basic, in immunity, 444
Substance abuse, 509-530; *see also* Chemical depen-
        dency(ies)
    in adolescence, 318-320
    causes of, 512
    family assessment for, 417-419
    ineffective family coping related to, 428-429
    issues and trends in, 510-511
    prevention of, school health nurse and, 618-619
Suicide
    in adolescence and young adulthood, prevention of,
        316
    in elderly, research on, *382*
    by men, 360
    prevention programs for, school health nurse and,
        617-618
Summative evaluation, 209
Summative evaluation, guidelines for, *241*
Supervisory evaluation in quality assessment and im-
        provement, 247
Support groups, 225-226
Symbolic-interactional framework for studying family,
        398
Synthesis, 180
Syphilis, 449t
Systems theory, 207-208
Systems theory framework for studying family, 398-399

T

T-4 cells in HIV, 455
Taste, disabilities of, in elderly, prevention of, 374t
Tax Equity and Fiscal Responsibility Act (TEFRA),
        68
Teacher, assessment of, 189
Teacher/educator, occupational health nurse as, 597
Teaching
    health, in community, 175-198; *see also* Health teach-
        ing in community
    methods for, selecting, 192-194
    principles of, 182, 183t
    process of
        assessment and, 185-189
        diagnosis and, 189
        evaluation and, 197
        implementation and, 194-197
        mistakes in, 196t, 197
        nursing process and, 182, 185-197
        planning and, 189-194
    theories of, 178-179

Teaching situation, teaching/learning process and, 188-189

Team, health, professional member of, occupational health nurse as, 597

Team playing as family response to health professionals, 493

Teleology, 667

Teresa, Mother, in history of community health nursing, 6, 8

Tertiary prevention, 27, 28, 128

Testicular cancer, 357-358

Tetanus, 448t

Theory X, 201-202

Theory Y, 201-202

Therapeutic play for children, 288

Therapeutic touch, 163-164

Tickborne encephalitis, immunization for, dosing schedule for, 450t

Time management, 210-211

Tinea capitis, 449t

Tobacco smoke as indoor pollutant, 656

Tolerance
  in physical dependence, 522
  to stimulants, 517

Total quality management, 237

Touch, disabilities of, in elderly, prevention of, 374t

Toxicology, 591-592

Tracers in quality assessment and improvement, 248

Trajectory in quality assessment and improvement, 248

Tranquilizers, abuse of, 519

Transcultural community health nursing, leading edge of, 62

Transmission, mode of, 131

Travis, John, health/wellness model of, 146-147

Treatment modalities, alternative or complementary, 162-164

Tremors in alcohol withdrawal, 526

Trisomy 21, 502

Trust
  versus mistrust in infant development, 287
  naive, as family response to health professionals, 492

Tuberculosis (TB), 461-466
  active, nursing interventions for persons with, 465-466
  contact investigation in, 464-465
  epidemiology of, 461-462
  immunization for, dosing schedule for, 450t
  incubation period for, 462
  mode of transmission of, 462
  multidrug-resistant, 465
  pathology of, 462-463

Tuberculosis (TB) — cont'd
  prevention of, 463, 464
  testing for anergy in, 463
  tuberculin skin test reaction for, in persons vaccinated with BCG, 463-464

Typhoid, immunization for, dosing schedule for, 450t

U

Underdeveloped nations, health service issues in, 81

Unfreezing in change process, 683-684

Uniform Needs Assessment Instrument (UNAI) for discharge planning, 558-559

United Kingdom, health care in, 78

Utilitarianism, 667

Utilization management in quality assessment and improvement, 249

V

Values in assessment of wellness behaviors, 158, 162

Varicella, 449t

Vehicular accidents, reducing injury from, 292-293

Venereal diseases, 449t

Very low birth weight, infant mortality and, 262, 263-264

Vicious communication cycle, 490-491

Victoria, Queen, in history of community health nursing, 9-10

Vietnam War in history of community health nursing, 14-15

Violence
  children and, 300-302
  family, 419, 420-422t, 422
    ineffective family coping related to, 429-432
  as family stressor, 415
  men's, 360-361
  women and, 341-342

Virtue ethics, 667-668

Virtuous communication cycle, 491

Vision, disabilities of, in elderly, prevention of, 375t

W

Wald, Lillian, in history of community health nursing, 10-12

Waste disposal
  hazardous, 640-645
  solid, 636-640

Water pollution, 645-646

Wellness
  in community, assessing level of, 28
  components of, 164-171
    environmental sensitivity as, 169-171

Wellness — cont'd
    inner harmony as, 167-169
    nutrition as, 165-167
    physical fitness as, 164-165
  definition of, 149
  models of, 149-162
    Community Wellness Program as, 157-158
    health behavior contract, 152, *153*
    health belief, 149-150
    holistic nursing, *157,* 158
    MATCH, 155-157
    self reliance, 152
    self-efficacy, 150-152
    social support, 152, 154-155
Wellness behaviors, assessment of, 158, *159-161,* 162
Wellness movement
  historical development of, 144-146
  prominent individuals in, 146-147
  terms used in, 147-149
Western Blot test for HIV, 455
Wheel model, 130, *131*
Withdrawal, alcohol, disorders associated with, 526-527
Withdrawal syndrome in chemical dependencies, 525
Women, 324-342
  abused, responses to, facilitative *vs.* inhibitive, *424*
  chemical dependencies among, 515
  entry of, into health care system, 327-329
  health care for
    historical factors influencing, 325-326
    legislative action on, 328t
    meeting needs for, in community, 330-331
    nursing process and, 329-330
    political factors influencing, 326-327
    preventive, 331-335
    secondary prevention for, 333-335
    social factors influencing, 326
    tertiary prevention for, 335
  health issues related to, *326*
  health of

Women — cont'd
  Healthy People 2000 objectives related to, *327*
    teen's guide to, *322*
  health resources for, *33*
  reproductive hazards for, 340-341
  self-concept and nurse's role in promoting positive self image, 335-337
  sexuality and, 337-341
  violence and abuse of, 341-342
Women's health care movement, 326
Women's Health Equity Act, 326
Workers' compensation laws, 585
Workplace
  hazards in, 588-594
    biologic, 592-593
    chemical, 589, 591-592
    ergonomic, 589, *590*
    physical, 588-589
    psychologic, 593-594
  health maintenance in, 587-588
World Health Organization (WHO), 78-81
  regional offices of, *82*
World War I in history of community health nursing, 14
World War II in history of community health nursing, 14

Y

Yellow fever, immunization for, dosing schedule for, 450t
Yin/Yang, treatment modalities related to, 162
Yoga, 164
Young adults, 307-322
  developmental tasks of, 313t
  emotional concerns of, 315-316
  emotional development of, 312
  health concerns of, 314-315
  recurrent infections and, 315
  social concerns relating to, 321
  spiritual development of, 312, 314
Youth, chemical dependencies in, 513